AF520898

Textbook of Agricultural Biotechnology

THE AUTHORS

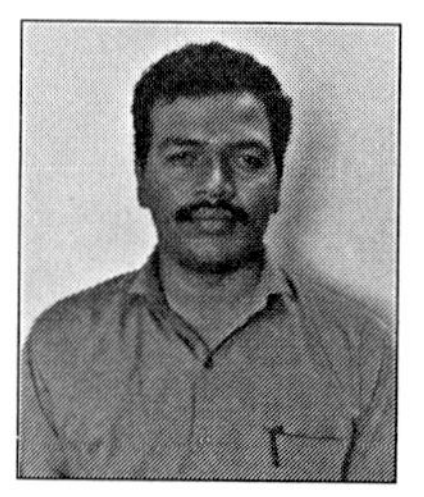

Dr. Sivaji Mathivanan, is presently working as Teaching Assistant (Biotechnology) in Agriculture College and Research Institute (AC and RI),Vazhavachanur, Tiruvannamalai, one of the constituent college of Tamil Nadu Agricultural University (TNAU), Coimbatore. He has started his under graduate programme B.Sc. Agriculture in Anbil Dharmalingam Agricultural College and Research Institute (ADAC and RI), Trichy, TNAU followed by Master Degree Programme M.Sc Agri. in Plant Biotechnology in Kerala Agriculture University (KAU) Thrissur, Kerala through DBT-JNU Fellowship and Ph. D in Biotechnology at AC and RI, Tamil Nadu Agricultural University, Coimbatore. He has qualified ICAR-SRF and ICAR-NET. He is having six year working experience in both research and teaching. He has published 6 Books, 35 national and international research paper, 10 book chapters and 25 popular article in various aspect of Biotechnology. He has Participated and presented 30 national and international seminar and symposium.

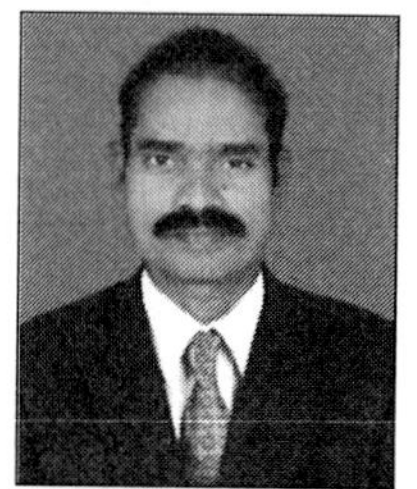

Dr. Muthaiyan Pandiyan, Ph.D, FNABS and FJPN, Professor, DEAN, Agricultural College and Research Institute, TNAU, Vazhavachanur, Tiruvannamalai, Tamil Nadu, India. TNAU, Tamil Nadu, India. He has completed his Ph.D in Plant Breeding and Genetics from Tamil Nadu Agricultural University, Coimbatore, Tamil Nadu, India. He is a notable breeder in national and international level. He is being developed MYMV durable resistant donor in mungbean with ricebean cross combination. He developed and released many varieties in pulses now all are ruling blackgram varieties VBN5 to VBN 8 and VBN3 and VBN4 greengram and VBN3 redgram popular among farmers, VBN7 in blackgram is national donor. Blackgram VBN 6 and VBN 8 occupied more area under cultivation. He has written ten books and 120 research articles both national and international journals. Apart from varieties, many technologies have been developed and released specifically says wild boar repellent for farming communities. He is reviewer for NISCAIR and Elsevier publications. He has registered plant materials in pulses and conserved the varietal seeds to NBPGR, New Delhi as plant Genetic Resources. He has guided more than five postgraduate and five Doctoral students and he published research,chapters and review articles at national and international repute journals like PLOS one, Crop evolution and Plant Genetic Resources, Applied genetics and Molecular Biology.

Textbook of Agricultural Biotechnology

— Authors —

Dr. M. Sivaji

Teaching Assistant
Agricultural Biotechnology
Department of Crop Improvement

Dr. M. Pandiyan

Dean
Agriculture College and Research Institute (AC and RI)
Vazhavachanur, Tiruvannamalai – 606 753
Tamil Nadu Agricultural University

2025

Daya Publishing House®
A Division of
Astral International Pvt. Ltd.
New Delhi – 110 002

ISBN: 9789359199238

Published by : **Daya Publishing House®**
A Division of
Astral International Pvt. Ltd.
– ISO 9001:2015 Certified Company –
4736/23, Ansari Road, Darya Ganj,
New Delhi-110 002
Ph. 011-43549197, 8130496929
E-mail: info@astralint.com
Website: www.astralint.com

Preface

Biotechnology is a science that has already established its impact on different fields such as Agriculture, Horticulture, Microbiology, Food Process Engineering, Pharmaceuticals, Bioenergetics, Information technology and Public Health. It has the potential to ensure food security, reduce hunger and malnutrition, and reduce rural poverty. Application of Biotechnology in agriculture mainly centres round in Tissue culture, Transgenic crops development and Molecular markers. ***Textbook of Agricultural Biotechnology*** covers all the fundamental aspects of these three important areas in agricultural biotechnology. It has been written in a very simple manner and explains the fundamental concepts and techniques in detail, so that they are very easily understood by students especially undergraduate students. It is expected that the readers will get an idea agricultural biotechnology and application of this in the field level.

This book comprises part I and part II, part I give brief about biotechnology. Part II contains of 34 chapters, chapter 1- 10 covers the basic introduction of Biotechnology and its aspects, and different types of tissue culture methods and its application in agriculture and its allied subjects. Chapter 11 - 19 describes about Basic molecular biology, structure and types of nucleic acids, Central dogma of life, gene structure and its regulation, PCR Blotting and DNA sequencing. Chapter 20 - 27 mainly covers genetic manipulation, rDNA construction, various genetic transformation methods, tools involved in development of transgenic crops, genetically modified crops for different characters, its regulation and biosafety. Chapter 28-34 explains about different types of molecular markers and marker assisted selection, QTL analysis, DNA finger printing, genomics, bioinformatics and its and application in biotechnology. Chapter 35and 35 covers about basics of nanotechchnology, nanomaterials and its application, nanobiotechnology and its application in agriculture. After completion of all these chapters important terminologies which is used in the agricultural biotechnology and repeatedly asking questions in the university exams are also included at the end of this book. This aspect will be more useful to the undergraduate students in exam point of view. This book will provide great assistance to the students to their understanding about the fundamentals concepts of agricultural biotechnology and their examinations.

We would like to thank all those who have contributed in making of this book, not least, the people, whose original investigations formed the basis of the book. This book can hardly claim any originality in content, the figures, illustrations, photographs used are collected from various books, different educational websites, journals and review papers published previously for which the authors are thankful. Key sources of this book are duly acknowledged in the reference section. We apologize unreservedly for any mistakes, all of which are ours, omissions or failure to acknowledge fully.

Dr. M. Sivaji

Dr. M. Pandiyan

Contents

Part I

Introduction to Biotechnology

The term Biotechnology was coined by a **Hungarian Engineer Karl Ereky in 1917**. "Bio" means life and "Technology" means the application of knowledge for practical use *i.e.*, the use of living organisms to make or improve a product. Synthesis of scientific and technical knowledge from many academic disciplines has produced the set of enabling technologies called as biotechnology.

Various Definitions of Biotechnology

- ☆ Biotechnology is defined as "the integrated use of biochemistry, Microbiology and engineering sciences in order to achieve technological (industrial) application of the capabilities of microorganisms, cultured tissue cells and parts thereof" **(European Federation of Biotechnology).**
- ☆ Biotechnology is defined as "a technology using biological phenomenon for copying and manufacturing various kinds of useful substances" **(Japanese Biotechnologists).**
- ☆ Biotechnology is defined as "the application of biological organisms, System or process to manufacturing and service industries" **(British Biotechnologists).**
- ☆ Biotechnology is defined as "the controlled use of biological agents, such as micro-organisms or cellular components for Beneficial use" **(US National Science Foundation).**
- ☆ Biotechnology is defined as "the application of scientific and engineering principles to the processing of materials by biological agents to provide agents to provide goods and service" **(The Organisation for Economic Co-operation and Development).**

- Biotechnology is defined as "the controlled and deliberate application of simple biological agents-living or dead, cells or cell components-in technically useful operations, either of productive manufacture or as service operation" **(J.D. Bu'Lock).**
- Biotechnology is defined as" the use of living organisms in systems or processes for the manufacture of useful products; it may involve algae, bacteria, fungi, yeast, cells of higher plants and animals or subsystems of any of these or isolated components from living matter" **(Gibbs and Greenhalgh).**
- Biotechnology is defined as" the application of biochemistry, biology, microbiology and chemical engineering to industrial process and products and on environment" **(The International Union of Pure and Applied Chemistry).**

Stages of Biotechnology Development

- Genetics-1900-1953
- DNA research, science explodes-1953 - 1976
- Biotechnology - 1977

Biotechnology is a collection of various technologies that enable us to improve crop yield and food quality in agriculture and to produce a broader array of products in industries. Biotechnology comprises various components

Various Components of Biotechnology

Tissue/Cell Culture Technology

Grow tissues/cells under laboratory conditions to produce an entire organism or to produce new products

Genetic Engineering (Recombinant DNA) Technology

The use of cellular enzymes to manipulate DNA and transferring manipulated DNA between unrelated organisms

Antisense or RNAi Technology

Block or decrease the production of certain proteins

Protein Engineering Technology

Improve existing/create novel proteins to make useful products

Bioinformatics Technology

Computational analysis of biological data, *e.g.*, sequence analysis macromolecular structures, high-throughput profiling data analysis

Functional Genomics (the -omics)

The use of genome-wide, high-throughput approaches to determine the biological function of all of the genes and their products

Transcriptomics (*e.g.* Microarray expression profiling)

Transcriptome is the complete set of RNA transcripts in a specific cell type or tissue at a certain developmental stage and/or under a specific physiological condition, including messenger RNA, transfer RNA, ribosomal RNA, and other non-coding RNAs. Transcriptomics focuses on the gene expression at the RNA level and offers the genome-wide information of gene structure, gene function and its importance in specific biological processes. With the development of next-generation high-throughput sequencing technology, transcriptome analysis has been progressively improving our understanding of RNA-based gene regulatory network.

Proteomics (*e.g.* Structures/modifications/interactions of proteins)

Proteins are responsible for an endless number of tasks within the cell. **The complete set of proteins in a cell can be referred to as its proteome and the study of protein structure and function and what every protein in the cell is doing is known as proteomics.** The proteome is highly dynamic and it changes from time to time in response to different environmental stimuli. The goal of proteomics is to understand how the structure and function of proteins allow them to do what they do, what they interact with and how they contribute to life processes.

Metabolomics (*e.g.* Metabolite profiling, chemical fingerprinting, flux analysis)

Metabolomics is one of the newest 'omics' sciences. The metabolome refers to the complete set of low molecular weight compounds in a sample. These compounds are the substrates and by products of enzymatic reactions and have a direct effect on the phenotype of the cell. Thus, metabolomics aims at determining a sample's profile of these compounds at a specified time under specific environmental conditions

Transgenomics (*e.g.* Knock-out, knock-in, gene tagging, mutagenesis)

Transgenomics is the process of introducing genomic clones from a donor species into a recipient species and then screening the resultant transgenic lines for phenotypes of interest. This method might allow us to find genes involved in the evolution of phenotypic differences between species as well as genes that have the potential to contribute to reproductive isolation: potential speciation genes.

Applications of Biotechnology

1. Plant/Agricultural Biotechnology

A. Crop Biotechnology

B. Horticultural Biotechnology
C. Tree Biotechnology
D. Animal Biotechnology
E. Food processing

2. **Environmental Biotechnology**

A. Environmental monitoring
- ✰ Diagnosis of environmental problems via biotechnology

B. Waste management
- ✰ Bioremediation: the use of microbes to break down organic molecules or environmental pollutants.
- ✰ Phyto remediation: the use of plants to remove pollutants (*e.g.* heavy metals) from
  - ❖ The environment.
- ✰ Pollution prevention
  - ❖ Renewable resources
  - ❖ Biodegradable products
  - ❖ Alternative energy sources

3. **Medical Biotechnology**

A. Diagnostics
B. Therapeutics
C. Vaccines
D. Medical research tools
E. Human Genome Research

4. **Evolutionary and Ecological Genomics**

- ✰ Finding genes associated with ecological traits and evolutionary diversification.
- ✰ Common goals: health, productivity

Plant Biotechnology/Agricultural Biotechnology

Tissue Culture

The technique of plant tissue culture is used for growing isolated plant cells, tissues and organs under axenic conditions (*in vitro*) to regenerate and propagate entire plants. 'Tissue culture' is commonly used as a blanket term to describe all types of plant cultures, namely callus, cell, protoplast, anther, meristem, embryo and organ cultures. It relies on the phenomenon of cell totipotency, *i.e.*, the ability of single cells to divide, to produce all the differentiated cells characteristic of organs and regenerate into a whole plant. The different techniques of culturing plant tissues may offer certain advantages over traditional methods of propagation.

Growing plants *in vitro* in a controlled environment, with in-depth knowledge of the culture conditions and the nature of the plant material, ensures effective clonal propagation of genetically superior genotypes of economically important plants. Tissue cultures represent the major experimental systems used for plant genetic engineering, as well as for studying the regulation of growth and organized development through examination of structural, physiological, biochemical and molecular bases underlying developmental processes.

Genetic Engineering/Recombinant DNA Technology

Manipulation of genes is called genetic engineering or recombinant DNA technology. Manipulation of genes would be done in two ways either gene(s) isolated from one organism and transfers them to another organism or puts them back in the original with a different combination. In agriculture it mainly involved to develop genetically modified plants.

A process to produce a genetically modified plant by removing genetic information from an organism, manipulating it in the laboratory and then transferring it into a plant to change certain of its characteristics. In Nutshell it's the manipulation of plants for the benefit of mankind

The plants are mainly manipulated for two major objectives:

A. Crop Improvement

- ☆ Herbicide tolerance (in use)
- ☆ Pest resistance (in use)
- ☆ Drought tolerance
- ☆ Nitrogen fixing ability
- ☆ Acidity and Salinity tolerance

B. Nutritional Value of Crops

- ☆ Improving food quality and safety
- ☆ Healthier cooking oils by decreasing the concentration of saturated fatty acids in vegetable oils
- ☆ Functional foods: foods containing significant levels of biologically active components that impart health benefits

Molecular Breeding

Traditional plant breeding involves cross-breeding of similar plants to produce new varieties with different traits. But it takes many generations to achieve desired result. By using various biotechnological tools, crop improvement can be achieved faster with more accurate manner.

Marker Assisted Selection (MAS)

Marker assisted genetic analysis involved in studying and analysis of DNA sequences to identify genes, QTLs (quantitative trait loci), and other molecular markers associate with organism functions, *i.e.*, gene identification. Marker-aided selection is the identification and tracing inheritance of previously identified DNA fragments through a series of generations.

History of Biotechnology

1797: First vaccination. Edward Jenner takes pus from a cowpox lesion, inserts it into an incision on a boy's arm.

1830: Proteins are discovered.

1833: First enzyme is discovered and isolated

1865: Gregor Mendel discovers the laws of inheritance by studying flowers in his garden and the science of genetics begins around 1900.

1915: Phages -viruses that only infect bacteria are discovered

1917: The term Biotechnology was coined by a Hungarian Engineer Karl Ereky

1927: Herman Muller discovers that radiation causes defects in chromosomes.

1944: DNA is proven to carry genetic information by Oswald Avery, Colin MacLeod and Maclyn McCarty.

1952: Hershey and Chase confirmed role of DNA as the basic genetic material

1953: James Watson and Francis Crick describe the double helical structure of DNA. They shared the 1962 Nobel Prize in Medicine or Physiology with Maurice Wilkins.

1955: The amino acid sequence of insulin is discovered by Frederick Sanger.

1958: DNA polymerase discovered and its action demonstrated

1958: DNA is made in a test tube for the first time. Sickle cell disease is shown to occur due to a change in one amino acid

1960: Genetic code deciphered

1971: The first complete synthesis of a gene occurs. Discovery of restriction enzymes that cut and splice genetic material very specifically occurs. This opens the way for gene cloning.

1973: Stanley Cohen and Herbert Boyer perfect genetic engineering techniques to cut and paste DNA using restriction enzymes.

1975: Georges Kohler and Cesar Milstein develop the technology to produce monoclonal antibodies - highly specific, purified antibodies derived from only one clone of cells that recognize only one antigen. They shared the Nobel Prize given at 1984 for Physiology or Medicine with Neils Jerne.

1977: A method is developed for rapidly determining the sequence of the bases that carry the genetic code in a DNA molecule

1981: The first transgenic animals are produced by transferring genes from other animals into mice.

1982: Krens, F.A., Molondijk, L. Williams G. J. and Schilperoort, R.A developed poly ethylene glycol method for the direct delivery of DNA into protoplasts.

1983: The polymerase chain reaction (PCR) technique, which makes unlimited copies of genes and gene fragments, is discovered by Kary Mullis, got Nobel Prize in Chemistry in 1993.

1983: Zambryski, P. Joos, H., Genetello, C., Leemans, J. Van Montagu M. and Schell Constructed Ti plasmid vector for the introduction of DNA into plant cells without alteration of their normal regeneration capacity.

1984: Watts, J. W. and King, J. M developed a simple method for large scale electrofusion of protoplasts.

1984: Brisson, N. Paszkowski, J. Penswick, J. R. Gronenborn, B. Potrykus, I. and Hohn, T Achieved transformation in which part of the cauliflower mosaic virus genome was replaced by selectable marker.

1985: Gheysen, G. Dahese, P., Van Montaque, M. and Schell, J developed very efficient gene transfer system using natural gene transfer mechanism of *Agrobacterium tumifaciens*.

1985: Cocking E. C exposed plasma membrane in the tips of root hairs of wide range of crop plants. The procedure enabled whole seedlings to have the plasma membrane at the tips of their root hairs exposed to foreign DNA and other microorganisms.

1985: Tabata, M. and Fujita, Y developed the technique of elucidation of the physical and chemical factors controlling the biosynthesis of the red napthoquinone pigments by *Lythospermum erythrorhizon*.

1986: First recombinant vaccine is approved for human use: hepatitis B. First anti-cancer drug is produced through biotech: interferon.

1986: Crossway, A. Oakes, J.V., Irvine, J.M., Ward B. Knauf, V.C. and Shewmaker, C.K developed a direct way of transferring cloned genes into protoplasts by microinjection of DNA directly into the nucleus of tobacco mesophyll protoplasts.

1986: Hamill, J. D. Parr, A. J., Robins, R. J. and Rhodes, M.J.C established hairy root cultures of Beta vulgaris and *Nicotinna rustica* following infection with *Agrobacterium rhizogenes* and the transformed cultures synthesized their characteristic secondary products at levels comparable with those of in vitro roots from the same variety.

1986: Abdullah, R., Cocking, E.C., and Thompson, J.A demonstrated that normal green rice plants can be regenerated efficiently and reproducibly from rice protoplasts via Somatic embryogenesis.

1986: Pirrie, A. and Power, J.B produced fertile, interspecific gametosomatic triploid hybrids of tobacco by fusing protoplasts of leaf (2n) and pollen tetrad (n).

1986: Kinsara A., Patnaik, S.N., Cocking, E.C. and Power, J.B produced somatic hybrids between *Lycopersicon esculentum* and *L. peruvianum.*

1987: First approval for field tests of a genetically modified food plant: virus-resistant tomatoes.

1987: Terada, R., Kyozuka, J., Nishibayashi, S., and Shimamoto, K regenerated plantlets form somatic hybrid cells of *Oryza sativa*, and *Echinochloa oryzicola.*

1987: Ethlenfelt, N.K. and Helgeson, J.P produced tetroploid and hexaploid somatic hybrids from protoplast fusions between *Solanum bravidens* (2x, non tuber bearing species) and 2x and 4x *S. tuberosum.*

1987: Neuhaus, G., Spangenberg, G. Mittelsten Sheid, O and Schweiger, H.G effected gene transfer by microinjecting the DNA into the cells of microspore derived proembryos.

1987: De la Pesa, A., Lornz, H., Schell, J developed transgenic rye plants obtained by injecting DNA into young floral tillers.

1988: Nomoru, K. and Komamine, A used single cells of carrot from a cell suspension instead of protoplasts, for microinjection and the microinjected carrot cells could divide and differentiated to embryos at a frequency of about 50 percent.

1988: Rhodes, C.A., Pierce, D.A., Mettler, I. J. Mascarenhas, D. and Detmer J.J produced transgenic maize plant by electrophoration.

1988: Toriyama, K., Arimoto, Y. Uchimiya, H, and Hinata K produced transgenic rice plant by electrophoration.

1989: Shimamoto, K., Terada, R., Izawa, T. and Fujimoto, H produced fertile transgenic rice plants regenerated from transformed protoplasts.

1989: Prioli, L. M. and Sondahl, M. R recovered fertile plants from protoplasts of maize.

1990: Milanova, V. and Zagorska, N. A succeeded in overcoming hybrid incompatibility between *Nicotiana africana* and *N. fricanam* and produced cytoplasmic male sterile plants by embryo culture.

1990: Iida, A., Seki, M. Kamada, M. YHamada Y. and Morikawa delivered genes into cultured plant cells by DNA-coated gold particles accelerated by a pneumatic particle gun.

1991: Kyozuka, J. Fujimoto, H., Izawa, T. and Shimamoto- K succeeded in getting tissue specific expression of maize alcohol dehydrogenase l gene in transgenic rice plants and their progenies.

1991: Spangenberg, G., Fredyl, E., Osusky, M. Nagel, J. and Potrykus, I developed a method for the predictable transfer of partial genomes predictable transfer of partial genomes by using sub protoplasts (cytoplasts and karyoplasts).

1991: Sautter, C., Waldner, H. Neuhaus, G., Galli, A. Neuhaus, G. and Potrykus developed a novel method for the acceleration of micro projectiles. The method is called as micro targeting.

1994: Genetically modified tomatoes are sold in the U.S. for the first time.

1990: The Human Genome Project an international effort to maps all of the genes in the human genome is launched.

2002: The draft version of the human genome is published.

1997: Scientists report the birth of Dolly, the first animal cloned from an adult cell.

1998: Human embryonic stem cell lines are established. They offer hope to many because they may be able to replace diseased or dysfunctional cells.

2003: The SARS (severe acute respiratory syndrome) virus is sequenced three weeks after its discovery.

2004: The first cloned pet a kitten is delivered to its owner. She is called Copy Cat (or Cc for short).

2006: A recombinant vaccine against human papillomavirus (HPV) receives FDA approval. The virus causes genital warts and can cause cervical cancer.

Landmarks in the Origin of Modern Biotechnology

Table 1.1. Milestones in Plant Biotechnology

Year	*The Breakthrough*
1983	Ti plasmid disarmed and first transgenic plants produced
1983	Selectable markers for plants
1986	Coat protein mediated virus resistance
1987	*Bt.*-based insect resistance
1987	Herbicide resistance
1987	Particle gun
1987	Cotton transformation
1988	Soybean transformation
1988	Rice transformation
1988	Ripening control in tomato
1988	Antisense in plants
1990	RAPD analysis
1990	Corn transformation
1990	Engineered male sterility

Year	*The Breakthrough*
1992	Wheat transformation
1992	Modified carbohydrate composition
1992	Engineered fertility restoration
1992	Modified fatty acid composition

Table 1.2. Landmarks in Commercialization of Modern Plant Biotechnology

Year	*Major Development*
1985	US allows plant patents
1986	First field trial of transgenic plant approved in the US and Europe
1987	USDA/APHIS proposed guidelines for field testing
1990	EC directive on deliberate release and commercialization of transgenics
1991	Revised UPOV convention accommodates biotech products
1992	Over four hundred field tests performed worldwide
1992	USDA/APHIS deregulates transgenic ripening controlled tomato
1992	USDA/APHIS proposes simpler procedure for field testing of six crop species
1992	FDA established frame work for food safety evaluation
1993	US patent on insect resistant plants issued

Part II

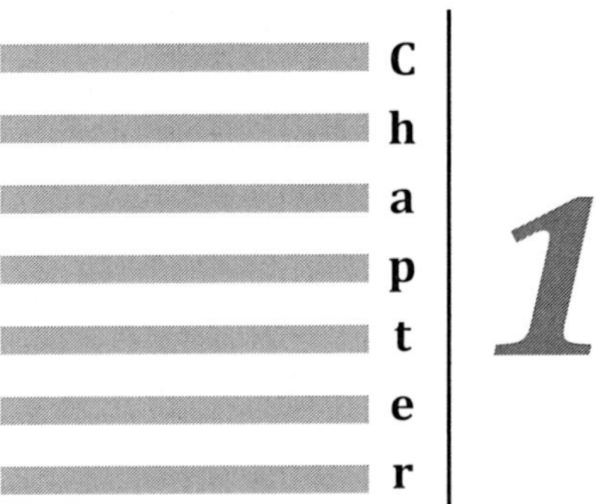

Chapter 1

Plant Tissue Culture: Concepts, History and Scope

Plant tissue culture broadly refers to *in vitro* cultivation of all plant parts *i.e.,* a single cell, a tissue or organ under aseptic conditions in artificial nutrient media. This new technique has enabled us to increase the knowledge in the following field of studies.

- Totipotency, nutrition, metabolism, division, differentiation and preservation of plant cells.
- Morphogenesis and plant regeneration from individual cells or tissues through the process namely organogenesis or somatic embryogenesis.
- Variations generated through *in vitro* culture.
- Evolution of haploids through anther, pollen culture and ovule culture.
- Wide hybridization programmes through ovule, ovary and embryo cultures to overcome both pre zygotic and post zygotic sterility mechanisms
- Micropropagation of plant materials
- *In vitro* selection of mutants tolerant to biotic and abiotic stresses.
- *In vitro* culture and secondary metabolite biosynthesis.
- Plant genetic engineering through *in vitro* culture methods and DNA transfer technique.

Cellular Totipotency

The inherent potentiality of a plant cell to give rise to a whole plant is described as cellular totipotency. **T.H. Morgan coined the term "Totipotency".** This is a capacity which is retained even after a cell has undergone final differentiation in the plant body. In plants, even highly mature and differentiated cells retain the ability to regenerate to a meristematic state as long as they have an intact membrane system and a viable nucleus. This is contradicting to animals, where differentiation is generally irreversible.

For a differentiated cell, to express its totipotency, it first undergoes dedifferentiation followed by redifferentiation.

- The phenomenon of a mature cell reverting to the meristematic state and forming undifferentiated callus tissue is termed 'dedifferentiation'.
- The phenomenon of conversion of component cells of callus tissue to whole plant or plant organs is called as 'redifferentiation'.

History of Plant Tissue Culture

1756: Duharmel du Monceau, H.L. discovered callus formation from the decorticated elm tree. This very old work was foreword for the discovery of plant tissue culture.

1839: Schwann, T.H expressed the view that each living cell of a multicellular organism would be capable of developing independently if provided with proper external conditions.

1878: Vochting, H. obtained very luxuriant callus from *Brassica rapa* and proposed the polarity in development of buds from the upper portion and roots or callus and from the lower portion of a stem piece.

1893: Rechinger, C. described callus formation on isolated stem fragments and root slices.

1901: Morgan, T.H. coined the term totipotency to describe the capability of a cell to form an individual plant.

1902: Haberlandt, G. a German plant physiologist, attempted to cultivate plant tissue culture cell *in vitro.* He is regarded as the father of plant tissue culture. He attempted culture of isolated single palisade cells from leaves in knop's salt solution enriched with sucrose. The cells remained alive for up to one month, increased in size, accumulated starch but failed to divide. He published a paper on "Experiments on the culture of isolated plant cells".

1904: Hanning attempted embryo culture of selected crucifers.

1922: Knudson reported asymbiotic germination of orchid seeds *in vitro*.

1922: Robbins, W.J. started cultivation of excised root tips and stem tips of maize under sterile conditions; however, the cultures did not survive independently.

1925: Liabach, F. demonstrated the most important application of the embryo culture by crossing *Linum perenae* with *L. austriacum* to get hybrid plants from shrivelled seeds.

1934: Gautheret, R.J made preliminary attempts with liquid medium for cultivating plant tissues but failed completely. Later he cultured the explants on medium solidified with agar, and got healthy calli from the explants.

1934: White, P.R obtained indefinite survival of cultured tomato roots on subculturing in liquid medium.

1939: White, P.R., Gautheret, R.J. and Nobecourt, P simultaneously announced the possibility of cultivating plant tissues for unlimited periods.

1941: Van Overbeek, J., Conklin, M.E. and Blackeslee, A.F established importance of coconut milk for growth and development of very young *Datura* embryos.

1944: Skoog, F started his work on organogenesis in tobacco callus.

1944: Skoog, F reported his work on adventious shoot formation in tobacco.

1946: Ball, E.A showed development of plantlets from sterile cultures of stem tips in *Tropaeolum* and *Lupinus.*He is considered as father of micropropagation.

1947: La Rue C.D initiated endosperm cultures of *Zea mays* and obtained subcultures.

1948: Skoog, F. and Tsui, C. studied the chemical control of growth and bud formation in tobacco stem segments and callus cultured in vitro and suggested that callus induction and shoot initiation can be regulated by making manipulations in the culture medium.

1952: Steward, F.C., Caplin, S.M. and Miller, F. K. discovered the synergistic action of 2, 4-D and coconut milk in a culture of potato tissue.

1952: Morel, G. and Martin, C. were the first to demonstrate that virus free plants can be recovered from infected plants through shoot meristem culture. Also they reported first application of micrografting.

1952: Routien and Nickel (Pfizer and Co. Inc., New York) got the US Patent on their claim that plant cells could be grown in liquid nutrient medium and has the potential to produce useful compounds.

1953: Muir, W.H. found out the cultural conditions favouring the isolation and growth of single cells from higher plants *in vitro* and established nurse culture technique.

1954: Muir, W.H. Hildebrandt, A.C. and Riker, A.J obtained the first suspension cultures by transferring callus fragments to agitated liquid medium

1954: Muir, W.H. Hildebrandt, A.C. and Riker, A.J. obtained first plant from a single cell.

1955: Miller, C.O., Skoog, F., Von Saltza, M. and Strong, F.M. identified a cell division factor *viz.*, 6-furfualamino purine commonly called kinetin.

1957: Skoog, F. and Miller, C.O. advanced the hypothesis that shoot and root initiation in cultured callus can be regulated by particular ratios of auxins and cytokinin.

1957: Maheshwari and Rangaswamy observed regeneration of somatic embryos *in vitro* from the nucellus of citrus ovules.

1957: Skoog, F. and Miller, C.O. discovered and introduced the idea of synergistic effects of auxins and cytokinins in promoting cell division in tobacco.

1958: Steward, F.C., Mapes, M.O. and Mears, K. observed the phenomenon of somatic embryogenesis in suspension culture of carrot. They also reported that cells in suspension derived from explanted roots of cultivated carrots were capable of forming unorganised cell clusters, which in turn could yield first roots, then shoots and ultimately whole plants.

1959: Reinert, J. observed the somatic embryo formation from callus clumps and suspension cultures of carrot.

1959: Gautheret published first handbook of Plant Tissue Culture.

1959: Melchers, G. and Bergmann, L. were first to culture haploid tissues other than pollen.

1960: Cocking, E.C discovered the technique of isolation and culture of protoplasts after digesting the cell walls enzymatically and demonstrated new cell wall regeneration on protoplasts from tomato fruit locule tissue.

1960: Bergmann, L. was first to obtain callus by plating cells from suspension cultures on to solid medium. This plating involved mixing cells with warm sugar medium just prior to gelation in petridish (Bergmann plating technique)

1960: Morel, G. discovered a technique to produce virus free progenies by meristem culture in Cymbidium.

1960: Cocking, E.C. discovered the technique of isolation and culture of protoplasts after digesting the cell walls enzymatically and demonstrated new cell wall regeneration on protoplasts from tomato fruit locule tissue.

1960: Bergmann, L. was first to obtain callus by plating cells from suspension cultures on to solid medium. This plating involved mixing cells with warm sugar medium just prior to gelation in petridish (Bergmann plating technique)

1964: Guha, S. and Maheshwari, S.C. cultured mature anthers of *Datura innoxia* to study the physiology of meiosis and accidentally noticed the development of embryoids from the anthers plated on basal medium supplemented with kinetin and coconut milk.

1965: Vasil, V. and Hildebrandt, A.C. described rearing of a mature tobacco plant from a single cell grown initially in microculture.

1966: Torrey, J.G. advanced the hypothesis that organogenesis in callus is initiated with the formation of clusters of meristematic cells called meristemoids.

1970: Kasha, K. J. and Kao, K.N. produced haploid plants of *Hordeum vulgare* by in vitro culturing of embryos obtained by cross *Hordeum vulgare* with *Hordeum bulbosum* in which elimination of bulbosum chromosome occurred.

1970: Steward pointed out, the plant tissue culture technique is another "Silent Revolution in Agriculture" having very good potentials to supplement conventional breeding approaches.

1970: Carlson reported the selection of biochemical mutants *in vitro* by the use of tissue culture derived variation.

1970: Power *et al.,* achieved protoplast fusion for the first time.

1971: Takebe, I., Labib, G. and Melchers, G. regenerated whole plants from isolated mesophyll protoplasts of tobacco.

1971: Bendich, A.J. and Filner, P. used the cells and tissues in culture for transformation studies.

1972: Withers, L. and Cocking, E.C. laid foundation for the protoplast fusion technique.

1974: Melchers, G. and Labib, G. proposed hybrids resembling the sexual hybrids by fusing protoplasts of two varieties of Nicotiana tabacum

1974: Murashige, T. developed the concept of developmental stages in cultures *in vitro*: Stage I: Explant establishment; Stage II: Multiplication of propagule and Stage III: Rooting and hardening for planting into soil.

1976: Mullin, R.H. and Schlegal, D.E. successfully employed cold storage to maintain *in vitro* virus free plantlets of strawberry.

1976: Seibert, M. established shoot initiation from carnation shoot apices frozen to -196°C.

1980: Gleba Y.Y. and Hoffmann, F. synthesized a new plant "Arabidobrassica by fusing the protoplasts *Arabidopsis* and *Brassica*.

1981: Larkin, P.J. and Scowcroft, W.R. developed the concept of somaclonal variation: A novel source of variability from cell cultures for plant improvement.

1981: Patnaik, G., Wilson, D. and Cocking, E.C. regenerated a whole plant from a single free cultured tobacco protoplast

Scope of Tissue Culture

1. Clonal Propagation or Vegetative Propagation

Most of the plants are sexually propagated. However, some plants reproduce asexually and some others can reproduce both sexually and asexually. While the sexually produced progenies show high degree of variability due to segregation and re-combinations, the vegetatively propagated progenies will be uniform with respect to all their characteristics and they will be identical to their mother plant. Thus, clonal propagation in many situations have greater advantages over the other.

Micropropagation is the method of clonal propagation of plants using *in vitro* techniques. This can be achieved by culturing apical or axillary buds which under favourable conditions of culture can grow and give rise to shoots which subsequently can be rooted to produce plantlets. Clonal plantlets can also be produced from plant parts like stem, leaf or root segments under culture. Here the explants may either directly or indirectly through an intervening callus give rise to shoots or somatic embryoids which ultimately produce plantlets. The most important advantage of micropropagation is the multiplication of superior genotypes. In unisexual plants selective multiplication of female plants can also be achieved by micropropagation.

2. Production of Disease Free Plants

Viral diseases can be a serious problem in some plants like potato, sugarcane *etc.* The propagation of virus infected plants causes a very serious problem in seeds as well as stem cuttings of such plants will harbour the viral population. Under this circumstance culturing the apical meristem and producing plants following tissue culture methods is the only means by which virus free plants can be obtained. Meristem culture coupled with rapid micropropagation is making a major contribution to the supply of quality planting materials in many crops where viral diseases are a serious problem.

3. Production of New Variants or Mutants

Variability is the fundamental basis of selection. Superior types can be selected from among the available variability. However, there are species where genetic variability is very little due to various reasons. Under such circumstances tissue culture technique offers an opportunity to create genetic variability in the population. One of the methods of achieving this is to resort to cell culture. By 1950's it was established that single cells under culture can give rise to full plants. Such plants showed variability which is commonly referred to as somaclonal variation. Techniques have also been developed to increase the magnitude of such variations by artificial means of mutagenesis. Since screening for characters like stress tolerance, disease resistance *etc.* can be carried out under the culture conditions itself selection of superior genotypes can be done using this method.

4. Production of Homozygous Plants

Pollen grains, the male sex cells of plants, can be made to grow and give rise to plants by culturing the anthers in artificial media. Since the pollen grains are haploid, the plants derived from them also will have only half the number of chromosomes. These plants can be made diploid by resorting to proper techniques and the plants thus produced will be homozygous for all the genes. Such homozygous plants though may not have immediate practical utility, will have far reaching uses in crop improvement programmes. Following the technique of anther culture the breeding time required can be reduced tremendously.

5. Production of Secondary Metabolites

Many plants produce secondary metabolites, which are having various uses. Many of the alkaloids, food flavours, sweeteners, vitamins, insecticides, enzymes *etc.* are some of the examples of such secondary metabolites. Usually such chemical compounds are extracted from various plant parts. However, it has been shown that in some plants such metabolites can be extracted from cultured tissues without going to the plants. In such cases, cell cultures are generally employed. The callus produced in culture are found to yield the secondary metabolites. This method has been put into practical use under many situations as a cheaper method of making available the chemical substance.

6. Overcoming Incompatibility Barriers

Hybridisation is a method of crop improvement where the favourable characteristics of two plants are combined into a single plant. In many cases conventional methods of hybridization may not be possible due to various incompatibility factors. This will be more so when the parents belong to different species, genera *etc.* Under such situations the incompatibility barrier and thus the production of hybrid is made possible. Some of the specific methods of tissue culture techniques that can be used for this are embryo culture (embryo rescue), ovule culture, pollen culture, *in vitro* pollination, protoplast culture and fusion *etc.*

7. Tissue Culture as a Tool for Genetic Engineering

Genetic engineering is the manipulation of the genetic material of plants at the DNA level. This is achieved by incorporating a desired gene to a plant which otherwise is lacking it. Use of tissue culture especially cell culture, protoplast culture, embryo culture *etc.* are the general techniques used for achieving this.

8. Germplasm Conservation and Exchange

The diverse germplasm of any species is normally maintained by using seeds or planting materials. However, this may become time consuming and expensive under many situations. The technique may be more labour intensive and require lot of space also. To overcome these difficulties the storage and maintenance of the germplasm can be done by using cultured materials like embryos, callus *etc.* Such materials will be easier for handling and storage. They can as well be used for exchange of germplasm.

Limitation of Tissue Culture

One of the most important limitations of tissue culture is the laborious and time consuming standardization procedure required to develop a proper protocol for culture. Unless an economically viable protocol is not available the technology cannot be implemented. This is especially true in case of micropropagation technique.

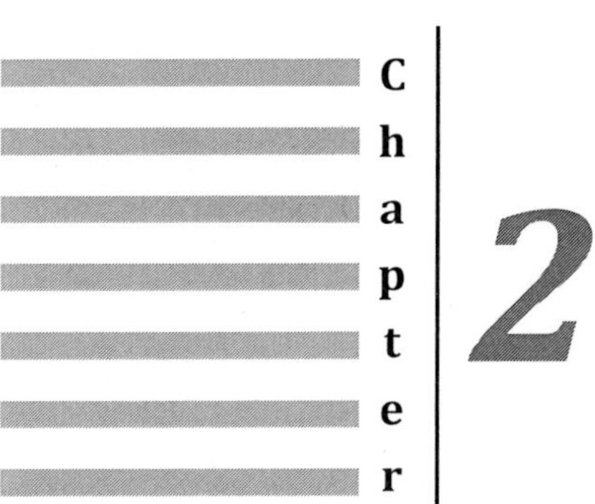

Media and Culture Conditions and Sterilization Techniques

The intact plants can make their own food but the *in vitro* culture of plant parts or cells requires a variety of nutrients and suitable physical conditions for their growth. The composition of medium for the tissue culture is the most important key factor in the successful culture of plant cells. The components of tissue culture media may be broadly grouped into basic/basal media and growth hormones. Basic medium provides the general requirements of growth of plants, plant parts and cultures. These are usually not species and purpose-specific. On the contrary, growth regulators are more specific for both purpose and species. For example, specific hormones are added for root induction and some other for multiple shoot production. Similarly, the hormonal mixture useful for one species will not be so for another, thus making it necessary for arriving at hormonal protocols for each plant species.

Basic Media

The components of basic media are the following:

1. Macronutrients: Always used
2. Micronutrients: Almost always used
3. Sugars: Almost always used
4. Vitamins: Generally used
5. Amino acids and other nitrogen supplements: Sometimes used
6. Undefined supplements: Sometimes used
7. Solidifying agent: Used when necessary

The medium should be accurately defined of inorganic and organic chemical additives so as to provide,

i) The nutrients for the survival of the plant cells, tissues and organs under culture

ii) The optimal physical condition of pH, osmotic pressure *etc.*

I. Media Composition

Nutrient Media

The composition of plant tissue culture medium depends upon the type of plant tissues or cells that are used for culture. No single medium can be used for all types of plants and organs, so the composition of the culture medium for each plant material has to be worked out.

A typical nutrient medium consists of the following components:

1. Inorganic Nutrients (Macro and Micro nutrients)

The six elements namely **nitrogen, phosphorus, potassium, calcium, magnesium and sulfur** are the essential macronutrients for tissue culture. The ideal concentration of **nitrogen, and potassium** is around **25 mmol L^{-1}**, while for **calcium, phosphorus, sulfur and magnesium, it is in the range of 1-3 mmol L^{-1}** Among the micronutrients **Iron, Managanese, Copper, Zinc, Molybdenum and Cobalt** requirement is very critical. Chelated form of **iron and copper** are commonly used in culture media (Table 2.1).

Table 2.1. Inorganic Plant Nutrition and their Physiological Function.

Element	*Function*
Nitrogen (N2)	Component of proteins nucleic acids some co-enzymes
Phosphorous (P)	Component of nucleic acids energy transfer component of intermediate in respiration and photosynthesis
Potassium (K)	Regulates osmotic potential principal in organic cation
Calcium (Ca)	Cell wall synthesis. Membrane function cell signalling
Magnesium (Mg)	Enzyme co-factor component of chlorophyll
Sulphur (S)	Component of some amino acids (Methionine cysteine) some co-factors
Iron (Fe)	Electron transfer as a component of cytochromes
Managanese (Mn)	Enzyme co-factor
Cobalt (Co)	Component of some vitamins
Copper (Cu)	Enzyme co-factor electron transfer reaction
Zinc (Zn)	Enzyme co-factor chlorophyll biosynthesis
Molybdenum (Mo)	Enzyme co-factor component of nitrate reductase.

2. Sugars

Sugar (usually **sucrose**) is used as a carbon and energy source in culture media. Plant cells and tissues in the culture medium are heterotrophic and therefore depend on the external carbon for energy. Among the various energy sources, sucrose is the most preferred. During the sterilization of the medium, sucrose gets hydrolysed to glucose and fructose and the plant cells utilize first the glucose and than the fructose. The other carbohydrates such as lactose, maltose, galactose *etc.* have been used in culture media but with limited success.

3. Vitamins

Vitamins (***e.g.* nicotinic acid, thiamine, pyridoxine and myo-inositol**) are growth regulatory substances that are derived from food in animals. The plant cells in culture are able to synthesize vitamins just like natural plants, but in suboptimal quantities which does not support proper growth of cells in culture. Therefore the medium is supplemented with vitamins to achieve good growth of cells. **The vitamins most commonly used are thiamine (B1), nicotinic acid (niacin) and pyridoxine.** MS, WPM, White's and SH media have all these three.

Myo-inositol is not a vitamin in the animal sense but is a common ingredient in bacterial and animal cell cultures. Its addition in plant tissue culture media has not been established to be essential but its presence has been found beneficial. **It is, therefore, called a plant vitamin.**

4. Amino Acids and other Nitrogen Supplements

Amino acids are added to the cell cultures to stimulate the cell growth and estabilish the cell lines. These are sources of N, but these cannot completely substitute inorganic sources. These were also found beneficial in some occasions; but wherever useful, the effects could be attributed to medium inadequacies. **Among the amino acids, the most commonly used is glycine. Some other sources are peptone, casein hydrolysate.**

5. Undefined Supplements

Many undefined supplements were employed in early tissue culture media. These were used mainly as sources of hormones. Over the years, their use is declining as the uses of hormones are being better understood even-though some of them are common even now. Some examples are coconut water, yeast extract, meat extract, malt extract fruit juices (banana and tomato).

6. Solidifying Agent

Tissues in static liquid medium are damaged by lack of oxygen if they sink and are often **gelled with gelling agents**. The most common gelling agent is agar, a polysaccharide obtained from sea weeds **(red algae, *Gelidium amansil*)** is added to the liquid medium for its solidification. **It melts at 100 °C and solidifies at 45°C.** It does not react with medium ingredient and is not digested by plant enzymes. It is usually added at **0.5 - 1 per cent.** Hardness depends on content of agar. Other gelling agents are gelatin, phytogel, gelrite, methocel, alginate *etc.*

7. Activated Charcoal

In some specific condition the addition of activated charcoal to culture media is reported to stimulate growth and differentiation in banana, orchids, carrot, ivy and tomato. It stimulates the growth by adsorption of inhibitory compounds and toxics.

II. Plant Growth Regulators

These are organic compounds, other than nutrients, which influence growth, differentiation and multiplication. They required in very minute quantity in the media. The requirement for these substances varies considerably with the tissue and it also depends on their endogenous level. There are many commercially available synthetic substances that mimics the PGR specific to certain species. There are different groups of PGRs commonly used in the media. They are auxins, cytokinins, gibberellins, ethylene and abscisic acid. Additional substances gaining recognition as hormones in plant tissue culture are: polyamines, jasmonates, salicylic acid and brassinosteroids.

a. Auxin

In nature, the hormones of this group are involved with elongation of stem, internodes, tropism, apical dominance, abscission *etc.*, In tissue culture auxins have been used for rooting, callus induction, somatic embryogenesis. The commonly used auxins in tissue culture are

1. Indole-3-acetic acid (IAA)(Natural)
2. Indole-3-butyric acid (IBA)(Natural)
3. Naphthalene acetic acid (NAA)
4. Dichlorophenoxyacetic acid (2, 4-D)

Among these IAA and IBA are natural auxins. Auxins are usually dissolved in either ethanol or dilute 0.5 N NaOH.

b. Cytokinins

These hormones are essential for cell division, modification of apical dominance, shoot differentiation *etc.*, In tissue culture media, cytokinins are incorporated mainly for cell division, differentiation of adventitious shoots from callus and organ and shoot proliferation. Commonly used cytokinins are

1. Benzylamino purine (BAP)
2. Isopentenyl adenine (2-ip)(Natural)
3. Furfurylamino purine (kinetin)(Natural)
4. Zeatin

Kinetin and Isopentenyl adenine are naturally existing cytokinins. Cytokinins are generally dissolved in dilute HCl or NaOH.

Auxin - Cytokinin Interaction (Skoog and Miller)

1. High auxin and low cytokinin ratio: **Initialize root formation, embryogenesis and callus formation.**
2. Low auxin and high cytokinin ratio: **Induce formation of adventitive or axillary shoots.**
3. The **auxin-cytokinin ratio is also essential for chloroplast formation** and other processes.

c. Gibberellins

Naturally occurring plant hormones involved in **internode elongation, enhancement of flower, fruit and leaf size, germination and vernalization in plants**. Among more than 100 known gibberellins, GA_3 is used widely in plant tissue culture. **Compared to auxins and cytokinins, gibberellins are used very rarely.** They stimulate normal development of plantlets from *in vitro* formed adventitious embryos. They are soluble in cold water.

d. Ethylene

A gaseous plant hormone involved in fruit maturation, abscission, and senescence. All kinds of plant tissue cultures produce ethylene and the rate of production increases under stress conditions. Use of ethylene precursor (2-Chloroethylphosphonic acid) in tissue culture may be promotory or inhibitory for the same process in different species. For example, it promoted somatic embryogenesis in *Zea mays* whereas the same process was inhibited in *Hevea brasiliensis.*

e. Abscisic Acid

A plant hormone involved in abscission, enforcing dormancy and regulating early stages of embryo development. It is required for normal growth and development of somatic embryos and promotes morphogenesis.

Physical Form of Plant Tissue Culture Media

To maintain the physical form of medium suitable for culturing, care should be taken to maintain the necessary (1) hydrogen ion concentration. (2) solidifying agent and (3) osmotic pressure of the medium.

1. Hydrogen Ion Concentration (pH)

The pH of the medium is usually adjusted between 5.0 and 6.0 prior to the addition of agar and autoclaving. The extremes of pH should be avoided as this will block the availability of some of nutrients to the cultures. **A pH of 5.8 is found to be optimum for plant tissue culture**. Generally, pH higher than 6.0 give a very hard medium and a pH below 5.0 do not allow satisfactory **solidification of agar**.

2. Osmotic Pressure

The cells cultured *in vitro* are mostly osmotically fragile and hence the osmotic pressure of the medium should be maintained at optimal level. This problem is serious one when liquid media are used. To adjust the osmotic pressure, stabilizers otherwise known as osmoticums *viz.*, **sorbitol and mannitol (sugar alcohol)** are used. These are non metabolisable sugars. The soluble sugars like sucrose, fructose, galactose, *etc.*, are also effective. **The sucrose is added to the medium not only to provide energy but also to maintain a suitable osmolarity in the medium.**

Preparation of Media and Major Types of Media Used in Tissue Culture Technique

The methodology for media preparation involves preparation of stock solutions (in the range of 10x to 250x concentrations) of highly purified chemicals and demineralized water. The stock solutions are stored in glass or plastic containers and frozen till further requirement. Now a days, plant tissue culture media are commercially prepared, and are available in the market as dry powders. The culture media is usually sterilized in an autoclave at 121°C and 15 psi for 20 minutes. Hormones and other heat sensitive organic compounds are filter sterilized and added to the autoclaved medium.

MS medium - formulated by Murashige and Skoog (MS) is most widely used for many types of culture systems (Table 2.3)

White's medium - is one of the earliest plant tissue culture media

B5 medium - developed by Gamborg for cell suspension and callus cultures and at present it's modified form used for **protoplast culture**

N6 medium - Nitsch's medium developed by **Nitsch and Nitsch and used for anther culture**

III. Sterilization

Plant tissue culture media which contain a high concentration of sucrose support the growth of many micro-organisms like fungi and bacteria. On reaching the medium, these microbes grow much faster than the cultured tissue and finally kill it. The contaminations may also give out metabolic wastes which are toxic to plant tissues. It is, therefore, essential to maintain a completely aseptic environment inside the culture vessels.

Medium

Microbial contaminations are present in the medium right from the start. To destroy them the mouth of the container is properly closed using a bacteria proof closure and the vial is autoclaved at **121° C for 15-40** min for the time the medium reaches the required temperature. The exposure time varies with the volume of the liquid as shown here (Table 2.2).

Table 2.2. Volume of the Material and Sterilization Time

Volume of Container (ml)	*Min. Sterilization Time (min)*
20-50	15
75	20
250-500	25
1000	30
1500	35
2000	40

Nutritive value of the culture medium may be reduced by prolonged sterilization. It also results in decomposition of chemicals present in the medium. If autoclave is not available a domestic pressure cooker may be used. Care must be taken while cooling. A rapid loss of pressure exceeding the rate of reduction in temperatures will make the liquid boil vigorously. The pressure gauge of the autoclave should be at zero before the autoclave is opened.

Some growth factors like GA_3, Zeatin, ABA *etc.* are thermolabile. These chemicals degrade on exposure to steam sterilisation. When using such a compound, the whole medium except the heat labile compound is autoclaved in a flask and kept in the sterilised hood to cool down. The solution of the thermolabile compound is sterilised by membrane filtration and added to the autoclaved medium when the latter is cooled down to 40°C (just before the setting of the agar) or to room temperature when using a liquid medium. **For filter sterilisation of the solutions, bacteria-proof filter membranes of pore size 0.45 micro meter (micron) or less are to be used**. The membranes are fitted into filter holders of appropriate size and autoclaved. The sterilised solution is added directly to the medium. Small volumes of solution can be sterilised by passing through the membrane filtration unit attached to a graduated syringe. Large filter assemblies are also available for larger volumes.

Glassware, Plastic-ware and Instruments

Glass culture vials are mostly sterilised together with the medium. The glassware may be sterilised by autoclaving. The objects to be sterilised are wrapped in aluminium foil before sterilisation. **The glassware can be sterilised by autoclaving or by heating in an oven at 160 - 180°C for 3 hrs.** Disadvantages of dry heat sterilisation are poor circulation and slow penetration. The instruments used for aseptic manipulations such as forceps, scalpel, needles and spatula are normally sterilised by dipping in 95 per cent ethyl alcohol followed by flaming and cooling. This is done at the start of the transfer work and is repeated several times during the operation. Autoclaving is not recommended for metal instruments because they may rust and become blunt.

Plant Material

Surface of plant parts carry a wide range of microbial contaminations. To avoid this source of infection, the tissue must be thoroughly surface sterilised before planting it in the nutrient medium. Tissues with systemic fungal or bacterial infection are usually discarded in tissue culture studies. To disinfect the plant tissues various sterilising agents have been used of which a few are listed below.

Sterilizing Agent	*Conc. Used*	*Duration*
1. Ethyl alcohol	70 per cent	10 seconds to 2 min.
2. Methyl alcohol	50 per cent	10 seconds to 2 min.
3. Chlorine water	3.5 per cent	10 seconds to 3 min.
4. Mercuric chloride($HgCl_2$)	0.1 per cent	3 min. to 15 min.
5. Sodium hypochlorite (Liquid bleach)	1.5 to3 per cent	3 min to 15 min
6. Calcium hypochlorite	25 to 100 g/l	3 min to 15 min
7. Isopropanol	80 per cent	30 min
8. Silver nitrate	1 per cent	30 min.

Most commonly used surface sterilant is mercuric chloride (0.1 per cent).

It is important to realise that the surface sterilant is also toxic to the plant tissues. Therefore the concentration of the sterilising agent and the duration of the treatment are chosen to minimise the tissue death. After sterilisation, the tissue is thoroughly washed with sterile distilled water to remove traces of the sterilant.

Ethyl alcohol is used as a surface sterilant for some plant tissue culture. After rinsing in ethanol for a few seconds, the material is left exposed in the sterile hood for evaporation of alcohol or can be washed with double distilled sterilized water. In general, if the explant is fairly hard and large enough to be easily handled, the inoculum can be directly treated with the disinfectant (seeds *etc.*). However, when immature ovules, embryos or endosperm are to be cultured, the ovary is sterilised and the explant is dissected out under sterile conditions (ovule, anthers, meristems *etc.*). In case when the explant carries a heavy load of micro-organism on its surface wash it in running tap water. Addition of surfactants like teepol to the sterilisation solution is also advised in such cases. Surfactants improve the efficiency of sterilisation by enhancing contact with the tissue. The choice of the sterilant and duration of sterilisation is standardised according to the explant. After sterilisation the plant material must be rinsed 3-4 times in sterile distilled water to remove all traces of the sterilant.

Table 2.3. Preparation of Stock Solutions for MS Medium

Ingredients	*Composition (mg/l)*	*Stock Solution (W/V) (g)*	*Final Volume of Stock Solution*	*Volume of the Stock Taken/Litre of Medium*
Macro Nutrients (10X)			500 ml	50 ml
NH_4NO_3	1650	16.50		
KNO_3	1900	19.00		
$CaCl_22H_2O$	440	4.40		
$MgSO_4.7H_2O$	370	3.70		
KH_2PO_4	170	1.70		
Minor Nutrients (100X)			250 ml	2.5ml
$MnSO_4.4\ H_2O$	22.3	2.23		
$ZnSO_4.4H_20$	8.6	0.86		
H_3BO_3	6.2	0.62		
Micro Nutrients (100 X)			100ml	1ml
$Na_2MoO_4.2H_2O$	0.25	0.025		
$CuSO_4.5\ H_2O$	0.025	0.0025		
$CoCl_2.6\ H_2O$	0.025	0.0025		
Iron Stock (50X)			250 ml	5ml
Na_2EDTA	37.25	1.863		
$FeSO_4.7H_2O$	27.85	1.393		
Kl (100X)			250 ml	2.5 ml
Kl	0.83	0.083		
MS Vitamins (100X)			100 ml	1ml
Nicotinic Acid	0.5	50 mg		
Pyridoxine. HCl	0.5	50 mg		
Thiamine. HCl	0.1	10 mg		
Glycine	2.0	200 mg		

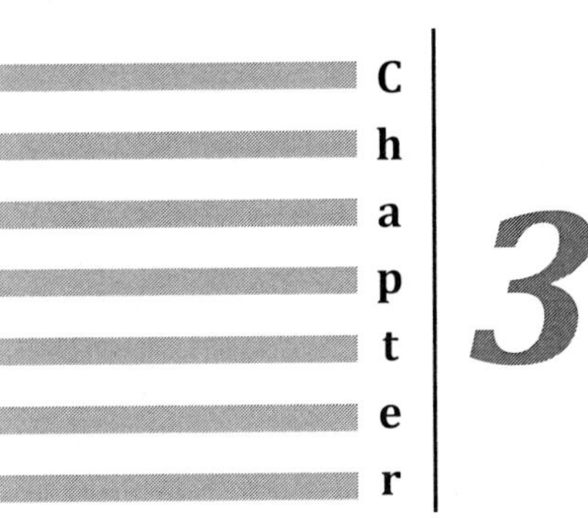

Regeneration Methods: Morphogenesis-Organogenesis and Embryogenesis

The process of growing an entire plant from a single and plant cell or group of cells *i.e.* callus, tissues and organs under defined physical and chemical condition based up on the principle of cellular totipotency is called plant regeneration. It is the major outcome of *in vitro* plant propagation and one of the important biotechnological application. Plant regeneration can be achieved by organogenesis and somatic embryogenesis (Figure 3.1).

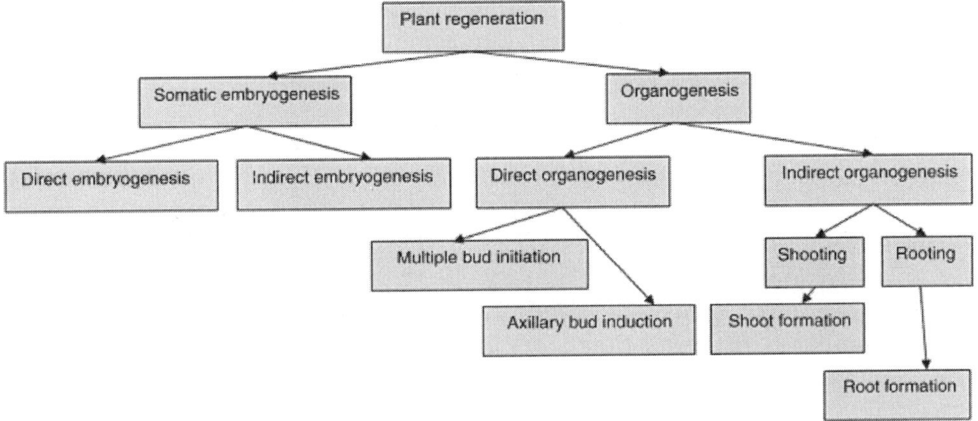

Figure 3.1. Different Routes of Plant Regeneration.

Development of organized structures such as shoots, roots, flower buds, *etc.*, from cultured cells or tissues under *in vitro* condition is called organogenesis. Organogenesis occurs in three distinct stages *viz.*, 1. Shoot bud formation 2. Shoot multiplication and elongation 3. Rooting of developed shoots. Regeneration through organogenesis is further classified in to direct and indirect organogenesis. **In direct organogenesis, *in vitro* organs are directly induced from explant tissues; in indirect regeneration, a *in vitro* organ is typically formed from not directly from explant tissue but an intermediate tissue, called callus**. Plant calli, are undifferentiated structures in which development of adventitious shoots from meristem like tissues called as **meristoemoids.** Meristemoid is a localized group of meristemic cells that may give rise to shoots and or roots. Meristemoids are considered to arise in areas that accumulate starch, which is believed to serve as an energy source for shoot bud differentiation. Shoot and root is usually developed from the shoot and root meristems present in the plumule and radicle respectively present in the zygote. But developing of shoots or roots from unusual points of origin, such as from callus, leaf, stem, flower buds *etc.*, other than zygotes or other than shoot and root meristem is called **adventitious shoots and roots**. In the process of either direct or indirect organogenesis, the cells and tissues are forced to undergo changes which lead to the production of a unipolar structure, whose vascular system is often connected to the parent tissue. The shoot buds or monopolar structures are formed by manipulating the ratio of cytokinin to auxin in the cultures.

In somatic embryogenesis, the totipotent cells may undergo embryogenic pathway to form somatic embryos (bipolar nature), which are grown to regenerate whole plants and each developing plant will be having its own vascular connections. It was first established in carrots (*Daucus carota*), where bipolar embryos developed from single cells. In 1939, regeneration using larger explant tissues from carrot and other species was successfully carried out in culture medium containing the critical phytohormone indole-3-acetic acid (auxin). **Auxins**, the first discovered plant hormone, containing an aromatic ring and a carboxylic acid group. Cytokinin is another phytohormone with a structure resembling to adenine is one of the nucleotide in nucleic acids. The identification of the major effect of auxin/cytokinin ratios on regenerated tissue type is one of the major breakthrough in the plant regeneration field. **In 1957, Skoog and Miller found that treating tobacco pith with high auxin/cytokinin ratios led to root formation**. In contrast, high cytokinin/auxin ratios induced shoot regeneration. When high concentrations of both hormones were added to explants, a mass of growing cells *i.e.* callus was induced. The 19th century observation stated that single, detached cells of lower plant forms could continue growth rise to the whole plant (theory of cell totipotency). In reality, the theory applies only to the cells capable of mitotic division; *i.e.* cells that are meristematic (*e.g.* embryos, stem/root tips, cambium) or otherwise relatively undifferentiated cells (*e.g.* parenchyma).

When plants are multiplied vegetatively by tissue culture or by cuttings from a single plants, those plants can be classified as a clone. This means that the genetic make-up of all offspring is identical to that of the single parent. On the other hand, plants propagated by seed, resulting from sexual reproduction, are not clones because each seed and the resultant plant has a unique genetic make-up-a mixture from two parents, different from either parent and different from one seed to another. The term "**cloning**", with respect to tissue culture is refers to the process of propagating culture in large numbers from selected plant with the same genotype as their mother plant. This process is also known as **micropropagation**. The process of growing an entire plant from a single cell or group of cells is called **plant regeneration**.

Morphogenesis

Attainment of biological organization or form is termed as morphogenesis (Figure 3.2).

The morphogenesis in a tissue culture system can be of two different ways (1) Organogenesis (2) Embryogenesis. **Embryos are developing from vegetative or somatic cells so termed as somatic embryogenesis**.

I) Organogenesis

In plant tissue culture, organogenesis means genesis of organs like shoots, roots, leaves, flowers, *etc.* The earliest report on induction of **shoot organogenesis *in vitro* was by White** (1939) using a tobacco hybrid; and the first observation of **root formation were reported by Nobecourt (1939)** using carrot callus. Till late 1950s, the basic regulatory mechanism underlying in organogenesis was not identified. Skoog and Miller (1957) were responsible to recognize the regulatory mechanism as a balance between auxin and cytokinin. As per their finding, a relatively high level of auxin to cytokinin favoured root formation and the reverse favoured shoot formation. Using this concept, it has now become possible to achieve organogenesis in a large number of plant species by culturing explants, calli and cell suspension in a defined medium. **Caulogenesis** is a type of organogenesis by which only adventitious shoot bud initiation takes place in the callus tissue. When organogenesis leads to root development, then it is known as **rhizogenesis**. Abnormal structures developed during organogenesis are called **organoids**. The localized meristematic cells on a callus which give rise to shoots and/or roots are termed as **meristemoids**. Meristemoids are characterized as an aggregation of meristem-like cells. These can occur directly on an explant or indirectly via callus.

Two kinds of organogenesis.

1. **Indirect organogenesis:** A developmental sequence involving an intervening callus stage is termed 'indirect' organogenesis (Figure 3.3).

   Primary explant → callus → meristemoid → organ primordium

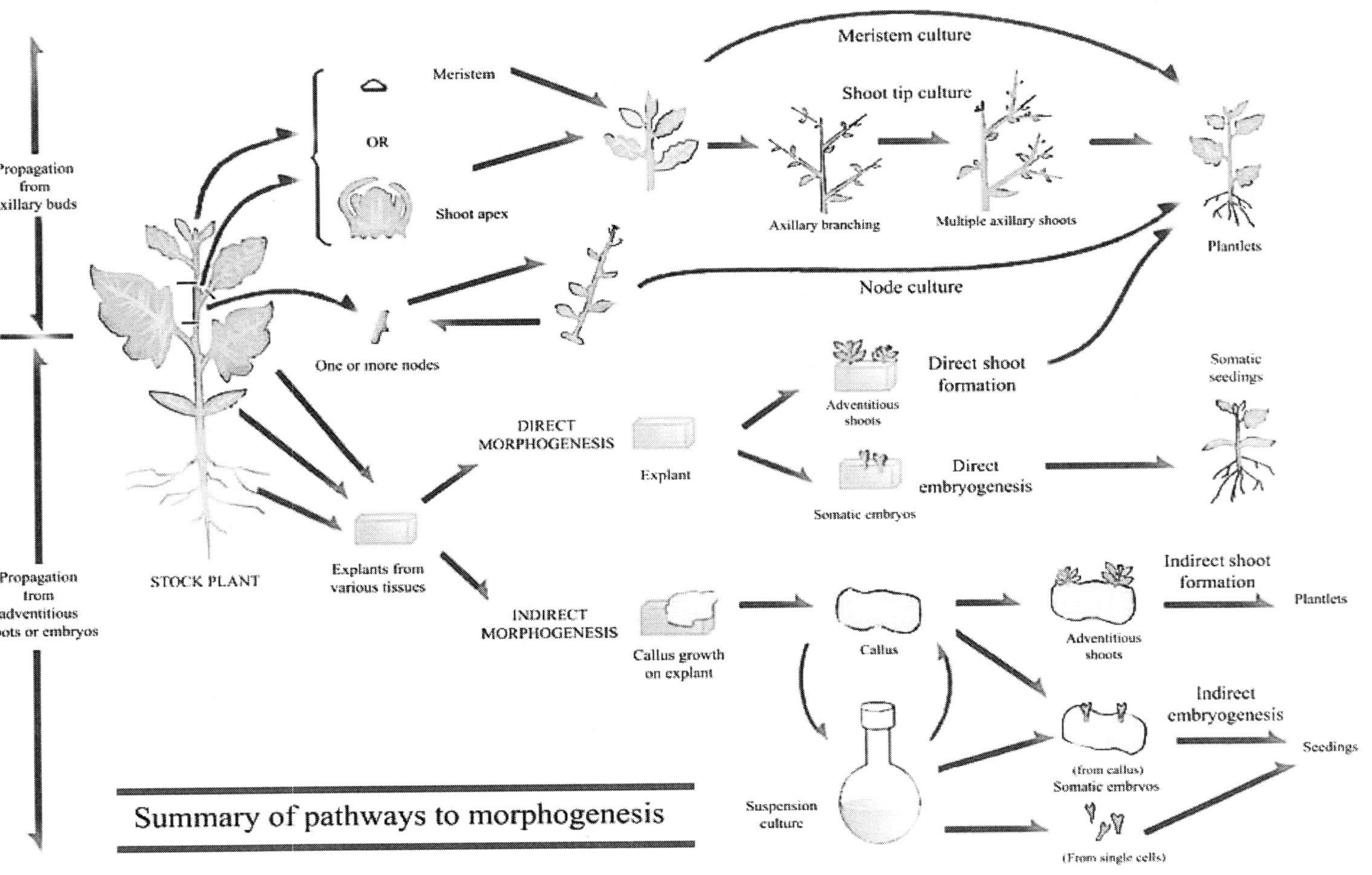

Figure 3.2. Different Routes of Morphogenesis.

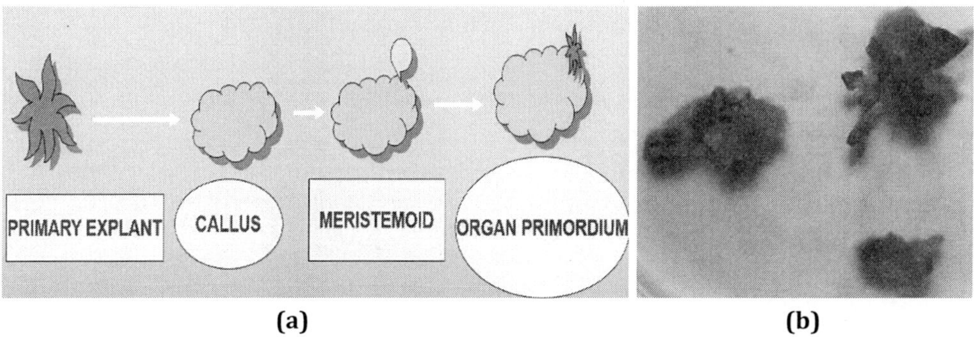

(a) (b)

Figure 3.3a. Indirect Organogenesis; b. Shoot Induction in Callus Tissue.

2. **Direct organogenesis:** Direct organogenesis is accomplished without an intervening proliferate callus stage (Figure 3.4).

   Primary explant → meristemoid → organ primordium

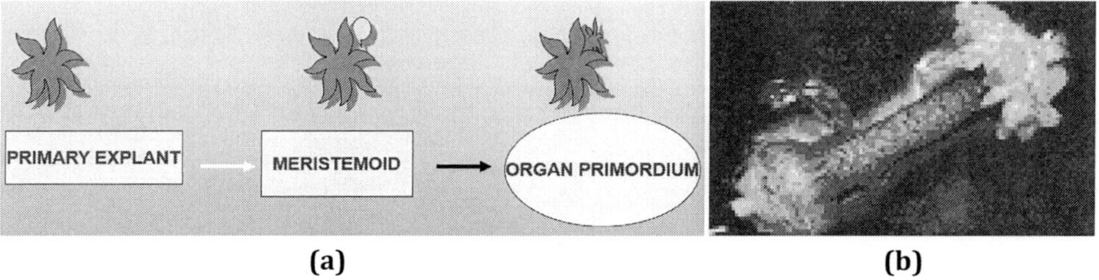

(a) (b)

Figure 3.4a. Direct Organogenesis; b. Shoot Induction Directly from Internode.

II) Embryogenesis

The capacity of flowering plants to produce embryos is not restricted only zygote, the genes coding for embryogenic differentiation and development are present in all the cells of plants. So the cells can be triggered in embryogenic pathway by specific induction. This phenomenon was first reported in detail by Steward and Reinert (1958) in cultured cells of carrot. Somatic embryogenesis can be defined as the developmental process producing a perfect embryo from simple cell without gametic fusion. Embryos have been classified into two categories: zygotic embryos and non-zygotic embryos.

Zygotic Embryogenesis

Embryos developing from zygotes (resulting from regular fusion of egg) are called as zygotic embryos or often simply embryos.

Non-zygotic Embryogenesis

Usually non-zygotic embryos are formed by cells other than the zygote.

a) **Parthenogenetic embryos** - formed from unfertilized eggs or a fertilized egg without karyogamy.

b) **Androgenetic embryos** – formed from microspores, micro-gametophytes or sperm.

c) **Somatic embryos** (also called as embryoids, accessory embryos, adventitious embryos and supernumerary embryos) – formed by somatic cells either *in vivo* or *in vitro.*

Somatic Embryogenesis

A somatic embryo is an embryo derived from a somatic cell, other than zygote, usually on *in vitro* culture. The process of somatic embryo development is called as somatic embryogenesis (Figure 3.5).

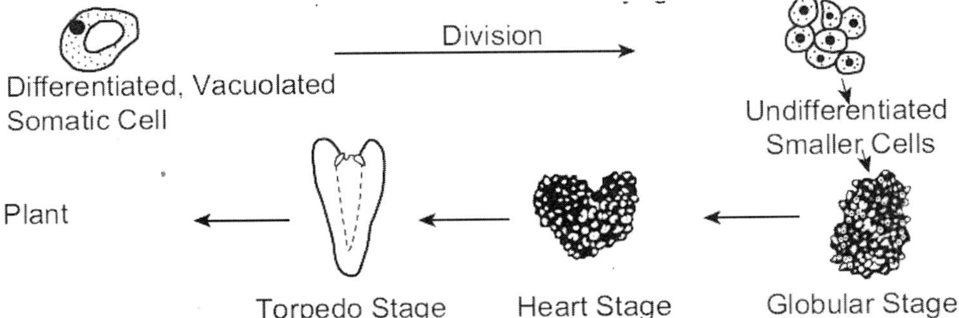

Figure 3.5. Sequence of Somatic Embryogenesis.

This is another major path of regeneration and development of plantlets for micropropagation or mass multiplication of specific plants. The cells, under a particular hormonal combination, change into the physiological state similar to zygotes (somatic zygotes) and follow an embryonic path of development to form somatic embryos. These somatic embryos are similar to normal embryos (seed embryos) developed from zygotes formed by sexual fertilization, then zygote converted in to **globular stage, heart stage, torpedo stage and finally cotyledonary stage** leads to develop into a complete plant (Figure 3.6). Since somatic embryos can germinate into a complete plant, these can be used for the production of artificial seeds. Somatic embryos developed by tissue or cell cultures can be entrapped in certain inert polymers such as calcium alginate and used as **artificial seeds.** Since the production of artificial seed is amenable to mechanization and for bioreactors, it can be produced in large numbers.

Stages in Development of Somatic Embryoids

Somatic embryos may arise *in vitro* by two different ways:

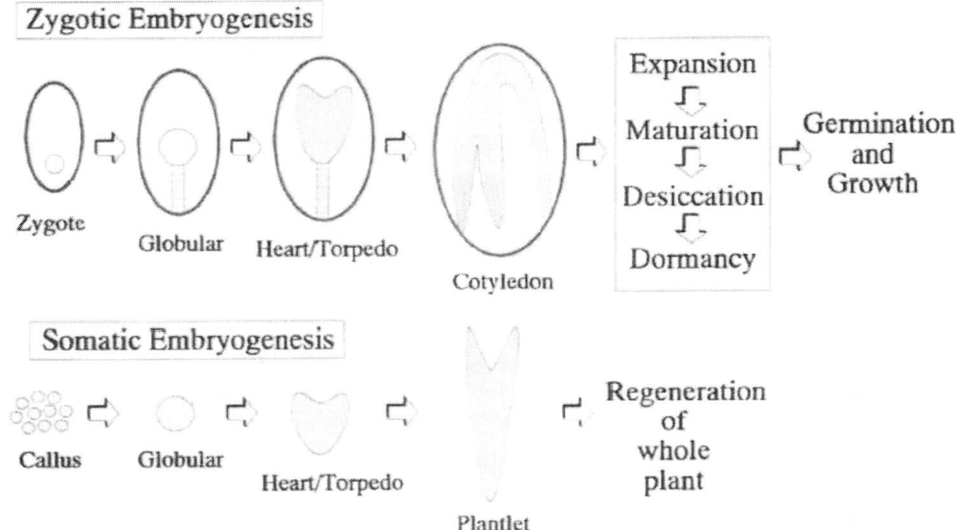

Figure 3.6. Variation between Zygotic and Somatic Embryogenisis.

1. Embryogenesis Directly from Pre-embryogenic Determined Cells (PEDC's)

Cells are already programmed for embryonic differentiation. These are cells those present nearer to the embryo such as hypocotyls, cotyledons, nuclear tissue *etc.* Usually embryoids will form directly on the explant. These PEDC's await either synthesis of an induced substance or removal of an inhibitor substance for the resumption of mitotic activity and embryogenic development.

2. Embryogenesis from Induced Embryogenic Determined Cells (IEDC's)

These cells otherwise follow the normal mitotic division and are fostered into embryogenic pathway by specific induction. Here the explant will divide at a faster rate to form an unorganised mass of cells (callus) and from this embryos will be differentiating. The embryo forming cells are characterised by isodiametric shape, thin cell wall, dense cytoplasmic contents, large starch grains, relatively larger nucleus, darkly stained nucleolus and high amount of RNA and protein. Plant regeneration via somatic embryogenesis for many species can be divided into two phases:

1. Selection and induction of cells with embryogenic competence,
2. Development of these cells into embryos.

Somatic embryos generally originate from single cells which divide to form a group of meristematic cells. Usually, this multi-cellular group becomes isolated by breaking cytoplasmic connections with the other cells around it and subsequently by cutinization of the outer walls of this differentiating cell mass. The cells of meristematic mass continue to divide to give rise to globular (round ball shaped), heart-shaped, torpedo and cotyledonary stages. Somatic embryo genesis begins with active division of cells which leads to increase in size but retains the spherical shape. At this stage the primary meristem (protoderm, ground meristem and procambium) becomes visible. Following this stage, the cell continues to divide and differentiate into a heart-shaped embryo, with initiation of cotyledon primordia. As the cotyledon develops the embryo passes into the torpedo-shaped stage. The cells inside the cotyledonary ring divide to form shoot and root apical meristem and procambium differentiation takes place. In general, the essential features of somatic embryo development, especially after the globular stage, are comparable to those of zygotic embryo.

Somatic embryogenesis leads to the production of a bipolar structure containing in root/shoot axis (radicle/plumule) with a closed independent vascular system. The radicular end is always sticks out from the cell mass. In contrast, a shoot bud is monopolar as it does not have a radicular end. Some times somatic embryos show abnormal developmental features, *e.g.* 3 or more cotyledons, bell-shaped cotyledon, larger size *etc.*; these problems are often overcome by the presence of ABA or a suitable concentration of mannitol.

Practical Application of Somatic Embryogenesis

The potential applications and importance of *in vitro* somatic embryogenesis and organogenesis are more or less similar.

i) Artificial or Synthetic Seeds Production

Synthetic seeds are "encapsulated somatic embryos which functionally mimic seeds and can develop into seedlings". Large scale production of somatic embryos and their encapsulation is referred to as artificial or synthetic seed production. It is an alternative to traditional micropropagation for production and delivery of cloned plantlets. Artificial or synthetic seed is a bead of gel containing somatic embryo or shoot bud. The first synthetic seeds were produced by Kitto and Janick in 1982 using carrot somatic embryos.

Artificial seeds may be produced by one of the two following ways

1. **Desiccated:**The desiccated synthetic seeds are produced from somatic embryos either naked or encapsulated in **polyoxyethylene glycol (Polyox)** followed by their desiccation. Desiccation can be achieved either slowly over a period of one or two weeks sequentially using chambers of decreasing relative humidity, or rapidly by unsealing the petri dishes and leaving them on the bench overnight to dry. **Such types of synthetic seeds are produced only in plant species whose somatic embryos are desiccation tolerant**.
2. **Hydrated:** Hydrated synthetic seeds are produced in those plant species where the somatic embryos are **recalcitrant and sensitive to desiccation**. Hydrated synthetic seeds are produced by encapsulating the somatic embryos in hydrogel capsules.

Procedure for Synthetic Seed Production

1. Establish somatic embryogenesis
2. Mature somatic embryos
3. Synchronize and singulate somatic embryos
4. Mass production of somatic embryos
5. Standardisation of encapsulation
6. Standardisation of artificial endosperm
7. Mass production of synthetic seeds and storage

Applications

1. Seed propagation of sterile plants.
2. High efficiency in multiplication.
3. Fixation of hybrid vigour, eliminate the need of inbred lines to produce F1 hybrids.
4. Elimination of the need of edible seeds or tubers for propagation.
5. Multiplication of genetically engineered individuals, which may be sterile and unstable during sexual production.
6. Protection of seedlings by incorporating useful chemicals in the encapsulation material.
7. Provide the advantages of true seed (case of handling and transportation) for vegetative propagation.

ii) Clonal Propagation

Since both the growth of embryogenic cells and subsequent development of somatic embryos can be carried out in liquid medium, it is possible to combine somatic embryogenesis with engineering technology to create large-scale mechanical or automated culture systems. Such systems are capable of producing propagules repetitively with labour input. In this process of repetitive somatic embryogenesis is initiated where by somatic embryos proliferate from the previously existing somatic embryo in order to produce clones.

iii) Raising Somaclonal Variants in Tree Species

Embryos formed directly from pro-embryogenic determined cells (PEDCs) appear to produce relatively uniform clonal material, whereas the indirect pathway involving induced embryogenic determined cells (IEDCs) generates a high frequency of Somaclonal variants. For clonal propagation of tree species, somatic embryogenesis from nucellar cells may offer only rapid means or obtaining juvenile plants equivalent to seedlings with parental genotype.

iv) Source of Regenerable Protoplast System

Embryogenic callus, suspension cultures and somatic embryos have been employed as source of protoplast isolation for a range of species. Cells or tissues in these system have demonstrated the potentiality to regeneration in culture and therefore, yield protoplast that are capable to forming whole plants.

v) Genetic Transformation

Repetitive embryos originate from single epidermal or sub epidermal cells which can readily be exposed to *Agrobacterium*. Thus the transformation technique applied to primary somatic embryos. Repetitive embryogenesis is also ideally suited to particle gun-mediated genetic transformation. Instead or recycling on *Agrobacterium* to mediate the transfer of genes into plant cells, the particle gun literally shoots DNA that has been precipitated onto particles of a heavy metals, into the plant cells. Embryogenic suspension cultures of the cotton and soybean, initiated cell lines following each firing of the gun. The transformed cell lines can then the induced to form an unlimited number of transformed somatic embryos through repetive embryogenesis.

vi) Synthesis of Metabolites

The repetitive embryogenesis system is of potential use in the synthesis of metabolites such as pharmaceuticals and oils. Borage contains high level of Y-Linoleic acid, used as precursor of post-glandins or in the treatment of atopic eczema. Somatic embryos of borage also produce this metabolite but through repetitive somatic embryogenesis a continuous supply of Y-lenolenic acid is ensured. Which otherwise would be limited to the growing season in the zygotic embryos.

vii) Protoplast Culture

Embryogenic cultures have proven to be especially valuable in providing a source of regenerable protoplasts. This also will provide a source for production of inter-specific and intergeneric somatic hybrid plants.

viii) In vitro Screening and Selection

The embryogenic process appears to be very sensitive to exogenous chemical compounds. High sensitivity to compounds that disturb metabolic processes may be an intrinsic characteristic of somatic embryos which are undergoing a delicate differentiation process. This sensitivity could potentially be exploited to identify plant genotypes resistant to certain factors such as Al, Fe toxicity or toxins produced by pathogens. Only the resistant ones will be regenerating. The *in vitro* screening of somatic embryo would be especially useful to a breeder trying to introgress a resistant trait into an adapted germplasm rather than screening large number of progeny for the presence of desired trait. Immature seed or embryos could be placed on regeneration medium containing the selective agent that is high levels of toxin. Only those containing resistance would proliferate others got eliminated from the population.

xi) Germplasam Preservation

Somatic embryos can be preserved within lesser space compared to other plant parts. This is advantageous in germplasm exchange. The somatic embryos can be preserved by desiccation directly or after making them synthetic seeds. These can be stored by omitting sucrose from medium or by addition of ABA to the medium.

Limitations

1. Besides the limitations imposed by genotypes on individuals within a given sp. there are species, genera and families that are more amenable to somatic embryogenesis than others. The families Umbelliferae, Rubiaceae, Ranunculaceae and Solanaceae as being especially amenable to somatic embryogenesis.
2. The embryogenic potential of a culture may decline over time.
3. Plants regenerated from somatic embryoids have in some instances been sterile or shown reduced fertility.
4. Although zygotic embryos are the desirable tissue for embryogenesis where the genotype to be multiplied is a heterotic F_1 hybrid or the progeny of selected parents. In many instances the aim is to clone a mature plant after performance evaluation. In these instances direct embryogenesis from mature plant parts is necessary as zygotic embryos represented developed variability.

Factors Affecting Somatic Embryogenesis

1. **Growth regulators:** In most species, an auxin is essential for somatic embryogenesis. Auxins are required for determination of IEDC's. But PEDC's either have no auxin requirement or require auxin only for onset of mitosis. Accumulation of protein, RNA and DNA in the embryogenic tissue is influenced favourably by the auxin level. After globular stage for further development either removal of auxin or at low level is found to be effective. Cytokinins are found to be effective in certain systems. ABA reduces abnormalities and induces maturity. GA promotes the germination of embryoids.
2. **Sucrose:** During the maturation of somatic embryos, they undergo biochemical changes to become more sturdy and hardy. This is achieved by culturing them on a high sucrose medium. High salt containing media such as MS, SH and B5, high sucrose content in the media *etc.* have a favourable effect on embryogenesis.
3. **Nitrogen source:** The form of nitrogen has marked effect on somatic embryogenesis. In carrot, NH^+_4 is essential during somatic embryo induction, while somatic embryo development occurs on a medium containing NO^-_3 as the sole nitrogen source. Glutamate, yeast extract *etc.*, also have positive effect on embryogenesis. Coconut milk is often used as organic supplement in certain systems.

4. **Genotype of explant:** Explant genotype may determine the regeneration of somatic embryo. Of the 500 varieties of rice screened, 19 showed 65-100 per cent embryogenesis, 41 showed 35-64 per cent embryogenesis and the remaining 440 cultivars were less efficient in regeneration. The most responding explant is the zygotic embryo that is cotyledons, hypocotyl, nucellar tissue *etc.*

5. **Other factors:** Polyamines (putrescine, spermidine and spermine) are required for embryo development *in vivo or in vitro.* High K^+ levels and low dissolved O_2 levels promote somatic embryo regeneration in some species. The need for reduced dissolved oxygen could be substituted by the addition of ATP to the medium, suggesting that, probably, oxygen tension enhanced the level of cellular ATP. In *Citrus,* some volatile compounds like ethanol inhibit somatic embryo regeneration.

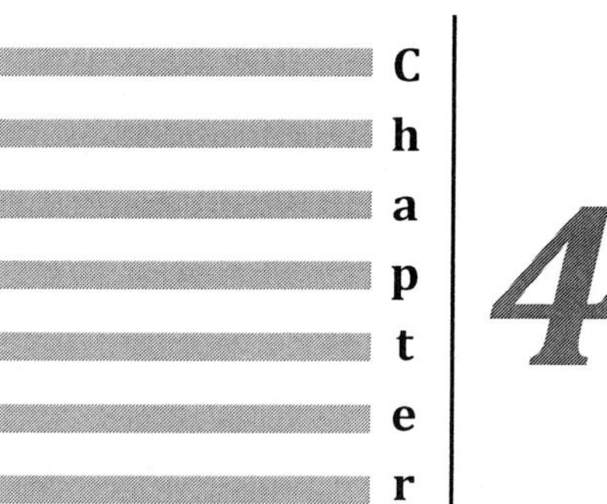

Chapter 4

Culture Types: Callus and Cell Suspension Culture, Shoot Tip and Meristem Tip Culture

Callus Culture

Callus is an undifferentiated mass of cells arising by the disorganised proliferation of cells (Figure 4.1). **The word callus is used to denote cells grown as a coherent mass of amorphous and loosely arranged parenchyma arising from explants.** Duhamel du Monceau discovered callus induction in 1756

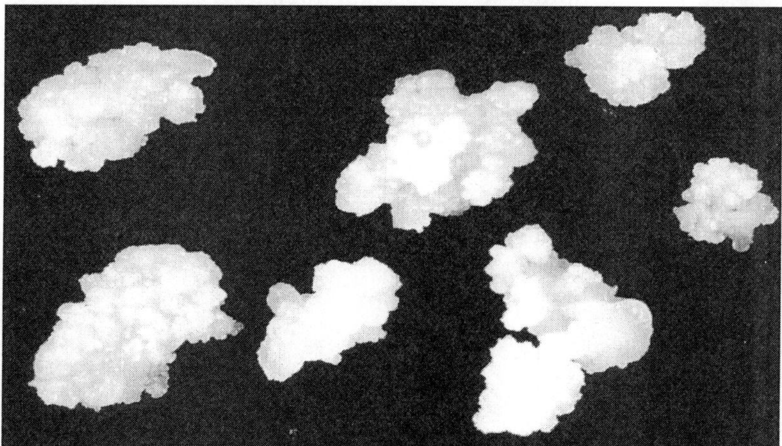

Figure 4.1. Proliferation of Cells.

but this discovery went largely unnoticed, since the techniques for asepsis were not known then. Based on this finding, Trecul (1853) and Vochting (1878) began the race and succeeded in finding the concept of cell totipotency. In culture, callus is induced by placing small pieces of explants on to a growth supporting medium under sterile conditions. With the stimulus of endogenous growth substances or growth regulating chemicals added to the medium cells are made metabolically active. The process of cell differentiation and specialisation occurring in the intact plant is reversed and the explanted tissue is said to become de-differentiated.

Successful callus cultures have been established in broad leaved dicotyledonous plants, monocotyledons, gymnosperms, ferns and mosses. Tissues from various organs have the potential to divide and proliferate when transferred to culture medium. But in most plants, tissues from some organs are more predisposed to rapid cell division than others. Thus in most cereals callus growth can only be obtained from tissues of certain organs such as zygotic embryos, germinating seeds, seed endosperm but it is difficult to induce callus from mature leaf tissue.

Callus induction from any explant is favoured by the application of **auxin (2,4-D)** to the nutrient medium. Discovery of growth factors *viz.*, auxins helped to obtain primary proliferation of plant tissues in culture and to maintain a high rate of non-differentiated tissues in culture. Callus induced from explants differ considerably in morphology: spherical, semi-spherical, plate like or amorphous. Their consistency may be compact, hard or loose, friable or dissociated. Based on the appearance of calli, they are classified as compact calli and friable calli. Generally the first category is heavily lignified and hard in texture, whereas the second type is easily separable into small fragments.

Method

For callus initiation, transfers the explants aseptically to the solid medium and gently press them into the agar in such a way that good contact has made. Radical tips laid horizontally on the agar whereas stem section placed vertically with one cut end in the agar, to confer good callus. Within 2-3 weeks, explants should show new growth as pustules or protuberances or as a fine mat across the surface depending on the distribution and mitotic activity of the parenchyma residing in the excised tissues. Some callus growths are heavily lignified and hard in texture, whereas others break easily into small fragments. Most explants have produced sufficient callus in an appropriate medium to allow for subculture within 3-7 weeks. When cultured for several weeks, callus will show signs of ageing. This can be noted as deceleration of growth, necrotic or browning and finally desiccation. The newly formed callus will be removed from the initial explant at this stage by cutting with the sterile scalpel. Once well established, most callus cultures will require regular subculture at approximately 4 week intervals.

Subculture of Callus

Callus induced from the explants can be isolated and maintained for any number of years by transferring the callus pieces to fresh medium supplemented with balanced auxin, cytokinin ratio and other additives. This step is termed as Subculture. Rapid subculture may improve the friability of the callus. A friable callus is found to be good than freshly induced callus for making suspensions. The subculture may be on solid medium or liquid medium (suspension culture). If liquid medium is used, constant agitations are to be provided. The morphological properties and consistency of callus tissues change easily during each subculture. Very frequently the tissue dies after three or four passage due to the exhaustion of some vital metabolites. However, the aging of callus affects proliferation after prolonged subculture. After the callus induction and proliferation in an induction medium, the calli have to be subcultured to maintain their viability. This subculture is determined by the rate of growth of tissues from the explants. Several methods are available to maintain the calli and are described below. The important methods are:

1. Callus culture on agar medium
2. Suspension culture or liquid culture
3. Special method of culture

1. Callus Culture on Agar Medium

Calli are excised under aseptic condition and divided into clumps of 3-4mm^3. The necrotic portions of calli formed due to lignification should be removed. The isolated callus pieces are transferred to fresh nutrient medium. Thus calli can be maintained by several passages. Passage time is determined by tissue growth, glassware size and the kind and amount of nutrient medium.

2. Cell Suspension Culture

When friable callus is placed into a liquid medium (usually the same composition as the solid medium used for callus culture) and then agitated single cells and/or small clumps of few to many cells are produced in the medium is called suspension culture. Liquid cultures may be constantly agitated generally by a gyratory shaker of 100-250 rpm to facilitate aeration and dissociation of cell clumps into small pieces. Suspension cultures grow much faster than callus cultures, need to be sub-cultured at every week, allow a more accurate determination of the nutritional requirement of cells and even somatic embryos.

The suspension culture broadly grouped as i) Batch culture ii) Continuous culture

i. Batch Cultures

Batch cultures are cultures grown in a fixed volume of culture medium. A small aliquot of the suspension is taken out and is continuously propagated by transferring to a fresh medium. In batch culture, the same medium and all the cells produced are retained in the culture vessel (*e.g.* culture flask 100-250 ml). During the incubation period, the biomass of the suspension cultures increases due to cell division and cell enlargement. This continues for a limited period after which the growth stops due to the exhaustion of some factors or the accumulation of certain toxic metabolites in the culture medium. If at this stage a small aliquot of the cell suspension, with uniformly dispersed cells and cell aggregates, is transferred to a fresh medium of the same composition (subculture), the cell growth is revived. Batch cultures are maintained by sub-culturing and are used for initiation of cell suspensions.

The cell number or biomass of a batch culture exhibits a typical sigmoidal curve. Initially, the culture passes through a lag phase, followed by a brief exponential growth phase during which active cell divisions occur. After three to four cell generations the growth declines and finally the culture enters the stationary phase. The duration of the lag phase would largely depend on the growth phase of the stock culture at the time of subculture and the size of the inoculum. Cultures can be maintained continuously in exponential phase by frequent (every 2-3 days) subculture of the suspensions. Prolonged maintenance of cultures in the stationary phase may result in extensive death and lysis of cells. Therefore, the suspensions are subcultured soon after they have reached their maximum dry-weight yield. For subculture of the suspension cultures a pipette or syringe with an orifice fine enough to allow single cells and small aggregates (2-4 cells) to pass through, but excluding larger cell clumps, is used. At the time of subculture the flask is allowed to stand for a few seconds to allow the large colonies to settle down, and suspension is taken from the upper part of the culture. The texture of a callus is genetically controlled and often it may be difficult to obtain a good dispersion of cells under any conditions. Generally, however, it has been possible to improve the tissue dissociation by manipulating the media composition and subculture routine. Addition of 2,4-D small amounts of hydrolytic enzymes such as cellulase and pectinase, or substances like yeast extract, had a promotory effect on cell dispersion.

Drawbacks of Batch Cultures

Batch cultures are not ideal for studies of cell growth and metabolism. Batch cultures are characterized by a constant change in the pattern of cell growth and metabolism, and the composition of the nutrient medium. In these cultures the exponential growth with a constancy of cell doubling time may be achieved for a short time but there is no period of steady-state growth in which the relative cell concentrations of metabolites and enzymes are constant. To a certain extent these problems are overcome by continuous cultures.

ii. Continuous Culture

These cultures are maintained in a steady state for a long period by draining out the used (or) spent medium and adding the fresh medium. Such subculture systems are either closed (or) open type. This culture used to study about cell growth and metabolism.

Closed Type

In this type addition of fresh medium is balanced by outflow of the old medium. The cells from the outflowing medium are separated mechanically and added back to the culture. Thus, in 'close continuous cultures' cell biomass continues to increase as the growth proceeds.

Open Type

In the 'open continuous cultures' the inflow of the medium is accompanied by a balancing harvest of an equal volume of the culture (medium and cells). The rate of inflow of medium and culture harvest are so adjusted that the cultures are maintained at a constant, submaximal growth rate indefinitely.

Open continuous culture again divided into two types 1.chemostat 2. turbidostat. In chemostat cultures, a steady state of cell growth is maintained by a constant inflow of the fresh medium in which the concentration of a chosen nutrient (nitrogen, phosphorus or glucose) would be adjusted. In such cases growth limiting nutrient are present at higher concentrations than that required to maintain the desired rate of cell growth. The increasing or decreasing level of the growth limiting factor corresponding increase or decrease in the growth rate of cells. Chemostat cultures offer the possibility of maintaining a steady-state of cell growth and metabolism, and to determine the effect of individual growth-limiting nutrients on cell growth. In turbidostat cultures, the input of fresh medium is intermittent, controlled by an increase in the turbidity of the culture from cell growth.

Application of Cell and Suspension Cultures

Micropropagation

For micropropagation suspension cultures can be used in two ways.

a. Somatic embryos are formed in suspension cultures
b. Cells from suspensions are plated on solid media where single cells or cell aggregates grow into callus colonies from which plants can be regenerated.

Mutant Selection

High degree of spontaneous variability occur in cell cultures. The frequency of variation can be increased by treating the cells with mutagens. Many cell lines resistant to amino acid analogues antibiotics, herbicides, fungal toxins *etc.* have been isolated from cell cultures.

Production of Secondary Metabolites

Production of secondary metabolites like alkaloids, antimicrobials, sugar derivatives, steroids *etc.* are possible by cell culure.

3. Special Method of Culture

An isolated cell or single cell separated from the suspension culture some times fails to divide when they plated directly on the medium used for callus cultures. But callus can be induced in these type of cells by following some of the special method like filter paper raft-nurse technique and microchamber technique.

1. The Filter Paper Raft-Nurse Technique

This method was developed by **Muir *et al.* (1954)** to culture single cells from suspension cultures and friable calli of tobacco and marigold. It involves cultivating individual cells on top of an actively growing callus separated by a piece of filter paper. Sterile 8 x 8 mm squares of filter paper are placed aseptically on top of the established callus of the same or different species before isolation of single cell. Individual cells are isolated from suspension cultures or a friable callus with the aid of a micropipette or microspatula. The filter paper is wetted with liquid exudates and nutrients produced from the nurse tissue piece.

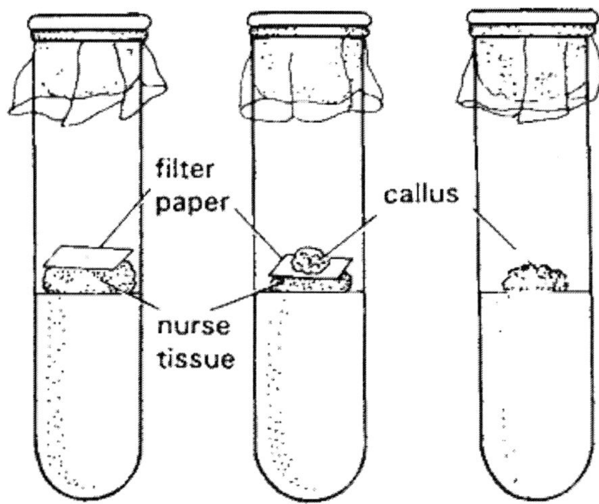

Figure 4.2. Nurse-Tissue Technique to Raise Single Cell Clones.

The isolated single cell is placed on the wet filter paper raft. Cell transfer should be rapid in order to avoid excessive drying of the cell and the raft. After a macroscopic colony develops from the cell it is transferred to agar medium for further growth and maintenance of the cell clone. An isolated cell which generally fails to divide when plated directly on the medium but divide under the nursing effect of the callus (Figure 4.2). Apparently, the callus supplies the cell with not only the nutrients from the culture medium and also some factor which is more critical for cell division. The cell division factor(s) can diffuse through the filter paper.

Feeder Layer Technique

The effect of callus tissue in stimulating the division of isolated cells can also be demonstrated by putting two callus pieces on an agar plate and seeding single cells around them. In such cultures cells close to the calli divide first. The beneficial effect of conditioned medium in single cell culture at low density is yet another evidence of the release of metabolites by growing tissues which are essential for cell division. The feeder layer technique for low density cell plating used is also based on the same principle as the raft-nurse technique.

2. The Microchamber Technique

This method was developed by Jones *et al.* (1960). They replaced the nurse tissue by a conditioned medium and grew single cells in a microchamber. In this method a drop of the medium carrying a single cell is isolated from suspension cultures, placed on a sterile microscope slide and ringed with sterile mineral oil. A drop of oil is placed on either side of the culture drop and a coverglass placed on each drop. A third coverglass is then placed on the culture drop bridging the two coverglasses and forming a microchamber to enclose the single cell aseptically within the mineral oil. The oil prevents water loss from the chamber but permits gaseous exchange. The whole microchamber slide is placed in a petri-dish and incubated. When the cell colony becomes sufficiently large the coverglass is removed and the tissue is transferred to fresh liquid or semi-solid medium. The microchamber technique permits regular observation of the growing and dividing cell (Figure 4.3). Vasil and Hildebrandt (1965) used the microchamber method and demonstrated that a complete flowering plant can be raised starting from an isolated single cell.

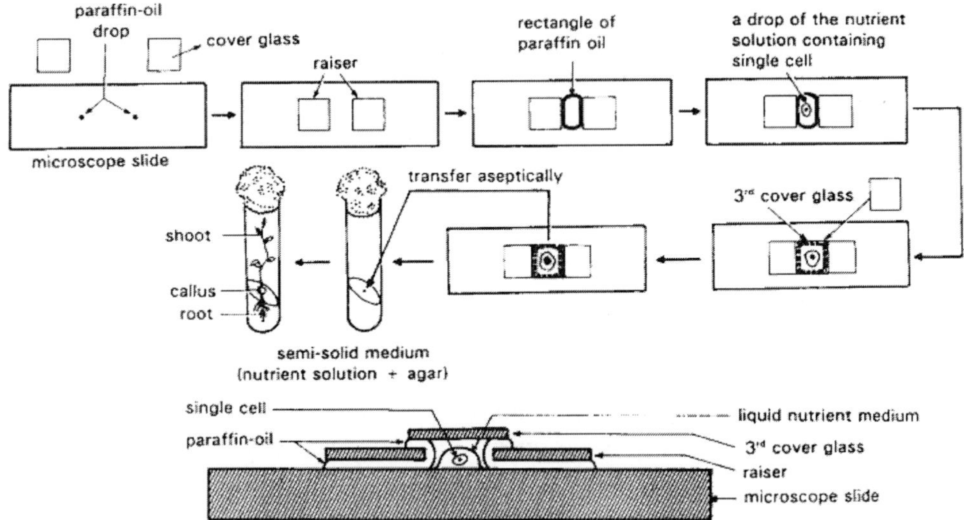

Figure 4.3. Different Steps Involved in the Microchamber Technique of Cell Cloning.

Meristem Tip/Shoot Tip Culture

Meristem

Meristem is a zone of cells with active divisions, situated in the top of buds and extremities of roots from which permanent tissue systems, *i.e.*, root, shoot, leaf, and flower, are derived.

Meristem Tip Culture

The shoot apical meristem is characterized as a dome of totipotent cell situated at the tip of the shoot, which is the center of activity for various developmental programs in the life of a higher plant. **The apical meristem together with one to three young leaf primordia, measuring 0.1-0.5mm, has been referred as meristem-tip. In contrast shoot tips are larger in the size from 0.5 to 5 mm.** Meristamatic cells are conserved and genetically stable, thus used for clonal propagation. Meristem-tip considered as a free from virus and other plant pathogens like mycoplasmas, bacteria, and fungi. So it can be used as a explant to produce virus free plants from virus infected plants. *In vitro* culture of a generally shiny, dome-like structure measuring less than 0.1 mm in length, most often excised from the shoot apex is used for elimination of virus. Though meristem culture technique is known since 1933 it was made successful only in **1965 byMorel and Martin**.

Shoot Tip Culture

Shoot tip explants are used for rapid *in vitro* propagation and the explant size will be vary from 0.5 - 5.0 mm. The size of the explant is bigger in case of shoot tip culture when compared with meristem tip culture (0.1-0.5mm) give better survival and establishment of explant. Eventhough the larger explants have better survivel and high regeneration capacity, these have higher the chances of virus contamination. Culture of smallest explants consisting of only the meristematic dome or with 2 or 3 leaf primordia would be ideal if the objective is virus elimination. So the ultimate aim to produce virus free plants either from virus infected plant or normal plants need to go for small explants (meristem culture) and for the mass multiplication of propagating material, shoot tip culture would be more beneficial.

The reasons proposed for the escape of the meristem from virus invasion are

a. Viruses readily move in plant body through the vascular system which is absent in meristem.

b. The alternate method of cell-to-cell movement of the virus through plasmodesmata is rather too slow to keep pace with the actively growing tip.

c. High metabolic activity in the actively dividing meristem cells does not allow virus replication.

d. The virus inactivating systems in the plant body has higher activity in the meristem than in any other region.

e. High endogenous auxin level in the shoot apices may inhibit virus multiplication.

Procedure of Meristem culture

Meristem tips are carefully dissected away from the apical or lateral shoot buds under a stereomicroscope under aseptic condition. After this though most meristem can be directly inoculated on a suitable culture medium without surface sterilization. Meristems are usually cultured on solid medium occasionally on liquid media supplemented with a low concentration of cytokinins and a moderate level of auxins. Further, this is transferred to root development media for root growth. After a period of 2-6 month the plants are transferred to greenhouse and sample plants are tested for the presence of virus by ELISA and PAGE techniques (Figure 4.3)

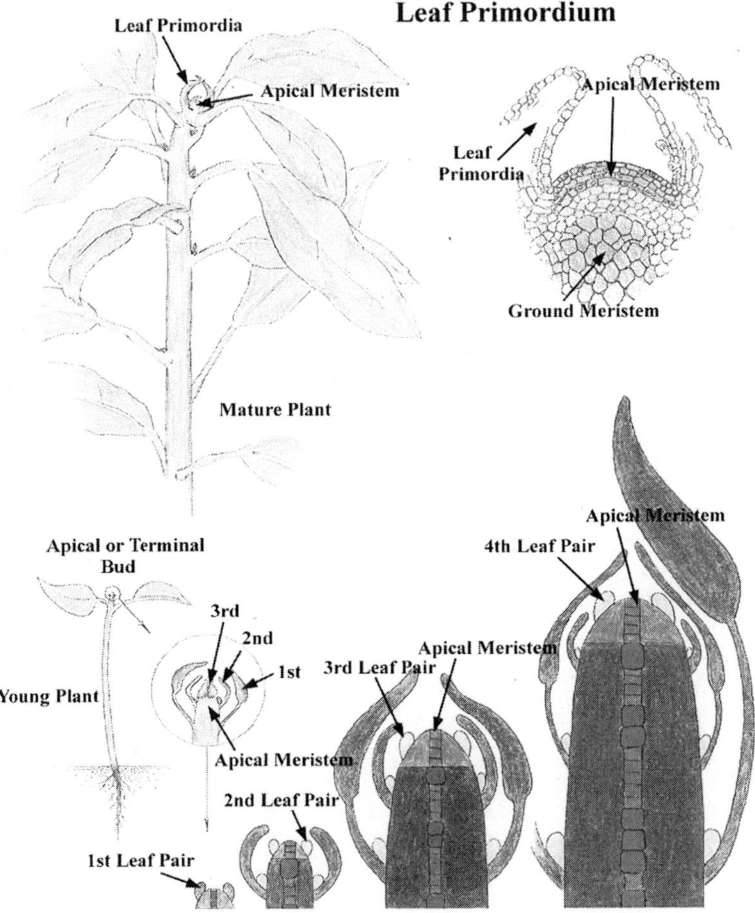

Figure 4.3. Components and Structure of Meristem in Plant.

Sometimes meristem tip cultures have failed to eliminate virus infection because the explant contains shoot apices with vascular tissue instead of true meristem. Meristem tip culture combined with heat treatment (thermotheraphy) or chemical treatment (chemotheraphy) has proved to be very effective in virus eradication.

Procedure of Meristem culture

Meristem tips are carefully dissected away from the apical or lateral shoot buds under a stereomicroscope under aseptic condition. After this though most meristem can be directly inoculated on a suitable culture medium without surface sterilization. Meristems are usually cultured on solid medium occasionally on liquid media supplemented with a low concentration of cytokinins and a moderate level of auxins. Further, this is transferred to root development media for root growth. After a period of 2-6 month the plants are transferred to greenhouse and sample plants are tested for the presence of virus by ELISA and PAGE techniques (Figure 4.4).

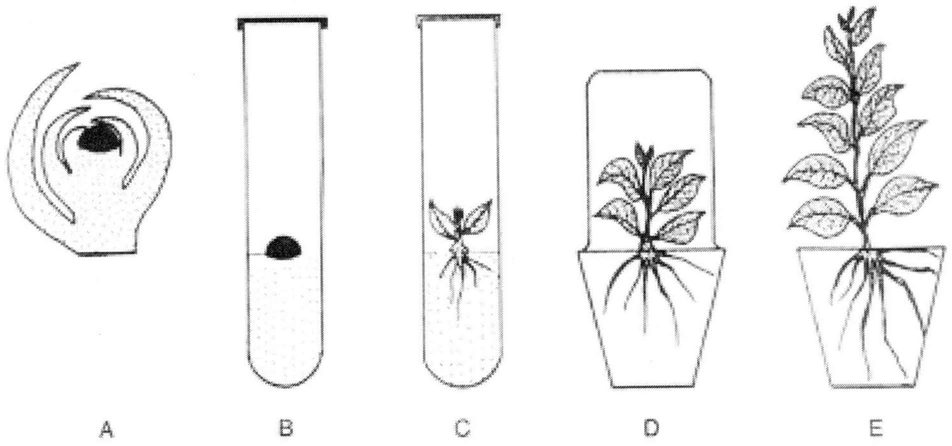

Figure 4.4. Various Stages of Meristem Tip Culture.

Thermotheraphy

Explants are exposed to the incidence of higher temperature(hot water/hot air) which is not lethal for viruses. Mostly used temperature range is 50-52° C with exposure for about 10-30 minutes. In case of whole plant, lower temperature has to be used (32-40° C) with exposure for 4 to 30 days. Potato Virus S (PVS) and Potato virus X (PVX) are difficult to eliminate by thermotherapy or meristem-tip culture alone. Virus-free plants obtained by combining meristem-tip culture with thermotherapy Potato Virus S (PVS) - 35° C several months.

Cryotherapy

More recently prolonged exposure to a low temperature (5° C), followed by shoot tip culture has proved quite successful in virus elimination; this is often called cryotherapy. Cold treatment is preferable to heat treatment as it is less injurious to the plants and often more effective in virus elimination.

Chemotherapy

Some of the chemical *viz.,* malchite green, ribavirin, Actinomycin D, DMEB (Deodecyl N methylephedrinecin bromide) and 2-thiouracil or virazole (50gm/l) are used to kill the virus in the explants. Sometimes the material is treated even for 30 days. Concentration of chemical compounds used for the chemotherapy assays are determined after phytotoxicity tests. Antiviral chemicals alone used to eliminate viruses or in combination with meristem culture or heat treatment are practiced to develop virus-free plants.

Electrotherapy

The apical meristem can be subjected to electrotherapy in electrotherapy chamber containing NaCl solution (1M). Pulses of 15V will be applied for 5-10 minutes would help to eliminate the virus.

Applications and Limitations

- ✰ Virus elimination generally improves the yield by 20-90 per cent over infected controls.
- ✰ Virus-free plants serve as excellent experimental materials for evaluating the detrimental effects of infections by various viruses.
- ✰ The virus free bulbs grew more rapidly, plants were more vigorous, and they produced a greater number of larger flowers that had richer colour than the virus infected stock.
- ✰ The virus-free plants are deliberately infected by known viruses, and effects of the infection on performance of the host are assayed.
- ✰ Meristem culture can also help eliminate other pathogens, *e.g.,* mycoplasmas, bacteria and fungi. Bacteria and fungi present in explants show up when they are cultured *in vitro*since tissue culture media provide excellent nutrition for the microbes.
- ✰ Meristem culture has been used to eliminate systemic bacteria form *Diffenbachia* and *Pelargonium,* and *Fusareum roseus* from carnations.

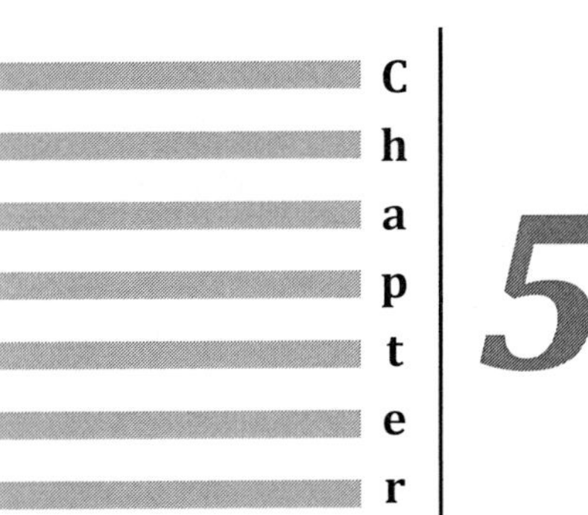

Anther and Pollen Culture, Ovule and Embryo Culture

Anther Culture

Haploid plants possess a single set of chromosomes (gametophytic no of chromosomes *i.e.* n) in the sporophyte in contrast to diploids which contain two sets of chromosomes (2n). The existence of haploid plants was reported by Bergner (1921) in *Datura stramonium*. Tulecke (1951) cultured the pollen grains of *Ginko biloba* (gymnosperm) and succeeded in inducing the development of haploid callus. **Guha and Maheswari (1964)** reported the direct development of haploid embryos and plantlets from microspores of ***Datura inoxia*** by the cultures of excised anthers. **In 1967, Bourgin and Hitsch** obtained the first **full haploid plants from *Nicotiana tabacum*.**

Haploid plants are very useful in:

a) Direct screening of recessive mutation because in diploid or polyploid screening of recessive mutation is impossible.
b) Development of homozygous lines in a short span of time.
c) The generation of exclusive male plants by the process of androgenesis using techniques to double the chromosome numbers.
d) Production of disease resistant plants by introducing disease resistant genes *e.g.* Barley accession Q 21681 resistant to stem rust, leaf rust, and powdery mildew.
e) Cytogenetic research which includes production of aneuploids, determination of origin and basic number of chromosome numbers, induction of genetic variability.

Androgenesis

In androgenesis, the male gametophyte (the microspore or immature pollen) produces haploid plants by stopping the development of pollen cell into a gamete and forcing it to develop into a haploid plant (Figure 5.1).

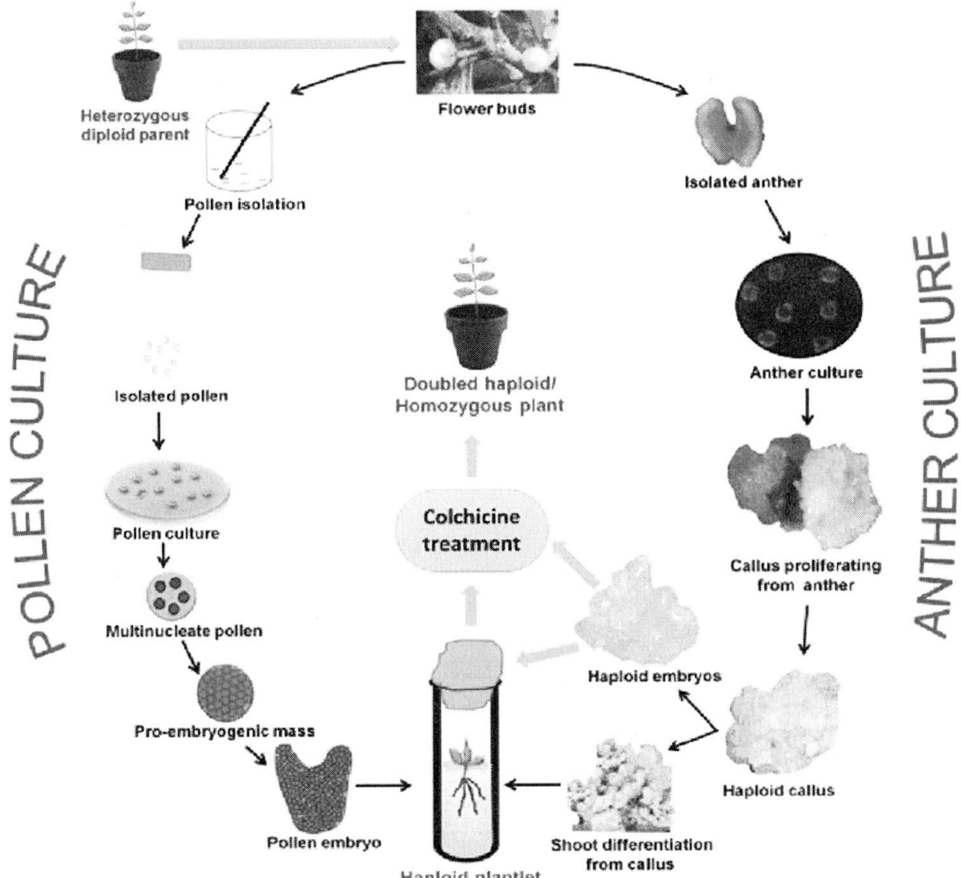

Figure 5.1. Anther Culture and Haploid Plant Development.

In vitro Androgenesis

In vitro androgenesis is the formation of sporophyte from the male gametophyte on artificial medium and is most commonly found in family Solanaceae and Poaceae (Graminae).

Direct Androgenesis

In the pollen derived embryogenesis, also called direct androgenesis, the pollen directly acts as a zygote and passes through various embryogenic stages similar to zygotic embryogenesis. Direct androgenesis is very common in many plants of the family Solanaceae and Brassicaceae.

Indirect Androgenesis

Indirect androgenesis is a process in which the pollen grains divide erratically to develop callus instead of forming normal embryo, *e.g.* in barley, wheat, Coffee *etc.*

The Technique of Anther Culture

Anther culture is the process of using anthers to culture haploid plantlets. The impact of haploid production in genetics and plant breeding has long been realized. However, their exploitation remained restricted because of the extremely low frequency with which they occur in nature. Spontaneous production of haploids usually occurs through the process of parthenogenesis (embryo development from unfertilized egg). Rarely, they reproduce male parent alone. This suggest that their origin through 'ovule androgenesis' (embryo development inside the ovule by the activity of the male nucleus alone).

The development of numerous plantlets in anther culture of *Datura innoxia*, firstreported by two Indian Scientists (Guha and Maheswari in 1964) was a major breakthrough in haploid breeding of higher plants. This technique of haploid production through anther culture (anther androgenesis or simply androgenesis) has been extended to numerous plant species including cereals, vegetables, oil and tree species.

Method

The anthers with their filaments are removed from the flower buds after surface sterilization. Under aseptic conditions, the anthers are excised and crushed in **1 per cent acetocarmine** to test the stage of pollen development. The anthers in correct stage of development are separated and inoculated on a nutrient medium. The anther cultures are maintained at 28°C and alternating photo periods of light (12-18 hrs) and darkness (6-12 hrs). The anthers proliferate and produce callus which forms an embryo and the embryo subsequently develops into a haploid plant.

The Technique of Pollen Culture

Isolation of Pollen

The pollens are extracted by pressing and squeezing the anthers with a glass rod against the sides of the beaker. The anther tissue debris is removed by filtering the pollen suspension and large and healthy pollen are washed and collected. These pollen are cultured on a solid or liquid medium and the callus or the embryo formed is transferred to a suitable medium to produce a haploid plant. The factors that affect androgenesis are the genotype and the physiological state of the donar plants, composition of the culture medium, the method adopted in the pretreatment of anthers to develop in to haploid plants and the stage of the microspore or pollen selected for culture. The haploid are identified by looking at their morphological features or by using genetic markers *e.g.* a1 marker for brown coloured aleurone to detect haploids in maize plant.

Pathways of Pollen Development

The early divisions in responding pollen grains may occur in one of the following four ways (Figure 5.2).

Pathway I: The uninucleate pollen grain may divide symmetrically to yield two equal daughter cells both of which undergo further divisions. (*Dature innotura*).

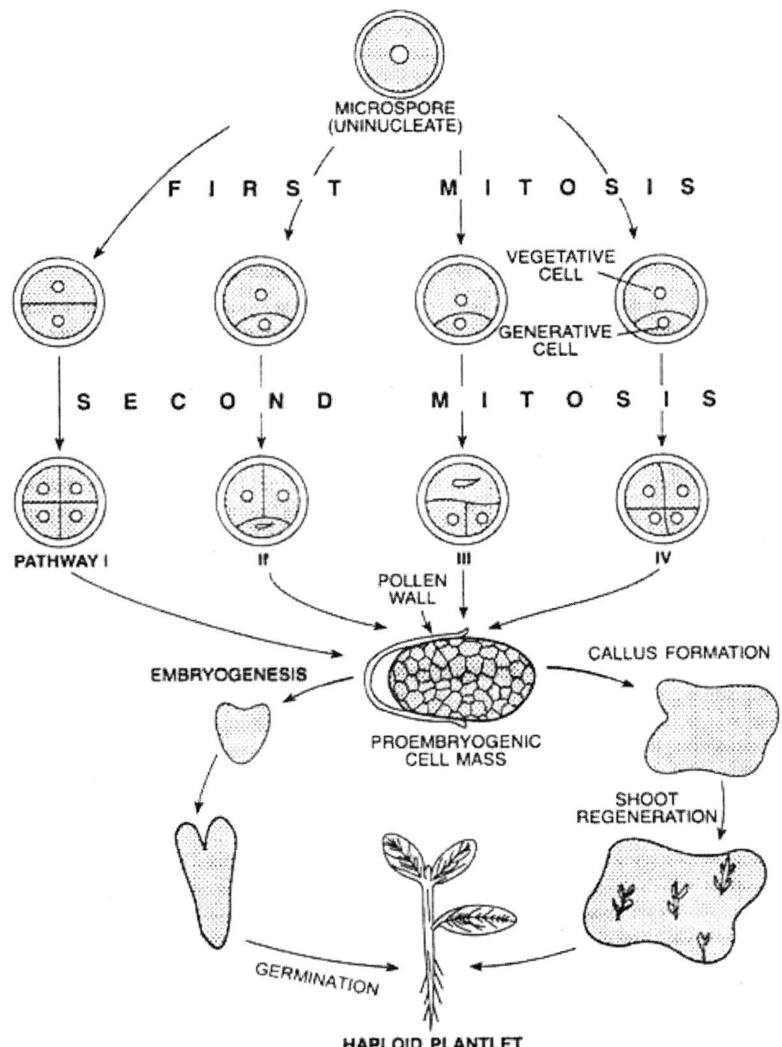

Figure 5.2. Pathways of Pollen Development and Haploid Plant Development.

Pathway II: In some other cases (*Nicotiana tabacum, Datura metel, Triticale*), the uninucleate pollen divides unequally (as it does in nature). The generative cell degenerates immediately or after undergoing one or two divisions. The callus/ embryo originate due to successive divisions of the vegetative cells.

Pathway III: But in some species like *Hyoscyamus niger,* the pollen embryos originate from the generative cell alone; the vegetative cell either does not divide or divides only to a limited extent forming a suspensor like structure.

Pathway IV: In certain species such as *Datura innoxia* the uninucleate pollen grains divide unequally, producing generative and vegetative cells, but both these cells divide repeatedly to contribute to the developing embryo/callus.

Factors Affecting Androgenesis

1. **Physiological status of the donor plants**- The age of the donor plants and the environmental conditions under which it has been grown significantly affects the androgenic process. Generally, the buds from the first flush of flowers show better response.
2. **Stage of pollen development**- The pollen grains around the first mitosis is most responsive. The uninucleate microspores produce haploids while the binucleate pollen form plants of higher ploidy.
3. **Anther wall factors**- the pollen from one cultivar of tobacco would successfully develop into an embryo even if transferred into the anthers of another cultivar.
4. **Genotype** – hybrids are more androgenic than their parents.
5. **Pretreatment of cultured anthers/pollen grains** – application of certain physical (temperature shock, centrifugation, γ irradiation) and chemical (auxins) treatments to cultured anthers or pollen grains prior to standard culture room conditions, has proved essential or promotory for *in vitro* androgenesis.
6. **Culture medium** – addition of etherel (2-chloroethylphosphonic acid), sucrose, agar and other nutrients specific to certain genotype found to increase the success rate of androgenesis.
7. **Effect of gaseous environment**- the composition of the gas mixture that surrounds the anthers has profound influence on the number of embryos produced in anther cultures. The removal of CO_2 from the culture vessel resulted in decline in anther culture response in *Nicotiana tobaccum.*
8. **Effects of light** – Isolated pollen cultures are more sensitive to light than anther culture.

Applications

1. **Production of diploids**- homozygous lines of the cross pollinating species and hybrids are highly desirable to increase the efficiency of selection and

production of homozygous plants. The conventional method to produce homozygous plants is lengthy and laborious, requiring 7-8 recurrent cycles of inbreeding. Moreover, this approach is impractical for self-incompatible and male sterile and tree species. On the other hand, homozygous plants can be obtained in a single generation by diploidization of the haploid. This kind of production of stable, homozygous dihaploids (DH) in a single generation equivalent to the F_8 generation of pedigree breeding and thus considerably shortens the breeding cycle.

2. **Haploids are extremely useful for detecting recessive mutants-** which may not express themselves in the heterozygous diploid background and therefore can be easily lost.
3. **Gametoclonal variation** –*in vitro* androgenesis provides a unique opportunity to screen the gametophytic variation caused by recombination and segregation during meiosis. For example, a gametoclone of tomato, which bears fruits with higher solid content than the parent cultivar, has been produced through anther culture.
4. **Mutagenesis-** Detection and isolation of recessive mutants in the haploid state and rapid obtainment of the mutated gene in a homozygous diploid state is a special merit of haploidy in higher plants. Application of mutagenic treatment at the microspore stage, which is a single celled structure, has the added advantage of obtaining solid mutants. Through, microspore mutagenesis, a mutant of *Brassica napus* with high oleic and low lanoleic acid content was obtained.
5. **Production of super male of *Asparagus officinalis*-** In *A. officinalis*, a dioecious crop species, an inbred population is produced through sib crosses between pistillate and staminate plants which yield 50 per cent males and 50 per cent females. However, the commercially desirable features of this crop are uniform male population with spears having low fibre content. Anther culture was used to produce haploids of this species and this was diploidized to raise homozygous males. These are called as super-males.

Limitations in Haploid Production

a) Due to the low frequency of haploid production the selection is very difficult.

b) Development of haploids with deleterious traits occurred frequently in cultures.

c) It is sometimes difficult to isolate haploids from the culture since the polyploids outgrow haploids.

d) The doubling of haploids (diploidization) does not always lead to the formation of homozygous plant.

e) The embryos derived from haploids often get aborted.

Ovule and Ovary Culture

Ovule culture is an experimental system by which ovules are aseptically isolated from the ovary and grown on a defined medium under controlled conditions. Pollination and fertilisation under *in vitro* conditions offer an opportunity for producing hybrid embryos among plants that cannot cross by conventional methods of plant breeding. An approach to overcome the barriers to pollen tube growth is direct pollination of cultured ovules (*in vitro* ovular pollination) or excised ovules together with placenta (*in vitro* placental pollination). This technique of *in vitro* pollination was developed at the University of Delhi by Maheshwari and Kanta (1964) to produce hybrids among species of the Papaveraceae and Solanaceae. **The technique of culturing excised ovaries under *in vitro* conditions is known as ovary culture.** Various steps followed in the ovary culture is given in Figure 5.3. This technique of ovary culture was developed by **Nitsch in 1951**. Ovary culture can be used to rear ovaries excised from pollinated flowers *in vitro* to develop into mature fruits. Another application of ovary culture is to overcome the barriers hindering the growth of the pollen tube on the stigma or style by intra ovarian pollination. In this technique the style or part of it can be excised and pollen grains either placed on the cut surface of the cultured ovary or transferred through a hole in the wall of the ovary. Some of the benefits of ovule and ovary culture are,

- ☆ **Gynogenesis:** Production of a haploid individual by the development of an unfertilised egg-cell as a result of delayed pollination resulting in parthenogenic haploids. **San Noem first reported the gynogenesis in barley in 1976.**

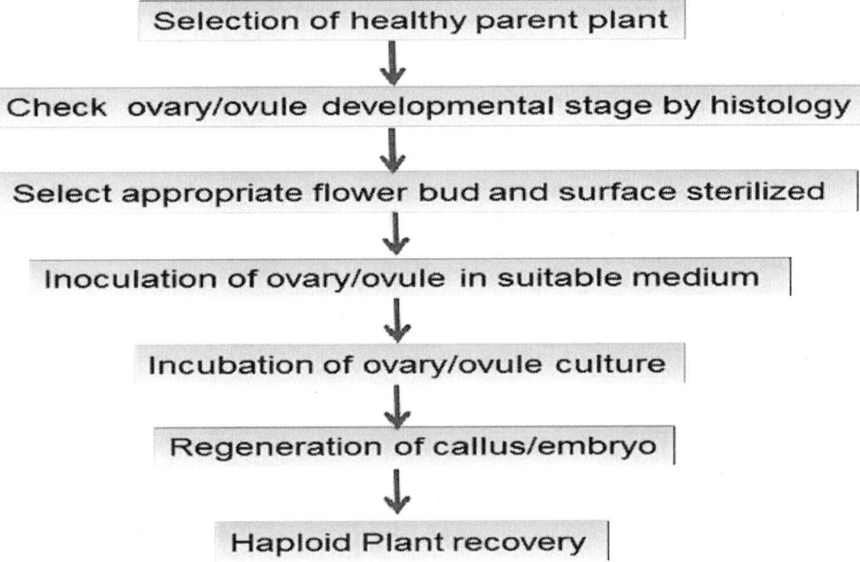

Figure 5.3. Steps of Ovary/Ovule Culture Haploid Development.

- ✰ Overcoming pre-fertilization incompatibility barriers such as self-incompatibility and cross-incompatibility.
- ✰ Raising Interspecific and intergeneric hybrids - Normally these hybrids fail to develop due to early embryo abortion and premature abscission of fruits. Ovule culture can be used to rescue them.

Embryo Culture

Embryo culture is an *in vitro* technique, which supplements the conventional breeding methods. Aseptic isolation of sexually produced (zygotic) immature or mature embryo *in vitro* with the goal of obtaining a viable plant called as embryo culture. In crop improvement programmes through hybridisation, one of the main problems is the failure of the hybrid embryo to develop and germinate normally. The hybrid embryo aborts at various stages of development. This is happening mainly because of the improper development of the endosperm. In normal seeds usually the endosperm provides nutrition to the developing embryo. In order to save these embryos, one of the best available option is embryo culture.

It involves the excision and *in vitro* culturing of zygotic embryos at different stages of development (Figure 5.4). **The first attempt to grow embryos of angiosperms under aseptic conditions was made by Hanning (1904) in *Raphanus*.** The practical application of the technique was demonstrated by Laibach (1925) in an interspecific cross between *Linune perenne x Linune austriacum*. The seeds formed were greatly shrivelled, very light and incapable of germination. But he was able to raise hybrid plants by embryo culture. He suggested to use this technique in the case of complex crosses in which seeds which are not viable.

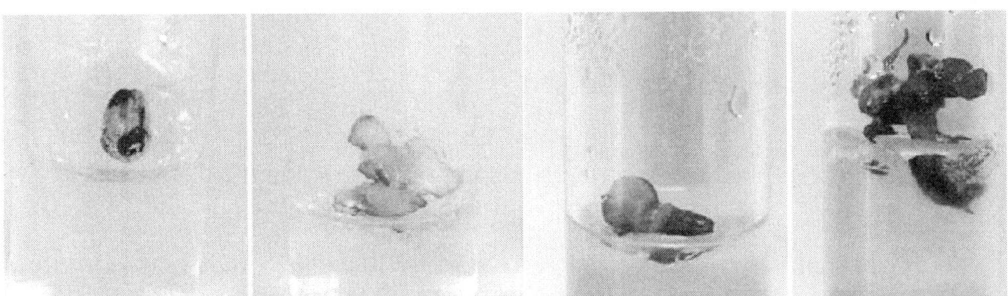

Figure 5.4. Different Stages in Embryo Culture.

Applications of Embryo Culture

1. Embryo Rescue

This technique is the only one method which can save rare hybrid embryos. The embryos can be extracted before they get aborted, then cultured on a suitable medium to get the hybrid seedling. So many successful examples are there.

Distant crosses (intergeneric and interspecific) may fail due to incompatibility, non-viability. It is because of poor development of endosperm causing embryo to starve and eventually abort resulting in shriveled seeds. Thus, embryo culture is used to recover hybrid plants and it is known as embryo rescue. In rice also interspecific crosses are done to incorporate resistance to adverse environmental conditions. In such cases also we can go for to rescue the hybrids *e.g. Hordeum* X *Triticum; Abelmoschus esculentus* X *A.manihot* hybrid; Hordeum x secale; Hordeum x Agropyron.

2. Haploid Production

Another novel advantage possible is in crosses where there is directional elimination of one set of chromosomes following distant hybridisation. This has been observed in one cross in

Horduem vulgare x *H. Bulbosum.* Fertilisation occurs normally but chromosomes of *H.bulbosum* get eliminated. So the embryo is haploid and it will exhibit only slow growth. The embryos of such seeds get disintegrated in 2-5 days. So it cannot be made to grow under natural conditions. Embryo culture is the only successful alternative to maintain and develop the functional embryo and produce haploid plants.

3. Shortening of Breeding Cycle

Usually the plant breeding programme is delayed because of the dormancy of seeds. In some plants, prolonged dormancy period is a problem. In such cases we can go for embryo culture and the breeding cycle can be reduced.

4. Rapid Seed Viability Test

Seed can be broken by embryo culture, it serves as a rapid technique for viability test and serves as a much reliable technique than staining technique.

5. Rare Plants Propagation

Embryo culture also helps in propagation of rare plants. In some coconut varieties rarely a soft tissue is found instead of liquid endosperm and such nuts are referred to as Makapunos and are highly priced and served as a delicacy in Philippines. The plants propagated from makapuno nuts will be true to type. But under normal conditions these seeds fail to germinate. But two scientists De Guzman and Del Rosario succeeded in raising seedlings from Makapuno nuts through embryo culture. Another example is of cultivated banana *M. balbisiana* seeds can not germinate naturally. They readily form plans when cultured *in vitro.* Rose normally takes two years to complete one generation. By embryo culture it can be reduced to one year. In orchids also fruits can be harvested before maturity (green pod culture) and embryos grown *in vitro.*

Embryo culture technique involves mainly 2 aspects

1. The preparation of the explant
2. The culture conditions

1. The Preparation of the Explant

As in any breeding methods, emasculation, bagging, tagging *etc.*, are necessary. Pollination is done by hand and the embryos are excised after some time, when it has reached a certain size. This period of necessary growth of the embryo inside the fruit varies considerably with the plant. It must be determined by a series of successive dissections. Usually the best stage is the heart shaped stage. The fruit is then collected, surface sterilised with sterilant and washed in distilled water. Further operations are carried out under a dissecting microscope on a slide, in a few drops of sucrose solution to prevent desiccation. The embryo is separated from the ovule by applying a slight pressure on ovules. The excised embryo is then transferred by a micropipette to a petridish containing agar medium. The mature embryos can be isolated with relatively ease by splitting open the seed. The seeds with hard seed coat are to be pre-soaked in H_2O so as to loosen the seed coat. Small embryos require careful dissection.

2. The Culture Conditions

Culture Medium

It is the most important aspect. The success of embryo culture to a great extent depends on the composition of media. The media should support the progressive orderly development of embryo excised at different stages of development. Since the earlier workers involved only in the development of plants from mature embryos the medium used were simple and contained only mineral salts and sugar. But the immature embryos fail to develop in such a simple medium. Their nutritional requirements are more complex so as to undergo pre-germinal development. With respect to nutrition, 2 phases of embryo development have been identified by scientists.

1. Heterotrophic

It is the early phase of embryo development, the embryo is dependent entirely on the endosperm of the surrounding maternal tissue for its nutrition.

2. Autotrophic Phase

The later phase in which the embryo is metabolically capable of synthesising the substance required for its growth from mineral salts and sugar. However, the critical stage at which the embryo comes out from the heterotrophic phase and enters the autotrophic phase varies with the species.

Mineral Salts

Requirement of the inorganic minerals salts vary greatly with the species as well as with the age of the embryo to be cultured. So all these are has to be standardised. Among the minerals **iron and calcium** were found to have a higher influence in the growth and development of the embryo.

Organic Nutrients

Among carbohydrates sucrose is the most important. It is added to give energy and suitable osmolarity of the medium. **Young embryos require a high concentration of sugar (8-12 per cent). Mature embryo grew fairly well with 2 per cent sucrose.** In long term experiments with the age of the cultures, the embryos need to be transferred to media with progressively lower levels of sucrose.

Amino Acids

The addition of amino acids either singly or in combination can stimulate embryo growth. **Aspargine and glutamine** have been proved to be most effective amino acids for the germination of excised embryo.

Vitamins

Their presence is not essential and can be added if necessary. Some are found to be inhibitory.

Growth Regulators

Exogenous application of growth regulators are not found to be necessary for the growth of embryo. However, in some cases if embryos exhibit dormancy. Some hormones are added to break dormancy.

Natural Plant Extracts

Coconut water, tomato juice, extracts of dates, banana *etc.* are found to be useful for the culturing of many young embryos. All these substances are reported to have prevented precocious germination in barley embryos.

Culture Conditions

- ☆ Temperature- 25-30°C
- ☆ Light- It is not critical for embryo culture
- ☆ pH- Varies with species, Rice - optimum pH is 5 where as Barley- 4.9 to 5.9.

Limitations of the Technique

1. This method cannot overcome barriers to crossability other than embryo abortion
2. The change from heterotrophic to autotrophic stage is not known exactly. And also it requires frequent subculturing
3. In some cases embryo abortion occurs at very early stage of development. For successful embryo culture the embryo should attain a certain size. So in many cases the technique fails.

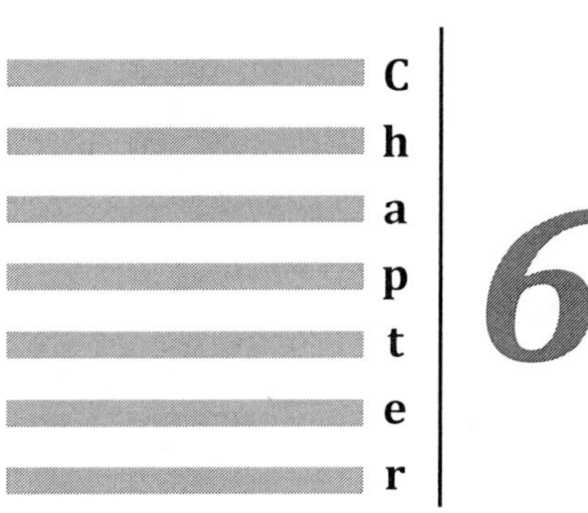

Micropropagation: Banana and Ornamental Plants

Generally, plants are propagated either sexually or asexually. Sexual propagation exhibits high heterogeneity unless the seeds are obtained from inbreds. Whereas, asexual propagation results in genetically identical progenies from the parent plant, known as clones. Method of production of such clones is known as clonal propagation. Advances in tissue culture techniques also aids in the rapid asexual clonal propagation of plants termed as micropropagation. Cultures are started with very small pieces of plants and hence referred as micropropagation. This means that only a small amount of space is required to maintain or multiply large number of plants. **Micropropagation is defined as "Multiplication of genetically identical copies of a parent plant under *in vitro* conditions, usually with an accelerated proliferation of shoots during subcultures". It can also be simply called as "*in vitro* clonal propagation".**

The major advantage of this technique over the conventional methods is that in a relatively short time and space, a large number of plants can be produced from a single individual in a cost effective manner. The speed with which the tissue culture technique has gained recognition in a very shorter period is because of its potentiality of commercialization. In 1946, E.A. Ball showed development of plantlets from sterile cultures of stem tips in Tropaeolum and Lupinus. **E.A. Ball is considered as Father of Micropropagation**.

Stages of Micropropagation

Micropropagation is a multistage complex procedure. Murashige in 1974, proposed a three (I to III) stage protocol for micropropagation of plants. Later, in

1981, Debergh and Maene added stage '02 . Currently, five stages procedure (0 to IV) is widely accepted and in practice (Figure 6.1).

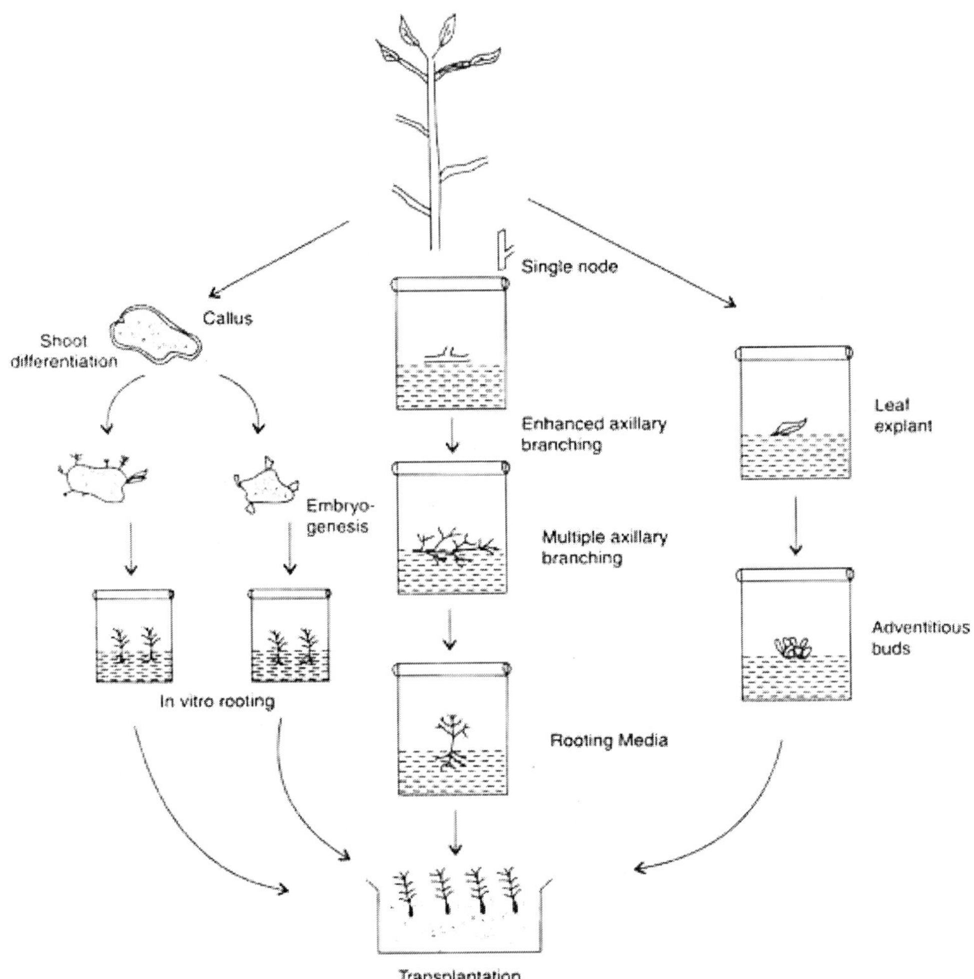

Figure 6.1. Overview of Micropropagation.

Stage 0. Mother Plant Selection

Before initiation of micro-propagation, selection of suitable mother plant is crucial in the whole exercise of propagation. Generally, disease free mother explant is selected for the micro-propagation to reduce contamination of cultures. Certain growth parameters of mother plant can be improved by pretreatment of mother explant before initiation of cultures.

Stage I. Establishment of Aseptic Culture

Micro-propagation begins with successful establishment of cultures of selected plant material. The initial steps of micro-propagation are generally associated with several hurdles such as rate of contamination and phenolic exudation. Plant tissues are commonly associated with bacteria and fungus.

In tissue culture media, presence of sucrose as a carbon source encouragies their growth and consequently kills inoculated tissues. Therefore, adequate sterilization methods are employed to eliminate microorganisms from explant. Several sterilizing agents or surface disinfectants such as sodium hypochlorite (2 per cent), calcium hypochlorite and saturated chlorine water are used.

Sodium hypochlorite is often used as 5-6 per cent commercial bleach. Examples are chlorox or javex. The plant segments are presoaked in 10-15 per cent commercial bleach for 10-12 minutes. High concentration is minimised to avoid tissue damage or cell death. To increase wettability, a small amount of (0.1 per cent) of surfactents such as tween 20, or teepol is added to the disinfecting chlorite (0.1 to 1 per cent) treatment. In addition, a quick dipping (5-30 sec) of explant in 70 per cent ethanol is frequently performed prior to bleach soaking. In certain cases, ethanol dipping may be followed by brief flaming. In the final treatment, sterile water is employed to remove traces of sterilizing agent *e.g.* mercuric chloride before inoculating explant. Beginning of micro-propagation encounters another barrier is phenolic exudation. During propagation of explant, high polyphenol oxidases are responsible for synthesis and release of phenolics, which can eventually kill plant tissues. Several chemicals can be employed to check exudation of phenolics. Adsorption property of activated charcoal can effectively reduce the problem. The most potential antioxidant chemical **polyvhenylpyrrolidine (PVP)** can effectively check phenolics exudation. Adding some other antioxidants like ascorbic acid into culture media and incubating the initial period of primary culture in **citric acid**, reduced light or dark incubation of culture can minimize the damage. In addition, liquid media and frequent sub culturing in liquid media are some of the promising methods in controlling phenolics.

Stage II. Multiplication of Shoots

The main objective of the stage II is the multiplication of organs like shoot and increasing their numbers considerably and shoot elongation. They are able to give rise to new individual plant. Multiplication of shoots through tissue culture involves three routinely used methods like:

(a) Callus mediated multiplication

(b) Adventitious shoots mediated multiplication

(c) By apical or axillary shoots

Callus Mediated Shoot Multiplication

Innumerable number of plants can be accomplished by callus culture (Figure 6.2). **Auxins in general favours callus induction in cultures.** Ratio of auxins to cytokinins could play a decisive role in re-differentiation of shoots from the callus. The callus system can be maintained for several weeks by sub culturing every 4 weeks. Callus mediated shoot multiplication involves certain drawbacks. There might be gradual decline or total loss of regeneration potential of callus cells. In addition, callus mediated regenerated plants generally exhibit genetic variations like euploids, aneuploidy, polyploid and other chromosomal abberation, which reflects on variations of morphological characters.

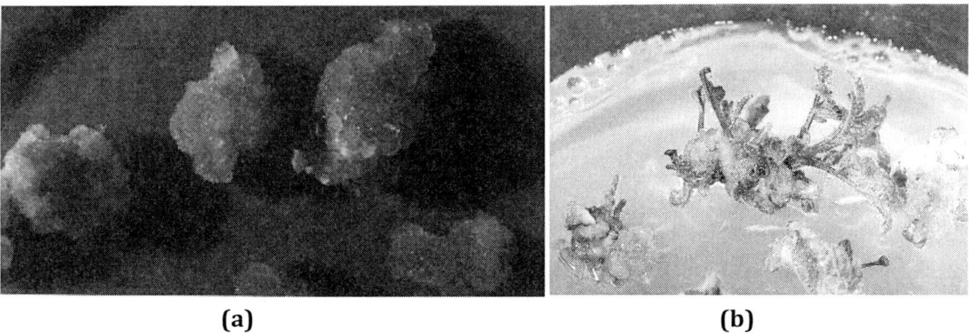

(a) (b)

Figure 6.2a. Shoot Initiation from Callus; b. Shoot Formation in Callus.

In vitro Multiplication of Adventitious Shoots

In this method, adventitious shoots arise directly from the tissues of the explant and does not involve callus mediated regeneration. The regeneration by direct organogenesis via adventitious shoot initiation refers to initiation of shoots directly from stem, tuber, bulb, leaf tissues other than leaf axils (Figure 6.3). Most of the commercial practical propagation involves adventitious bud formation. The main advantage of micro-propagation by direct adventitious shoot regeneration produce numerous small shoots rapidly from each explant, so propagation ratio

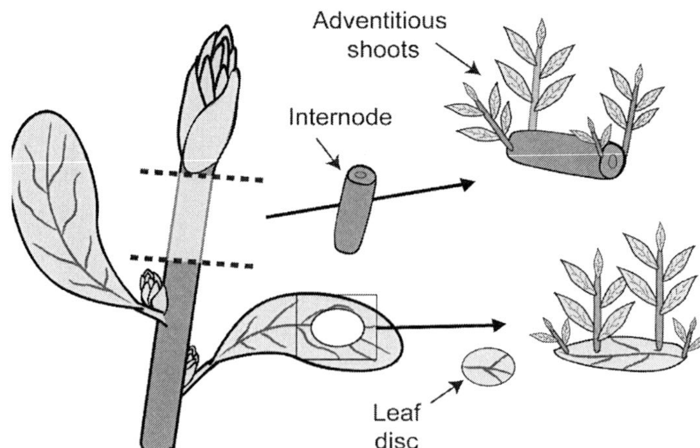

Figure 6.3. Multiplication of Adventitious Shoots from Internode and Leaf Explant.

is very high. In nature, several examples of initiation of adventitious buds from leaf or stem cutting which are not propagated vegetatively as in case of flax and *Brassica* members. Several Plantlet obtained directly from explant and the plants obtained from adventitious bud induction maintain genetic uniformities which is advantageous for commercial ornamental industry.

Axillary Shoot Proliferation

Axillary shoots developed from axillary buds present in the axils of each leaf (Figure 6.4). In leaf axils unsprouted status of axillary buds is due to apical dominance exhibited by growing shoot tip region at the top. Synthesis of auxin in apical shoot meristem is probably responsible for apical dominance. However, apical dominance can be reversed by synthesis of cytokinin in axillary buds or entry of cytokinin into the buds. In micro-propagation strategy mass multiplication of plants can be accomplished by enhanced axillary branching, which involves placing nodal explant containing 1 to 2 axillary buds on the media in horizontal position (*in vitro* layering) for enhanced branching. The culture media are generally enriched with very high concentration of cytokinin. Synthetic cytokinin like BAP and kinetin play a prominent role in releasing unsprouted axillary buds and its further proliferation. The concentration of BAP or kinetin can be used between 2 and 10 mg/L or some cases upto 40 mg/L yield desirable results. High cytokinin overcomes apical dominance and release axillary buds to develop into new shoots. Thus, mass of miniature, shoots are produced in the culture vessels. These miniature shoots are separated and transferred to fresh set of media. The shoot multiplication cycle can be repeated for several times until millions of shoots are produced.

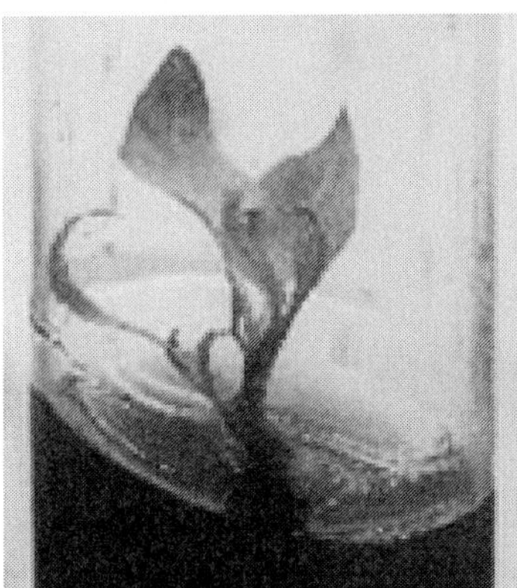

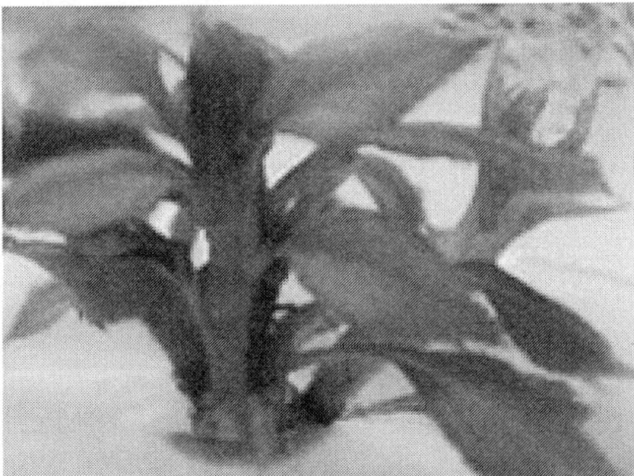

Figure 6.4. Multiplication through Axillary Shoot.

Stage III. *In vitro* Rooting

Shoots or plantlets obtained during stage II are very small and do not contain roots enable to grow in soil, even fails to utilize soil nutrients. Therefore, adequate steps are taken in stage III to grow individual plantlets that can carry out photosynthesis and survive without external supply of carbohydrate. Therefore, *in vitro* grown shoots must be transferred to a rooting media. There is a clear distinction between rooting media from shooting media. *In vitro* rooting can be accomplished by adding auxins to the culture media. Generally, addition of cytokinin is totally restricted due to its total inhibition role. Root induction takes place readily in many herbaceous species, but it can be very difficult or recalcitrant in most woody species. *In vitro* rooting can be both *in vivo* and *in vitro*. In addition to the favourable role of auxins in root induction, strength of media is very important. Media containing half or quarter strength of the salts can be useful in the induction of roots *in vitro*. Supplying riboflavin and other adjuvants enhances root induction process in stage III (Figure 6.5).

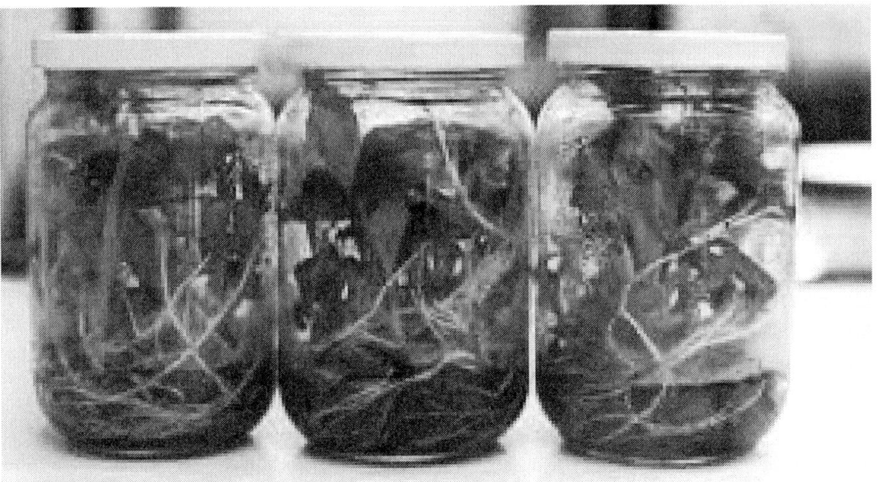

Figure 6.5. Root Formation in Tissue Culture Plants.

Stage IV. Transplantation or Hardening

Once *in vitro* rooting process completes, plantlets are ready to be transferred from the aseptic tissue culture container into the soil. Immediate transfer of tissue culture plants into soil is detrimental for survival of regenerated plants due to desiccation, infection, and light temperature shock. Tissue culture plants generally lack protective cuticle layer and hairy roots, therefore are subjected for light and temperature shock. Excess of water loss was noticed from the leaves of plants immediately after transplantation. High rate of water loss due to lack of protective cuticle layer and root hairs, therefore every chances of exposure of seedlings to light and temperature shock. Plantlets are not developed on their own. The photosynthetic minimum period (7 days) is required for them to be capable of producing their own source of carbon. In addition to these problems, *in vitro* grown roots are highly tender and their vascular systems are poorly developed. In order to compound these problems regenerated plants are subjected to hardening and is carried out by removing test tube grown plantlets and washed under distilled water to remove media sticking to the basal portion of the shoots, plantlets are then placed in sterilized soil or humus soil plus sand (1: 1) or vermiculate soil. These are completely covered by plastic sheet or directly placed in greenhouse to provide 90 to 100 per cent humidity for upto 15 days. Humidity is gradually reduced to 90 per cent then to 80 per cent and finally to 70 per cent. The acclimatized plants are then transferred to the field.

Micropropagation of Banana

Banana is an important fruit crop, widely grown in developing countries. Bananas are generally propagated by vegetative means, which has many disadvantages attributed to low quality of planting material (pest and disease infested), fidelity and easy availability. Micropropagation in banana is feasible with advantages of high multiplication rates and production of high quality planting materials with high genetic fidelity.

Banana Shoot Tip Culture

A. Initiation of Shoot Tip Culture

- ✰ Shoot tips can be extracted from the pseudostem, suckers, peepers or lateral buds which contain a shoot meristem and they are taken from healthy disease free mother plants for shoot tip culture.
- ✰ The suckers are carefully cut to expose the shoot tip of 10 cm^3 and cut further to about 3 cm diameter and 5 cm length (Figure 6.6).

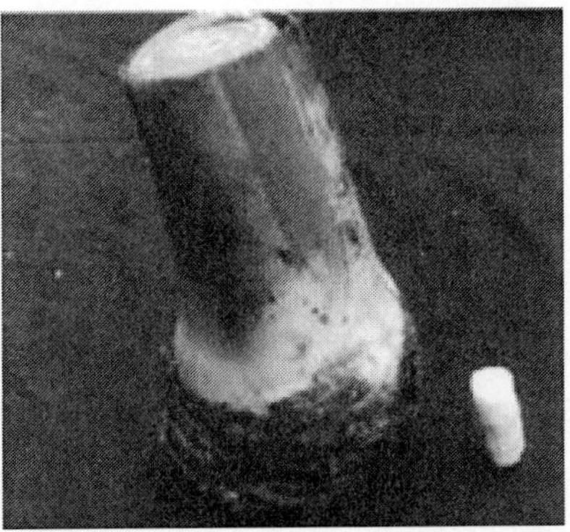

Figure 6.6. Banana Sucker and Shoot Tip Explant taken from Sucker.

- ✰ To prevent browning of shoot tips, they are stored in antioxidant solution (100 mg Ascorbic acid + 150 mg Citric acid per litre of sterile water), till they are moved to laminar airflow chamber.

- Afterwards, the shoot tips are disinfected with 70 per cent ethanol for 30 seconds and later with 0.1 per cent mercuric chloride for 10 minutes. Surface sterilized shoot tips are washed three times using sterile water. The outer surface of explant exposed to sterilizing agent is removed and the explants trimmed using surgical blade to bring the final size to about 3-4 cm length and 1-2 cm diameter.
- Decapitation and wounding of shoot tips are carried out to overcome apical dominance and to encourage axillary bud proliferation. The explants are inoculated under sterile conditions inside Laminar Airflow Chamber.
- The optimum incubation temperature should be in the range of 24-26 °C. Generally the light intensity is maintained at 1,500-3,000 lux. Initially, the cultures are maintained at 16 h light/8 h dark cycle.

B. Shoot Multiplication

- First subculture is done after 20-25 days of initiation when the explants turn green in colour. For subculturing, the outer dead tissue from the base of explant is removed and one or two leaf bases are peeled till the fresh meristematic tip gets exposed.
- During the second subculture, the central meristem produces clusters of proliferating buds and 1-3 axillary buds get regenerated from the basal parts of explants around the central apical meristem.
- In further subculturing, the explant is cut into three to four pieces and each slice with two to three proliferating clusters is inoculated to individual culture bottles.
- During fourth and fifth subcultures, a single clump contains about 15-25 proliferating shoots (Figure 6.7).

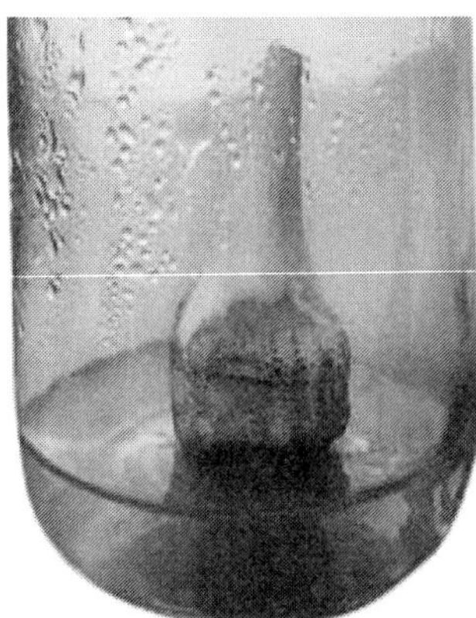
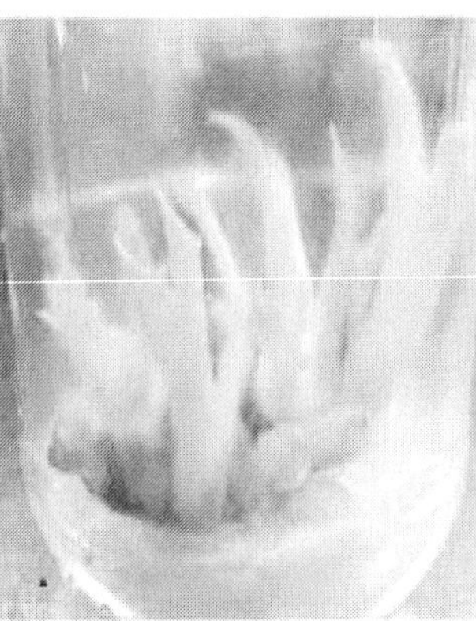
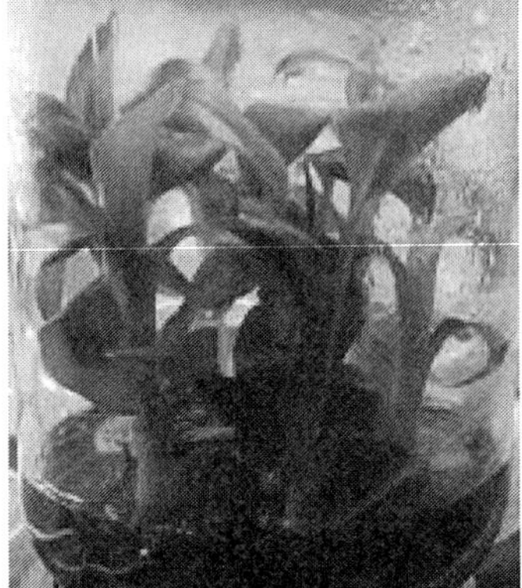

Figure 6.7. Banana Shoot Tip Establishment and Shoot Multiplication.

- ✰ To minimize somatic variation, the subculturing is restricted to a maximum of seven cycles when each bottle contains 25-30 plantlets with well developed shoots and roots.

C. Rooting

- ✰ After 5-6 subculture cycles, the proliferated buds are transferred to rooting medium containing auxin and activated charcoal. After a month, the rooted plantlets are ready for hardening (Figure 6.8).

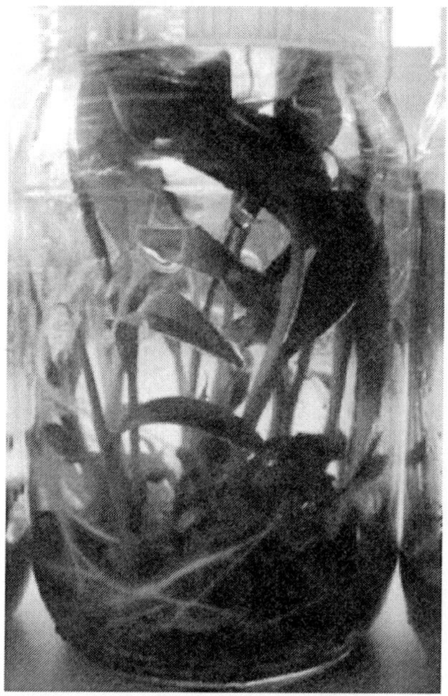

Figure 6.8. *In vitro* Rooting of Shoot Elongated Tissue Culture Banana.

D. Hardening

- ✰ Once the plantlets are ready for shifting outside the laboratory, they are carefully acclimatized to adapt to the greenhouse and later to least protected field conditions. During hardening, the plantlets undergo physiological adaptation to changing external factors like water, temperature, relative humidity and nutrient supply (Figure 6.9).
- ✰ The hardened plantlets are carefully maintained in greenhouse until transportation.

Advantages of Micropropagation

- ✰ Production of large number of plantlets in short duration, thus helping in rapid introduction and dissemination of new varieties.

Table 6.1. Micropropagation Protocols for Ornamental Crops

Crop	*Explant*	*Initiation and Proliferation*	*Rooting*	*Authors*
Rose (*Rosa* spp.)	Nodal Segments	MS + 3mg/L BAP	½ MS + 1mg/L NAA	Oo *et al.*, 2008
Carnation (*Dianthus caryophillus*)	Apical and nodal meristems	**Initiation** - MS + 4mg/L BAP **Proliferation** - MS + 1mg/L BAP	MS + 1mg/L NAA	Ali *et al.*, 2008
Lilium (*Lilium regale*)	Buds	MS + 2mg/L BAP + 1mg/L IBA + 1mg/L IAA	½ MS + 1mg/L NAA + 2mg/L Activated Charcoal	Saifullah *et al.*, 2010
Gerbera (*Gerbera jamesonii*)	Stem apices	MS + 1 mg/L BAP + 1 mg/L kinetin	quick dipping the shoot bases for 3–5 s in 2,000 mg/L IBA	Minerva and Kumar, 2012
Orchids (*Dendrobium fimbriatum*)	Seeds	***In vitro* germination** – PM Medium **Shoot Elongation** - MS + 2mg/L BAP + 0.01 mg/L IBA **Proliferation** – MS + 1mg/L BAP + 0.5 mg/L Picloram	MS + 1mg/L NAA	Kabir *et al.*, 2013
Anthurium (*Anthurium andraeanum*)	Leaf	**Callus induction** -1/2 MS + 0.6 mg/L 2,4-D + 1 mg/L BAP **Shooting** - Modified ½ MS (Low NH_4NO_3) + 0.1 mg/L 2, 4-D + 1 mg/L BAP	Modified ½ MS + 1mg/L IBA + 0.04 per cent Activated charcoal	Atak *et al.*, 2009

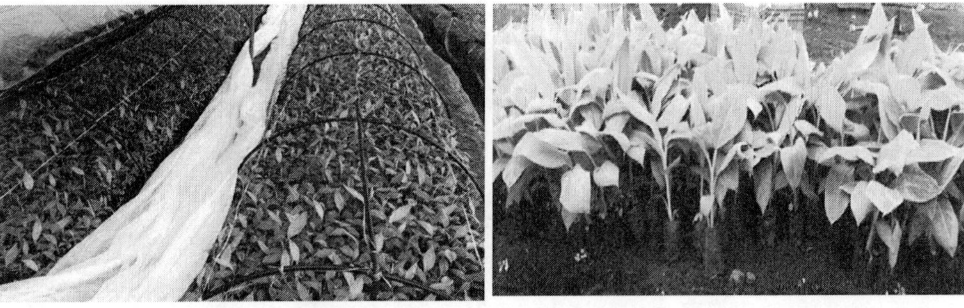

Figure 6.9. Hardening of Tissue Culture Banana.

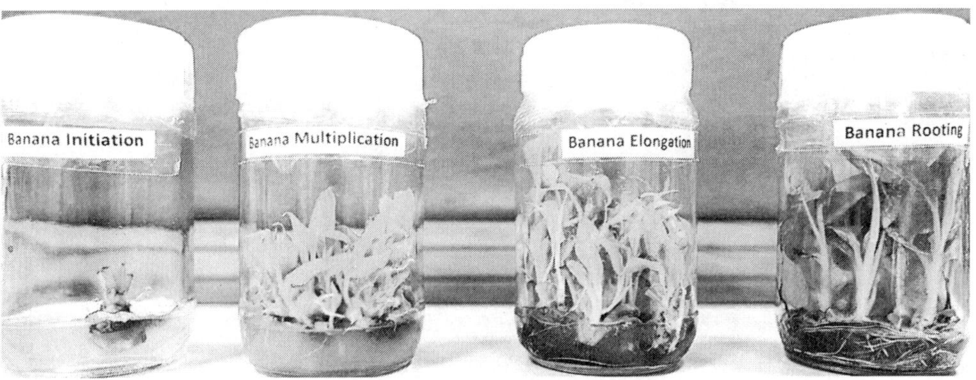

Figure 6.10. Sequences of Shoot Tip Culture in Banana Plant Multiplication.

- A high degree of genotypic and phenotypic uniformity of the progeny plants can be maintained.
- Season independent production of planting material can be achieved.
- Micropropagated plants exhibit uniform growth and maturity.
- Production of disease free planting material can be achieved.
- Micropropagation enables growers to increase the production of plants that normally propagate very slowly such as *Narcissus* and other bulbous crops.
- A more flexible adjustment of factors influencing vegetative regeneration is possible such as nutrient and growth regulator levels, light and temperature. The rate of propagation is therefore much greater than in macropropagation. This would enable newly selected varieties to be made available quickly and widely, or large numbers of plants to be produced in a short while.
- It would be possible to rapidly multiply endangered species and those that are difficult to propagate vegetatively through conventional methods.

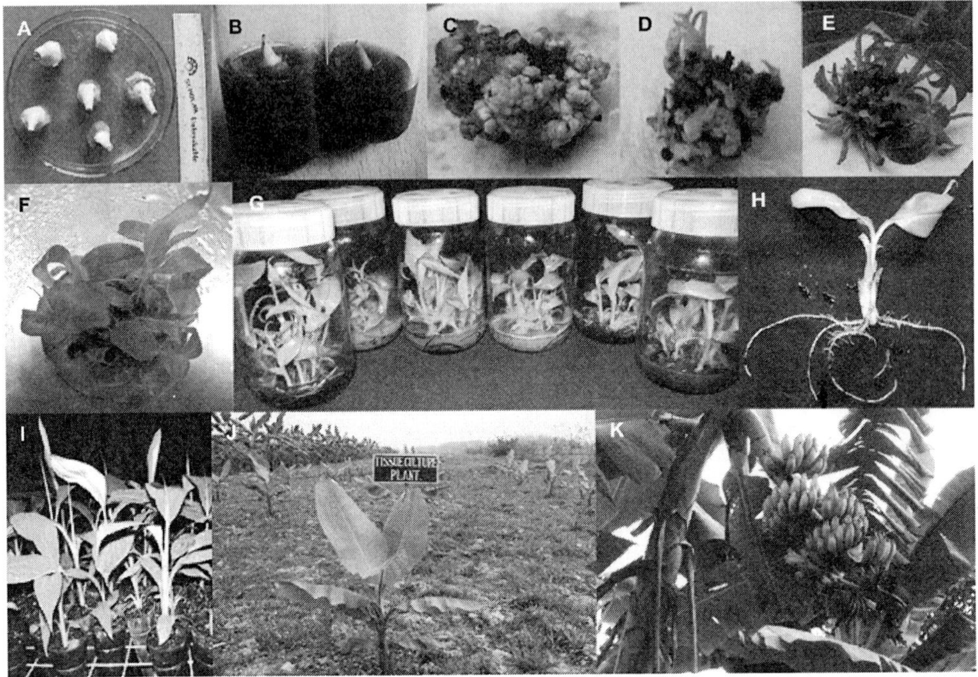

Figure 6.11. Whole Process in Micropropagation of Banana Regeneration through Shoot Tip Culture and Multiple Shoot Formation. (A) Meristematic shoot tips. (B) Initiation of meristematic shoot tips. (C-E) Different stages of multiplication after 8 weeks. (F-G) Elongation of multiplied shoots. (H) Rooting of in vitro shoot. (I) Hardening of in vitro rooted plants in greenhouse. (J) Acclimatized plant in the field after 15 days of transplantation. (K) Fruiting of in vitro plants

Disadvantages of Micropropagation

- ✰ Expensive laboratory equipment and service
- ✰ No possibility of using mechanization
- ✰ Plants are not autotrophic
- ✰ Poor Acclimatization to the field is a common problem (hyperhydricity)
- ✰ Mass propagation cannot be done with all crops to date. In cereals much less success is achieved.
- ✰ Regeneration is often not possible, especially with adult woody plant material.

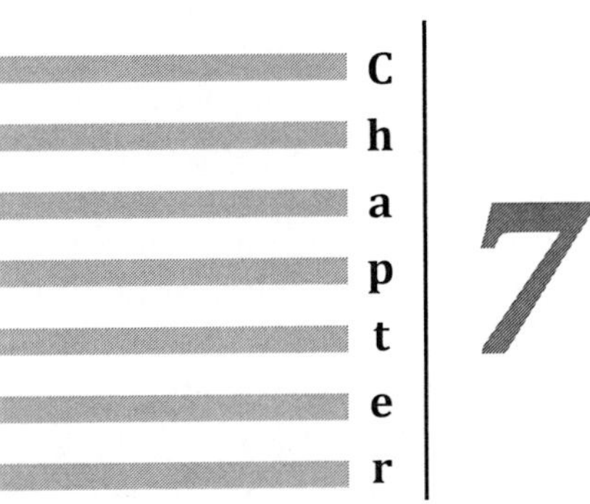

National Certification System for TC Plants

Conventional propagation method which includes sowing of seeds, propagation by cutting, layering *etc.*, suffers from the inherent limitations in the number that can be produced, non-uniformity of quality and incidence of diseases. Plant Tissue Culture Technology offers great promise for the rapid production of quality planting material on account of disease free and true to type plants produced through micropropagation techniques in the laboratory irrespective of the season. In India the tissue culture industry is growing at a rate of 15 per cent per annum. Demand for high quality, high yielding, disease free planting stock of agricultural, plantation and horticulture crops, has been increased significantly over the last two decades. However, the tissue culture propagation, does not exclude the infection of viruses, viroids, phytoplasmas and bacteria unless the parental material used for tissue culture production and stock cultures are tested and maintained free from above mentioned pathogens. The need for a certification programme for the tissue culture plants is more important since inadvertent micropropagation of virus infected plants will not only result in its poor performance, but also in undesirable spread of viruses wherever such plants are grown. Also,failure to use prescribed standard protocols will result in variations in the plants produced. The most deleterious variants in tissue culture raised plants are those that effect yield, genetic fidelity/ uniformity and carry infection of viruses, and other fastidious pathogens, which are difficult to diagnose. This is an area of great concern, and requires a well-structured system be put in place to provide support to the tissue culture industry for the commercialization of virus free and high quality planting material.

Government of India established the National Certification System for Tissue Culture Raised Plants (NCS-TCP) in 2006, authorizing Department of Biotechnology, Ministry of Science and Technology under the Seeds Act, 1966 for ensuring production and distribution of quality tissue culture planting materials. NCS-TCP is a unique quality management system, first of its kind in the world which ensures recognition of tissue culture production facility for the production of quality planting material and certification of end products. For the successful implementation of NCS-TCP; DBT has identified NCS-TCP Management Cell (NMC), Referral Centers (RCs) and Accredited Test Laboratories (ATLs). Tissue culture production facilities get recognition under this quality management system based on compliance with technical capabilities, infrastructure, package of practices and documentation/record keeping. Once the tissue culture production facility is recognized, they become eligible to get quality certificate for tissue culture raised planting material from accredited test laboratories. The certified batches of tissue culture raised plants are provided with certification labels enabled with barcode. This barcode provide end users to trace back history of plants from where the tissue culture raised planting material are derived.

NCS-TCP has made significant impact in the last one decade of its implementation. **Currently, around 79 Companies are recognized. Two Referral Centre's and five Test Laboratories are accredited under this system**. The recognized companies are eligible for getting their planting material certified from the Accredited Test Laboratories. So far, more than 275 million Tissue Culture plants have been certified through this system.

Organization Structure of NCS TCP

For implementing the NCS-TCP, DBT has established a well-defined operational structure consisting of NCS-TCP Management Cell, Referral Centres,Accredited Test Laboratories, an Appellate Authority, A high level Apex Committee and Project Monitoring and Evaluation Committee for close monitoring and review of the activities related to NCS-TCP (Figure 7.1).

Role and Responsibilities

1. Apex Committee (AC)

Role of this committee is to provide technical advice and guidance on policy matters relevant to NCSTCP and approval of guidelines/SOPs established under NCS-TCP.

2. Appellate Authority (AA)

An **Appellate Authority** under the Chairpersonship of Secretary, DBT established to review the decision taken with regard to accreditation of test laboratories, recognition of tissue culture production facilities and also for certification of tissue culture material. The Nodal Officer designated by the

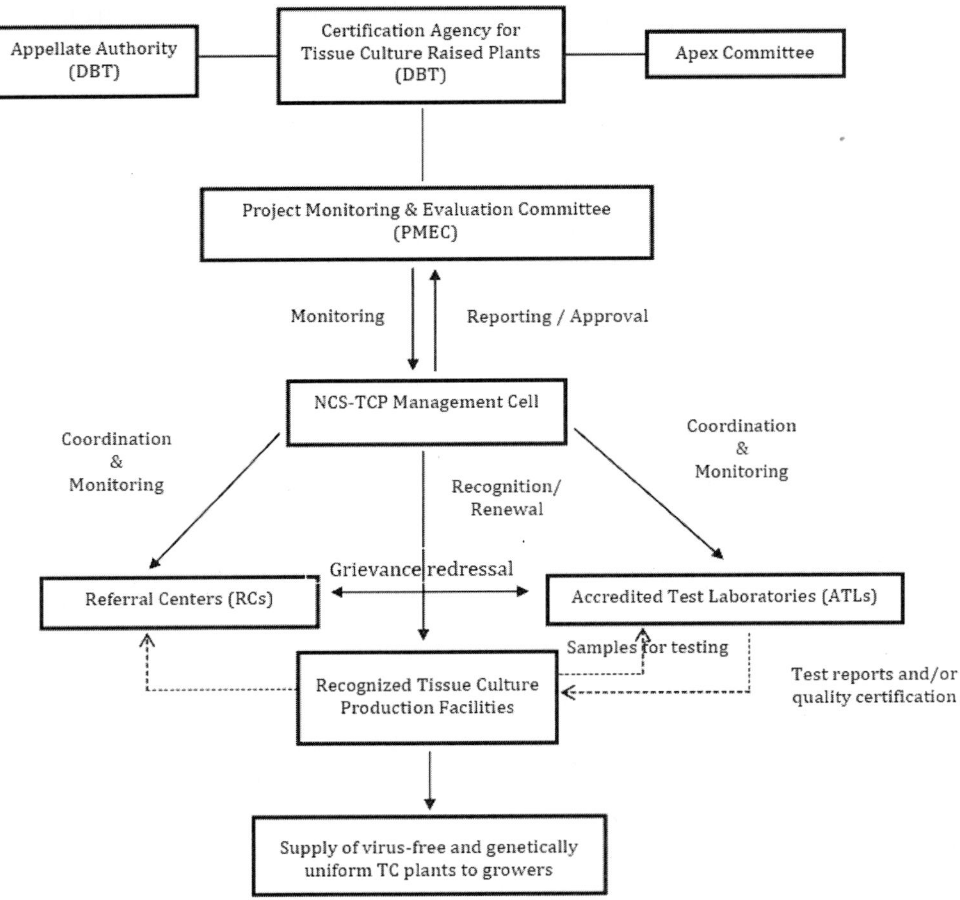

Figure 7.1. Organizational Setup of NCS-TCP.

Tissue Culture Certification Agency will act as Member Secretary. The members represented in the appellate panel will include:

1. Chairman - Secretary/Additional Secretary, DBT or his nominee
2. Two or more experts in the area of Virus Indexing and Genetic fidelity/ uniformity Testing and or expertise in the field concerned
3. Representative from Ministry of Agriculture, Govt. of India
4. Nodal Officer designated by the Certification Agency of NCS-TCP would act as Member Secretary

3. Tissue Culture Certification Agency (TCCA)

The Tissue Culture Certification Agency (DBT) is responsible for implementing the National Certification System for Tissue Culture raised Plants (NCS-TCP) in the Country. A NCS-TCP Management Cell (NMC) has been setup for managing the NCSTCP in accreditation of test laboratories for testing of virus and genetic fidelity/uniformity and also recognition of tissue culture production facilities, based on the established guidelines and criteria and assisting DBT in implementation of NCS-TCP in the country. Referral laboratories have been identified for carrying out confirmatory tests, if required, and also for developing standard protocols, validating protocol and diagnostic reagents, maintenance of referral material, training of technical personal working at accredited test laboratories (ATLs), providing diagnostic reagents to ATLs *etc.* The certification agency is overall responsible for developing standard tests, production protocols/guidelines and manuals.

4. NCS-TCP Management Cell (NMC)

NMC has been established by the Tissue Culture Certification Agency (TCCA) at Biotech Consortium India Limited (BCIL), New Delhi, for assisting DBT in implementation of NCS-TCP in country. NMC is also responsible for assisting DBT in accreditation of test laboratories for virus diagnosis and genetic fidelity/uniformity testing of tissue culture raised plants and recognition of tissue culture production facilities and its renewal. NMC is also responsible for advisory services to DBT for new initiatives, updation of SOPs, guidelines and management of information.

5. Accreditation Panel (AP)

The NCS-TCP Management Cell maintains a panel of experts to undertake assessment of test laboratories for virus diagnosis and genetic fidelity/uniformity testing for accreditation and/or periodical auditing of accredited facilities for granting renewal/revalidation/reinstatement. The accreditation panel also makes an assessment of the tissue culture production facilities. The panel comprises experts specialized in plant tissue culture, plant biotechnology, plant virology, plant bacteriology, molecular biology and phytosanitary. The accreditation panel submits its assessment report based on established criteria/guidelines to the NMC for grant of accreditation/recognition. The NMC should ensure that the essential criteria are met with prior to assessment of facility for accreditation/recognition through application/self assessment report.

6. Referral Laboratory (RL)

The referral laboratory is responsible for carrying out confirmatory tests in the event of dispute or nonconformity of test results, developing standard protocols, validating protocol and diagnostic reagents, maintenance of referral material, training of technical personal working at accredited test laboratories (ATLs), providing diagnostic reagents to ATLs. The Referral Laboratory will not involve in routine virus diagnosis/genetic fidelity/uniformity testing of tissue culture raised plants, however as per the decision of the DBT, the referral laboratories will undertake random testing of samples at different test laboratories.

The DBT has designated Referral laboratory or center for virus diagnosis/ genetic fidelity testing of tissue cultures plants.

1. Referral Center for Virus Diagnosis – Indian Agriculture Research Institute (IARI), New Delhi.
2. Referral Centers for Genetic Fidelity/Uniformity – National Research Center on Plant Biotechnology (NRCPB), New Delhi.

7. Accredited Test Laboratories (ATLs)

Test laboratories are accredited entities, responsible for testing the tissue culture material for virus diagnosis and genetic fidelity/uniformity, for the purpose of certification. The Test laboratory prepares a test report based on tests conducted in conformity with the standards/protocols/guidelines. Based on the test report, each accredited test laboratory (ATLs) is authorized to issue the Certificate of Quality for the Tissue Culture Plant (CQ-TCP) along with certification label on behalf of the tissue culture certification agency. ATLs are responsible for maintaining/ procuring all diagnostic kits, primer, probes *etc.* required for routine testing. Each ATL would perform both tests-for virus diagnosis and true-to-type. At present five ATLs have been identified by DBT under NCS-TCP to testing and certification of Recognized TCPFs. Those are,

- ☆ National Research Centre for Banana(NRCB), Trichy.
- ☆ University of Agricultural Science (UAS), Bangalore.
- ☆ Vasantdada Sugar Institute (VSI), Pune.
- ☆ Indian Institute of Sugarcane Research(IISR), Lucknow.
- ☆ Central Potato Research Institute (CPRI), Shimla.

8. Recognized Tissue Culture Production Facility

Commercial Tissue Culture Production Facility with minimum production capacity of 0.5 million plants per annum may get recognition based on their compliance with NCS-TCP guidelines which is assessed by the accreditation panel (AP). All the activities of tissue culture production facility including hardening facility needs to be operational at the time of comprehensive assessment by the accreditation panel. Comprehensive assessment report prepared by accreditation panel includes observation on infrastructure, technical/scientific expertise and package of practices. Recognized tissue culture production facilities are eligible to get there planting material certified from accredited test laboratory. Recognized tissue culture production facility should adopt standard operating procedure (SOP) and maintain all relevant records. Recognition of tissue culture production facility is granted for a period of two years thereafter it would be re-assessed for "Renewal of Recognition". Till date 79 commercial tissue culture production units have been identified as 'Recognized Tissue Culture Production Units" by (DBT), under (NCS-TCP) in all over India. Among those Tamil Nadu has owned 10 units.

Guidelines and Tissue Culture Standards for Crops under NCS-TCP

In the year of 2020 the guidelines and tissue culture standards for Potato, Banana, Sugarcane, Apple, Citrus, Vanilla, Black Pepper and Bamboo have been notified by Ministry of Agriculture and have been approved by Central Seed Certification Board. Tissue culture standards for Anthurium, Teak, Strawberry, Lillium, Cardamom, Mangium, Gerbera, Fig, Jatropha, Carnation, Grape, Turmeric, Ginger, Orchids and Date palm are under development process and will be available soon.

Services Rendered by NCS-TCP

1. Process of accreditation of Test Laboratories
2. Recognition of Tissue Culture Production Facilities in India
3. Capacity Building/Training
4. Certification of Tissue Culture Raised Plants

1. Process of Accreditation of Test Laboratories

NCSTCP give accreditation to the test laboratories, which are responsible for testing the tissue culture material with good quality, for the purpose of certification (Figure 7.2).

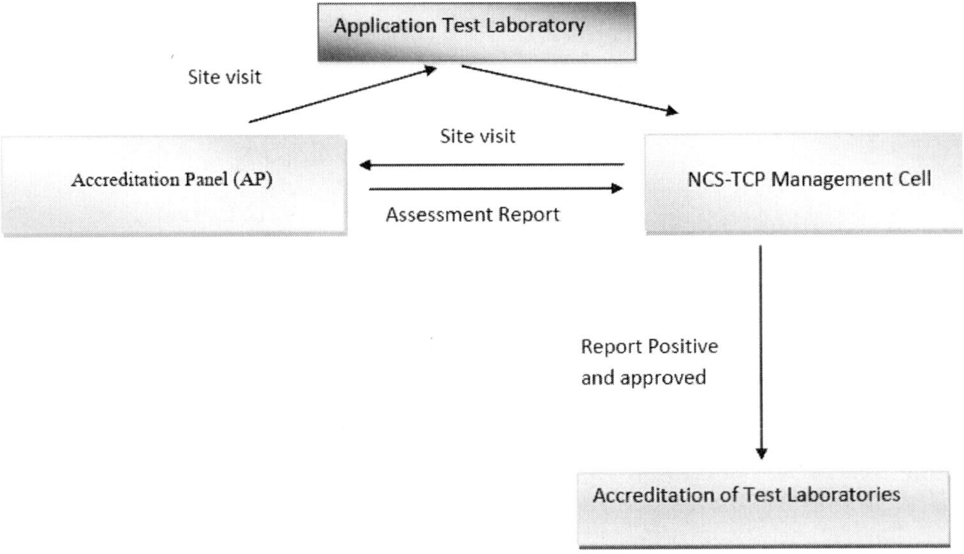

Figure 7.2. Process to get Accreditation of Test Labs by NCS-TCP.

2. Recognition of Tissue Culture Production Facilities in India

Eligibility Criteria for Recognition of Tissue Culture Production Facilities are,

1. Any tissue culture production facility (Public sector, Private sector, NGO and others) engaged in production of tissue culture plants with minimum production capacity of 0.5 million (5 Lakhs) plants per annum.
2. Tissue culture production facility should be fully operational (including all areas of laboratory and hardening facility) at the time of application and site visit.

Process of Recognition/Renewal of Recognition of Tissue Culture Production Facilities (TCPFs)

Application form for recognition/renewal of recognition is available at www.dbtncstcp.nic.in. The NMC would adhere to time frame for site visit of accreditation panel for recognition/renewal of recognition of TCPFs *i.e.* 30 working days from the time of complete application from TCPFs. In case of non-conformities, verification visit would be organized within30 working days day after formal communication from TCPFs of their corrective actions and receipt of verification visit fee (Figure 7.3).

So far seventy nine commercial tissue culture production units have been approved as a recognized tissue culture production units from seventeen states of India *i.e.*, Andhra Pradesh, Bihar, Chattisgarh, Gujarat, Haryana, Himachal Pradesh, Karnataka, Maharashtra, Madhya Pradesh, Odisha, Punjab, Rajasthan, Tamil Nadu, Telangana, Uttar Pradesh and West Bengal by the Department of Biotechnology (DBT), Govt. of India under the "National Certification System for Tissue Culture Raised Plants (NCS-TCP)".

Among seventy nine, ten tissue culture production facilities have been recognized in the year 2020 in Tamil Nadu. They are as follows;

1. Annai Meenashi Biotech, Hosur, Tamil Nadu
2. Genewin Biotech, Hosur, Tamil Nadu
3. Growmore Biotech Ltd., Hosur, Tamil Nadu
4. Hi-Fi Biotech India Private Limited, Salem, Tamil Nadu
5. Hosur Hortitech, Hosur, Tamil Nadu
6. Jay Blossom Biotech, Hosur, Tamil Nadu
7. Jayasree Biotech, Hosur, Tamil Nadu
8. SPIC Agro Biotech Centre, Coimbatore, Tamil Nadu
9. Sree Visal Biotech, Hosur, Tamil Nadu
10. Thulasi Biotech, Jolarpet, Tamil Nadu

3. Capacity Building/Training

Ultimate goal of NCS-TCP is the production and distribution of quality planting materials. To achieve this goal, two level programme would be organized time to time.

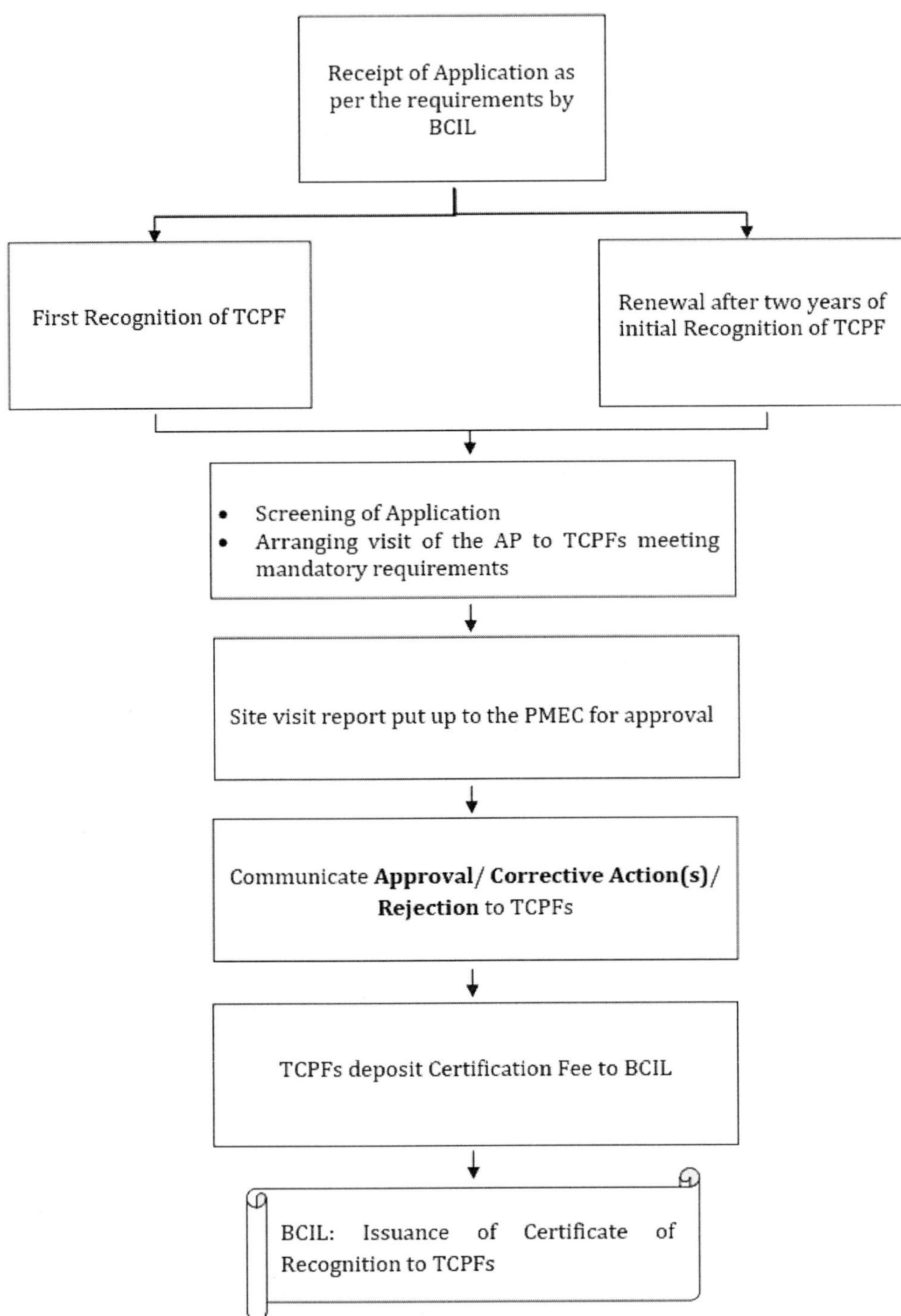

Figure 7.3. Process of Recognition/Renewal of Recognition of TCPFs.

1. Training and capacity building for the tissue culture production facilities.
2. Time to time training of the technical persons form the Accredited Test Laboratories (ATLs).

4. Certification of Tissue Culture Raised Plants

Test Laboratories have been accredited for different plant species which are being multiplied by the tissue culture companies. Only the recognized tissue culture production facilities are eligible to get their material tested and certified by the Accredited Test Laboratories (ATLs) (Figure 7.4). For example the detailed procedure of getting certificates for tissue culture banana is given below.

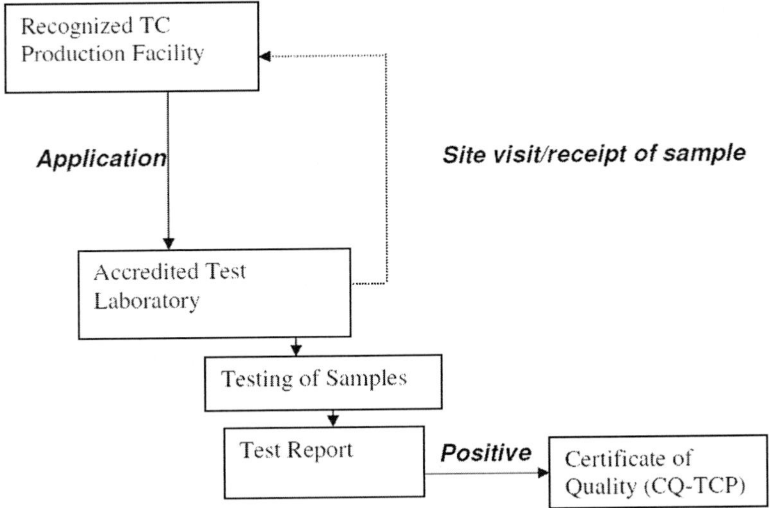

Figure 7.4. Steps for getting Certification of Tissue Culture Raised Plants.

Procedures and Standard Parameters for Production of Banana by Tissue Culture

In tissue culture it is well known that lesser the number of subcultures, lower will be the chances of somaclonal variation. However, it must also be realized that if the number of passages are far too small then the entire production process becomes economically unviable. Therefore, efforts should be made to optimise the shoot multiplication process and extend the number of passages only till the clonal uniformity of the progenies is maintained. However, in banana under no circumstances shoots should be subcultured for more than 8 passages.

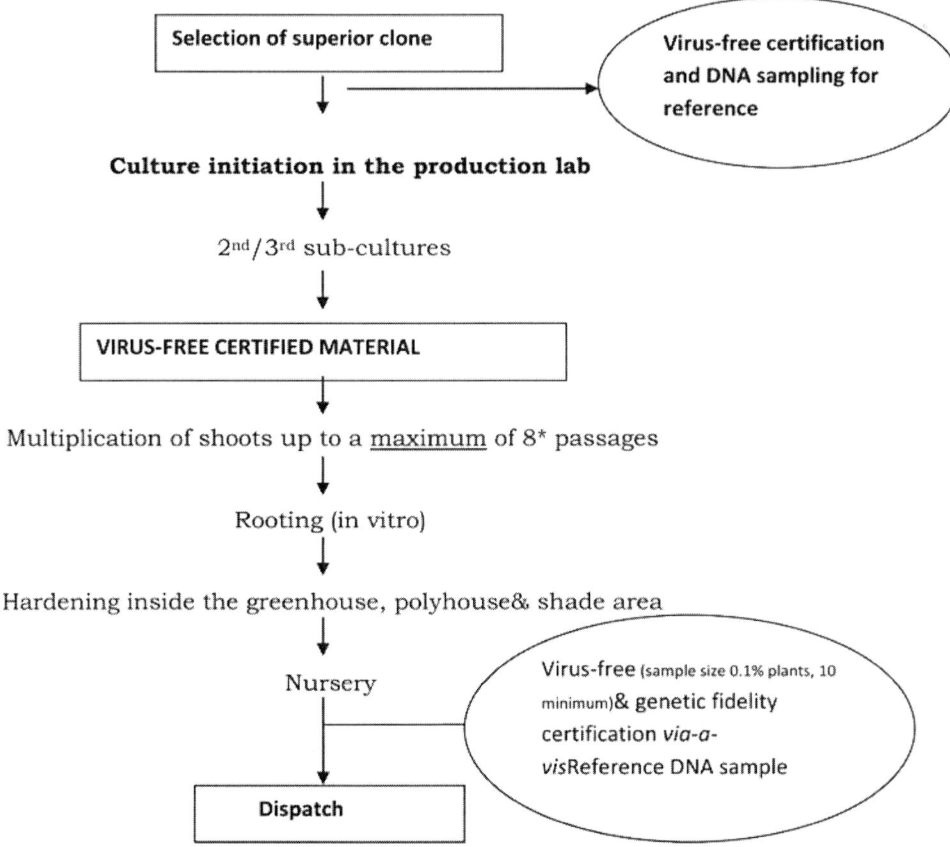

Figure 7.5. Procedures and Standard Parameters of Certified Tissue Culture Banana Plant Production.

Labelling Banana-Tissue Culture (BTC)

1. BTC shall be supplied in containers. A paper-lined label of 12cm x 6 cm containing following information shall be affixed on the container (Figure 7.6).
2. Certified tissue culture raised quality plants/Propagules label shall be rubber stamped with signature, name and designation of the concerned Agency.
3. Colour of the label shall be diagonally yellow No. 356 (IS 5-1978) and opaline green (IS No. 275)
4. The container should also have printed on it the kind, variety and name of Institution'

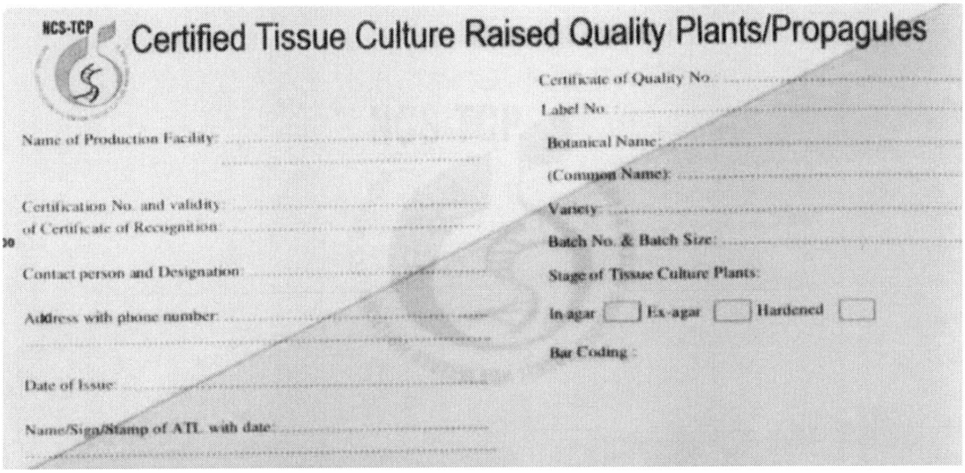

NCS-TCP

Certified Tissue Culture Raised Quality Plants/Propagules

Name of Production Facility: ....

Certification No. and validity of Certificate of Recognition: ....

Contact person and Designation: ....

Address with phone number: ....

Date of Issue: ....

Name/Sign/Stamp of ATL with date: ....

Certificate of Quality No.: ....

Label No.: ....

Botanical Name: ....

(Common Name): ....

Variety: ....

Batch No. & Batch Size: ....

Stage of Tissue Culture Plants:

In agar [ ] Ex-agar [ ] Hardened [ ]

Bar Coding :

Figure 7.6. Tissue Culture Banana Plant Certification Label.

5. BTC producing agency shall maintain the account of labels printed and issued. The above tissue culture standard is available at NCS-TCP official website (www.dbtncstcp.nic.in) alongwith approved tissue culture standards for other 7 plant species *i.e.* bamboo, apple, black pepper, vanilla,citrus, potato and sugarcane.

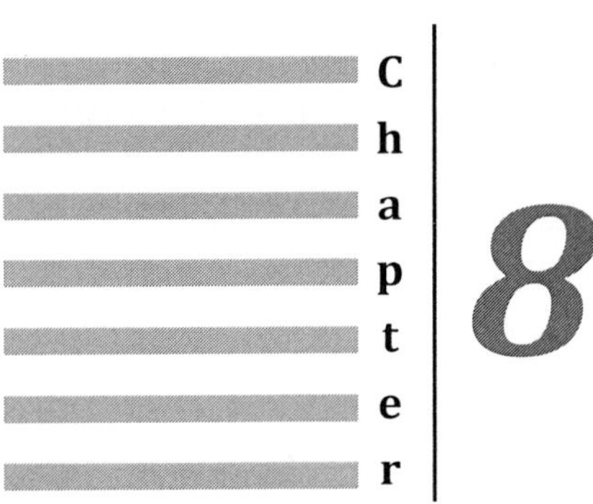

Meristem Tip Culture (Virus Free Plants) and Anther Culture (Double Haploids)

Most of the crop plants, especially those propagated by vegetative methods are systemically infected with one or several pathogens. The death of the plant does not always result from the attack of pathogens. Many viruses may not even show visible symptoms. The presence of viruses in the plants can reduce the yield and/or quality of crops. Yield increases upto 30 per cent have been reported consequent to the replacement of virus-infected stock with specific pathogen free plants. Thus, eradication of viruses and other pathogens helps in optimising the yields and also to facilitate the movement of living plant materials across the international boundaries. It is virtually impossible to eliminate the plant of these internal pathogens by the use of chemicals. Virus multiplication could be suppressed by the use of relatively expensive compounds such as virazole and vidarabine in the nutrient medium. However, the concentrations of these antimetabolites at which they are effective may be phytotoxic to the plant tissue.

Around 600 plant viruses are known of which about 80 can be transferred through seed and the rest through vegetative propagation. Hence virus free starting material is of absolute importance when vegetative propagation is used. Virus free is used to mean free from those viruses that have been identified and whose presence is discernible.

The Methods of Producing Virus Free Plants are as follows

1. Heat treatment 2. Meristem culture 3. Heat treatment followed by meristem culture 4. Adventitious shoot formation followed by meristem culture 5. Grafting of meristems on virus free (seedling) rootstocks (micrografting).

1. Heat Treatment

The entire plant or parts of the plant from which explants are taken are subjected to prolonged exposure to temperatures around 37°C. A temperature and treatment time should be chosen which allow the plant to just survive while the virus is inactivated. Usually warm air treatment is used for establishing a virus-free nuclear stock which is then propagated under conditions preventing reinfection.

2. Meristem Culture

Morel and Martin (1952) were the first to isolate the apical meristem of a systemically infected plant *in vitro* in order to obtain virus free plants, genetically identical to the mother plant by isolating meristems from dahlia and growing them on various nutrient media.

The meristem is a dome of actively dividing cells about **0.1 mm in diameter and 0.25 mm** long. The reason why the meristematic regions are free of viruses is still not clear. It is believed that there is competition in or around meristem between production of virus particles on the one hand and cell production on the other. In meristematic tissue during cell division, the capacity for nucleic acid synthesis is being utilised for cell production to the detriment of virus multiplication. In cells below the meristem which increase in size rather than dividing, virus multiplication takes place. Alternatively, the absence of vascular elements in the meristem is thought to hinder the transport of virus particles. The possible absence of plasmodesmata in the meristem and the absence of vascular elements are thought to be the other reasons for the low concentration of viruses in meristems. Another probable reason proposed by some scientists is that the high concentrations of auxin and cytokinin in meristematic cells might be inactivating the virus particles (Figure 8.1).

Meristems of apical and axillary buds can be used. The meristems are protected by developing leaves. The chances of obtaining virus free plants are increased if the isolation is restricted to the apical dome. However, in such cases, the chances of growth are comparatively reduced. Hence with the meristem one or two leaf primordia are also excised which increase the chance of developing but reduce the possibility of complete virus elimination.

Meristems are isolated from growing shoots for better chances of eliminating the virus. Shoots are well cleaned and the leaves removed before subjecting to surface sterilisation. After rinsing in sterile water, the meristems are isolated under stereo microscope, the stage of which has been thoroughly cleaned with ethanol. The meristems are isolated by removing the leaves and the leaf primorida one by one by using a needle or narrow scalpel blades. When the meristem is practically free, it, along with one or two leaf primordia is cut out, usually as a cube of material and inoculated on a nutrient medium.

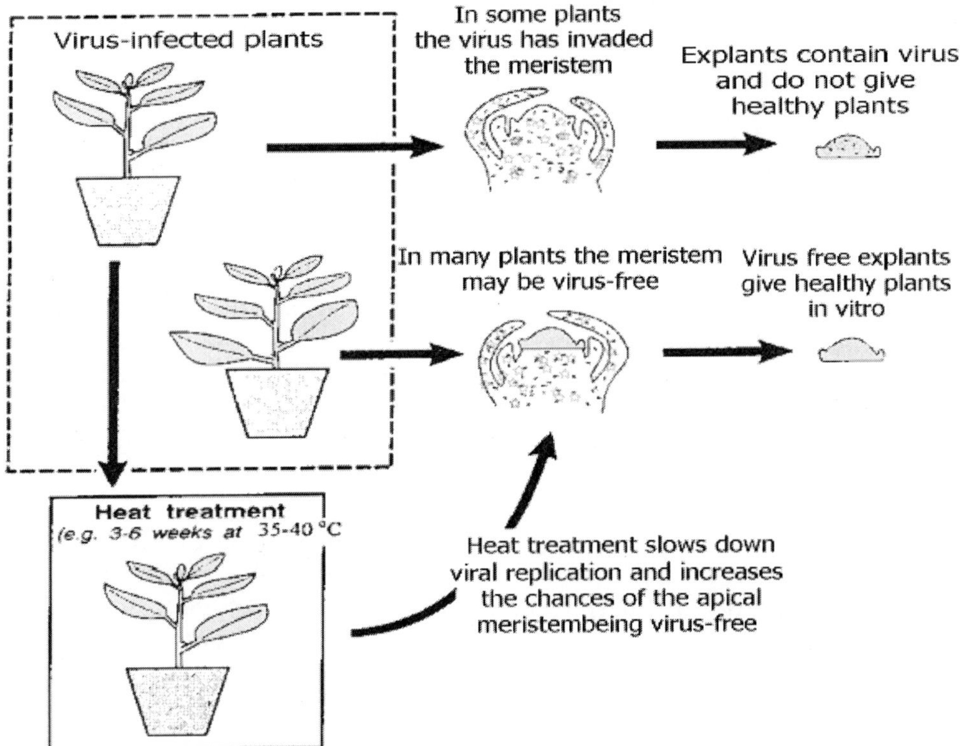

Figure 8.1. Strategies for Obtaining Virus-Free Plants by Meristem Culture.

Meristems are usually isolated on solid media, although liquid media may be used utilising paper bridges. **Sucrose is commonly used as the carbon source (2-5 per cent w/v)**. The vitamins that are commonly used are thiamine, pyridoxin, panthothenic acid and nicotinic acid. Growth regulators are generally used at low concentration (0.1 - 0.5 mg/l). Auxin and cytokinin may be necessary for stimulating cell division and auxin for root formation. GA_3 is sometimes added to obtain shoot extension. In certain cases, the meristems are first cultured on basal medium and later on transferred to medium with cytokinin to prevent the brown discolouration of the meristems. For most plants, 16 h illumination and temperatures around 21-25° C are ideal. Bulbous plants may require lower temperatures.

The explant size may also affect the rooting of the plantlets. Stone (1963) found that carnation shoot tips smaller than 0.2mm were unlikely to root and those larger than 0.75 mm produced plantlets that still contained mottle virus. Tips between 0.2 and 0.5 mm had the best chance of producing virus free plants. In cassava, only explants exceeding 0.2 mm formed complete plants while those less than 0.2 mm in length produced either callus or callus with roots.

3. Heat Treatment and Meristem Culture

To increase the chances of obtaining virus free plants in difficult cases, especially when more than one virus is present, heat treatment is often given at the beginning of the meristem culture. Thus the virus concentration is lowered and/ or the virus free zone enlarged. The length of the heat treatment (35-40°C) varies from 5-10 weeks and the procedure has been successfully used with potatoes, chrysanthemum, carnation and strawberry.

4. Adventitious Shoot Formation followed by Meristem Culture

Adventitious shoots produced from virus infected explants could be used for isolation of meristems and virus free plantlets produced from them. In some plant species, such as petunia and tobacco particular areas of the leaf are virus free while the plant as a whole is infected with the virus. Isolation of virus free zones and regeneration of adventitious shoots results in the production of virus free plants.

5. Micrografting

This is a relatively new technique and consists of grafting a meristem taken from a mother plant on to a decapitated seedling grown under *in vitro* conditions. This method is particularly useful when it is not possible to induce a meristem to grow or a shoot obtained from meristem culture will not form roots. The virus free seedling (rootstock) is grown under *in vitro* conditions and after decapitation, the apical dome is grafted on to it. Successful micrografting has been carried out in Citrus, Grape, Apricot, Peach, Apple *etc.*

Virus Identification

Visual determination whether the plant is virus free(free of known viruses) is difficult since there are many latent virus infections. The potential virus free plant must be assayed which can be carried out as follows:

1. Test Plants

The sap from one of the plants to be assayed is smeared onto the leaf of a test plant which has been injured with sand paper. If virus is present in the sap, then after a few days, the test plant begins to show characteristic symptoms: Test plants used are *Chenopodium amaranticolor, C. quinea, Gomphresa globona* and different species of *Nicotiana*. Disadvantages of this method are the length of time needed and the requirement for growth facilities.

2. Electron Microscopy

The plant material could be examined directly under the electron microscope to detect the presence of viruses. However, the electron microscope being expensive, facilities for use of the same are available only in a few places.

3. Serology

Serological techniques such as the **ELISA (Enzyme Linked Immuno Sorbent Assay**) can be used for the assay. The basis for the assay is the development of specific antibodies in the blood of rabbits when inoculated with a plant virus. If a drop of the centrifuged plant sap is added to a drop of antiserum from the blood of the rabbit, if virus is present, precipitation takes place. The ELISA is a sensitive method for determining the accumulation of virus antigen in the plant tissue.

The test is conducted in wells of microtitration plates which are first coated with anti-viral antibody. Test samples are added to the coated wells. Virus particles present in the sample react with the virus specific antibody and are detected by the subsequent addition of a second anti-viral antibody labelled with peroxidase. Labelled antibody, present only in the wells to which virus has adhered is then revealed by the addition of an appropriate substrate which changes colour on reaction with peroxidase. Under appropriate conditions and within certain limits, the intensity of the colour which develops is proportional to the amount of enzyme - linked antibody present and hence to the amount of virus. The virus free material can be re-infected and hence procedures to prevent the same should be adopted

1. The plants should be grown in greenhouses that are free of infections and vectors (aphid free) or in a place where there are naturally no carriers of viruses.
2. Carriers of diseases (mainly insects and nematodes) should be controlled. The sources of infection should be continuously removed.
3. Strict hygiene is necessary in handling the plants. Grafting and other knives as well as hands and clothes of the staff should be disinfected to prevent mechanical transfer of the viruses.
4. The pots and the potting mixers should be sterilized.
5. Continuous selection visually and by assays should be carried out.

Anther Culture (Double Haploid Production)

Haploids are plants with a single set of chromosomes (n). Ordinarily in normal plants somatic cells contain 2 copies of each chromosome (2n) whereas in haploids only one copy of each chromosome is present. Haploid plants can be produced through *in vitro* culture of male gametophytic cells at the microspore or immature pollen developmental stage by redirection of gametophytic development to sporophytic development. These cells respond *in vitro* by undergoing embryogenesis or haploid callus proliferation. Plants can be regenerated through shoot and root induction from haploid callus or haploid embryos. It is possible to produce homozygous, doubled haploid, pure breeding lines through chromosome doubling treatments applied to haploid cells or plants. The allelic simplicity of haploid plants or their corresponding doubled haploids facilitates genetic studies and hybrid breeding strategies. Since they contain only one copy of each gene, all the genes will be expressed irrespective of whether dominant or recessive. By doubling the chromosome number of haploids, homozygous diploids can be obtained. Haploids are very important in genetical studies and in plant breeding programmes. Doubled haploid cultivars of self pollinating crops, such as wheat and barley, have been released directly following field trials. For cross pollinating crops, doubled haploids have been used as parents of hybrid cultivars because it produce uniform hybrid population without segregation. Alternatively, haploid plants can be obtained *in vivo* through parthenogenesis after wide hybridization (Figures 8.2 and 8.3). The *in vivo* techniques employed to induce haploid production include.

a. **Gynogenesis:** Production of a haploid individual by the development of an unfertilised egg cell as a result of delayed pollination.
b. **Androgenesis:** Production of haploid individual by the development of an egg cell containing the male nucleus. In this case elimination or inactivation of the egg nucleus occurs before fertilisation.
c. Genome elimination by distant hybridisation
d. Semigamy
e. Chemical treatment
f. Irradiation treatments
g. Temperature shocks

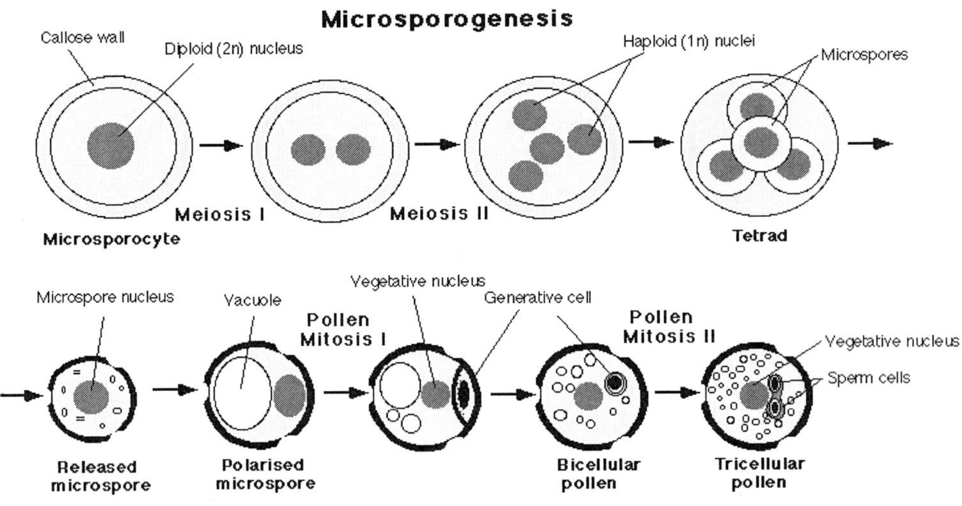

Figure 8.2. Process of Microsprogenesis and Microgametogenesis.

In vivo methods yield a low frequency of haploid production. On the contrary the success achieved using *in vitro* methods has been spectacular. Indian scientists Guha and Maheswari published the first report showing that isolated anthers of *Datura innoxia* were able to form haploid embryos *in vitro* in 1964. Subsequently

Bourgin and Nitsch (1967) obtained the first haploid plants from isolated anthers of *Nicotiana*.

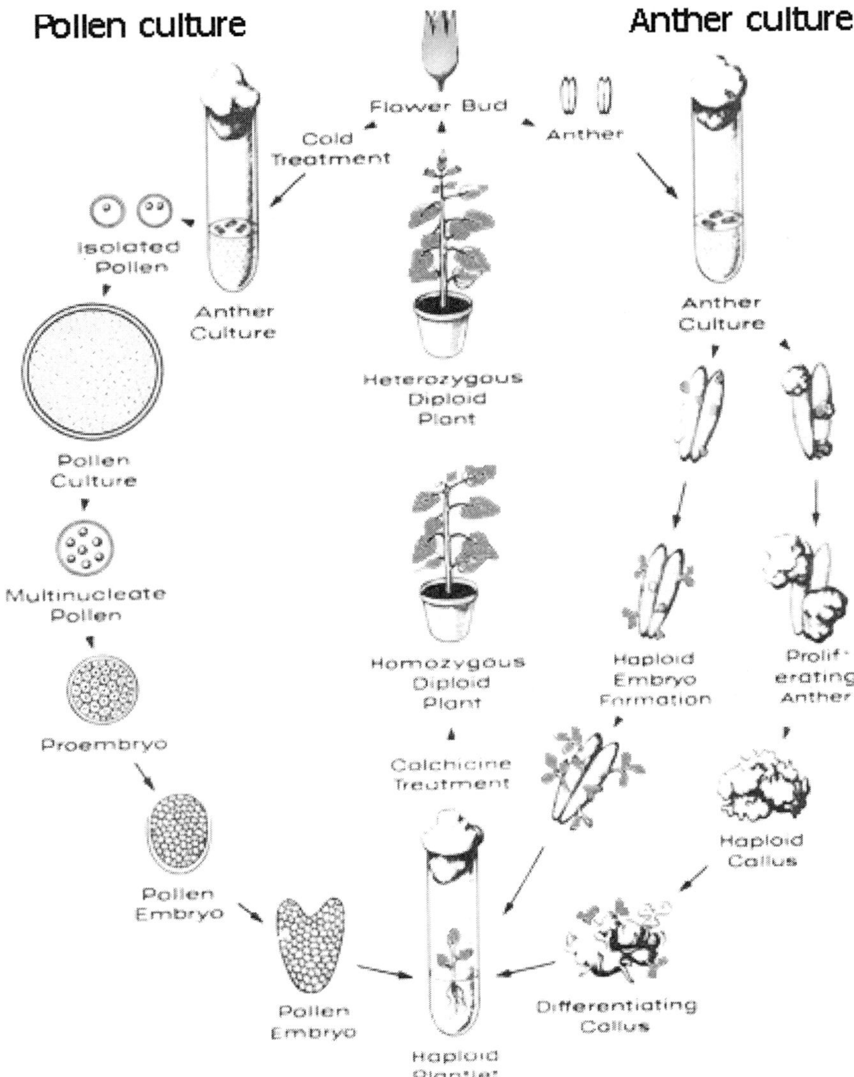

Figure 8.3. Various Modes of Haploid Plant Formation by Anther and Pollen Culture.

Technique of Anther Culture

Young plants grown under controlled conditions of temperature, humidity and light are used as experimental material for anther culture. Anthers should be taken from young plants. With the increasing age of donor plant anther culture redponse declines and abnormalities may appear. Since the stage of pollen is a critical factor for successful anther culture it is important to use the bud of the right stage.

The selected buds are surface sterilised. Anthers along with their filaments are exised under aseptic conditions and tested for the correct stage of pollen development by crushing one of them in 1 per cent acetocarmine. If it is found to be of the correct stage, anthers of the remaining stamens are detached and placed horizontally on the medium. Adequate care should be taken that the anthers are not injured during the entire operation because wounding often stimulates callusing of the anther wall tissues. Another approach is to isolate pollen from anther and prepare pollen suspension cultures.

The anther cutlures are maintained in alternating periods of light (12-18 hr, 5000-10000 lux/m^2) at 28°C and darkness (12-6hr) regimes depending on individual systems. In responsive anthers, the wall tissues gradually turn brown and after 3-8 weeks burst open due to the pressure exerted by the growing pollen callus or pollen plants. Individual plants or shoots are then transferred to a medium which supports a good root system. The rooted plants are ultimately transplanted to soil in small pots or seed trays and maintained under controlled environmental conditions in greenhouse (Figure 8.4).

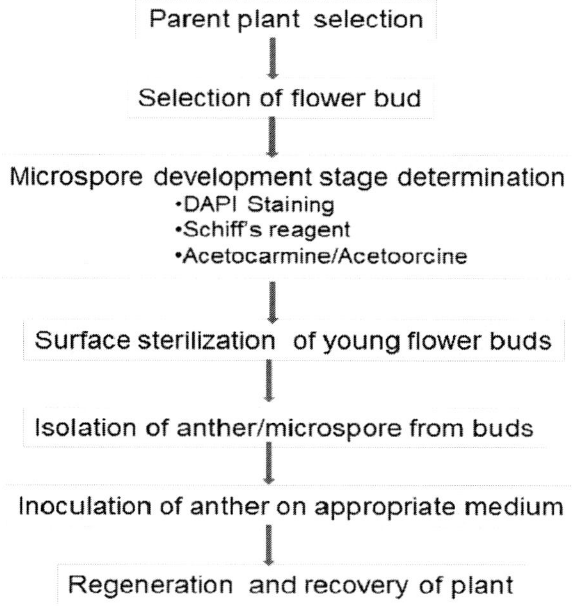

Figure 8.4. Steps in Anther Culture Technique.

Factors Influencing Anther Culture

1. Genotype of Donor Plant

The genotype of the donor plant plays a significant role in determining the frequency of pollen plant production. In cereals, the induction frequency of pollen callus and subsequent green plantlet formation is controlled by many genes. Therefore it is worthwhile to select only highly responsive genotypes for anther culture.

2. Anther Wall Factor(s)

There is a nursing effect of whole anthers for andeogenic development of isolated pollen for number of plant species. An extract from anther also stimulates pollen-embryo production. In henbane, embryogenic pollen are restricted to the peripherry of the anther locule, and it indicates that wall factor is important in the induction of embryogenic division in pollen grains. However, there are reports that glutamine alone or in combination with serine and myoinositol could replace the anther wall factor(s) for isolated pollen cultures.

3. Physiological Status of the Donor Plant

Age of the donor plant and the environmental conditions under which it is grown also influence anther culture response. Generally anthers from young plants are more responsive. Anthers excised towards the end of flowering season exhibit a delayed response. Also the frequency of responding anthers will be low in such case. Seasonal variations also influence the frequency of responding anthers. Therefore, it is recommended that only materials grown under controlled environmental conditions, be used for anther culture.

4. Stage of Pollen Development

Androgenesis occurs when a pollen is induced to shift from a gametophytic pathway to a sporophytic pathway of embryo formation. The shift may occur prior to division of the microspore (premitotic) that forms the binucleate pollen grain or after microspore mitosis (post mitotic) wherein either vegetative cell or generative cell (or both) divide to undergo androgenesis. For maximum production of pollen plants, the appropriate stage of microspore development varies with plant species. Anthers of some species (*e.g. Datura*) give the best response if pollen is cultured at the binucleate stage whereas in most others (*e.g.* wheat, rice, barley) anthers are most productive when cutlured at the uninucleate microspore stage. *Brassica* species show better response when mature anthers or pollen are isolated from them and cultured.

5. Effect of Temperature and Light

Temperature shocks enhance the induction frequency of androgenic plants. Induction of androgenesis has been found very effective when the panicle of cereals like maize, rye are stored at low temperatures prior to anther culture. Pretreatments of anthers at elevated temperatures (35°C) stimulate androgenesis in some *Brassica* and *Capsicum* species. The frequecny of haploids formed and the growth of plantlets is generally better in light although pollen plants from some genotypes grow both in the light and in the dark.

6. Culture Medium

The available reports do not suggest an anther culture medium applicable to all systems since the requirement vary with genotype, age of anther and the conditions under which donor plants are grown. Androgenic development of microspores from *Nicotiana tabacum and Datura innoxia* can be induced on simple agar plates containing only sucrose. On such a medium the development proceeds upto the globular stage. Further growth of embryos is possible only when mineral salts are added to the medium. Most solanaceous species exhibit androgenesis on a complete nutrient medium of Nitsch or MS. Of the various minerals, iron seems crucial for pollen embryo development. In majority of the non-solanaceous species known to exhibit androgenesis, pollen embryo formation occurs only when the medium is fortfied with growth regulator. Sucrose is another essential constituent of the medium. It is generally used at a concentration of 2-4 per cent but some species such as *Brassica* require a higher (10 per cent) concentration. Incorporation of activated charcoal into the medium stimulate androgenesis in some systems.

Diploidisation of Haploid Plants

Hapolid plants obtained from anther culture grow normally under *in vivo* conditions upto the flowering stage but viable gametes are not formed due to the absence of one set of homologous chromosomes and consequently there is no seed set. Therefore it is necessary to diploidise the haploid plant. Usually for chromosome doubling colchicine is used. Pollen derived plants are immersed in filter sterilised solution of **colchicine (0.4 per cent)** for 2-4 days followed by their transfer to culture medium for further growth. Alternatively the treatment is given in the form of a lanolin paste. It is applied in the axils of the upper leaves and the main axis is decapitated to stimulate the axillary buds to grow into diploid and fertile branches.

Application of Hapoids

Haploids are useful in hybrid development programmes. The first step in the production of any hybrid is the development in inbreds to be used as parents in hybrid production. Conventional method of inbred development involve several years of selfing and selection till homozygosity is achieved which is a time consuming and labourious process. By anther culture haploids can be obtained and by doubling the chromosome number of haploids completely homozygous diploids can be obtained in 2 generations with considerable saving of time, money and labour. Since haploids contain only one copy of each gene all the genes will be expressed whether dominant or recessive. So haploids can be used in the selection of mutants.

Limitations

1. Though the technique of anther culture has been exploited for the production of haploids in large numbers in several species, it is not applicable to all genotypes of crop species. Success so far achieved is restricted to three families- Solanaceae, Cruciferae and Gramineae.

2. When we culture the anther as a whole, resulting plants will be a mixture of haploids and diploids. This necessitates cytological analysis for the isolation of haploids. Chromosome doubling is time consuming and may not always result in the production of homozygote. Doubled haploids sometimes exhibit segregation in their progeny.

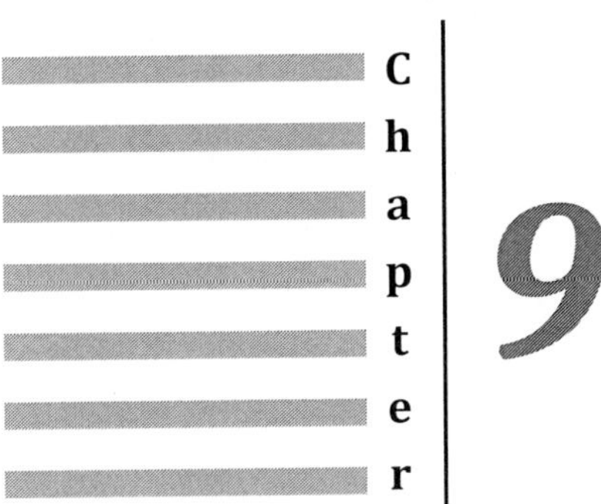

Protoplast Isolation and Fusion, Somaclonal Variation, Synthetic Seeds

One of the significant developments in the field of plant tissue culture is the isolation, culturing and fusion of plant protoplasts. **The term protoplast refers to all the components of a plant cell excluding the cell wall. Hanstein in 1880 introduced the term protoplasts.** Isolated protoplasts are naked plant cells or cells with cell wall removed by mechanical or enzymatic methods. **Protoplasts were first isolated by Klercker in 1892 by mechanical removal of cell wall of plasmolysed cells. Today protoplasts are isolated in large numbers by enzymatic removal of cell walls which was first achieved by Cocking in 1960 from tomato root tips**. The totipotency or regeneration potential of isolated protoplasts was first demonstrated by **Takabe *et al.* (1971)** by regenerating plantlets from isolated tobacco protoplasts. Since then a number of crops of commercial importance like potato, tomato, rice, linseed, alfalfa, cucumber, egg plants, lettuce, cassava and *Brassica* species *etc.* have been routinely regenerated.

1. Protoplasts are valuable experimental material for physiological, genetic and biochemical studies.
2. They can be induced to undergo intra and inter specific fusion to form a somatic hybrid.
3. They can be used for the isolation of cell organelles.

4. Protoplasts can be induced to take up foreign organelles and genetic material.
5. Protoplasts can be stored through immobilisation and cryopreservation.

The plant cell wall offers support, prevents the cell membrane from bursting when osmotic pressures are altered and prohibits entry of infecting microorganisms. The three primary components of the plant cell wall have been identified as cellulose, hemicellulose and pectic substances.

Protoplast Isolation Involves the Following Steps

1. Incubation or enzyme treatment to release the protoplasts from the source tissue.
2. Purification to recover the protoplasts from the cell debris and enzyme.
3. Determination of protoplast viability and density.

Protoplasts are Isolated by Two Methods

1. **Mechanical method**: The cells are kept in a suitable plasmolyticum and cut with a fine knife and gently tweezed using dissecting needles (Figure 9.1). It has the disadvantages of being tedious and low yield of protoplasts.

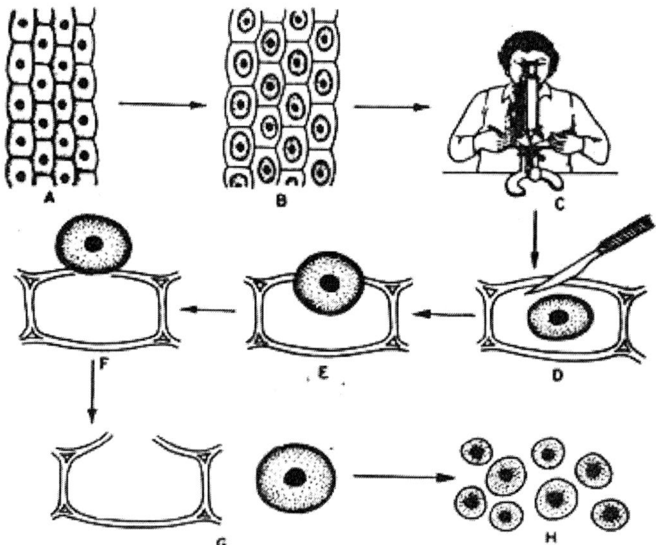

Figure 9.1. Mechanical Method of Protoplast Isolation.

2. **Enzymatic method**: This is commonly used. Two types of enzymes are needed for protoplast isolation.
   (a) Pectinases - remove the cementing material between cells and separate the cells by degrading the middle lamella.

(b) Cellulases and hemicellulases - degrade the cell wall and releases the protoplasts.

The enzymatic isolation of protoplasts can be performed in two different ways.

a. The one step or simultaneous method
b. The two step or sequential method.

In the first, the tissue is subjected to a mixture of enzymes including pectinase and cellulase. This method is faster and results in a higher yield of uniform protoplasts and also reduces the chances of microbial contamination. In the sequential method the tissue is first treated with pectinase to separate the cells. The separated cells are then treated with cellulase which releases the protoplasts. The one step method is mostly followed (Figure 9.2).

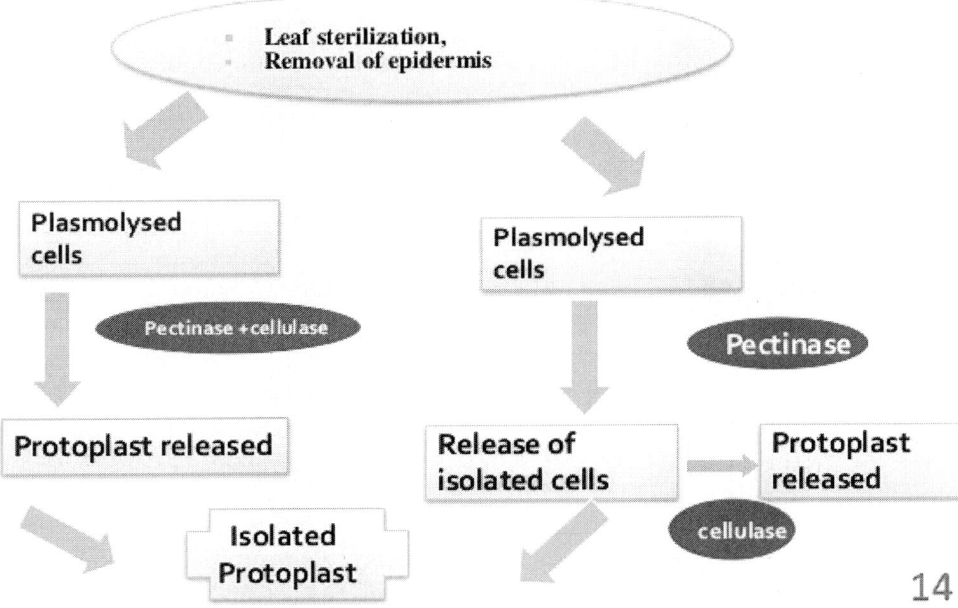

Figure 9.2. Simultaneous and Sequential Enzymatic Method of Protoplast Isolation.

Enzymes

Most of the enzymes used for protoplast isolation are extracted from fungi

Cell Wall Degrading Enzymes

Cellulases	Organism
1. Cellulase	*Aspergillus niger*
2. Driselase	Basidia mycetes
3. Cellulysin	*Trichodermia reesi*

Hemicellulases

1. Hemicellulase	*A. niger*
2. Rhozyme HP 150	*A. niger*

Pectinases

1. Macerase (Macerozyme)	*Rhizopus* sp.
2. Pectinase	*A. niger*
3. Pectolyase Y.23	*A. japonicus*

The release of protoplasts is very much dependent on the nature and concentration of enzymes used. The optimum concentration of enzymes, osmoticum duration of enzyme treatment *etc.* are to be decided after several trials. The incubation period in the enzyme solution may be as short as 30 minutes or as long as 20 hrs. Generally 10 ml of enzyme solution is needed for 1 g tissue. In dicots like tobacco 0.1 to 0.2 per cent macerozyme and 1 per cent cellulase is used for isolation of protoplasts from leaves while in cereals 2 per cent cellulase, 0.5 per cent macerozyme and 1 per cent hemicellulase is used.

The Yield and Viability of Protoplasts Depends on Several Factors

1. Source Tissue

Protoplasts can be isolated from all cells except vascular bundles. Leaves, cell cultures and hypocotyl are mostly used and give higher yield of protoplasts where as roots and cotyledons give lower yield of protoplasts. Most convenient and popular source of plant protoplasts is leaf. The age of the plant and conditions under which it is grown is important. *In vitro* growing shoots are better as it has controlled growth condition and they do not require surface sterilisation. Glass house plants kept under high humidity, low light intensity, short day conditions temperature range of 20-25°C, 60-80 per cent RH and a good supply of nitrogen fertiliser give better results. Because of the difficulty in isolating culturable protoplasts from leaf cells of cereals and some other species their cultured cells (callus) have been used as source material. Then the yield of protoplasts depends on growth rate and growth phase of the cells. Frequently subcultured suspension cultures and cells taken from early log phase are most suitable. In the case of non sterile explants surface sterilisation has to be done. When leaf tissues are used for protoplast isolation the lower epidermis is peeled off or the leaf is sliced into this pieces or pricked with needles followed by slicing.

2. Osmotic Conditions

Protoplasts are isolated by treating tissues with a mixture of wall degrading enzymes in solution with other chemicals. These include a mixture of salts, or a complete culture medium, a buffer and an osmotic stabiliser. Protoplast released directly into standard cell culture medium will burst. The wall presence must be replaced by osmotic pressures in the isolation mixture and also later in the culture medium. The optimum osmotic potential varies with the sources of cells and tissues used. In general a suitable osmotic potential can be generated by 0.3 to 0.7 M sugar solutions. The most widely used osmotica are **sorbitol and mannitol** either alone or in combination in the range **450-800 m mol l^{-1}**. Salts are not recommended as osmotic stabilisers because they reduce the activity of wall degrading enzymes. **Low concentration of $CaCl_2$ (0.1 to 0.5 mM) is recommended which improves the stability of the plasma membrane**. Protoplasts are more stable in a slightly hypertonic rather than isotonic solution. In a solution of proper osmolarity freshly isolated protoplasts appear completely spherical. The enzyme solution may also include a phosphate of MES buffer (2 (N-Morphilino) ethane solfonic acid) to minimise the shift to acidic pH that may occur during protoplast isolation. PDS or Potassium Dextran Sulphate (0.5 per cent) is also added to enzyme solution to remove the detrimental effects of contaminating proteins present in crude enzyme preparations.

3. Incubation Conditions

Isolation conditions are very important for the successful release of protoplasts without impairing cell viability. Activity of enzymes is pH dependent. It is mostly adjusted between 5.4 - 6.2. Protoplasts are usually isolated in the dark or low light intensity and temperature in the range of 25.-30 °C is found adequate. Agitation of incubation mixture improves release of protoplasts from cell suspension cultures. The incubation period in the enzyme solution may be as short as 30 minutes or as long as 20 hrs.

Purification

After enzyme treatment a mixture of undigested cells, components of broken or burst cells and protoplast is obtained. This should be purified to eliminate broken and undigested cells. Different techniques are available. The most frequently used purification technique is filtration and centrifugation. The protoplast mixture is passed through a filter of 40-100 micron pore size followed by centrifugation at 100 run per minute. The protoplats are precipitated while cell fragments float which can be decanted. The centrifugation and decantation step is repeated to recover a purified protoplast preparation which is resuspended and cultured in protoplast medium.

Flotation technique is used for extremely delicate protoplast A concentrated solution of sucrose (15-20 per cent) or sorbitol may be combined with the enzyme protoplast mixture and using appropriate speed of centrifugation, protoplasts are recovered at the tip of the centrifuge tube.

Protoplast Viability and Density

The most frequently used staining methods for assessing protoplast viability are using **FDA (fluorescencein diacetate) phenol safranine, calcofluor white**

and Evan's blue. FDA accumulates in the cell membranes of viable protoplasts which fluorescence yellow green within 5 minutes. In the dye exclusion method using phenol safranine and Evan's blue, viable protoplasts exclude the stains while broken and dead protoplasts are permeable to them. Calcofluor White (CFW) binds to the B-linked glucoside in the newly synthesised cell wall giving a ring of white fluorescence in viable protoplasts. Other methods to assess protoplast viability include observations of cyclosis, oxygen uptake studies and photosynthetic activity. The concentration of protoplasts in a given preparation can be determined by the use of a haemocytometer. Protoplasts should be cultured at a density of at least 5 x 10 ^{4} protoplasts per ml.

Culture of Protoplast

The first step in the protoplast culture is the development of a cell wall around the membrane of isolated protoplast. This is followed by induction of division in the protoplast derived new cell giving rise to a small cell colony. By manipulation of the nutritional and physiological conditions in the nutrient media, cell colonies may be induced to grow callus continuously or to regenerate whole plants (Figure 9.3).

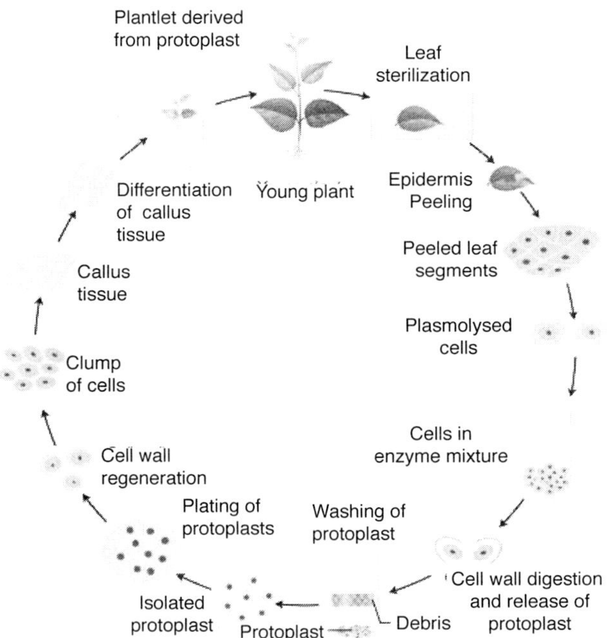

Figure 9.3. Protoplast Culture.

Protoplast Fusion

Protoplasts fusion or somatic hybridization is one of the most important uses of protoplast culture. This is particularly significant for hybridization between species or genera, which cannot be made to cross by conventional method of sexual hybridization (Figure 9.4).

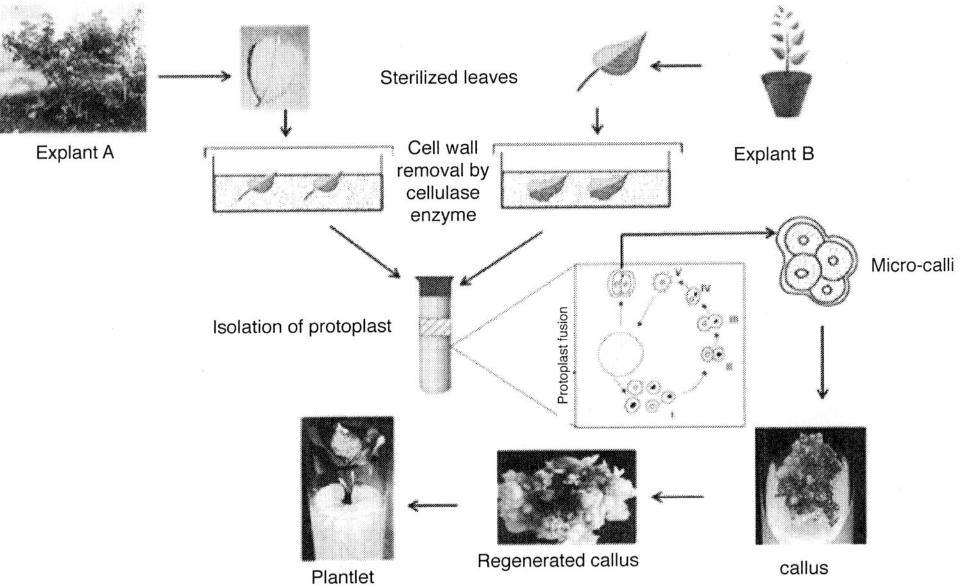

Figure 9.4. Protoplast Fusion.

Somatic Hybridization

In vitro fusion of plant protoplasts derived either from somatic cell of somatic plant or from two genetically different plant is called somatic hybridization

Methods of Protoplasts Fusion

1. Spontaneous fusion
2. Induced fusion

1. Spontaneous Fusion

Protoplasts during isolation often fuse spontaneously and this phenomenon is called spontaneous fusion. Simply physical contact is sufficient to bring about the spontaneous fusion among similar parental protoplasts. Spontaneous fusion usually gives rise to homokaryon usually intraspecific.

2. Induced Fusion

For achieving interspecific and intergeneric fusion *i.e.* hybrid protoplast produced by fusion between protoplasts of two species resulting in a heterokaryon various methods (chemical, electric, mechanical) are followed.

A. Chemical Method (Chemofusion)

Chemofusion requires a fusing agent called fusogen. Most commonly used fusogen is Poly Ethylene Glycol (PEG), Fusogen first brings the protoplasts together and then causes them to adhere to one another for bringing about fusion. The following chemicals are used as fusogen (Figure 9.5).

1) Poly Ethylene Glycol (PEG) (1 ml of protoplasts suspended in a culture medium with 1ml of 50 per cent of PEG) $NaNO_3$ and Calcium ions (Ca^{++}) should be taken in the tube and shake well for 5 seconds.
2) The protoplasts are allowed to sediment for 10 minutes washed with growth medium and examined for successful agglutination and fusion.

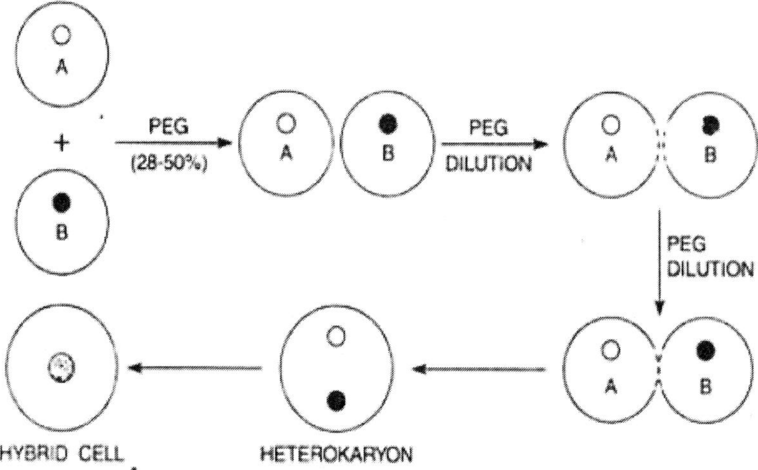

Figure 9.5. Chemofusion Technique of Protoplast Fusion.

Electric Fusion

If protoplasts are placed into a small vessel containing electrodes and a potential difference is applied then the protoplasts will line up between the electrodes. Afterwards an extremely short square wave electric shock is applied protoplasts can be induced to fuse.

Mechanical Fusion

The isolated protoplasts are brought into intimate physical contact mechanically under microscope using micromanipulator and perfusion micropipette.

Cybrids

The cytoplasmic hybrids where the nucleus is derived from only one parent and the cytoplasm is derived from both the parents are referred as cybrids. The process of formation of cybrids is called cybridization. During the process of cybridization and heterokaryon formation, the nuclei are stimulated to segregate so that one protoplast contributes to the cytoplasm while the other contributes nucleus alone. The irradiation with gamma rays and X-rays and use of metabolic inhibitors makes the protoplasts inactive and non-dividing. Some of the genetic traits in certain plants are cytoplasmically controlled. This includes certain types of male sterility, resistance to certain antibiotics and herbicides. Therefore cybrids are important for the transfer of cytoplasmic male sterility (CMS), antibiotic and herbicide resistance in agriculturally useful plants. Cybrids of *Brassica raphanus* that contain nucleus of *B. napus*, chloroplasts of atrazinc resistant *B. capestris* and male sterility from *Raphanus sativas* have been developed (Figure 9.6).

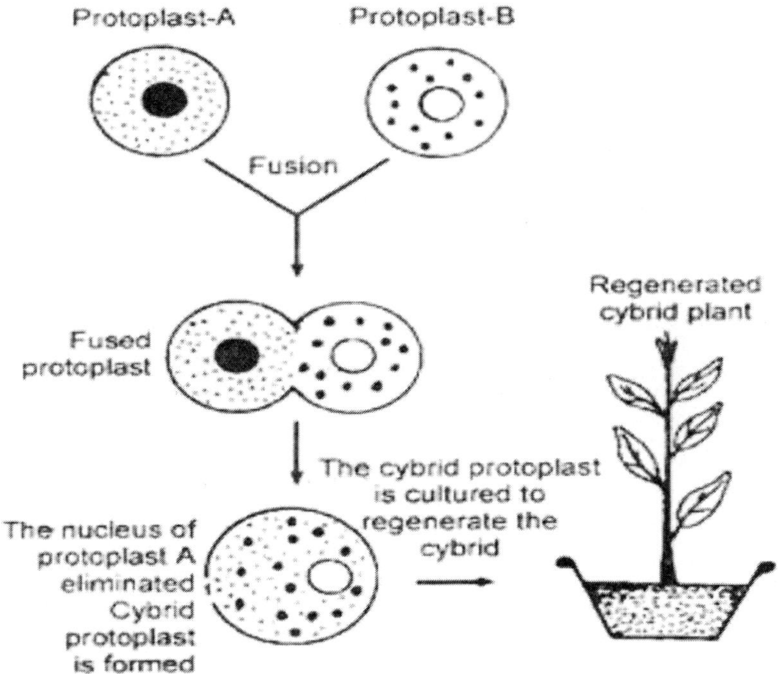

Figure 9.6. Production of Cybrids.

Cybrids can be produced in the following methods:

1. Fusion of normal protoplasts from one parent with enucleated protoplasts from the other parent. Enucleated protoplasts can be obtained by high speed centrifugation (20,000 – 40,000g for 45 – 90 minutes) of protoplasts or by irradiation treatment
2. Fusion of normal protoplasts form one parent and protoplasts containing non viable nuclei from the other
3. Selective elimination of one of the nuclei from the heterokaryon.
4. Selective elimination of chromosomes of one parent at a later stage after fusion of the nuclei (Figure 9.7).

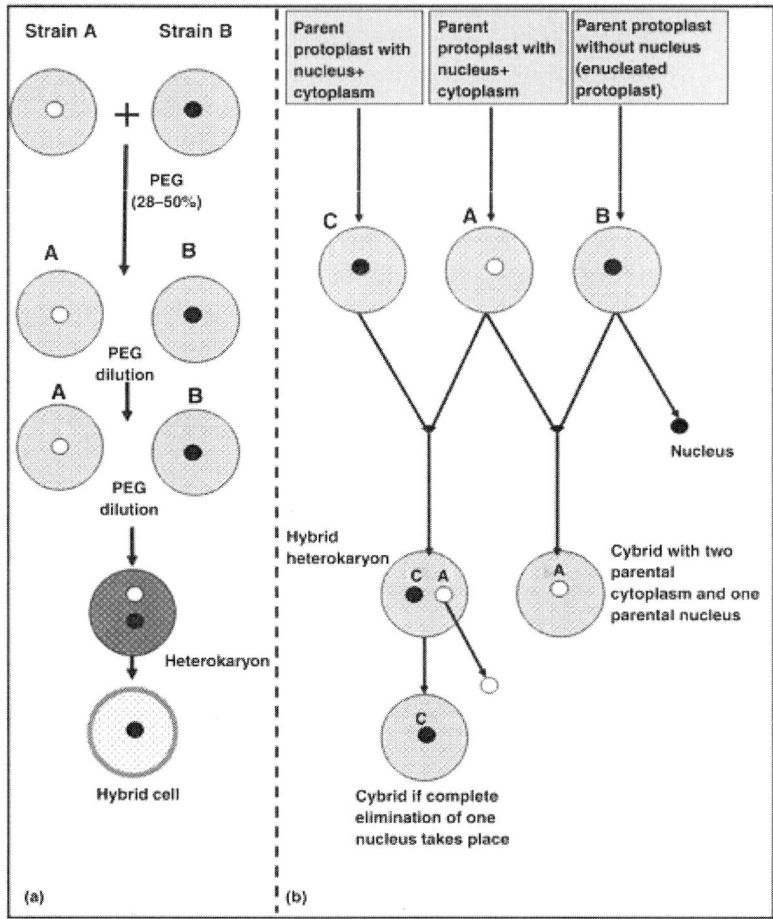

Figure 9.7. Two different Route of Cybrid Production.

Somaclonal Variation

Somaclonal variation is the genetic variation seen in plants that have been produced by plant tissue culture. This term is introduced by **Larkin and Scowcroftin 1981**. However first report of morphological variation in plants regenerated from cell culture was made by **Heinz in 1971 in sugarcane.** Larkin and Scowcraft proposed the term **Somaclonal variation** to describe all those variations which occurs in plants regenerated from any form of cell culture. The plants derived from cell and tissue cultures are termed as somaclones and the plants displaying variation as somaclonal variants. The first generation somaclonal variants are denoted as SC_1 and subsequent selfed generations as SC_2, SC_3, SC_4, *etc.* The somaclonal variation may be epigenetic or genetic. Only the genetic variation is transmitted to the next generation and is thus important for crop improvement.

The epigenetic changes are expressed at cell culture stage but usually disappear when plants are regenerated to reproduce sexually.

Types of Somaclonal Variation

Based on the tissue from which variation originate somaclonal variation can be divided into the following types;

1. **Gametoclonal variation:** Variation observed among the plants regenerated from gametic cultures
   a. **Androclonal variation** observed among the plants regenerated from anther (or) pollen culture
   b. **Gynoclonal variation** observed among plants generated from ovule (or) ovary culture
2. **Protoclonal variation:** Variation observed among the plants regenerated from protoplast cultures
3. **Calliclonal variation**: variation observed among the plants from callus cultures

Genetic Mechanisms Causing Somaclonal Variation

1. Change in chromosome number (Karyotype changes)
2. Changes in chromosome structure (Deletion/Duplication/Inversions)
3. Single gene mutations
4. Cytoplasmic genetic changes (Changes in mitochondrial DNA)
5. Mitotic crossing over
6. Gene amplification due to tissue culture stress
7. Transposable elements
8. DNA Methylation

Methods for Obtaining (or) Isolating Somaclonal Variants

1. *In vitro* Culture without Selection Pressure

Prolonged or continuous subculture of callus to many generation in tissue culture method produce somoclonal variation. Variants can be screened with desired or improved character once callus got regenerated in to plants. There is no invitro selection to the specific characters under in this method (Figure 9.8).

Examples

a. Sugarcane cv. Pindar – Pindar (70-31) – Resistance to Fiji disease and downey mildew.
b. Potato cv. Russet Burbank - Protoplast culture regenerants - Resistance to early blight and late blight.
c. Geranium 'Pelargonium' species – Velvet Rose – Improved Scent.

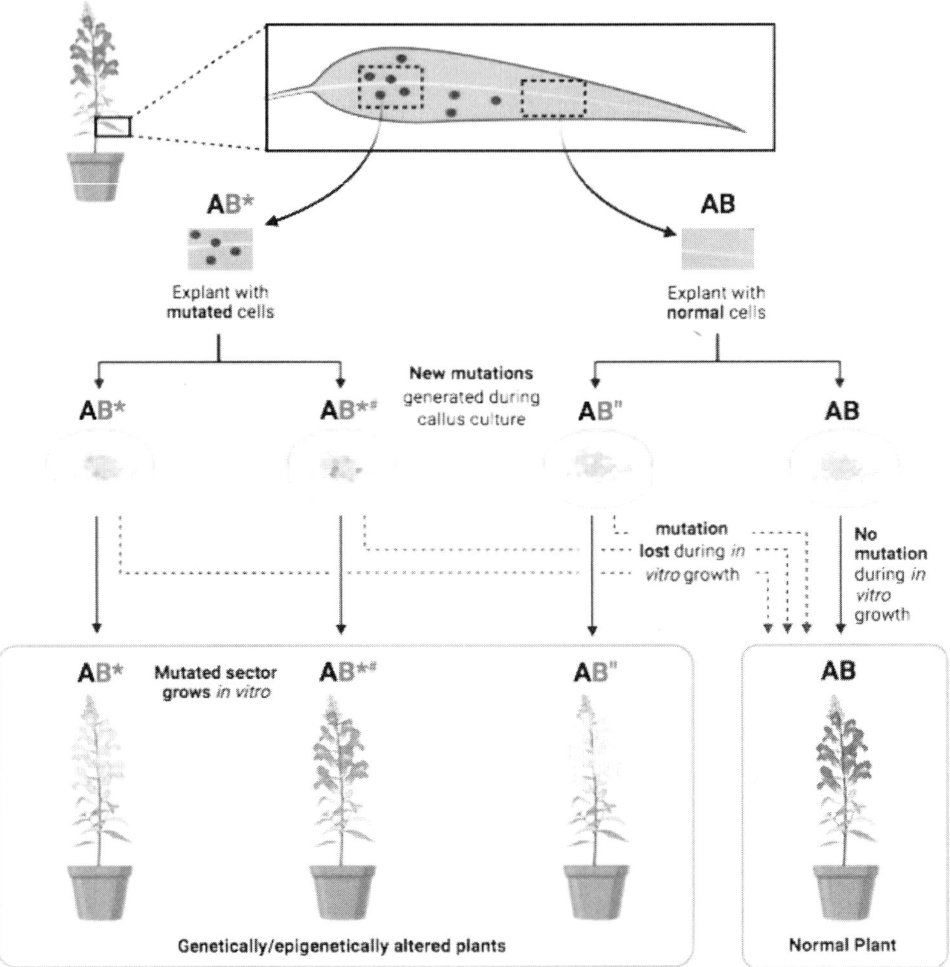

Figure 9.8. Generation of Somaclonal Variation in *In vitro* Culture Plant.

2. *In vitro* Culture with Selection Pressure

Somaclonal variants for a particular character are selected with an appropriate selective pressure, undergoing few selection cycles under *in vitro* conditions. It is done by exerting selection pressure using particular chemicals in the media (Figure 9.9).

- **Disease resistance:** Selection for disease resistant lines can be done by mixing the toxin produced by the pathogen in media (*Phytophthora* resistance in potato).
- **Herbicide resistance:** Herbicide resistant lines can be screened by adding the target herbicide for which resistance is needed, to the media at appropriate concentration (Paraquat resistant tobacco cell lines)

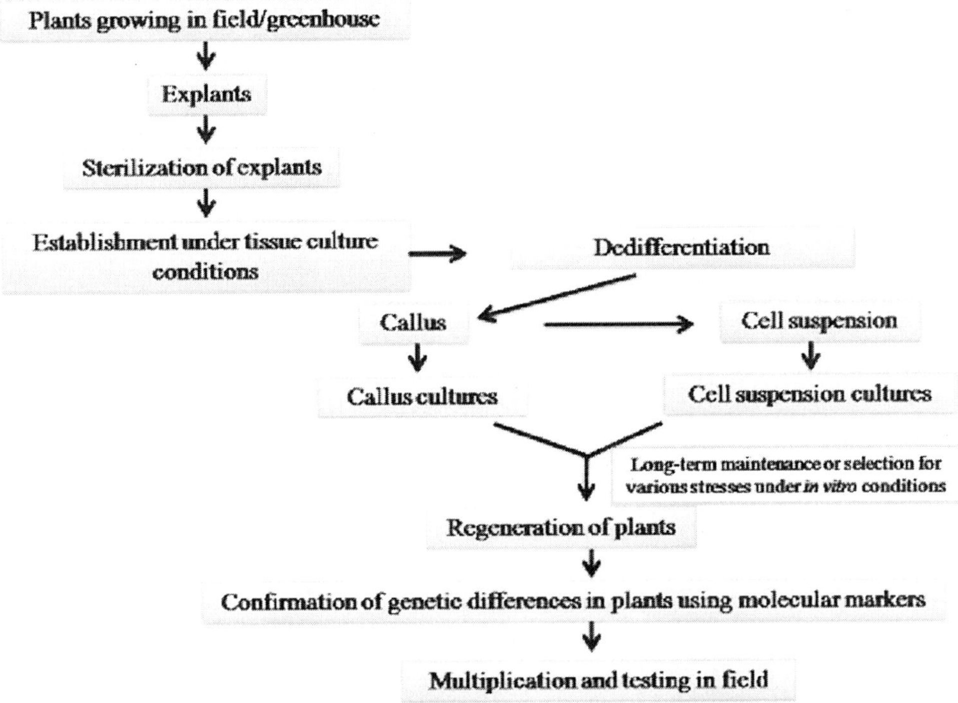

Figure 9.9. Somaclonal Variation in under *In vitro* Culture with Selection Pressure.

- ☆ **Salinity Tolerance:** Salt tolerant variants are obtained by adding NaCl to the medium (BTS 24 a rice somaclone tolerant to salinity developed from Pokkali).
- ☆ **Drought Tolerance**: Drought/water logging tolerance is obtained by adding PEG (R 111 is a sorghum somaclone with drought tolerance)
- ☆ Temperature stress/chilling response of the variants are tested by exposing the culture to very high or low temperature (tobacco for chilling response, pear for temperature stress).

Table 9.1. Applications of Somaclonal Variation

	Character	*Examples*
1.	**Novel variants**	a. An improved scented Geranium variety (Velvet Rose)
		b. Thrornless blackberries (Rubus)
		c. Pusa Jai Kisan mustard
2.	**Disease resistance**	a. Fungal disease - Rice brown spot disease– *Helminthosporium oryzae*
		b. Bacterial disease – Bacterial wilt of Tomato – *Pseudomonas solanacearum*
		c. Viral disease - Sugarcane Fiji Disease Virus

	Character	*Examples*
3.	**Abiotic stress resistance**	a. Drought tolerance – R111 - Sorghum
		b. Salt tolerance - BTS24 – Rice
		c. Cold (Freezing) tolerance – Norstar – Winter wheat
		d. Aluminium tolerance – Carrot, sorghum, tomato.
4.	**Herbicide resistance**	a. Glyphosate tolerant tobacco
		b. Imidazoline tolerant cotton
		c. Difenzoquat tolerant wheat
5.	**Insect resistance**	a. Aphid resistance – "Stephens" – Wheat
		b. Armyworm resistance – Brazos R-3 – Bermuda grass
6.	**Seed quality**	Bio L 212 - *Lathyrus sativa* – Low ODAP (Neurotoxin) content

Factors Influencing Somoclonal Variation

1. Genotype

The genotype of plans used for somoclonal variation is an important variable. Genotype can influences both frequency of regeneration and the frequency of somoclones.

2. Explant Sources

The sources of explants has been considered a critical viable for somoclonal variation. *e.g.* Variants in Geranium has been recovered from in *vivo* root and petiole cuttings, but not stem cuttings.

3. Duration of Cell Culture

Chromosome variation has been reported for many established plant cell cultures. It is widely accepted that most long term cultures are chromosomally variable. Polyploidy and aneuploid plants have been frequently recovered in large number of species. *e.g. Geranium, Nicotiana*, tomato, alfalfa and *Saccharum*.

4. Culture Conditions

It has been known that growth regulator composition of the culture medium can influence frequency of karyotypic alterations in cultured cells. The growth regulators such as 2,4-D, NAA and BAP have been most frequently considered to be responsible for chromosome variability.

5. Selection Agent and Technique

In vitro selection of cell lines against appropriate inhibitor (selection agent) is critical. Also, the standardized concentration of inhibitor that will kill 70-90 per cent of wild type cells is necessary. Low level doses and less selection cycles may allow cells to escape for pure physiological reasons which may outnumber true mutants.

Limitations of Somaclonal Variation

1. Variation is cultivar dependent.
2. Variations are not always heritable and stable.
3. Frequencies of variation vary.
4. Many changes are undesirable.
5. Many changes are not novel.

Synthetic Seeds

The techniques of tissue culture have made it possible to culture and clone plants in labs, conserve specific genes, and allowed for the mass propagation of plants. Among various techniques, somatic embryogenesis gained much popularity because of the formation of an embryo from any somatic cells of the plant. The introduction of somatic embryogenesis increased the demand for artificial seeds and led to the concept of synthetic seeds. **Synthetic seeds are defined as encapsulated plant tissues, such as somatic embryos, shoot buds, axillary buds, shoot tips, cell aggregates, and any other micro propagules that have the potential to grow like a plant, under *in-vivo* or *in-vitro* conditions when sown as seeds.** Usually large scale production of somatic embryos and their encapsulation is referred to as artificial or synthetic seed production. It is an alternative to traditional micropropagation for production and delivery of cloned plantlets. Artificial or synthetic seed is a bead of gel containing somatic embryo or shoot bud (Figure 9.10). The first synthetic seeds were produced by **Kitto and Janick in 1982** using carrot somatic embryos.

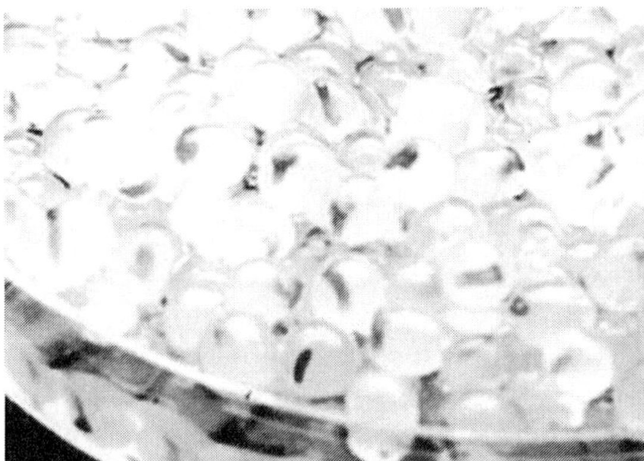

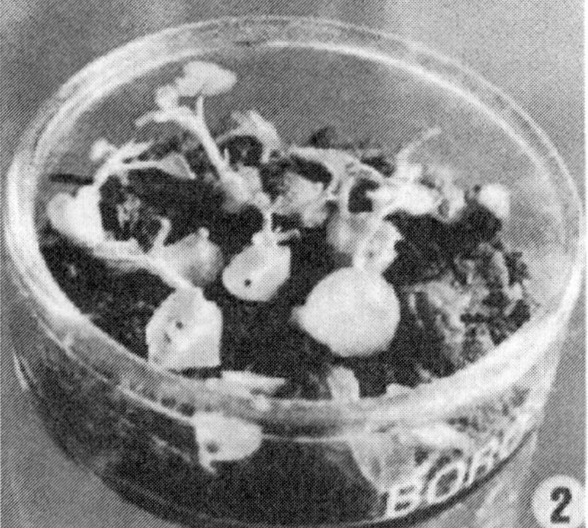

Figure 9.10. Synthetic Seeds and Germination of Synseeds into Plantlets.

Why Synthetic Seeds?

In some of the horticultural crops seeds propagation is not successful due to;

- ☆ Heterozygosity of seeds particularly in cross pollinated crops

- Minute seed size *e.g.* orchids
- Presence of reduced endosperm
- Some seeds require mycorrhizal fungi association for germination *e.g.* orchids
- No seeds are formed

Characteristics of Synthetic Seeds

1. High volume and large scale propagation method
2. Maintains genetic uniformity of plants
3. Direct delivery of propagules to the field, thus eliminating transplants
4. Lower cost per plant let
5. Rapid multiplication of plants

Procedure for Synthetic Seed Production

1. Establish somatic embryogenesis
2. Mature somatic embryos
3. Synchronize and singulate somatic embryos
4. Mass production of somatic embryos
5. Standardisation of encapsulation
6. Standardisation of artificial endosperm
7. Mass production of synthetic seeds and storage

Artificial or synthetic seeds may be produced by one of the two following ways

1. Desiccated

The desiccated synthetic seeds are produced from somatic embryos either naked or encapsulated in **polyoxyethylene glycol (Polyoxr)** followed by their desiccation. This material doesn't allow for the growth of the microorganisms and is non-toxic to embryos. In this case, a mixture is prepared by using equal volumes of embryo suspension and a 5 per cent (w/v) solution of polyox to give a final concentration of 2.5 per cent polyox. Then by using a pipette the suspension is dispensed as 0.2 ml drops on to Petri plates or teflon sheets. Then the drops are dried either slowly over a period of one or two weeks sequentially using chambers of decreasing relative humidity, or rapidly by leaving them on the bench overnight to dry. Desiccation can be achieved and desiccated synthetic seeds are produced only in plant species whose somatic embryos are desiccation tolerant.

2. Hydrated

Hydrated synthetic seeds are produced in those plant species where the somatic embryos are recalcitrant and sensitive to desiccation. This involves the encapsulation of a single somatic embryo in hydrogel capsules. The most popular method of forming hydrated synthetic seeds is using **Ca-alginate encapsulation**. The procedure followed to produce hydrated synthetic seed involves the mixing of somatic embryos with a 2 per cent (w/v) solution of Na-alginate. Then, the embryo is dropped into a 100 mM solution of $Ca(NO_3)_2$ or 75 mM $CaCl_2.2H_2O$ by using a plastic pipette.

Encapsulation with Alginate Matrix

Alginate hydrogel is frequently selected as a matrix for synthetic seed because of its moderate viscosity and low spinnability of solution, low toxicity for somatic embryos and quick gellation, low cost and bio-compatibility characteristics. Alginate is a straight chain, hydrophilic, colloidal polyuronic acid composed primarily of hydro-β-D-Mannuronic acid residues. The major principle involved in the alginate encapsulation process is that the sodium alginate droplets containing the somatic embryos when dropped into the $CaCl_2.2H_2O$ solution form round and firm beads due to ion exchange between the Na+ in sodium alginate with Ca^{2+} in the $CaCl_2.2H_2O$ solution. The hardness or rigidity of the capsule mainly depends upon the number of sodium ions exchanged with calcium ions. Hence, the concentration of the two gelling agents *i.e.*,**sodium alginate and $CaCl_2.2H_2O$,** and the complexing time should be optimized for the formation of the capsule with optimum bead hardness and rigidity. **In general, 3 per cent sodium alginate upon complexing with 75 mM $CaCl_2.2H_2O$ for half an hour gives optimum bead hardness and rigidity for the production of viable synthetic seeds** (Figure 9.11).

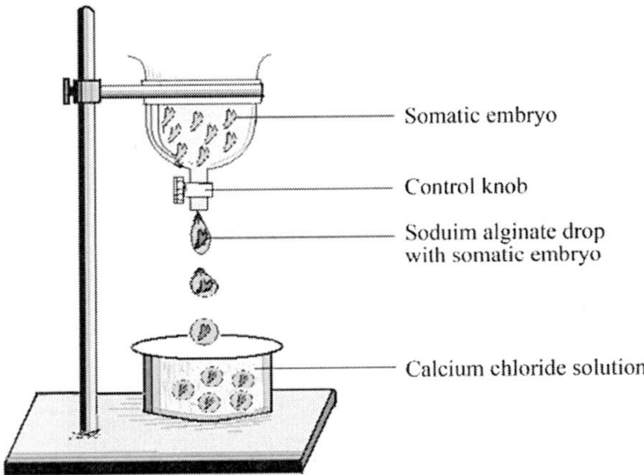

Figure 9.11. Method of Somatic Embryo Encapsulation (Hyderated synthetic seed).

Factors that Affect a Synthetic Seed's Production

1. Selection of Plant Materials

The synthetic seeds can be produced by using somatic embryos or other plant propagules, However, a specific plant species supports a specific plant material for the production of synthetic seeds. For example, somatic embryos have been successfully used to produce synthetic seeds in several plant species that include *Oryza sativa, Dalbergia sissoo, Curcuma amada, Hemidesmus indicus, etc.* Whereas, some plants support the production of synthetic seeds when nodal segments are used. It includes *Eclipta alba, Cannabis sativa, Solanum tuberosum, Gossypium hirsutum, etc.*

2. Selection of Encapsulation Matrix

The encapsulation of seeds is an essential factor that determines the production of synseeds. So, there are some qualities that the encapsulating material should have if it's going to be used for the production of synseeds. It includes:

1. It must not damage the embryo.
2. The coating should be mild to protect the embryo.
3. The coating should be durable for rough handling during manufacture, storage, transportation, and planting.
4. The coat must contain all the essential growth materials such as nutrients and growth regulators.
5. The formed synseeds should be transplantable using the existing techniques.

The most widely used encapsulating material is sodium alginate. However, there are some other agents as well that are used with sodium alginate for encapsulation. It includes gelatin, potassium alginate, sodium pectate, and carrageenan.

The advantages of synthetic seeds production are given below:

1. Easy handling.
2. Short- and long-term storage capacity.
3. Genetic uniformity.
4. Low-cost quality plant materials are required.
5. It allows the transportation and exchange of germplasm between national and international laboratories.

Applications

1. The production of synthetic seeds facilitates the growth of several plants that have low seed viability, seedless fruit, and poor germination rates, and that depend on mycorrhizal–fungal symbiosis for germination.
2. It is very useful when it comes to genotypes selection, germplasm preservation, and *in vitro* propagation of endangered, rare, and commercially important plants
3. It also allows the conservation of plant species through short- and medium-term preservation.

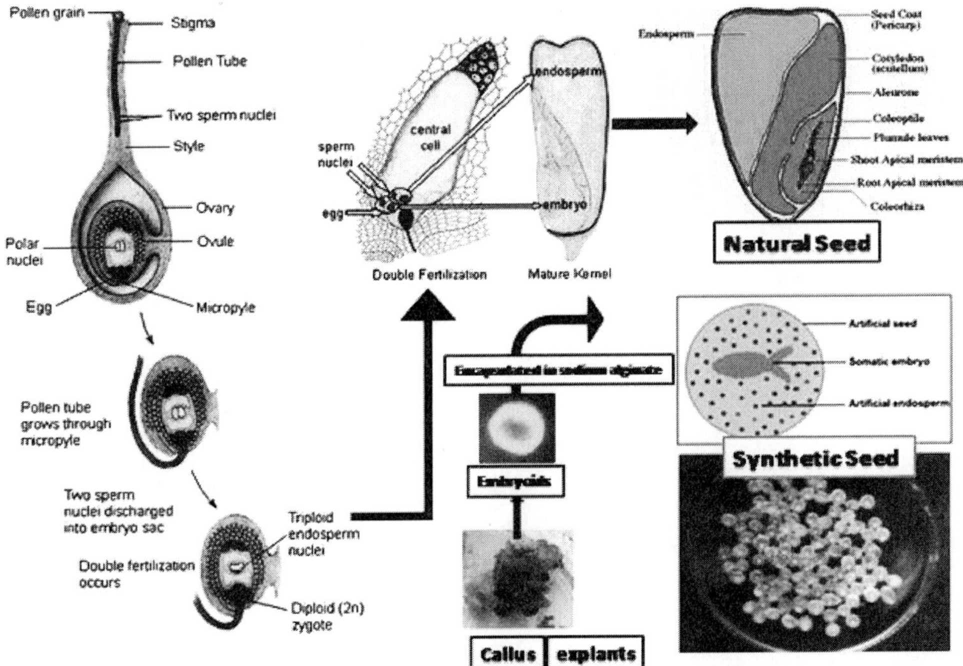

Figure 9.12. Difference between Natural Seed and Synthetic Seed.

4. Multiplication of Genetically engineered individuals, which may be sterile and unstable during sexual production.
5. Protection of seedlings by incorporating useful chemicals in the encapsulation material.
6. Provide the advantages of true seed (case of handling and transportation) for vegetative propagation.

Limitations

1. Large scale production of high quality somatic embryos is a costly affair
2. Poor germination of synthetic seeds due to lack of supply of nutrients, sufficient oxygen, microbe invasion and mechanical damage of somatic embryos.
3. Possible occurrence of somaclonal variation.
4. Special skills are required to carry out the work.

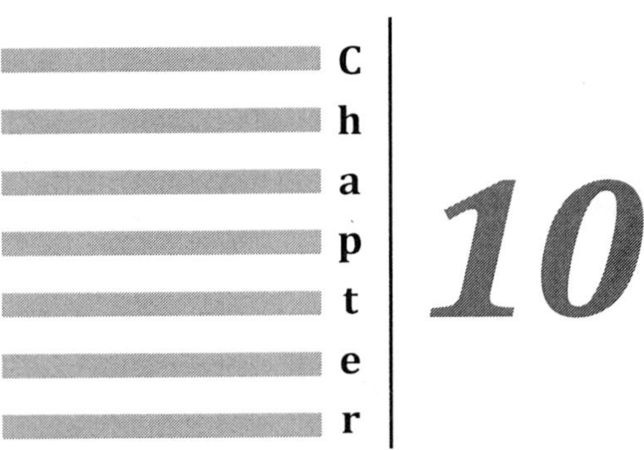

Secondary Metabolites Production: *In vitro* Germplasm Conservation

Plants produce several secondary metabolites that are of importance in the healthcare, food, flavor and cosmetics industries. Many natural products, pharmaceuticals, food products *etc.* are produced from the plant secondary metabolites, which are obtained solely from massive quantities of whole plant parts. Secondary metabolism in plants is activated only in particular stages of growth and development or during periods of stress, limitation of nutrients or attack by micro-organisms. Moreover secondary metabolites produced by the plants are specific to an individual species, genus and are produced during specific environmental conditions only. The source plants are cultured in tropical, subtropical, geographically remote areas, which are subject to drought, disease, changing land use patterns and other environmental factors makes them difficult to use as a source of many secondary metabolities. Because of these reasons the quantity of economically important secondary metabolities production is low and processing costs like extraction and purification is very high. As a result, commercially available secondary metabolites, used as pharmaceuticals, flavours, fragrances and pesticides *etc.* are generally considered high value products (since production low)fetching high price. Because of these, important products of secondary metabolities are high cost and economically unaffordable. Plant tissue culture can be defined as the *in vitro* manipulation of plant cells and tissues and is a keystone in the foundation of plant biotechnology. Whole plants can be regenerated under *in vitro* conditions using plant organs, tissues or single cells, by inoculating them in an appropriate nutrient medium containing specific growth regulators under sterile environment. So Plant cell cultures would be an attractive source for the production of high-value secondary metabolites and best alternative to the secondary metabolites production through whole plants under natural condition (Figure 10.1).

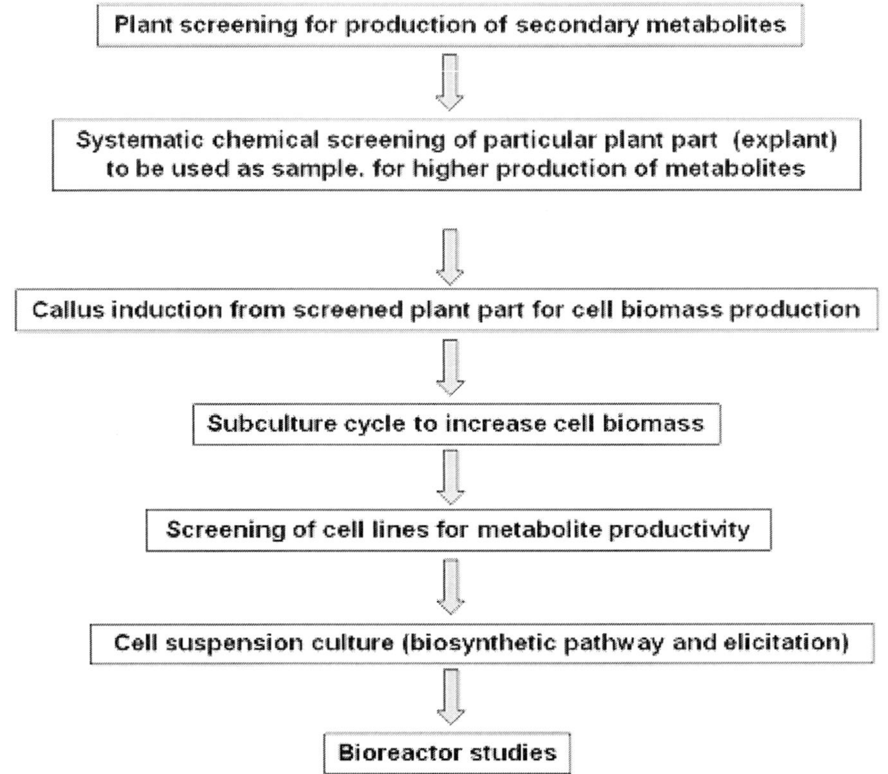

Figure 10.1. Steps Involved in the Production of Secondary Metabolites from Plant Cell Culture.

Plant Secondary Metabolites

Plant products can be classified into primary plant metabolites and secondary metabolites. Primary plant metabolites are essential for the survival of the plant. It consists of sugars, amino acids and nucleotides synthesized by plants and are used to produce essential polymers. Primary metabolites are widely distributed and are vital for basic cell metabolism. They are referred to as high volume low value compounds. Secondary metabolites are the chemicals, which are not directly involved in the normal growth and development, or reproduction of an organism. But these are playing a significant role in plant defense mechanisms. Primary metabolites are providing the basis for normal growth and reproduction, while secondary metabolites are for adaptation and interaction of the plant with the environment. These chemicals are extremely diverse; many thousands have been identified in several major classes and are limited in distribution, restricted to a particular taxonomic group. Hence, they can sometimes be used as taxonomic characters in classifying plants. Secondary metabolities are present in small quantities as they have only adaptive roles and they are metabolically expensive to produce, hence referred as low volume and high value compounds. The economic importance of secondary metabolites lies in the fact that they can be used as sources of industrially important natural products like colours, insecticides, antimicrobials, fragrances and therapeutics. Therefore, plant tissue culture is getting more importance for secondary metabolite production.

Definition

Primary Metabolites

Chemical compounds that mainly participate in metabolism of plants, growth, photosynthesis, reproduction, or other primary functions such as amino acids, nucleic acids *etc.*, are called as **primary metabolites**.

Secondary Metabolites

The metabolites produced by plants are not directly involved in the physiological metabolism or primary functions of those plants are called as **secondary metabolites**.

These secondary metabolites include alkaloids, glycosides (steroids and phenolics), terpenoids, latex, tannins *etc.* It has been observed that as the cells undergo morphological differentiation and maturation during plant growth, some of the cells specialize to produce secondary metabolites. Humans use some of these compounds as pharmaceuticals, flavours, fragrances, cosmetics, food additives, feed stocks, antimicrobials and recreational drugs. So biotechnologists have special interest in plant tissue culture for the large scale production of commercially important compounds. These chemicals are extremely diverse; many thousands have been identified in several major classes. They have been classified into terpenes (composed entirely of carbon and hydrogen), phenolics (composed of simple sugars, benzene rings, hydrogen and oxygen) and nitrogen and/or sulphur containing compounds (Table 10.1). It has been observed that each plant family, genus and species produces a characteristic mix of these bioactive compounds.

A simple classification includes three main groups:

1. Terpenoids
2. Phenolics (including polyphenols and tannins)
3. Nitrogen and/or sulphur containing compounds

Table 10.1. Classification of Secondary Metabolites

Terpenes		Phenols		Nitrogen and /or sulphur containing compounds	
Type	Example	Type	Example	Type	Example
Monoterpenes	Farnessol	Lignan	lignan	Alkaloids	Nicotine
Sespuiterpenes	Limonene	Tannins	gallotannin	Atropine	
Diterpenes	Taxol	Flavonoids	anthocyanin	Glucosinolates	Sinigrin
Triterpenes	Digitogenin	Coumarins	Umbelliferone		
Tetraterpenoids	Carotene				
Sterols	Spinasterol				

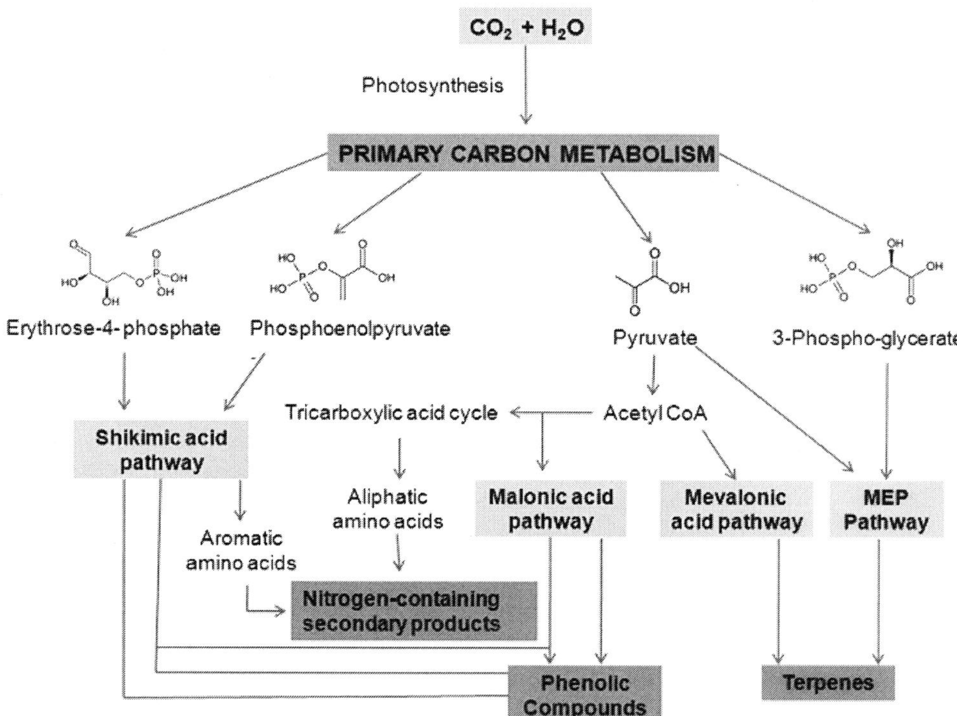

Figure 10.2. The Production of Secondary Metabolites Associated with the Pathways of Primary Metabolism.

Applications of Secondary Metabolites

Many of these secondary products especially various alkaloids are of immense use in medicine. The yield of these chemicals in cell culture, is though generally lower than in whole plants, it is substantially increased by manipulating physiological and biochemical conditions.

Shikonine is a dye produced by the cells *Lithospermum erythrorhizon* on a commercial scale. Besides this there are a number of secondary metabolite products that are being widely used for various purposes. Vincristine is used as anticancer agent, digoxin controls cardiovascular disorders, pyrithrins is an insecticide *etc.* Some important secondary metabolite, source plant and its uses is given in Table 10.2.

1. As pharmaceuticals *e.g.* Anticancerous alkaloid vincristine form *Catharantus*
2. As aromatic compounds *e.g.* Menthol from *Mentha* spp.
3. As plant derived proteins *e.g.* Papain from *Carica papaya*
4. As pesticides *e.g.* Pyrethrum from *Chrysanthemum*
5. As plant based dyes *e.g.* Shikonin from *Lithospermum*

Table 10.2. Plant Species and Secondary Metabolites Obtained from them Using Tissue Culture

Product	*Plant Source*	*Uses*
Artemisin	*Artemisia spp.*	Antimalarial
Azadirachtin	*Azadirachta indica*	Insecticidal
Berberine	*Coptis japonica*	Antibacterial, anti inflammatory
Capsaicin	*Capsicum annum*	Cures Rheumatic pain
Codeine	*Papaver spp.*	Analgesic
Camptothecin	*Campatotheca accuminata*	Anticancer
Cephalotaxine	*Cephalotaxus harringtonia*	Antitumour
Digoxin	*Digitalis lanata*	Cardiac tonic
Pyrethrin	*Chrysanthemum cinerariaefolium*	Insecticide (for grain storage)
Morphine	*Papaver somniferum*	Analgesic, sedative
Quinine	*Cinchona officinalis*	Antimalarial
Taxol	*Taxus spp.*	Anticarcinogenic
Vincristine	*Cathranthus roseus*	Anticarcinogenic
Scopolamine	*Datura stramonium*	Antihypertensive

Bioreactors

A bioreactor may be referred to as any manufactured or engineered device that supports a biologically active environment. Bioreactors are widely used for industrial production of microbial, animal and plant metabolites as by allowing large-scale cultivation of cells. A simple diagram of a bioreactor is shown in Figure 10.3.

Bioreactors for Plant Cell Culture

Mass culture of plant cells under *in vitro* condition has been proposed as a viable alternative for the production of vast arrays of high value, low volume phytochemicals. Therefore, during the past two decades considerable work has been done to design bioreactors for plant cell culture. A bioreactor is a glass or steel vessel in which organisms are cultured. Ideally, bioreactors are fitted with probes to monitor the pH, temperature and dissolved oxygen in the culture and have provisions to sample the cultures, add fresh medium, adjust pH, air supply, mixing of cultures and controlling the temperature, without affecting the aseptic nature of the culture.

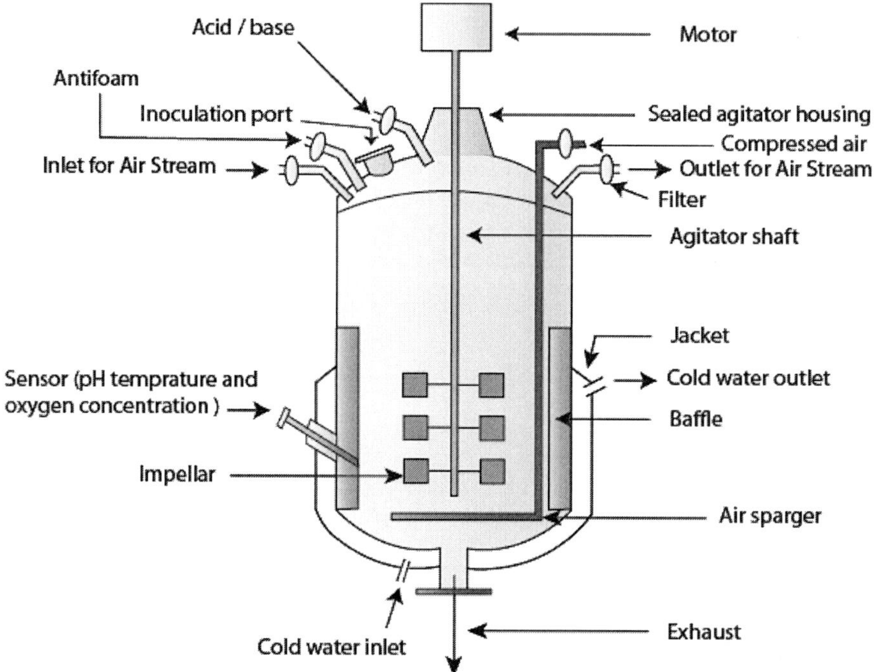

Figure 10.3. Diagram of a Typical Bioreactor.

Although the basic requirements for suspension cultures of plant cells are similar to those of submerged microbial cultures, the fermentors used for microbial cell cultures are not suitable for plant cell cultures because of striking differences in the nature and growth pattern of the two types of cells. Efficient mixing of plant cells cultured on large scale is extremely important to provide uniform physiological conditions inside the culture vessel. Mixing promotes better growth by enhancing the transfer of nutrients from liquid and gaseous phases to the cells and by break-off and dispersion of air bubbles for effective oxygenation. Although, plant cells have higher tensile strength in comparison to microbial cells, their large size, rigid cellulosic wall and extensive vacuole make them sensitive to the shear stress restricting the use of high agitation for efficient mixing. Plant cells are, therefore, often grown in modified stirred-tank bioreactors at very low agitation speeds. Air-lift reactors may provide even better and uniform environmental conditions at low shear.

All plant cells are aerobic and require continuous supply of oxygen. However, plant cells require less oxygen than micro-organisms because of their slow metabolism. In some cases, high oxygen concentration is even toxic to the metabolic activities of cells. Air is normally sparged or blown at the base of the bioreactor. Plant cells in suspension culture tend to form aggregates of 2-200 cells. During the late exponential phase of growth, cells become more sticky because of increased excretion of polysaccharides into the culture vessel. This leads to the adhesion of plant cells to the reactor wall, probes and stirring device and the formation of larger aggregates. Mixing is affected, as the aggregates tend to sediment or stick to the reactor surface, forming extensive wall growth. Large aggregates also create dead zones in the culture vessel and can block the opening and pipe lines of the reactor. Cell aggregation adversely affects the operation of the probes used to monitor culture conditions during growth and product formation. In spite of these effects, certain degrees of cell aggregation (cell-cell contact) and cell differentiation seem to be essential for secondary metabolite production.

Selection of a Bioreactor

The suitability of a particular bioreactor for plant cell cultivation could be evaluated by considering the following factors: 1. capacity of oxygen supply and intensity of air bubble dispersion in broth 2. intensity of hydrodynamic stresses generated inside the reactor and their effect on the plant cell system 3. adequacy of mixing of culture broth at high cell concentration 4. ability to control temperature, pH, and nutrient concentration inside the reactor 5. ability to control aggregate size (which may be helpful for increasing product formation); 6. ease of scale-up 7. simplicity of aseptic operation for long durations.

Different Types of Bioreactor Used for Secondary Metabolite Production form Free Suspension Cell Culture and Immobilized Cell Culture

The major types of bioreactors currently in use for suspension culture of plant cells are stirred-tank, bubble column, air-lift, and rotating-drum reactors (Figure 10.4).

(i) Stirred-Tank Reactor

The stirred-tank reactor (Figure 10.4A), in which air is dispersed by mechanical agitation, represents the classical bioreactor for aerobic fermentations. Its behaviour has been well studied in a number of biological systems. Temperature, pH, amount of dissolved oxygen, and nutrient concentration can be controlled better within this reactor than any other reactor. A major drawback of the stirred-tank reactor is the shearing stress generated by its stirring device to which plant cells may be sensitive. Despite this, most existing laboratory and commercial bioreactors are of the stirred-tank design which have been suitably modified for plant cell culture, such as: (1) the impeller speed is reduced and in some cases the turbine impeller is replaced by a marine screen or paddle; (2) removal of baffles, pH probe and other probes not required; and (3) the sample ports are enlarged to about 1 cm to reduce blockage caused by cell aggregates. For the first industrial plant cell culture process, in which shikonin was produced from *Lithospermum erythrorhizon*, stirred-tank reactors of 200 liter and 500 liter capacities were used. Cells of *Catharanthus roseus* have been grown in stirred-tank reactors. Some other disadvantages of stirred-tank reactors are their high energy requirements and complexity of construction and the fact that they are difficult to scale up.

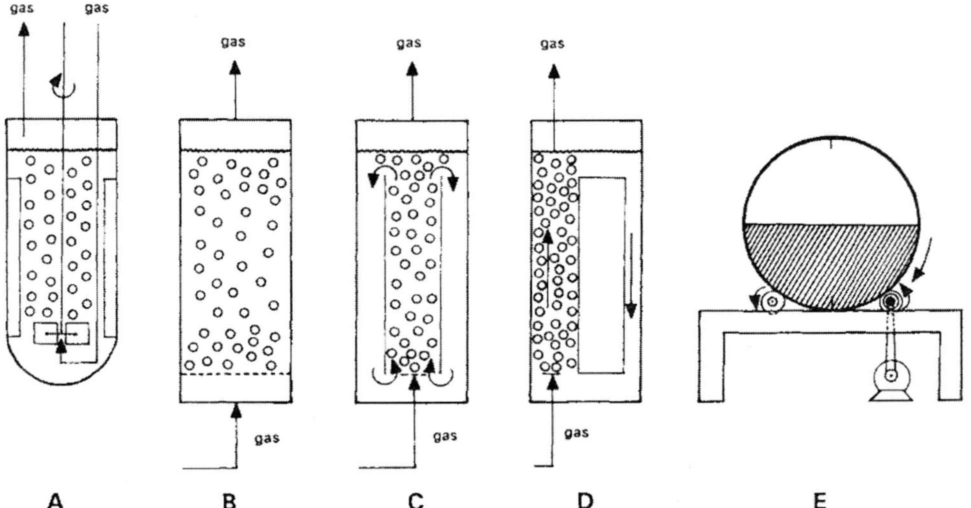

Figure 10.4. (A) Stirred-Tank Reactor; (B) Bubble-Column Reactor; (C) Air-Lift Reactor with Draft-Tube; (D) Air-Lift Reactor with Outer Loop; (E) Rotating-Drum Reactor.

(ii) Bubble-Column Reactor

The bubble-column reactor (Figure 10.4B) is one of the simplest types of gas-liquid bioreactors used for aerobic fermentation. It consists of a cylindrical vessel aerated at the bottom. In such a system the gas is dispersed pneumatically through a deep pool of liquid by means of nozzles or perforated plates. Some of the merits of bubble-column reactor are: (i) it facilitates sterile operation because of the absence of moving parts and the fact that nonsealing parts are required, (ii) it provides high mass and heat transfer areas without the input of mechanical energy and may, thus, be suitable for shear-sensitive systems such as plant and animal cell culture, and (iii) the scale-up is relatively easy, and the reactor requires minimum maintenance. The disadvantages of the bubble-column reactor are the undefined fluid flow pattern inside the reactor and its non-uniform mixing.

(iii) Air-Lift Reactor

In air-lift reactor, as its name implies, compressed air is used for aeration and mixing of the contents of the reactor vessel. Its operation is based on the draught tube principle. Air sparged into the base of the reactor lowers the density of the medium which rises up the draft tube pulling fresh medium in at the base and, therefore, a flow is achieved. Schematic diagrams of the draught tube (inner loop and outer loop) air-lift vessels are given in Figure 10.4C and Figure 10.4D. A more uniform flow pattern is achieved in the air-lift reactor compared with the bubble column reactor, where a random flow pattern exists. Air-lift reactors up to 100 liter capacity have been used extensively by Fowler and his co-workers for cultivation of *C. roseus* cells. The cells of *Berberis wilsoneae, Cinchona ledgeriana, Cudrania tricuspidata, Dioscorea deltoidea, Digitalis lanata, Morinda citrifolia, Tripterygium wildordii* and, recently, *L. erythrorhizon* have also been cultured in air-lift reactors. In all cases, the reactor configuration gave favourable results in terms of biomass and product formation. The air-lift reactor is one of the most suitable bioreactor types for cultivation of plant cells on a large scale. It provides reasonable mixing and oxygen transfer at low shear, and less contamination occurs because there are no moving parts and no intrusion of impeller shaft. The operating cost, compared to the stirred-tank reactor, is low because of its simple design and it does not require power input for the stirrer. Despite these advantages air-lift reactors have not been used as extensively as stirred tank reactors. The disadvantages of air-lift reactors are the development of dead zones inside the reactor and insufficient mixing at high cell densities.

(iv) Rotating-Drum Reactor

The rotating-drum reactor consists of a horizontally rotating-drum on rollers connected to a motor (Figure 10.4E). The rotating motion of the drum facilitates good mixing and aeration without imposing a high shear stress on the cultured cells. Baffles in the inner wall of the drum help to increase oxygen supply. This type of reactor has the capacity to promote high oxygen transfer to cells at high density. It has been used to grow cultures of *C. roseus* and *L. erythrorhizon* up to 1000 liter in volume. In a comparative study of the performance of rotating-drum and stirred-tank reactors for the cultivation of *Vinca rosea* the former was found to be superior on the basis of increased oxygen transfer at high cell densities. The rotating-drum reactor facilitates better growth and imparts less hydrodynamic stress. In the stirred-tank reactor growth rate was low at low agitation speed because of insufficient oxygen supply, while at high agitation speed the cells died. Hence, for cultivation of cells at high densities, the rotating-drum reactor was preferred. The rotating-drum reactor has also been shown to be superior to air-lift and modified stirred-tank reactors for the cultivation of *L. erythrorhizon*. The major disadvantage of this reactor type is the restriction in scaleup.

(v) Immobilized Plant Cell Reactors

Different types of free cell culture reactors is not suitable for immobilization plant cells culture for the production of industrially important phytochemicals. So for that specialized bioreactor need to be designed as an alternative to free cell culture reactors. Entrapment in natural (alginate, agar, agarose, carrageenan) or synthetic (polyacrylamide)polymers, adhesion to reticulate polyurethane foam, and confinement behind semi-permeable membranes have been employed to immobilize plant cells. Alginate has been the most popular polymer used to immobilize plant cells. Cell suspension in 4 per cent sodium alginate solution is allowed to fall as 2 mm drops in a beaker containing 0.2 M solution of $CaC1_2$. Ca-alginate is formed by ion exchange reaction and the drops harden as beads within 20-30 min. Alginate entrapped cells can be cultured in packed-bed (Figure 10.5A), fluidized-bed (Figure 10.5B) or polyurethane draft tube reactor (Figure 10.5C). Polyurethane foam has been used to immobilize a range of cell lines. The cells are immobilized in these matrices by flowing cells and medium through the foam or by adding sterile foam to growing cultures.

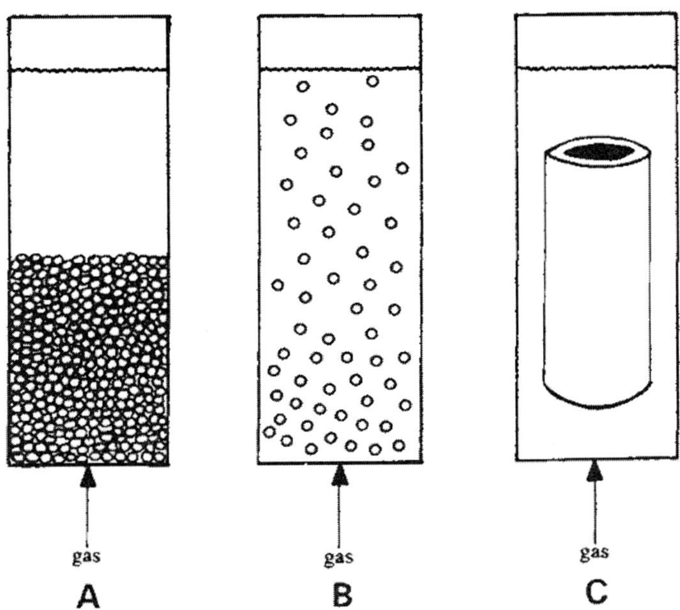

Figure 10.5. (A) Packed-Bed Reactor; (B) Fluidized-Bed Reactor; (C) Polyurethane Draft Tube Reactor.

Secondary Metabolites Production through *In vitro* Tissue Culture Methods

1. Plant Cell Cultures

Once interesting bioactive compounds have been identified from plant extracts, the first part of the work is collecting the largest genetic pool of plant individuals that produce the corresponding bioactive substances. However, a major characteristic of secondary compounds is that their synthesis is highly inducible. Therefore, it is not certain, given extract is a good indicator of the plant potential for producing the compounds. The ability of plant cell cultures to produce secondary metabolites came quite late in the history of *in vitro* techniques. For a long time, it was believed that undifferentiated cells, such as callus or cell suspension cultures were not able to produce secondary compounds, unlike differentiated cells or specialized organs.

2. Callus Culture

Callus is a mass of undifferentiated cells derived from plant tissues for use in biological research and biotechnology. In plant biology, callus cells are those cells that cover a plant wound. To induce callus development, plant tissues are surface sterilized and then plated onto *in vitro* tissue culture medium. One of the auxin growth regulator 2,4-D, supplemented into the medium to initiate callus formation. It is well known that callus can undergo somaclonal variations, usually during several subculture cycles. This is a critical period where, due to *in vitro* variations, production of secondary metabolite often varies from one subculture cycle to another. When genetic stability is reached, it is necessary to screen the different cell (callus) lines according to their aptitudes to provide an efficient secondary metabolite production. Hence, each callus must be assessed separately for its growth rate as well as intracellular and extracellular metabolite concentrations. This allows an evaluation of the productivity of each cell line so that only the best ones will be taken for further studies, for example, for production of the desired compound in suspensions cultures.

3. Cell Suspension Cultures

Cell suspension cultures represent a good biological material for studying biosynthetic pathways. They allow the recovery of a large amount of cells from which enzymes can be easily separated. Compared to cell growth kinetics, which is usually an exponential curve, most secondary metabolites are often produced during the stationary phase. This lack of production of compounds during the early stages can be explained by carbon allocation mainly distributed for primary metabolism when growth is very active. On the other hand, when growth stops, carbon is no longer required in large quantities for primary metabolism and secondary compounds are more actively synthesized. However, some of the secondary plant products are known to be growth-associated with undifferentiated cells, such as betalains and carotenoids.

4. Organ Cultures

Plant organs are alternative to cell cultures for the production of plant secondary metabolites. Two types of organs are generally considered for this objective: hairy roots and shoot cultures. A schematic representation of various organized cultures, induced under *in vitro* conditions, is given in Figure10.6.

4.1. Shoot Cultures

Shoots exhibit some comparable properties to hairy roots, genetic stability and good capacities for secondary metabolite production. They also provide the possibility of gaining a link between growth and the production of secondary compounds.

4.2. Hairy Root Cultures

Hairy roots are obtained after the successful transformation of a plant with ***Agrobacterium rhizogenes.*** They have received considerable attention of plant biotechnologists, for the production of secondary compounds. They can be subcultured and indefinitely propagated on a synthetic medium without phytohormones and usually display interesting growth capacities owing to the profusion of lateral roots. This growth can be assimilated to an exponential model, when the number of generations of lateral roots becomes large.

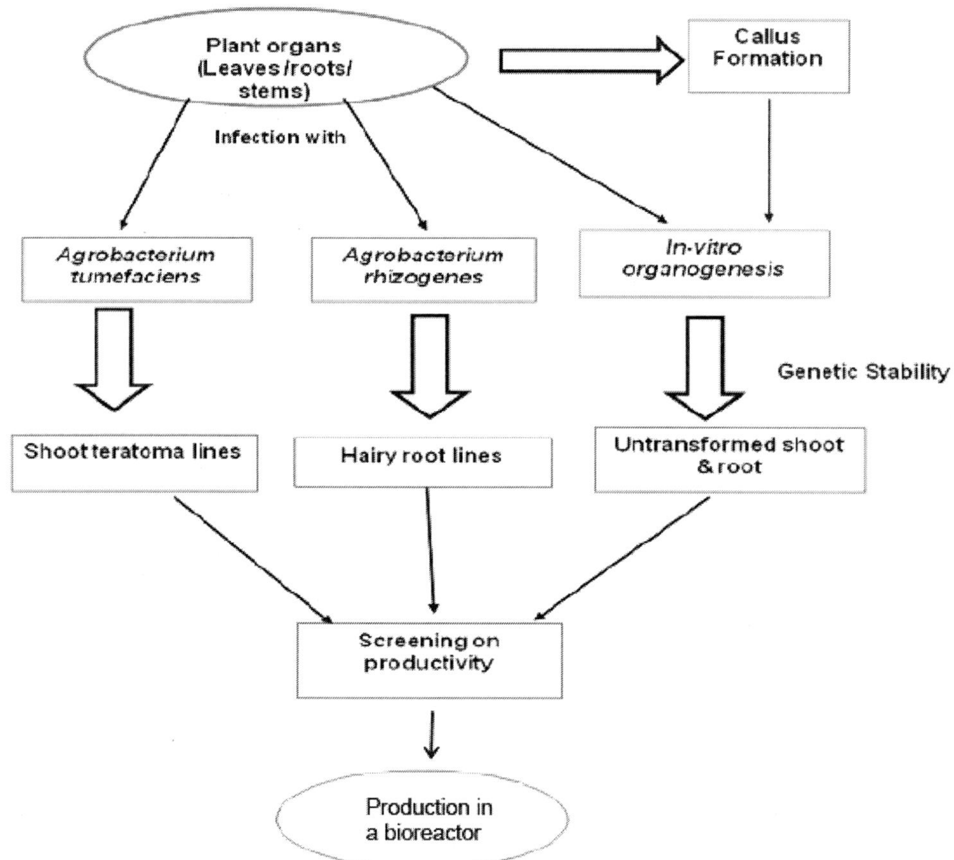

Figure 10.6. Possible Ways for the Production of Secondary Metabolites from Plant Organ Cultures.

Strategies for Enhanced Production of Secondary Metabolites in Plant Cell Cultures

Secondary Metabolites Production

Although the native plants are capable of producing the secondary metabolites of commercial interest, tissue culture systems are preferred for higher production in a short time with minimum interference of environmental factor. The production process of secondary metabolites from tissue culture comprises of seven aspects, those are: (1) Selection of cell lines for high yield of secondary metabolites (2) Medium composition and effect of nutrients (3) Large scale cultivation of plant cells (4) Elicitor-induced production of secondary metabolites (5) Biotransformation using plant cell cultures (6) Effect of environmental factors (7) Secondary metabolite release and analysis.

1. *Selection of Cell Lines for High Yield of Secondary Metabolites*

The fore most importance of secondary metabolites production through tissue culture is to produce high amounts of secondary metabolites. Some special techniques have been devised to select cell lines that can produce higher amounts of desired metabolites. The heterogeneity within the cell population will be screened by selecting cell lines capable of accumulating higher level of metabolites (Figure 10.7). The techniques commonly employed for cell line selection are cell cloning, visual or chemical analysis and selection for resistance.

2. *Medium Composition and Effect of Nutrients*

The *in vitro* growth of the plant cells occurs in a suitable medium containing all the required elements. The ingredients of the medium effect the growth and metabolism of cells. For optimal production of secondary metabolites, a two-medium approach is desirable. The first medium is required for good growth of cells (biomass growth) while the second medium, referred to as production medium promotes secondary metabolite formation. The effect of nutrients (carbon and nitrogen sources, phosphate, growth regulators, precursors, vitamins, metal ions) on different species in relation to metabolite formation are variable. For *e.g.* if **sucrose concentration is increased from 3 per cent to 5 per cent, production of rosamarinic acid is increased by five times. In case of shikonin production, IAA enhances the yield whereas 2,4-D and NAA are inhibitory.**

3. *Large Scale Cultivation of Plant Cells*

In order to achieve industrial production of the desired metabolite, large scale cultivation of plant cells is required. Plant cells (20-150 μm in diameter) are generally 10-100 times larger than bacterial or fungal cell. When cultured, plant cells exhibit changes in volumes and thus variable shapes and sizes. Further, cultured cells have low growth rate and genetic instability. All these aspects have to be considered for mass cultivation of cells.

The following four different culture systems are widely used:

1. Free-cell suspension culture
2. Immobilized cell culture
3. Two-phase system culture
4. Hairy root culture

1. *Free-Cell Suspension Culture*

Mass cultivation of plant cells is most frequently carried out by cell suspension cultures. Care should be taken to achieve good growth rate of cells and efficient formation of the desired secondary metabolite. Stirred-tank reactor, bubble-column reactor, air-lift reactor and rotating-drum reactors are some of the example for culturing of free cell suspension bioreactors for production of secondary metabolities.

Two important aspects have to be considered for good success of suspension cultures.

a. Adequate and continuous oxygen supply.
b. Minimal generation of hydrodynamic stresses due to aeration agitation.

2. *Immobilized Cell Cultures*

Plant cells can be made immobile or immovable and used in culture systems. Cell cultures encapsulated by gel like substances or entrapped in membranes are called immobilized plant cell cultures. Immobilization of plant cells allows better cell to cell contact and the cells are also protected from high shear stresses. These immobilized systems can effectively increase the productivity of secondary metabolites in a number of species.

The common methods adopted for entrapment of cells are,

a. *Entrapment of Cells in Gels*

The cells or the protoplasts can be entrapped in several gels *e.g.*, alginate, agar, agarose, carrageenin. The gels may be used either individually or in combination. The techniques employed for the immobilization of plant cells are comparable to those used for immobilization of microorganisms or other cells.

b. *Entrapment of Cells in Nets or Foams*

Polyurethane foams or nets with various pore sizes are used. The actively growing plant cells in suspension can be immobilized on these foams. The cells divide within the compartments of foam and form aggregates.

c. *Entrapment of Cells in Hollow-Fibre Membranes*

Tubular hollow fibres composed of cellulose acetate silicone polycarbonate and organized into parallel bundles are used for immobilization of cells. It is possible to entrap cells within and between the fibres. Membrane entrapment is mechanically stable. However, it is more expensive than gel or foam immobilization.

Bioreactors for Use of Immobilized Cells

Fluidized bed or packed bed bioreactors are employed to use immobilized cells for large scale cultivation. In the fluidized-bed reactors, the immobilized cells are agitated by a flow of air or by pumping the medium. In contrast, in the packed-bed bioreactor, the immobilized cells are held stationary (not agitated) and perfused at a slow rate with an aerated culture medium.

3. *Two-Phase System Culture*

Plant cells can be cultivated in an aqueous two phase system for the production of secondary metabolites. In this technique, the cells are kept apart from the product by separation in the bioreactor. This is advantageous since the product can be removed continuously. Certain polymers (*e.g.* dextran and polyethylene glycol for the separation of phenolic compounds) are used for the separation of phases.

4. *Hairy Root Culture*

Hairy root cultures are used for the production of root-associated metabolites. In general, these cultures have high growth rate and genetic stability. For the production of hairy root cultures, the explant material (plant tissue) is inoculated with the cells of the pathogenic bacterium, *Agrobacterium rhizogenes.* This organism contains root-inducing (Ri) plasmid that causes genetic transformation of plant tissues, which finally results in hairy root cultures. Hairy roots produced by plant tissues have metabolite features similar to that of normal roots. Hairy root cultures are most recent organ culture systems and are successfully used for the commercial production of secondary metabolites.

Bioreactors for Hairy Roots

While designing a suitable bioreactor for hairy root cultures the physiology and morphology of the hairy roots should be taken into consideration. The major problem in bioreactor cultivation of hairy roots is their tendency to form clumps resulting from the bridging of primary and secondary roots. This results in densely packed root beds and reduces transfer of oxygen and nutrients. Root thickness, root length, the number of root hairs and root branching frequency are some of the factors which should be taken into consideration for hairy root cultures in bioreactors. Immobilization of hairy roots by horizontal or vertical meshes as well as by cages or polyurethane foam promotes their growth in submerged stirred bioreactors, bubble columns, air lift reactors and drum reactors where the roots are immersed in the culture medium.

4. *Elicitor-Induced Production of Secondary Metabolites*

The production of secondary metabolites in plant cultures is generally low and does not meet the commercial demands. **Elicitors are the compounds of physical or chemical or biological origin which stimulate the production of higher secondary metabolites, and the phenomenon of such stimulation is referred to as elicitation.** Addition of these elicitors to the medium in low concentration enhances the production of secondary metabolites. Elicitors produced within the plant cells are endogenous elicitors *e.g.* pectin, pectic acid, cellulose, other polysaccharides. **Elicitors are not produced by the their own, added from the outside are referred as exogenous elicitors *e.g.* chitin, chitosan, glucans.** All the elicitors of biological origin are biotic elicitors. **The term abiotic elicitors is used to represent the physical (cold, heat, UV light, osmotic pressure) and chemical agents (ethylene, fungicides, antibiotics, salts of heavy metals)** that can also increase the product formation.

5. *Biotransformation Using Plant Cell Cultures*

The conversion of one chemical into another (*i.e.,* a substrate into a final product) by using biological systems (*i.e.* cell suspensions) as biocatalysts is regarded as biotransformation or bioconversion. The biotechnological application of plant cell cultures in biotransformation reactions involves the conversion of some less important substances to valuable medicinal or commercially important products. In biotransformation, it is necessary to select such cell lines that possess the enzymes for catalysing the desired reactions. Bioconversions may involve many types of reactions *e.g.* hydroxylation, reduction, glycosylation. For example, amino acids have been added to suspension culture media for production of tropane alkaloids, indole alkaloids. The amount of precursors is usually lower in callus and cell cultures than in differentiated tissues. **Phenylalanine acts as a precursor of rosmarinic acid; addition of phenylalanine to *Salvia officinalis* suspension cultures stimulated the production of rosmarinic acid and decreased the production time as well.** Phenylalanine also acts as precursor of the N-benzoylphenylisoserine side chain of taxol; supplementation of *Taxus cuspidata* cultures with phenylalanine resulted in increased yields of taxol. The timing of precursor addition is critical for an optimum effect. The effects of feedback inhibition must surely be considered when adding products of a metabolic pathway to cultured cells.

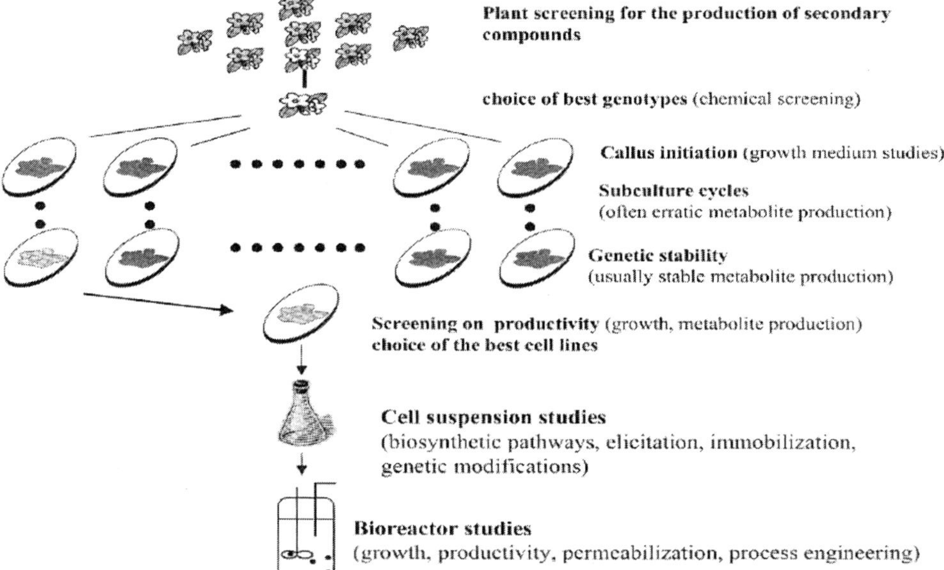

Figure 10.7. Method of Selection of High Yielding Cell Lines.

6. Effect of Environmental Factors

The physical factors namely light, incubation temperature, pH of the medium and aeration of cultures influence the production of secondary metabolites in cultures.

7. *Secondary Metabolite Release and Analysis*

The methods employed for the separation and purification of secondary metabolites from cell cultures are the same as that used for extraction of secondary metabolites from plants which is produced naturally. Sometimes, the products formed within the cells are released into the medium, making the isolation and analysis easy. For the secondary metabolites stored within the vacuoles of cells, two membranes (plasma membrane and tonoplast) have to be disrupted. By manipulating the permeability of cell membrane, they can be secreted out to the media. Permeabilisation can be achieved by electric pulse, UV, pressure, sonication, heat, *etc.* Even charcoal can be added to medium to absorb secondary metabolites. Some times **Dimethyl Sulfoxide (DMSO)** is used as a permeabilizing agents for the release of products.

In general, separation and purification of products from plant cell cultures are expensive, therefore every effort is made to make them cost-effective. Two approaches are made in this direction:

1. Production of secondary metabolite should be as high as possible.
2. Formation of side product(s) which interfere with separation must be made minimal.

Once a good quantity of the product is released into the medium, separation and purification techniques (*e.g.* extraction) can be used for its recovery. These techniques largely depend on the nature of the secondary metabolite.

Advantages of *In vitro* Secondary Metabolites Production

1. Compounds can be produced under controlled conditions as per market demands.
2. Culture systems are independent of environmental factors, seasonal variations, pest and microbial diseases and geographical constraints.
3. Cell growth can be controlled to facilitate improved product formation.
4. The quality of the product will be consistent as it is produced by a specific cell line.
5. Recovery of the product will be easy.
6. Plant cultures are particularly useful in case of plants which are difficult or expensive to be grown in the fields.
7. Mutant cell lines can be developed for the production of novel compounds of commercial importance, which are not normally found in plants.

8. Biotransformation reactions (converting specific substrates to valuable products) can be carried out with certain cultured cells.
9. The production control is not at the mercy of political interference.
10. The production time is less and labour costs are minimal.

Considering the advantages listed above, about 25-30 per cent of medicines for human use, and the various chemical materials for industrial purposes are obtained from plant tissue cultures. In general, tissue culture production of natural materials is cheaper compared to synthetic production. However, there are certain limitations associated with tissue cultures.

Limitations/Disadvantages

1. In general, *in vitro* production of secondary metabolites is lower when compared to intact plants.
2. Many a times, secondary metabolites are formed in differentiated tissues/ organs. In such a case, culture cells which are non-differentiated can produce little.
3. Cultured cells are genetically unstable and may undergo mutation. The production of secondary metabolite may be drastically reduced, as the culture ages.
4. Vigorous stirring is necessary to prevent aggregation of cultured cells. This may often damage the cells.
5. Strict aseptic conditions have to be maintained during culture technique: Any infection to the culture adversely affects product formation.

Some Secondary Metabolites Produced in Cell and Root Culture

Shikonin

Shikonin and its derivatives such as acetyl shikonin and isobutyl shikonin accumulated in roots of *Lithospermum erythrorhizon*. They are reddish purple pigments and have been used in traditional dyeing. The plant has also been used as a herbal medicine. Because of a shortage of this plant, Scientists in Japan investigated mass cultivation of *L. erythrorhizon* cells to produce shikonin compounds. Using the cell line established by Tabata's laboratory of Kyoto University, they optimized its culture conditions extensively to increase the level of the products using flasks and various types of fermentors including a rotating cylindrical fermentor.

They found that *L. erythrorhizon* produced shikonins in White's medium but the cell growth was poor in the same medium. On the other hand, Linsmair-Skoog's (LS) medium was recognized to support the growth but not shikonin production. Therefore, they used a two-stage culture for mass production of shikonin compounds. Namely, to proliferate the cells, LS medium was used at the first stage of the fermentation, and then the cells were transferred into White's medium for production of shikonin compounds (Figure 10.8).

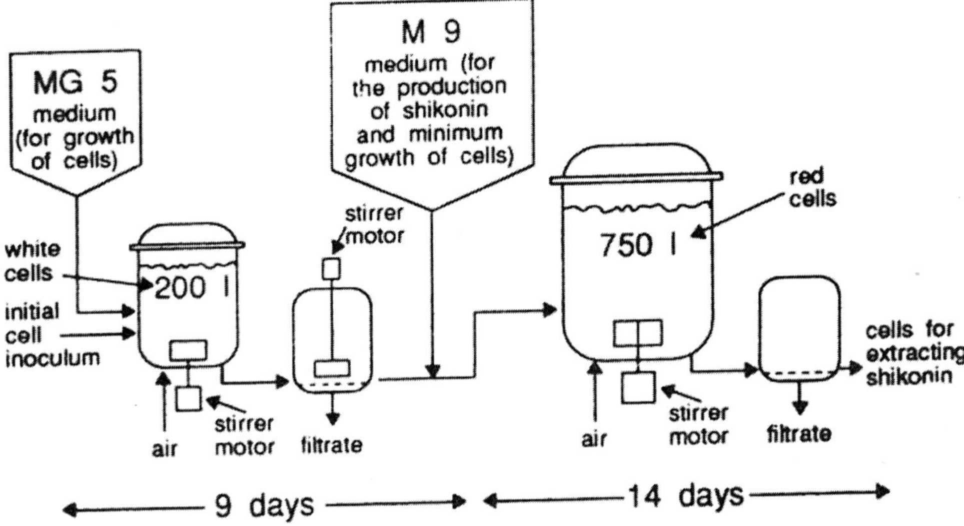

Figure 10.8. Shikonin Production from Cell Culture.

Shikonin Production

1st Stage: Cells of high producing strain M-18 were propagated in a growth medium MG-5 (Modified LS Medium) without producing shikonin derivatives.

2nd Stage: The cells from the growth medium are transferred to M-9 medium (White's medium) for shikonin production. The components of LS and M-9 medium are more suitable for shikonin production. The shikonin yield also increased when both the initial cell density and medium concentration were doubled.

The concentration of dissolved oxygen is also vital. It should be adjusted to 6.4 and 6.0 ppm for the first and the second culture stage. Cells of the stock culture are grown in a jar fermenter are inoculated in the first stage tank (200 L) with MG-5 medium for cell growth and incubated for 9 days and subsequently transferred to filtering apparatus. The production medium M-9 is poured into the tank and cell in this medium are pumped into 2nd tank (750 L) for shikonin production. After incubating the cells for 14 days in the 2nd tank, the pigmented cells are harvested by filtering off the medium. The extracted and purification can be carried by treating the cells with n-hexane from the cultured cells and subsequently hydrolysis with 2 per cent KOH and recrystallized to give a pure shikonin.

Uses

Anti-inflammatory

Antibacterial

Antitumor

In the treatment of haemorrhoides or piles.

Taxol

Taxol (plaxitaxol), a complex diterpene alkaloid found in the bark of the *Taxus* tree, is one of the most promising anticancer agents known due to its unique mode of action on the micro tubular cell system. In 1989, Christen *et al.,* reported for the first time the production of taxol (placlitaxel) by *Taxus* cell cultures.

Morphine and Codeine

Latex from the opium poppy, *Papaver somniferum*, is a commercial source of the analgesics, morphine and codeine. Callus and suspension cultures of *P. somniferum* are being investigated as an alternative means for production of these compounds. Production of morphine and codeine in morphologically undifferentiated cultures has been reported

Ginsenosides

Ginseng has been recognized as a miraculous promoter of health and longevity. The primary bioactive constituents of ginseng were identified as ginsenosides, a group of triterpenoid saponins. Among them, ginsenoside Rg1 is one of the major active molecules from *Panax ginseng* obtained by ginseng root callus cultured on a chemically defined medium.

L-DOPA

L-3,4-dihydroxyphenylalanine, is an important intermediate of secondary metabolism in higher plants and is known as a precursor of alkaloids, betalain, and melanine, isolated from *Vinca faba, Mucuna, Baptisia* and *Lupinus.* It is also a precursor of catecholamines in animals and is being used as a potent drug for Parkinson's disease, a progressive disabling disorder associated with a deficiency of dopamine in the brain.

Berberine

Berberine is an isoquinoline alkaloid found in the roots of *Coptis japonica* and cortex of *Phellondendronamurense*. This antibacterial alkaloid has been identified from a number of cell cultures, notably those of *Coptisjaponica, Thalictrum* spp. and *Berberis* spp.

In vitro Germplasm Conservation

Plant genetic resources are the most valuable and essential basic raw materials to meet the current and future needs of crop improvement programme. The diversity comprises native land races, local selections, elite cultivars and wild relatives of crop plants. **The sum total of hereditary material or genes present in a species is known as the germplasm of that species.** So germplasm collection is a collection of a large number of genotypes of a crop species and its wild relatives.

The principle of any technology designed for germplasm conservation should be to preserve the maximum possible genetic diversity of a particular plant of genetic stock for future use. Broadly speaking, there are two basic approaches to genetic resources conservation, namely *in situ* and *ex situ* conservation (Figure 10.9).

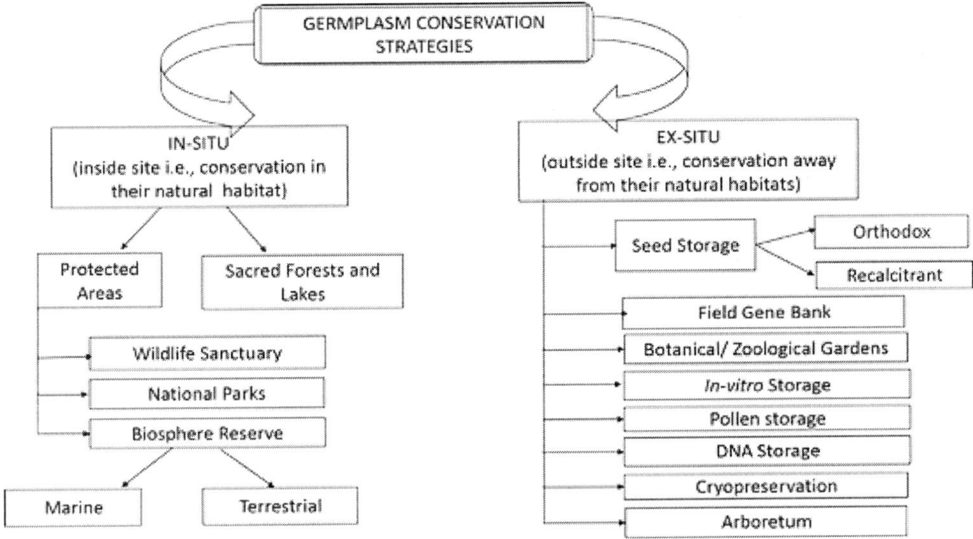

Figure 10.9. Methods of Germplasm C.onservation.

1. *In situ* Conservation (In its original place)

This method of conservation mainly aims at preservation of land races with wild relatives in which genetic diversity exists and/or in which the weedy/wild forms present hybridise with related cultivars.

Limitations

1. There is a risk of the material being lost due to environmental hazards.
2. The cost of maintaining a large proportion of available genotypes in nurseries or fields may be extremely high.

In *in situ* conservation the plant materials are conserved in their natural environment without any manipulation of ecosystem.

e.g. Natural biospheres, gene sanctuaries.

2. *Ex situ* conservation

Ex situ conservation is the chief mode for preservation of genetic resources, which may include both cultivated and wild material. In *ex situ* conservation the plants are taken out from their natural habitat and grown in the field or they are kept under controlled storage conditions.

Ex situ conservation involves both *in vivo* and *in vitro* methods of conservation.

I. *In vivo* Method

The plants are taken out from their natural habitat and the available varieties are followed to grow in the normal way.

e.g. Botanic gardens (living gene banks), Field gene banks - in field gene banks the plant materials are maintained as living collection in a field or orchard or plantation, generation after generation.

Draw Backs

1. Potential risk of germplasm being lost due to disease, stress or disaster - that means FGB are open to various risks.
2. Large amount of space and labour are required to maintain a small proportion of diversity, so they are costly to maintain.

Advantage

The crop sp. which produce recalcitrant seeds and those which cannot be even multiplied vegetatively can be preserved as living collection only. They can be continuously evaluated and desired accessions can be directly used.

Seed Gene Banks

Seed gene banks aim to provide ideal storage conditions so that the mean viability period of the seed is greatly extended by reducing the life process to a low level. Germplasm conservation in the form of seeds is most convenient since seeds occupy a relatively small space. Their transport to various introduction centres and gene banks is also economical.

Draw Backs

a. Loss or viability over the passage of time and susceptibility to insect or pathogen attack.
b. Inability to maintain distinct clones except for inbred and apomictic species and
c. Non-applicability to vegetatively propagated crops like Dioscorea, Ipomoea, Potato *etc.*

II. *In vitro* Conservation

The limits of conventional methods can be overcome by *in vitro* methods. *In vitro* methods are the most useful for conservation of vegetatively propagated plants, species with recalcitrant seeds *i.e.* those seeds which cannot be desiccated beyond a relatively critical moisture content. They are killed if the moisture content goes below 12 and 35 per cent) *e.g.* cocoa, rubber, most tropical fruits and many timber species and genetically engineered material.

The potential advantages of *in vitro* conservation include

a. Requirement for little space for preservation of a large number of clonally multiplied plants.

b. Maintenance of the material in an environment free of pests or pathogens.

c. Protection against dangers of natural environmental hazards.

d. Availability of nucleus stock to propagate a large number of plants rapidly whenever necessary and

e. Minimising the obstacles generally imposed by quarantine systems on the movement of live plant across national boundaries since they are raised and maintained in an aseptic environment.

Application of Plant Cell and Tissue Cultures in Germplasm Conservation

Materials Used for Conservation

The materials stored *in vitro* may be isolated protoplasts, cells from suspension or callus cultures, meristem tips, propagules at various stages of development or organised plantlets. The cultured cells or shoots can be maintained by serial subcultures at 4-8 weekly intervals for virtually unlimited periods. The storage of germplasm by repeated cultures has some disadvantages. These include the risk of germplasm loss due to human error or the failure in maintenance of *in vitro* security resulting in invasion by a pathogen. Genetic stability is also affected during serial subculturing of the plant material, especially in the case of materials in an undifferentiated phase (cell or callus cultures). Maintenance of the material as plantlets and subsequent propagation from their nodal cuttings reduces the risk of genetic instability. Prolonged storge of somatic embryos also ensures a high degree of genetic stability.

Basically two types of *in vitro* conservation techniques can be devised. They are minimal growth storage and cryopreservation.

Minimal Growth Storage

It is a method of *in vitro* germplasm conservation, where the material that is to be conserved is stored at low and non freezing temperature. It can be followed in several ways like reduced temperature or light, incorporation of sub lethal levels of growth retardants, induction of osmotic stress with sucrose or mannitol and maintenance of cultures at a reduced nutritional status particularly reduced carbon reduction of gas pressure over the cultures, desiccation and mineral oil overlay.

Principle employed in this care is the manipulation of normal culture conditions in such a way that the cultures are maintained in a viable condition, at the same time the growth rate is very low, so that the interval between subsequent subculturing can be prolonged and the variation can be reduced. The advantage of this approach is that cultures can be readily brought back to normal culture conditions to produce plants on demand. The first successful report of minimal growth storage was by Galzy (1989) at 9°C for 290 days.

Cryopreservation

The principle underlying cryopreservation basically involves bringing the culture to a state of non-dividing and zero metabolism, which is achieved by subjecting it to super low temperatures in the presence of cryoprotectants. Strictly speaking any storage which utilises a temperature less than zero is a cryopreservation.

Definition

Cryopreservation is the preservation of material by storage in liquid nitrogen at -196°C. The process of cryopreservation is less laborious and the material is cooled slowly to low temperature of -30 to - 40 °C. Cooling rate is as slow as 2 °C/hr. It is maintained at this temperature for a few hours, the time varies for each and every species and then gradually immersed in liquid nitrogen. In cryopreservation the stored material will be in a viable state but all the metabolic activities are totally arrested. It facilitate prolonged storage for indefinite period. Any material can be subjected to this storage.

First successful report of cryopreservation was **by Quatrano (1908) in which he preserved the suspension culture of Flax at -50°C and subsequently** in 1973 Sakai and Sugiwara reported the successful freezing of the callus of *Populus euramericana* at -196°C. Embryogenesis from this was done by Nag and Street (1973).

If the materials need to be stored in cryopreservation, then those meterials should be allowed for some pre and post freezing treatments, so that the cells will be protected from ultra low temperature thus reducing the damage caused by freezing injury. For this purpose specific protocols have been standardised, which is specific for each and every species and also for particular plant parts.

The protocols developed for two types species 1.cold hardy species 2. non cold hardy species.

1. Cold Hardy Species

These crops can tolerate freezing to some extent and their natural ability is exploited by this. After sufficient period of storage the material can be subcultured. For this the material is warmed slowly and regenerated in media.

2. Non Cold Hardy Species

These crops cannot tolerate low temperature and the protocol is much more complicated and a series of steps are there. Various stages in a freeze preservation protocol can be followed:

1. Pre growth treatment/pre treatment

2. Cryoprotectant treatment/cryoprotection
3. Freezing
4. Storage
5. Thawing for reculturing and
6. Regrowth

1. Pre Growth Treatment/Pre Treatment

It is done prior to storage at ultra low temperature. These pretreatments are supposed to bring about certain physiological changes in the material which increases freeze tolerance. Pre growth manipulations involve cold hardening by exposure to low temperature. Pre treatment can be done before the collection of explant *i.e.*, to the stock plant or to the explant itself. *e.g.* keeping stock plants at 4°C.

a. Dehydration of the Material to a Safe Level

The internal water should not crystallise, so during pre treatment if we dehydrate the material to safe levels the rewarming temperature becomes less critical.

b. Exposure to Low Temperature

This practice was found beneficial in majority of the cases. In the case of *Solanum tuberosum* a cold treatment given to the stock plant itself increased survival. 4°C for 3 days and low temperature survival was upto 30 per cent.

c. Hormonal Manipulation

In the embryogenesis of carrot callus 2, 4-D withdrawal at the later stages has been found to increase the freeze tolerance.

2. Cryoprotectant Treatment/Cryoprotection

Cryoprotectants are chemicals added to media to protect the material from ultra low temperature damage. Presence of cryoprotectants in small amounts in the initial stages is found to be beneficial *e.g.* In the case of maize a 10 per cent proline treatment during pre growth stage has been found to be beneficial. **Common cryoprotectants used are - Dimethyl sulphoxide (DMSO) - 5-8 per cent, proline - 10 per cent, glycerol and glucose in proper concentration in some cases.**

a. The cryoprotectants help to lower the freezing point of intracellular water and prevent the formation of large ice crystals.
b. Cryoprotectants increase the permeability of cell membrane and aids in the dehydration of cells.
c. Cryoprotectants have a protective mechanism against the toxic solution effect.

   e.g. Proline - protects plant cells against accumulation of high solute concentration during stress condition.

Application of Cryoprotectants

Cryoprotectants are added to the medium after sterilization by passing through a microfilter of 0.4 M, the material along with the medium and the cryoprotectant solution is put in the cryovial (1.5 ml) and then plunged into liquid N.

Points to be noted while adding cryoprotectants

a. It is always better to add cryoprotectants as mixtures

   e.g. DMSO + glycerol will help to increase the effectiveness of the cryoprotectant and decrease the toxic effect.

b. Addition of cryoprotectant is to be done over a period of time

   e.g. For half an hour at intervals of 5-10 minutes, so as to reduce the osmotic shocks

c. The culture has to be maintained at 0° C while the cryoprotectant is added (keep them in ice bath) to reduce the toxic effect.

3. Freezing

The cryoprotected specimen is dispersed in sterile polypropelene cryovials (flame sealed) along with the medium and cryoprotectant and then subjected to freezing. Different types of freezing methods are adopted.

A. Slow Freezing

The material is cooled slowly at a rate of 0.5 - 4°C per minute, at this slow cooling rate the material is cooled upto -100° C it is dipped in liquid nitrogen of -196°C. *e.g.* Rice suspension culture slow rate of 0.1°C/minute is better.

B. Rapid Freezing

Material is directly dipped in liquid nitrogen. The advantage suggested is that the critical temperature zone for ice crystal growth will be passed very quickly so that the formation of large ice crystals can be avoided. It has been observed that the size of ice crystal is more important rather than presence or absence of ice crystals.

C. Two Step Freezing

This type of freezing is found to be beneficial in majority of the cases. The material is first cooled at a slow cooling rate of 30 to -50°C and then kept for 30 minutes, then rapidly plunged into liquid N. The slow freezing at the initial stages tend to reduce the intracellular ice crystal formation.

D. Dry Freezing

Prior to liquid nitrogen storage some amount of dehydration is brought about by using an air stream or desiccator. Then the material is subjected to slow freezing.

E. Droplet Freezing

Adopted in the case of Cassava meristems. Cryoprotectanct treated meristem is frozen in small quantity of cryoprotectant solution, 2-3 ml of cryoprotectant along with meristem is placed in Aluminium (Al). foil which is placed in a petriplate and is subjected to liquid N storage. Al. being an efficient conductor of heat, homogeneous dispersion of heat and hence uniform cooling.

4. Storage

Liquid Nitrogen (LN) storage tanks are used for storage. 650 liter storage tank can hold about 5000 cryovials of 1 ml size. The LN has to be changed at 30-120 days. Storage can also be done in LN refrigerators, here weekly changes of LN and can be recultured as and when required.

5. Thawing/Rewarming

Rapid thawing is the best for maximum survival. They are plunged in warm water at 37- 40°C for 1 to 2 minutes with a warming rate of 500 - 750°C per minute. Then the material is transferred to ice bathe till it is taken out for culturing. While reculturing the thawed material is highly sensitive to light and should be done under low light intensities and also a semi solid medium is the best. The removal of the cryoprotectant is not advised; because cryoprotectants like DMSO has beneficial effect, that is free radical seavenger effect. When the cryoprotectant is removed some other vital salts may also be washed away (leached out). Also there is changes of deplasmolysing injury. The viability of the material can be tested using Evans blue test, FDA test, TTA *etc.*

Factors Affecting Cryopreservation

1. Nature of the Plant Material

It is of atmost importance, plant material is selected in such a way that genetic stability is maintained maximum. For suspension culture it is better to use cultures in the late lag phase or exponential phase. For embryo - globular stage. The stage should be standardised for each and every crop.

2. Moisture Content of the Material

The material should be sufficiently dehydrated so that the ice crystals of lethal size should be avoided.

3. Cooling/Freezing Rate

A cooling rate slow enough to cause sufficient dehydration, but fast enough to avoid solute toxicity should be adopted. Two step freezing is the best.

4. Thawing Rate

Rapid thawing (warming 500 - 750°C per minute) is best to avoid recrystallization of ice.

5. Storage Temperature

Storing in -196°C is ideal for long term strorage of material.

Advantages

1. Aseptic storage is possible
2. Space saving - 800 events of grapes each of 6 replication could be stored in a space of $2m^2$ (1 ha in the field)
3. Protection from natural calamities
4. Large no. of plants can be evolved and stored
5. 100 per cent perfect storage condition

Limitations

1. Initial cost involved is high
2. A continuous supply of LN is very necessary
3. Once the *in vitro* techniques are standardised, then only it can be applied
4. Callus formation increases the genetic variability and the very aim is spoilt.

Applications

The principle objectives of germplasm conservation using cell and tissue cultures have been:

1. Conservation of Somaclonal and gametoclonal variation in cultures.
2. Maintain of recalcitrant seeds.
3. Conservation of cell lines producing medicines.
4. Storage of pollens for enhancing longevity.
5. Conservation of rare germplasm arsing through somatic hybridization or other methods of genetic manipulations.
6. Delaying the process of ageing.
7. Storage of meristem culture for micropropagation, micro grafting and production of disease free plants.
8. Conservation of plant material from enhanced species.
9. Establishment of germplasm bank.
10. Exchange of information as well germplasm at the international level.

Works Going on in India

1. NBPGR - NFPTCR - National Facility for Plant Tissue Culture Repository (1986) A project funded by DBT
2. CPCRI - Central Potato Research Institute - 300 accession of *S. tuberosum* - meristem and shoot tips mostly under minimal growth.
3. CRRI, Cuttak - Anther culture of rice.
4. IIHR, Bangalore - pollen storage
5. CTCRI - Medium storage of cassava (6 months) and sweet potato (12 months)

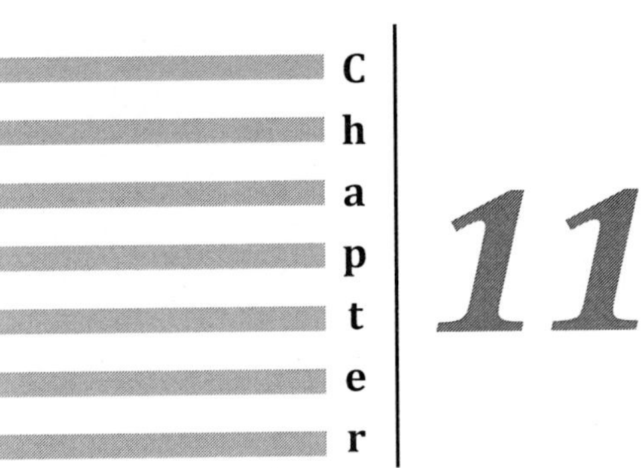

Genome Organization – Prokaryotes and Eukaryotes

Gene and Genome

A gene is the basic physical and functional unit of heredity. Genes, which are made up of DNA, act as instructions to make molecules called proteins. The conventional definition of genome is number of chromosomes representing haploidy (Figure 11.1). The first genomes studied in depth at the molecular level

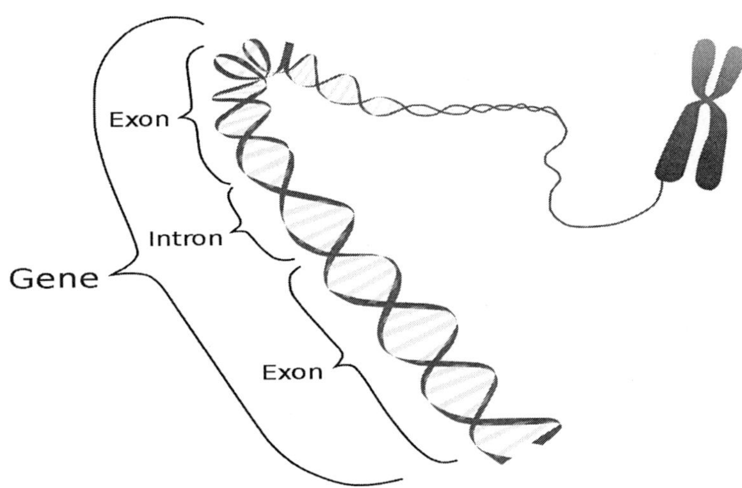

Figure 11.1. Place of Gene in Chromosome.

were the bacterium *Eschercia coli* and its bacteriophage. The second group of genomes studied in great detail at the molecular level were mitochondria and chloroplasts.

Genome Organisation

- Strasburger (1875) found chromosomes as thread like structures during cell division and size varies from 0.25 μm to 3.0 μm.
- Chromosomes made up of DNA, RNA, proteins, histones and non-histones proteins.
- The fundamental structural unit of chromatin is an assemblage, called the **nucleosome**, composed of five types of histones (designated H1, H2A, H2B, H3, and H4) and DNA.
- Nucleosomes are the fundamental packing unit particles of the chromatin and give chromatin a **"beads-on-a string**" appearance in electron micrographs that unfold higher-order packing.
- All histones are rich in basic amino acids – **lysine and arginine**.
- A nucleosome consists of **approximately 1.8 turns of DNA** wound around a core particle of histone proteins.
- The core particle is a roughly heart-shaped octamer of 4 types of histones: each proteins two molecules (H2A, H2B, H3 and H4).
- Approximately **166 base pairs are bound to the nucleosome: 146 (±1) base** pairs are tightly bound to the core particle and the **remaining 20 base pairs are associated with the H1 histone.** This nucleosome structure is closely similar in all eukaryotes.
- The DNA between two nucleosomes is called the **linker DNA.** This linker DNA gives unfolded chromatin a beads-on-a-string appearance (the nucleosomes are the beads). Thus, linker DNA joins two neighboring nucleosomes.
- The average linker length is variable in different species and for different cells within the same species, but they range from 8bp to 114 bp base pairs depending on the species. Wolfe suggests that linker lengths tend to be shortest in the lower eukaryotes (*e.g.* yeast), intermediate in plants, and longest in the higher eukaryotes (*i.e.* animals).
- Usually the linker length is related with greater transcriptional activity. That is, the average repeat length of the chromatin usually increases as the level of transcriptional activity increases.
- When chromatin is isolated from cells under conditions similar to those expected in a cellular environment, chromatin does not have a beads-on-a-string structure.
- Instead, the majority of the chromatin appears to be composed of relatively smooth fibers about 25 to 35 nm in diameter.

- ☆ The folding mechanism and higher-order structure of the chromatin fiber is uncertain. But in one of the more widely accepted models, beads-on-a-string chromatin winds into a regular coil called the **solenoid** (Figure 11.2).

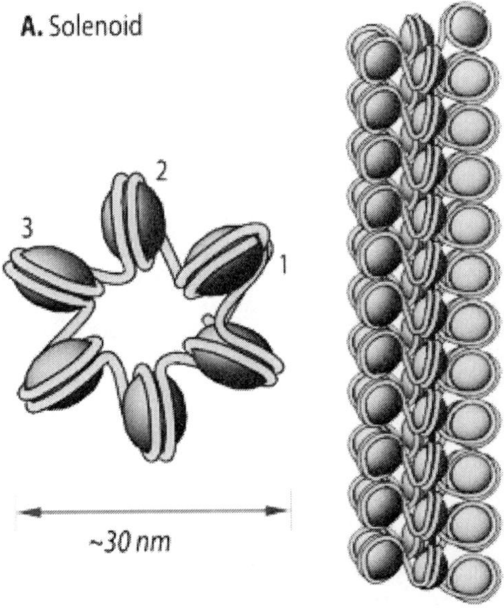

Figure 11.2. Solenoid Model of DNA Coiling with Histone Octamer.

- ☆ The solenoid model of the chromatin fiber is proposed to contain six to eight nucleosomes per turn and has a total outside diameter of about 34 nm.
- ☆ Although chromatin is organized at levels beyond the chromatin fiber (solenoid), the molecular arrangement of the highest levels of chromatin organization is not well understood.
- ☆ However, it has been suggested that chromatin fibers are divided into functional units called domains, and when the chromatin condenses, groups of proteins link these chromatin domains together and arrange the chromatin fibers into loops.
- ☆ When DNA is stained, for example, with a fluorescent compound, it can be visually divided into condensed chromatin or unfolded chromatin (Figure 11.3).
- ☆ Comprised of most active portions of chromosomes that stain lightly are only partially condensed; this chromatin is termed **euchromatin**. The condensed regions of chromatin are referred to as **heterochromatin** (Figure 11.4).

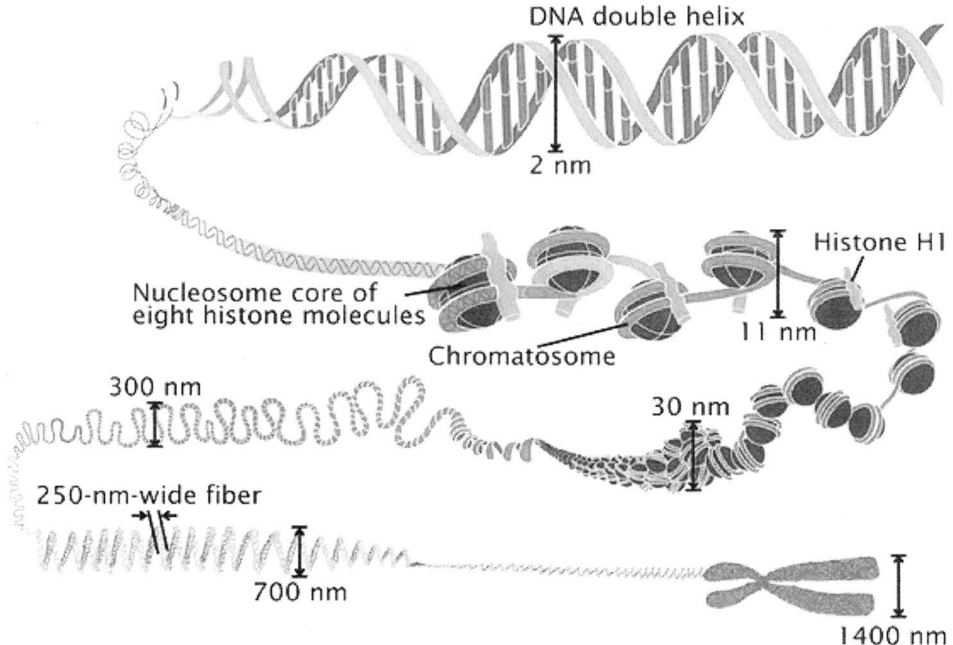

Figure 11.3. DNA Packaging in Eukaryotes.

- Important biochemical processes occur in euchromatin but are absent or proceed very slowly in heterochromatin.
- Euchromatin is the lightly packed from chromatin that is rich in gene concentration. It is often under active transcription.
- It represents most of the chromatin that disperse after mitosis has been completed.
- Euchromatin contains structural genes which replicate and transcribe during G_1 and S phase of interphase.
- Euchromatinis to be considered as genetically active chromatin, since it has a very important role in the expression phenotype of the genes.
- Euchromatin participates in the active transcription of DNA to mRNA products.
- In the dark-staining regions, the chromatin remains in the condensed state and is called heterochromatin.
- Heterochromatin is characterized by its especially high content of repetitive DNA sequences and contains very few, if any, structural genes.
- It is late replicating (*i.e.*, it is replicated when the bulk of DNA has already been replicated) and is not transcribed.

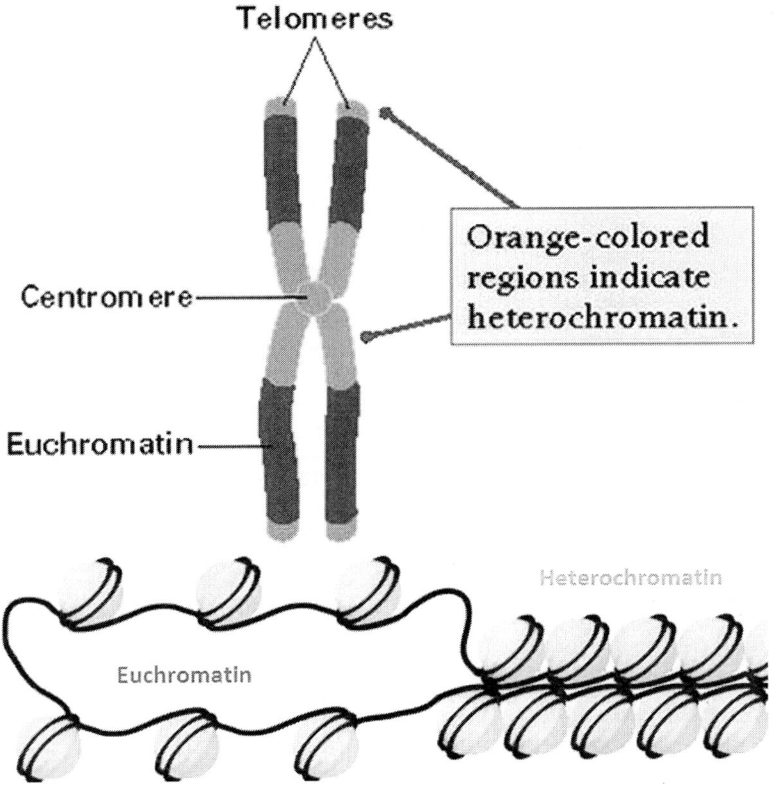

Figure 11.4. Euchromatin and Heterochromatin Regions in Chromosome.

- It is thought that in heterochromatin the DNA is tightly packed in the 30 nm fibre
- There are two types of heterochromatin: constitutive heterochromatin and facultative heterochromatin.
- Facultative heterochromatin is essentially euchromatin that has undergone heterochromatinization which may involve a segment of chromosome or a whole chromosome, or one whole haploid set of chromosomes.
- Constitutive heterochromatin remains permanently in the heterochromatic state, *i.e.*, it does not revert to euchromatic state, *e.g.* centromeric regions. It contains short repeated sequences of DNA, called **satellite DNA**.
- The bulk of constitutive heterochromatin is composed of non-coding DNA sequences that are repeated hundreds of thousands or even millions of times.

Table 11.1. Difference between Euchromatin and Heterochromatin

Characters	*Euchromatin*	*Constitvitive Heterochromatin*	*Facultative Heterochromatin*
Relation to bands	In R bands	In C bands	In G bands
Location	Chromosome arm	Usually centromeric	Chromosome arms
Condition during interphase	Usually dispersed	Condensed	Condensed
Genetic activity	Usually active	In active	Probably inactive
Relation to chromosomes	Inter chromomeric	Centromeric chromosomes	Intercalary chromosomes

Chromosome (Chroma – color; Soma – body)

In the nucleus of each cell, the DNA molecule is packaged into thread-like structures called **chromosomes**. Each chromosome is made up of DNA tightly coiled many times around proteins called histones that support its structure. Chromosomes were first described by **Strasburger (1815**), and the term **'chromosome' was first used by Waldeyer in 1888**. They appear as rod shaped dark stained bodies during the metaphase stage of mitosis when cells are stained with a suitable basic dye and viewed under a light microscope. In eukaryotes the chromosomes are multiple large, linear and are present in the nucleus of the cell. It is helps to the inheritance (through gene transmission) of characters from one generation to next generation.

Chromosome structure and size varies from 1 to 30 micron length and diameter from 0.2 to 2 micron. In each chromosome contains the following structure (Figure 11.5)

1. Chromatid,
2. Chromonema,
3. Chromomeres,
4. Centromere,
5. Secondary constriction or Nucleolar organizer,
6. Telomere and
7. Satellite.

1. Chromatid

At mitotic metaphase each chromosome consists of two symmetrical structures called chromatids. Each chromatid consists of a single DNA molecule. Both chromatids are connected to eachothersolelyby way of the centromere and come to be separated at the commencing of anaphase when the sister chromatids of a chromosome migrate to the opposite poles.

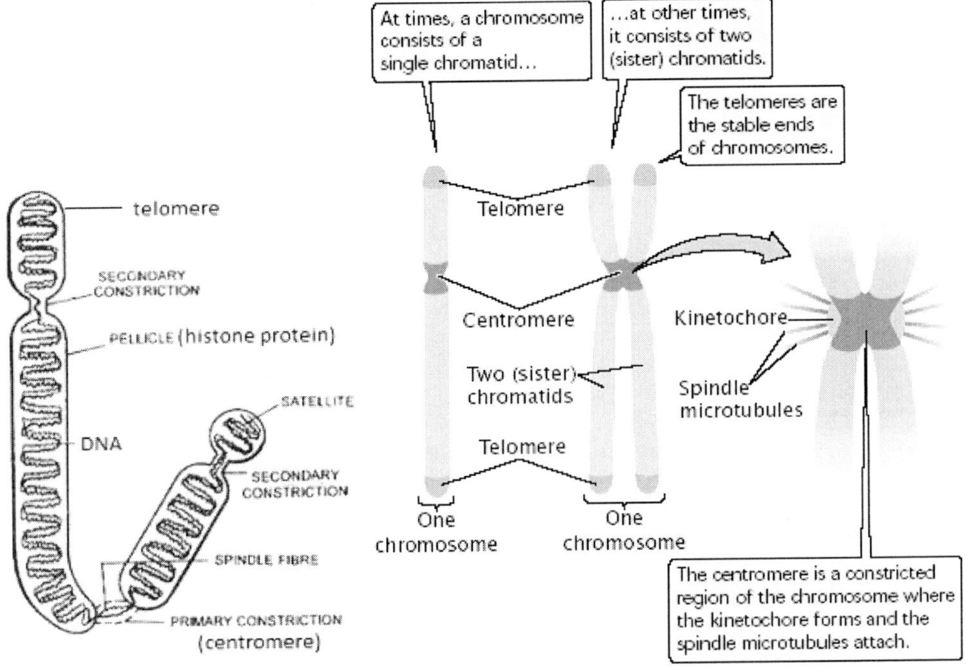

Figure 11.5. Structure of a Eukaryotic Chromosome.

2. Chromonema

In each chromatid, there are two longitudinal chromonemata coiled with each other.

3. Chromomeres

Chromomeres in the form of small dense masses are observed at regular intervals on the chromonemata. Chromomeres are areas of tightly folded DNA and are believed to correspond to the units of genetic characteristic in the chromosomes (Figure 11.6).

4. Centromere

A section of the chromosome is recognized as permanent. It is a small shape in the chromonema and is marked with the aid of a constriction. At this point the two chromonemata are joined together. This is recognized as centromere or kinetochore or main constriction. Non stainable component of chromosome making foremost construction. The chromosomes are connected to spindle fibres at this locationat some stage in cell division is referred to as kinetochore. The section of the chromosome which lies on both side of the centromere represents arms which can also be equal or unequal depending upon the role of centromere.

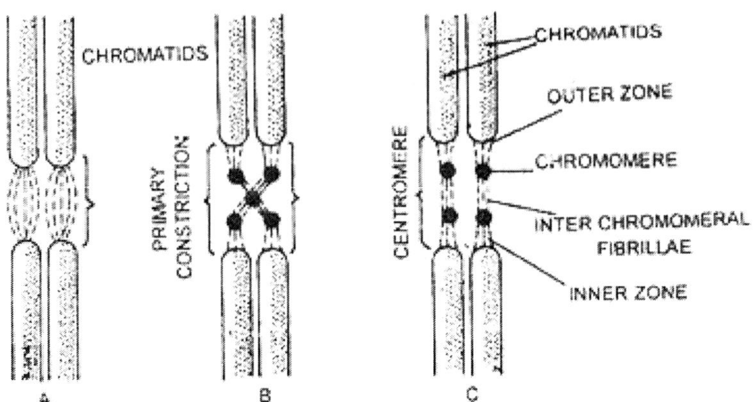

Figure 11.6. Structure of Chromomeres and Centromere.

5. Secondary Constriction or Nucleolar Organiser

Secondary constrictions can be unique from main constriction or centromere, due to the fact chromosome bends only at the function of centromere at some point of anaphase.

Nucleolus is constantly related with the secondary constriction of sat-chromosomes. Therefore, secondary constrictions are additionally known as **Nucleolus Organiser Location (NOR)** and sat-chromosomes are frequently referred to as nucleolus organiser chromosomes. NOR of every sat-chromosome carries numerous hundred copies of the gene coding for ribosomal RNA (rRNA).

6. Telomeres

The chromosomal ends are recognised as the **telomeres.** If a chromosome breaks, the damaged ends can fuse with every other chromosome end due to lack of telomeres. Telomeres are the buildings at the ends of linear eukaryotic chromosomes. They consist of a sequence of special DNA sequences and specialised proteins that bind to them. Telomerase provides a special sequence on the ends of eukaryotes chromosomes.

7. Satellite

The chromosome location distal to the secondary constriction *i.e.* the location between the secondary constriction and the nearest telomere is recognized as **satellite**. Therefore, chromosomes having secondary constrictions are known as **satellite chromosomes or sat-chromosomes**. The number of sat-chromosomes in the genome varies from one species to the other.

Chemical Composition

Chromatin is composed of DNA, RNA and protein. The protein of chromatin is of two types: the histones and the non-histones. Purified chromatin from interphase nuclei consists of about **30-40 per cent DNA, 50-65 per cent protein and 0.5-10 per cent RNA**,however there is a big variant due to species and tissues of the identical species.

DNA

The quantity of DNA existing in ordinary somatic cells of a species is steady for that species; any variant in DNA from this value is strictly correlated with a corresponding variant at the chromosome level. Gametes of a species comprise solely 1/2 of the quantity of DNA present in its somatic cells. The quantity of DNA existing in somatic cells additionally relies upon on the segment of cell cycle.

Protein

Proteins connected with chromosomes might also be categorized into two wide groups: (i) basic proteins or histones and (ii) non-histone proteins. Histones represent about 80 per cent of the whole chromosomal protein, they are existing in an almost 1:1 ratio with DNA (weight/weight). Their molecular weight levels from 10,000-30,000 and they are absolutely devoid of **tryptophan**. **Histones** are a enormously heterogenous type of proteins separable in 5 specific fractions distinctive as H1 H2a, H2b, H3 and H4 after ewin (1975).Fraction H1 is lysin-rich, H2A and H2B are slightly lysine rich, while H3 and H4 are arginine-rich. Histones play a predominant feature in chromosome organisation the place H2a, H2b, H3 and H4 are involved in the structural organization of chromatin fibres, while fraction H1 holds together the folded chromatin fibres of chromosomes. Non-histone proteins make up about 20 per cent of the whole chromosome mass, however their quantity is variable and there is no specific ratio between the quantities of DNA and non-histones present in chromosomes (Table 11.2).There may additionally be 12 to greater than 20 different kinds of non-histone proteins which exhibit variant from one species to the different and even in different tissues of the equal organism. This category of proteins consists of many vital enzymes, such as DNA and RNA polymerases *etc.*

Table 11.2. Details of Histone Protein

Histone Type	*Common Basic Residuces*	*Molecular Weight*
H1	Lyine rich	23 kDa protein
H2A	Slightly serine rich more lysine rich	13,960 Da protein
H2B	Slightly serine rich more lysine rich	13,744Da protein
H3	Arginine rich	15,242 Da protein
H4	Arginine rich	11, 282 Da protein

Chromosome Numbers and Genome

The chromosomes comprised of DNA and proten molecules. Eukaryotic gene contains **exons and introns**. DNA coils histone protein and form chroantins. Basic structure of chromatins are bead and string structure. In this bead is nucleosome and string is linker DNA. So the nucleosome is a structure in which histone protein is wrapped up two times with linker DNA (Figure 11.7).

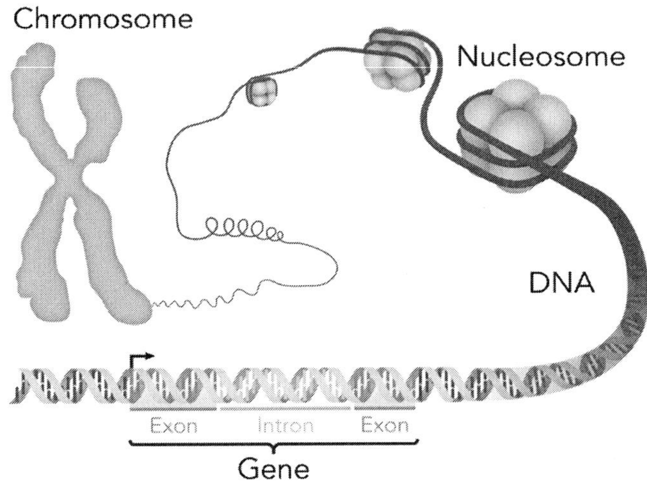

Figure 11.7. Gene, DNA, Nucleosome and Chromosome.

Each eukaryotic species has a characteristic number of chromosomes per cell: potatoes have 48 chromosomes, fruit flies have 8, and humans have 46. There appears to be no special significance between the complexity of an organism and its number of chromosomes per cell.

In most eukaryotic cells, there are two sets of chromosomes. One set is inherited from the male parent and the other from the female parent together constituting a **homologous pair**. Each cells has chromosome in one set and corresponding chromosome in the other set, for example, human cells have 46 chromosomes, comprising 23 homologous pairs.

With this variation in chromosome structure, the number of chromosomes in each organism, (otherwise called as ploidy level) also varies. Double the dose of a genome (haploidy (n) - single set of chromosomes) is expected as the normal ploidy level and the ploidy of an organism having two sets of chromosomes is called as **diploid (2n)**. The organisms having chromosome numbers deviating from the diploid numbers, are heteroploid. Organisms are classified as diploids and polyploids depending upon their chromosomes number (Table 11.3).

DNA sequences can be divided into three groups depending on the number of times a sequence appears in the genome.

1. **Low or single copy DNA:** These are sequences encoding most enzyme functions. In general, these can constitute upto 50 per cent of the total DNA.

Table 11.3. Various Ploidy Level in Eukaryotes

Diploids	Individuals having chromosomes double the number of haploidy
Heteroploids	Individuals with chromosomes deviating the diploid number
Polyploids	Individuals with chromosomes multiples of haploid number, but more than diploid number (*3n, 4n, 5n...*)
Aneuploids	Individuals with chromosomes deviating from the exact multiples of the basic number (*x+1, x+2, x-1, x-2*)

2. **Middle repeat DNA:** These sequences code for most of the structural components of a cell. Thirty to forty per cent of the genome may comprise middle repeat DNA
3. **Highly repetitious DNA:** This is simple sequence DNA and is frequently non-coding. In mammals, this can constitute 20-50 per cent of the genome, but in many plants this figure can exceed upto 80 per cent (In general, DNA in the genome is arranged with single copy sequences interspersed with either repetitive or middle repeat DNA)

The complexity of any genome is assessed based on the proportion of above-mentioned sequences. Some sequences present in DNA are said to be mobile. These mobile elements are known as transposons. These are able to excise from one locus and inserted into another locus thus making inactivation of active genes.

Microsatellites

Microsatellites are also known as **Short Tandem Repeats (STR)or Simple Sequence Repeats (SSR)**, because a repeat unit consists of only **1 to 6 bp** and the whole repetitive region spans less than **150 bp**. Similar to minisatellites, the number of repeats for a given microsatellite may differ between individuals. Therefore, microsatellites can also be used for DNA fingerprinting. In addition, both microsatellite and minisatellite patterns can provide information about paternity.

Minisatellites

The size of a minisatellite ranges from **1 kb to 20 kb**. One type of minisatellites is called Variable Number of Tandem Repeats(VNTR). **Its repeat unit ranges from 9 bp to 80 bp**. They are located in non-coding regions, and thus the number of repeats for a given minisatellite may differ between individuals. This feature was first discovered by **A. J. Jeffreys in 1985**, and used for DNA fingerprinting (= DNA profiling/DNA typing), which has found many applications.

Repetitive DNA Sequences are just a junk?

- ☆ The existence of large amounts of repetitive DNA sequences in eukaryotes led to explore their role in eukaryotic genome organization and expression. In humans, up to 97 per cent of the genome remains as repetitive DNA which are non-coding.
- ☆ The recent studies indicated that the repetitive DNA sequences have some major role in genome organization and gene expression.
- ☆ The repetitive DNA sequences bind nuclear proteins and show characteristics of a specific DNA-protein interaction. What functions these DNA-protein interactions exhibit has not been determined.

Major Difference in Prokaryotes and Eukaryotes Genome Organization

A major difference between prokaryotic and eukaryotic cells is that a eukaryote has a nuclear envelope,which surrounds the genetic material to form a nucleus and separates the DNA from the other cellular contents. In prokaryotic cells, the genetic material is in close contact with other components of the cell, a property that has important consequences for the way in which genes are controlled.

Another fundamental difference between prokaryotes and eukaryotes lies in the packaging of their DNA. In eukaryotes, DNA is closely associated with a special class of proteins, the histones, to form tightly packed chromosomes. This complex of DNA and histone proteins is termed chromatin, which is the stuff of eukaryotic chromosomes. Histone proteins limit the accessibility of enzymes and other proteins that copy and read the DNA but they enable the DNA to fit into the nucleus. Eukaryotic DNA must separate from the histones before the genetic information in the DNA can be accessed.

Table 11.4. Difference in Prokaryotes and Eukaryotes Genome Organization

Sl.No.	*Characteristic*	*Prokaryotes*	*Eukaryotes*
1	Genome	Usually one circular DNA molecule	Usually several linear DNA molecule
2	Location of Genetic information	Nuclear area (Nucleoid) (region where the genome present)	Membrane bound nucleus
3	Genome size	600kb to 9.5 Mb	3 Mb to 140000 Mb
4	Amount of DNA	Relatively small	Relatively large
5	DNA	Not complexed with histone in eubacteria; some histones in archaea	complexed with histones
6	Nucleolus	Absent	Present
7	Average gene size/ number	950bp/4300	2500bp/19000

Sl.No.	*Characteristic*	*Prokaryotes*	*Eukaryotes*
8	Extra chromosal DNA	In plasmids	In mitochondria, chloroplasts
9	Operon-like regulatory unit	General	No
11	Rate of non-coding sequences	Low	High
13	Intron	Rare	General
15	Ploidy level	Haploidy	Haploidy to Polyploidy
16	Chromosome number	One	More than one
17	Genetic information	Found in single chromosome	In paired chromosome

However, prokaryotes do not possess histones, so their DNA does not exist in the highly ordered, tightly packed arrangement as found in eukaryotic cells. The copying and reading of DNA are therefore simpler processes in prokaryotes. Genes of prokaryotic cells are generally on a single, circular molecule of DNA, the chromosome of the prokaryotic cell. In eukaryotic cells, genes are located on multiple, usually linear DNA molecules. But some important bacterial genes are frequently found on other DNA molecules called plasmids. Furthermore, in some eukaryotes, a few genes are located on circular DNA molecules found outside the nucleus (Table 11.4).

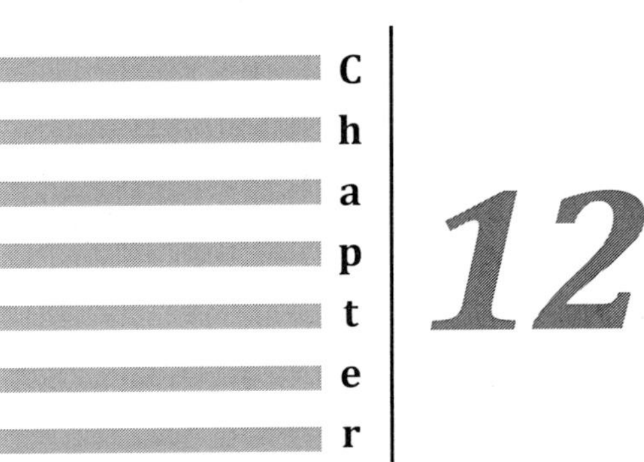

Central Dogma of Life: Structure of Nucleic Acids

The Central Dogma

Central dogma of genetics, involves information flow from DNA to RNA via transcription in the nucleus, followed by RNA transport into the cytoplasm, where it is translated into protein (Figure 12.1). **Central Dogma** concept was put forward by Francis Crick (a physicist) in 1958. The Central Dogma of molecular biology is that DNA directs its own **replication** and its **transcription** to yield RNA which, in turn, directs its **translation** to form proteins.

The Central Dogma of Molecular Biology

The Central Dogma sets out a hierarchy of information. DNA is the information store because both strands contain a complete set of information. During replication both DNA strands can act as templates for the generation of two daughter double helix that is identical to the parent. When this information is used to direct the synthesis of a protein, the relevant section of DNA is copied into messenger RNA through the transcription process. This contains the same information but in a form of mRNA that can be read by the protein synthesis machinery. Finally, a protein is produced by concatenating amino acids according to the sequence specified by the mRNA (Translation). These dominant processes correspond to the solid arrows in Figure 12.2.

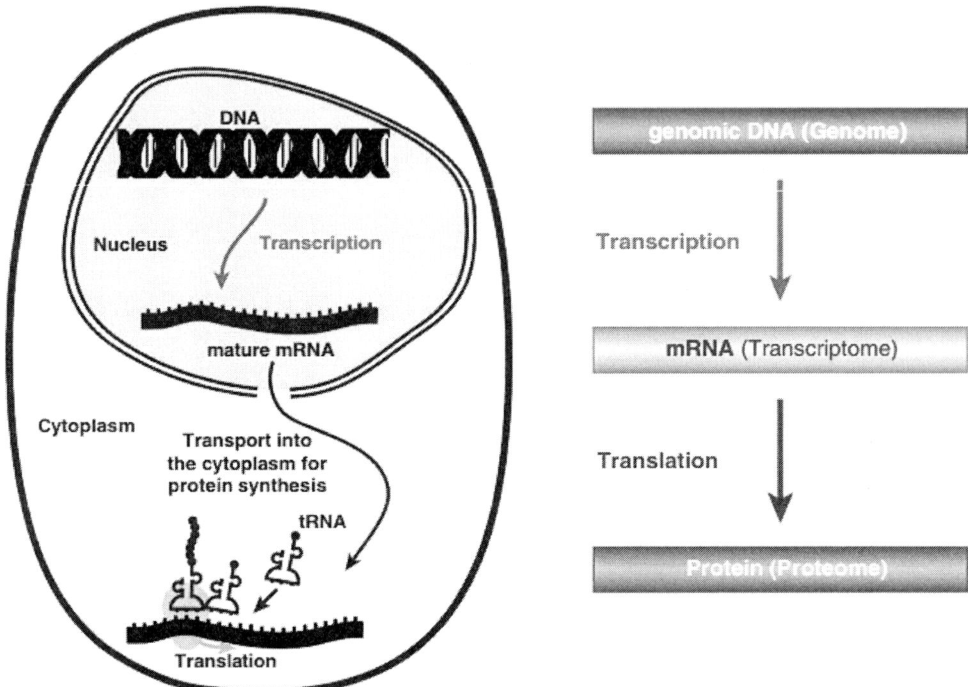

Figure 12.1. Concept of Central Dogma.

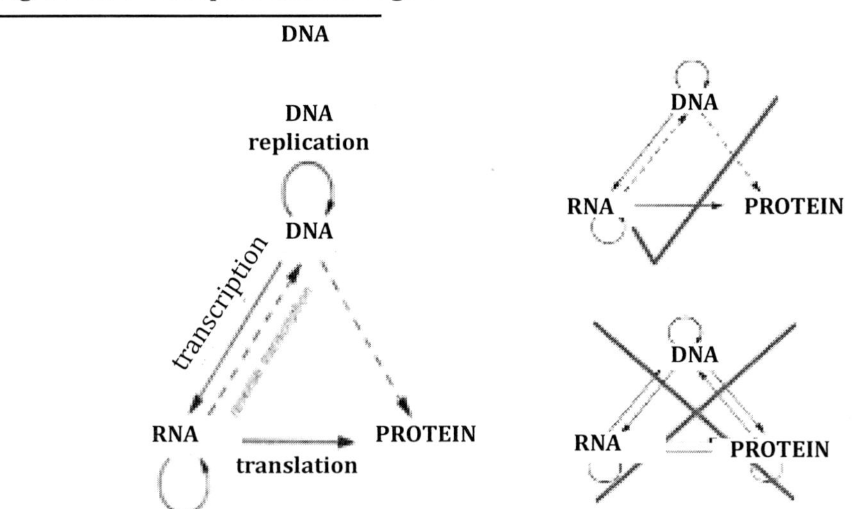

Figure 12.2. DNA makes RNA makes Proteins.

Some viruses store genetic information in RNA, and use an enzyme called reverse transcriptase to make a DNA copy from the RNA in order to make use of the protein synthesis machinery of the infected cell, this involves information flow in the opposite direction to the normal process. Some RNA viruses and plants have RNA-directed RNA polymerases, as the name implies, they can replicate RNA directly. There is no known process in which DNA is used directly to determine protein synthesis but this would not invalidate the Central Dogma. What is important is the absence of certain arrows: proteins never direct the synthesis of DNA or RNA (Figure 12.2).

Structure of Nucleic Acids

Nucleic acids are large biomolecules, essential for all known forms of life. Nucleic acids, which include DNA (Deoxyribonucleic acid) and RNA (Ribonucleic acid), are made from monomers known as **nucleotides**. In biological systems, they serve as information-carrying molecules.

Bases, Nucleosides and Nucleotides

Nucleotides are the building blocks of all nucleic acids. Nucleotides have a distinctive structure composed of three components covalently bound together (Figure 12.3).

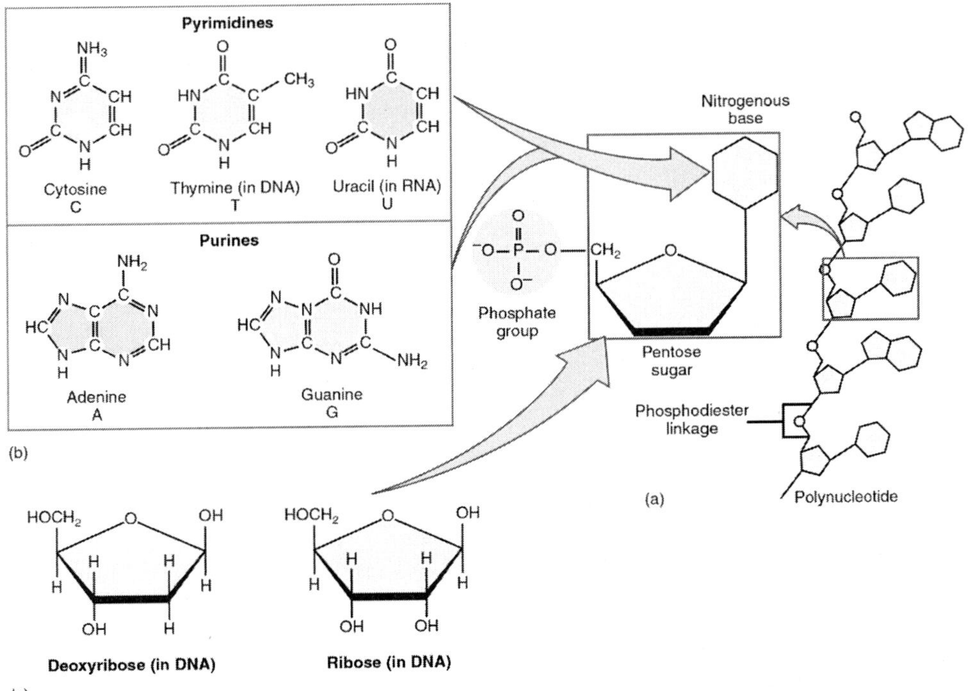

Figure 12.3. a. Nucleotide; b. Nitorgenous Bases; c. Pentose Sugar of DNA and RNA.

- A nitrogen-containing "base" either a pyrimidine (one ring) or purine (two rings)
- A 5-carbon sugar - ribose or 2'- deoxyribose sugar
- A phosphate group

5-carbon Sugar (Pentose sugar)

In DNA molecule, 2' carbon atom of pentose sugar contain only 'H' that lacks the oxygen (O) atom, so this is called as 2-deoxy ribose suger. In case of RNA, 2' carbon atom pentose sugar contain OH group so this sugar is called ribose sugar.

Nitrogenous Bases - In DNA, there are four heterocyclic bases: **adenine (A)** and **guanine (G)**are purines; **cytosine (C)** and **thymine (T)** are pyrimidines. In RNA, thymine is replaced by the structurally very similar pyrimidine, **uracil (U)** **(Figure 12.4)**.

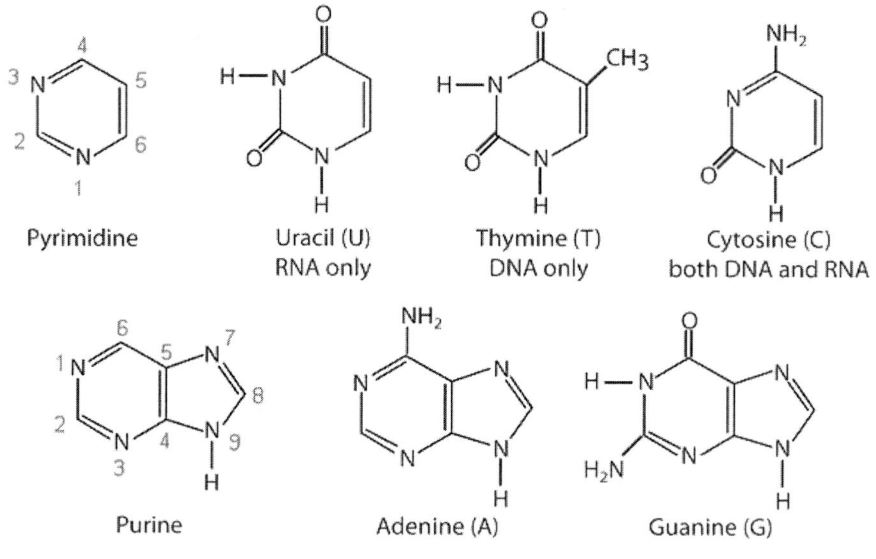

Pyrimidine

Uracil (U)
RNA only

Thymine (T)
DNA only

Cytosine (C)
both DNA and RNA

Purine

Adenine (A)

Guanine (G)

Figure 12.4. Nitrogenous Bases of DNA and RNA.

The combination of a base and sugar is called a **nucleoside.** The bond between the bases and the sugars is the glycosylic bond. In DNA the sugar is 2'-deoxyribose and the compounds are 2'-deoxyribonucleosides, whereas in RNA the sugar is ribose, and the nucleosides are named ribonucleosides.

A **nucleotide** is a nucleoside with a phosphate group (base+sugar+phosphate) covalently bound to it. If the sugar is 2'-deoxyribose, then the nucleotide is called a **2'-deoxynucleotide**; if the sugar is ribose, the nucleotide is a **ribonucleotide** (Table 12.1).

Table 12.1. The Bases and their Corresponding Nucleosides and Nucleotides

Base	*Abbr.*	*Nucleoside*	*Nucleotide*	*Nucleic Acid*
Adenine	**A**	Deoxyadenosine	Deoxyadenosine monophosphate	DNA
		Adenosine	Adenosine monophosphate	RNA
Guanine	**G**	Deoxyguanosine	Deoxyguanosine monophosphate	DNA
		Guanosine	Guanosine monophosphate	RNA
Cytosine	**C**	Deoxycytidine	Deoxycytidine monophosphate	DNA
		Cytidine	Cytidine monophosphate	RNA
Thymine	**T**	Deoxythymidine	Deoxythymidine monophosphate	DNA
Uracil	**U**	Uridine	Uridine monophosphate	RNA

The nucleotides are joined to one another in a chain by **phosphodiester linkage** between the sugar of one nucleotide and the phosphate of the next, resulting in a "sugar-phosphate backbone". The polarity of the nucleic acids showing two distinctive ends: the 5′ and 3′ ends is mentioned as 5′ → 3′ based on the moieties at the 5′ and 3′ carbons of the sugar molecule (Figure 12.5**)**. The 5' carbon has an attached phosphate group, while the 3′ carbon has a hydroxyl group. The sequence of the four bases along the backbone encodes biological information.

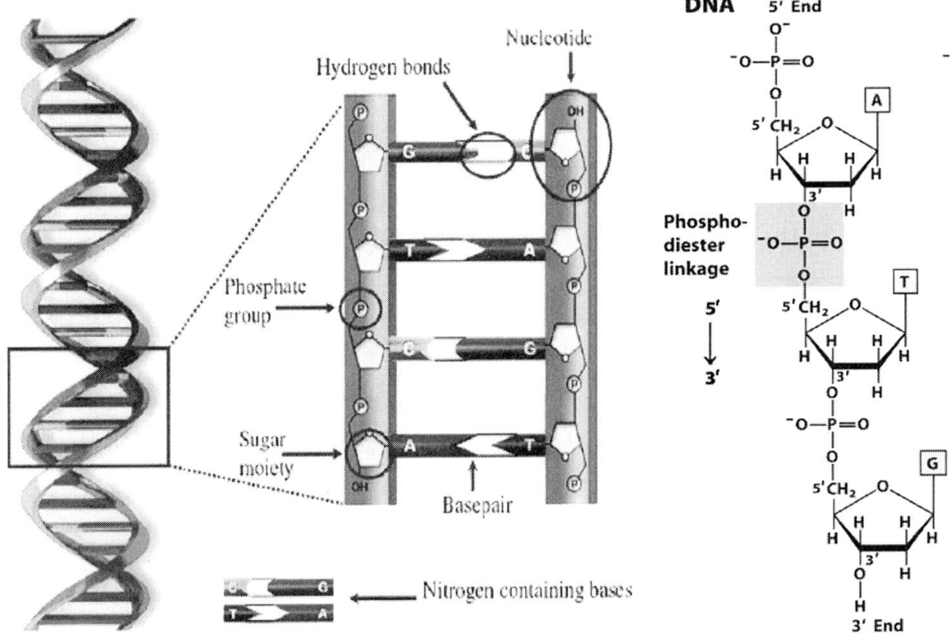

Figure 12.5. Structure and Backbone of DNA Strand.

Double Helical Structure of DNA

DNA stands for Deoxyribo Nucleic Acid which is a molecule that contains the instructions an organism needs to develop, live and reproduce. These instructions are found inside every cell and are passed down from parents to their progeny. It is a nucleic acid and is one of the four major types of macromolecules that are known to be essential for all forms of life. DNA is found in the nucleus, with a small amount of DNA also present in mitochondria in the eukaryotes. The most widely accepted model for the structure of DNA molecule was proposed by **Watson and Crick in 1953 (Nobel Prize for Medicine in 1962).** According to their model, the DNA has the following structural characteristics.

- ✰ The DNA molecule is a double helix.
- ✰ The molecule is formed by two separate antiparallel polynucleotide strands which are spirally coiled round each other in a right-handed helix. One strand runs in 5′ → 3′ while other one runs in 3′ → 5′.
- ✰ The two strands are held together by **hydrogen bonds**.
- ✰ The double stranded helical molecule has alternate major (or deep) and minor grooves. DNA binding proteins attach to these grooves.
- ✰ It is 20 Å (2 nm) wide and extends 34 Å (3.4 nm) per 10 bp of sequence and each base with 0.34 nm.
- ✰ The double helix makes one complete turn about its axis every 10.4-10.5 base pairs.
- ✰ The two strands are complementary to each other with regards to the arrangement of the bases in the two strands.
- ✰ **The purines and pyrimidines exist in base pairs *i.e.* (A with T) and (G with C). G-C base pairs have 3 hydrogen bonds, whereas A-T base pairs have 2 hydrogen bonds** (Figure 12.6).
- ✰ Sum of purines (A and G) always equal with sum of pyrimidines (C and T) called stoichiometric equality (Chargaff's rule)
- ✰ Adenine is always equivalence with Thymine and Cytosine with Guanine
- ✰ AT type : Sum of A + T is larger than the sum of G+C
- ✰ CG type : sum of C + G is larger than the sum of A + T (More common in micro organisms)

Forms of DNA

- ✰ A number of different forms of nucleic acid double helix have been observed and studied, all having the basic pattern of two helically-woundanti parallel strands. They are A-DNA, B-DNA and the Z-DNA. The structure identified by Watson and Crick, and described above, is known as B-DNA.

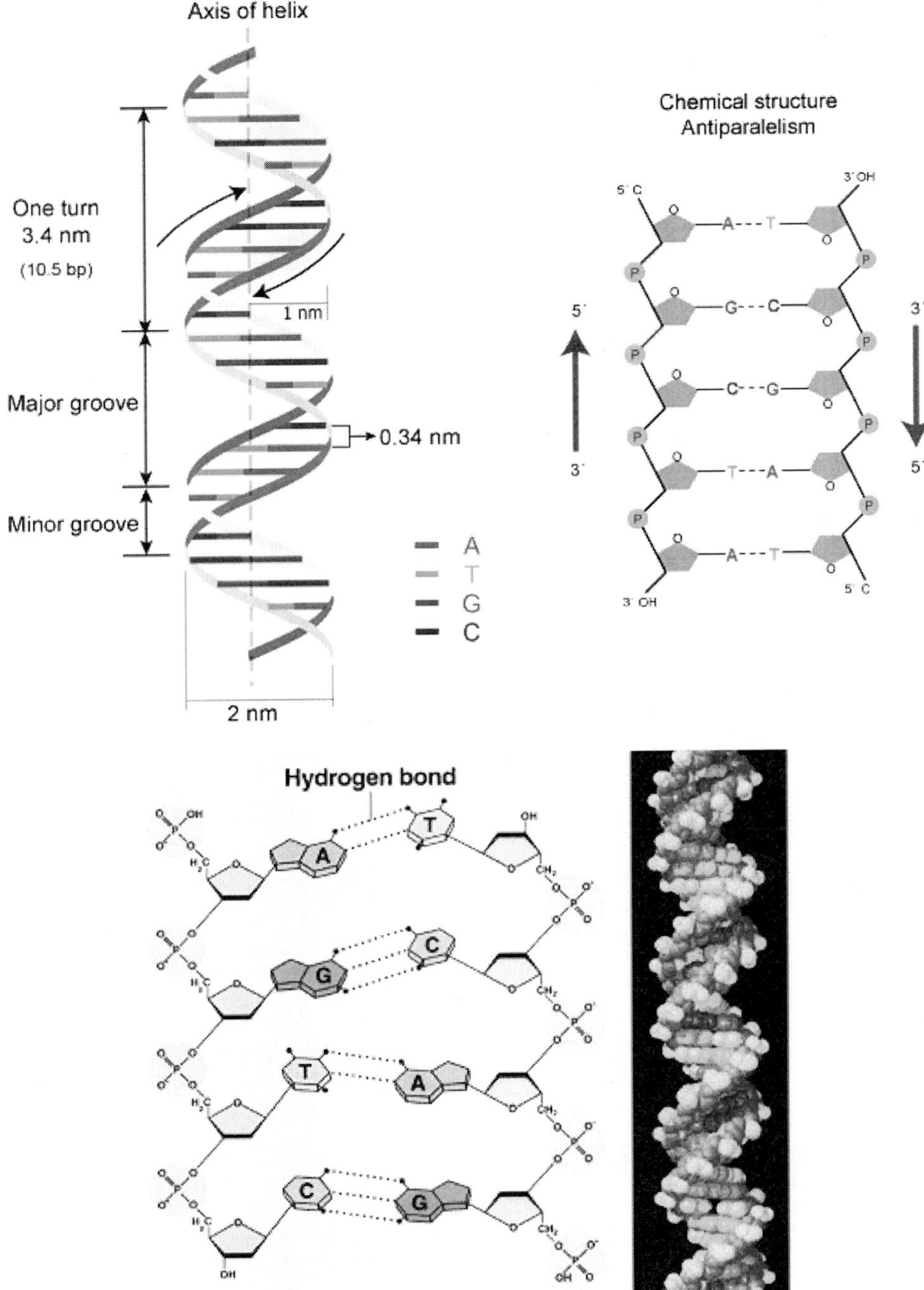

Figure 12.6. Double Helical Structure of DNA.

- A-DNA is the helix formed by RNA-RNA, and by DNA-RNA hybrids having a shorter, wider helix than B. The diameteris about 26 Åand has 11 base pairs per helical turn
- C-DNA is one of the many possible double helical structures of DNA. Right-handed with the axial rise of 3.32A° per base pair. 33 base pairs per turn. Formed at 66 per cent relative humidity and in presence of Li+ and Mg^{2+} ions. Has a diameter of 19 A°, smaller than that of A and B DNA. This form of DNA is not very stable and not very common
- Z-DNA is a relatively rare left-handed double-helix. Given the proper sequence and superhelical tension, it can be formed *in vivo* but its function is unclear. It has a more narrow, more elongated helix than A or B. The most obvious distinction is the left-handed helical rotation.

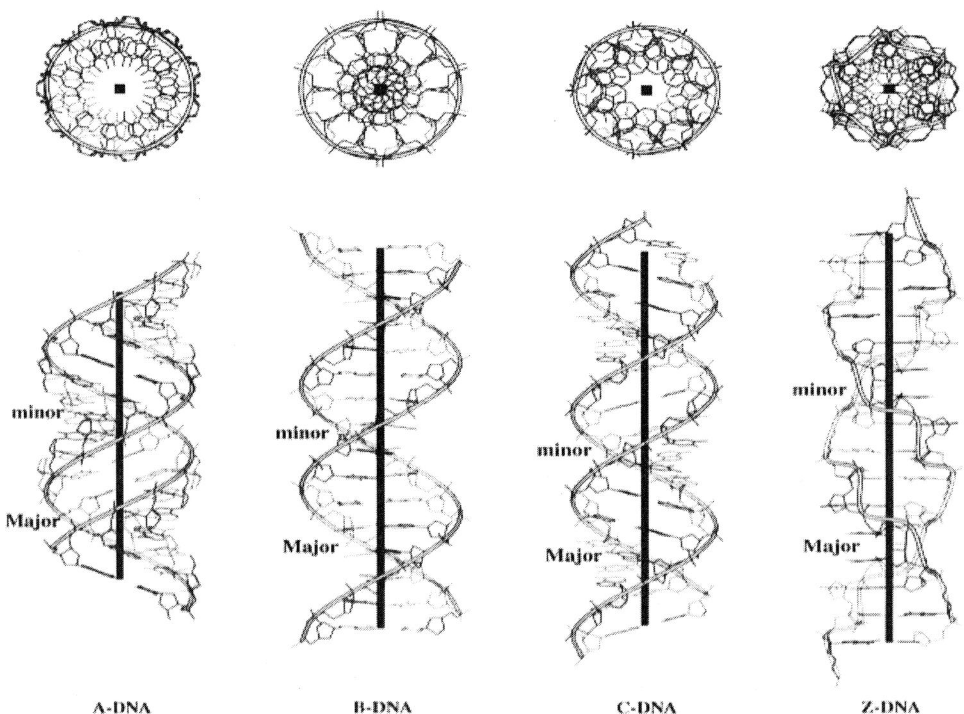

Figure12.7. Different Form of DNA Exist in Biological Organism.

Ribonucleic Acid (RNA)

Ribonucleic acids (RNA) are biological molecules that perform multiple vital roles in the coding, decoding, regulation, and expression of genes. Like DNA, RNA is assembled as a chain of nucleotides, but is usually single-stranded. RNA contains ribose sugar molecule. The complementary nitrogenous base to adenine (A) is uracil (U) (Figure 12.8).

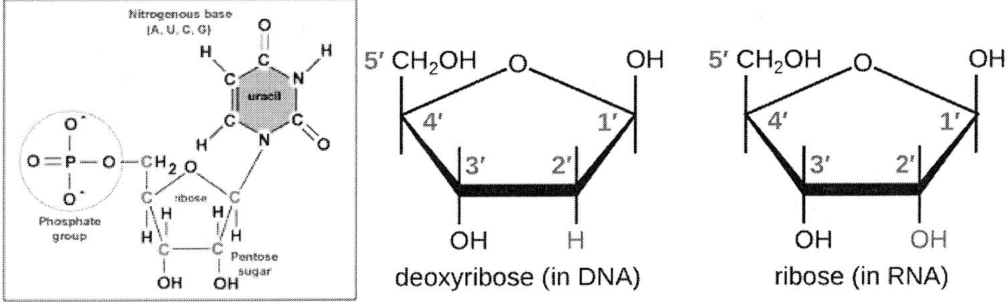

Figure 12.8. Structure of a Ribonucleotide and a Ribose Sugar.

Structure of RNA

Like **DNA**, RNA is a long polymer consisting of nucleotides (Figure 12.9).

- RNA is a single-stranded helix.
- The strand has a 5′ end (with a phosphate group) and a 3′ end (with a hydroxyl group).
- It is composed of ribonucleotides.
- The ribonucleotides are linked together by $5' \rightarrow 3'$ phosphodiester bonds.
- The nitrogenous bases that compose the ribonucleotides include adenine (A), guanine (G), uracil (U) and cytosine (C). Thus **thymine in DNA is replaced by uracil in RNA**, a different pyrimidine. However, like thymine, uracil can form base pairs with adenine.
- The sugar in RNA is ribose rather than deoxyribose as in DNA.
- The corresponding ribonucleosides are adenosine, guanosine, cytidine and uridine. The corresponding ribonucleotides are adenosine 5'-triphosphate (ATP), guanosine 5'-triphosphate (GTP), cytidine 5'-triphosphate (CTP) and uridine 5'-triphosphate (UTP).

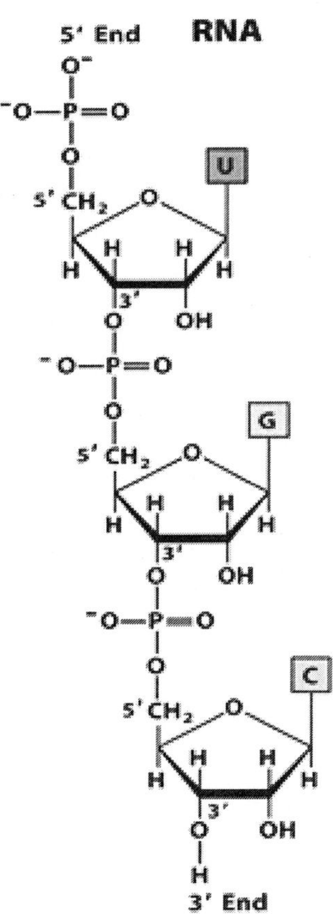

Figure 12.9. Structure of a RNA Strand.

RNAs form globular conformations in which local helical structures are formed by intra-molecular hydrogen bonding base stacking with in the single nucleic acid chain. These regions can form where one part of the RNA chain is complementary to another. This conformational variability is reflected in the more diverse forms and roles of RNA (mRNA, tRNA, rRNA, siRNA, *etc.,*) in the cell, when compared with DNA.

Types of RNA

1. Genetic RNA; 2. Non-genetic RNA

1. Genetic RNA

Some of the virus particle is not having DNA. So those having either single strand or double strand RNA as a genetic material *e.g.,* Tobacco Mosaic Viruses

2. Non-genetic RNA

The non genetic RNA is synthesised form DNA of respective genes and all are involved in protein synthesis. There are three major types.

i) Messanger RNA (mRNA)
ii) Ribosomal RNA (rRNA)
iii) Transfer RNA (tRNA)

i) Messenger RNA (mRNA)

It constitutes a small fraction (5-10 per cent) of the total RNA present in the cell. Most heterogeneous of the 3 types of RNA in terms of both base sequence and size. They are short lived M.W. 5,00,000 to 20,00,000. mRNA's are synthesised in nucleus during transcription from one strand of DNA. **The enzyme is used to synthesize mRNA is RNA polymerase II.** It carries the genetic code copied from the DNA during transcription in the form of triplets of nucleotides called codons. It takes part in protein synthesis. Since it brings the message of protein synthesis from DNA, it is called as messenger RNA.As part of post-transcriptional processing in eukaryotes, the 5' end of mRNA is capped with a guanosine triphosphate nucleotide, which helps in mRNA recognition during translation or protein synthesis. Similarly, the 3' end of an mRNA has a poly A tail or multiple adenylate residues added to it, which prevent enzymatic degradation of mRNA. Both 5' and 3' end of an mRNA imparts stability to the mRNA (Figure 12.10).

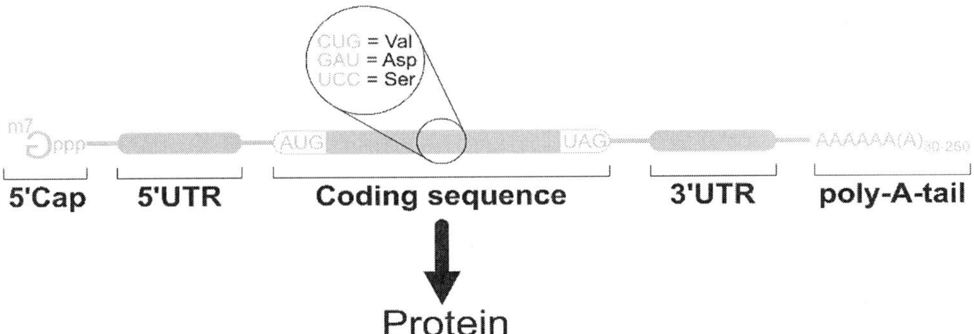

Figure 12.10. Structure of mRNA Strand.

ii) Ribosomal RNA (rRNA)

It is normally found in the ribosomes along with ribosomal proteins and account for **85-90 per cent** of the total RNA present in the cell. Ribosomes consist of two major components: the small ribosomal subunits, which read the RNA, and the large subunits, which join amino acids to form a polypeptide chain. rRNA is the most stable type of RNA. The eukaryotic ribosome is composed of two subunits: a large subunit (60S) and a small subunit (40S). The 60S subunit is composed of the 28S rRNA, 5.8S rRNA, 5S rRNA, and 50 proteins. The 40S subunit is composed of the 18S rRNA and 33 proteins. The bacterial ribosome is composed of two similar subunits, with slightly different components. The bacterial large subunit is called the 50S subunit and is composed of the 23S rRNA, 5S rRNA, and 31 proteins, while the bacterial small subunit is called the 30S subunit and is composed of the 16S rRNA and 21 proteins. rRNA take part in translation process of protein synthesis (Figure 12.11).**The synthesizing enzyme of rRNA is RNA polymerase I**.

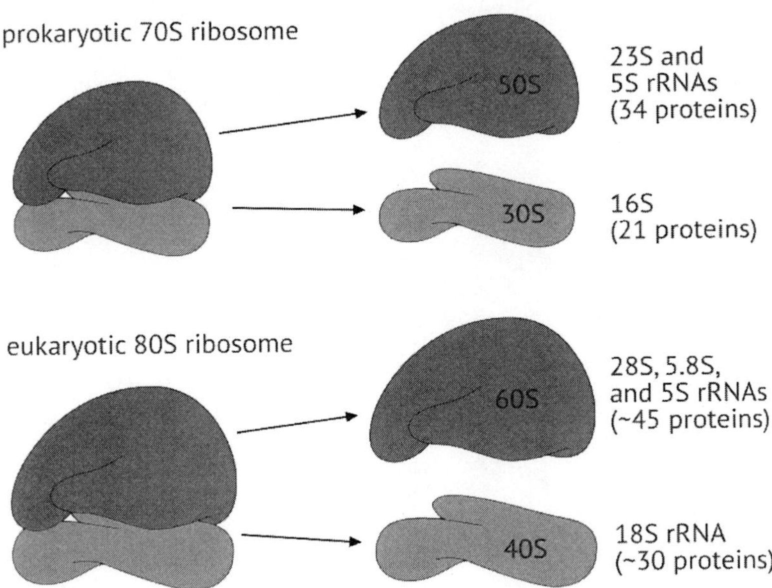

Figure 12.11. Structure Eukaryotic Ribosomes and rRNA Composition.

iii) Transfer RNA (tRNA)

tRNA is the smallest of the 3 types of RNA having about 75-95 nucleotides. Transfer RNA brings or transfers amino acids to the ribosome that correspond to each three-nucleotide codon of rRNA. The amino acids then can be joined together and processed to make polypeptides and proteins. Therefore they are called transfer RNA (tRNA). Each of the 20 amino acids has a specific tRNA that binds with it and transfers it to the growing polypeptide chain. tRNAs also act as adapters in the translation of the genetic sequence of mRNA into proteins. Therefore they are also called adapter molecules. tRNAs have a **clover leaf structure** which is stabilized by strong hydrogen bonds between the nucleotides. Apart from the usual 4 bases, they normally contain some unusual bases mostly formed by methylation of the usual bases, for example, methyl guanine and methylcytosine (Figure 12.12). **The synthesizing enzyme of tRNA is RNA polymerase III.**

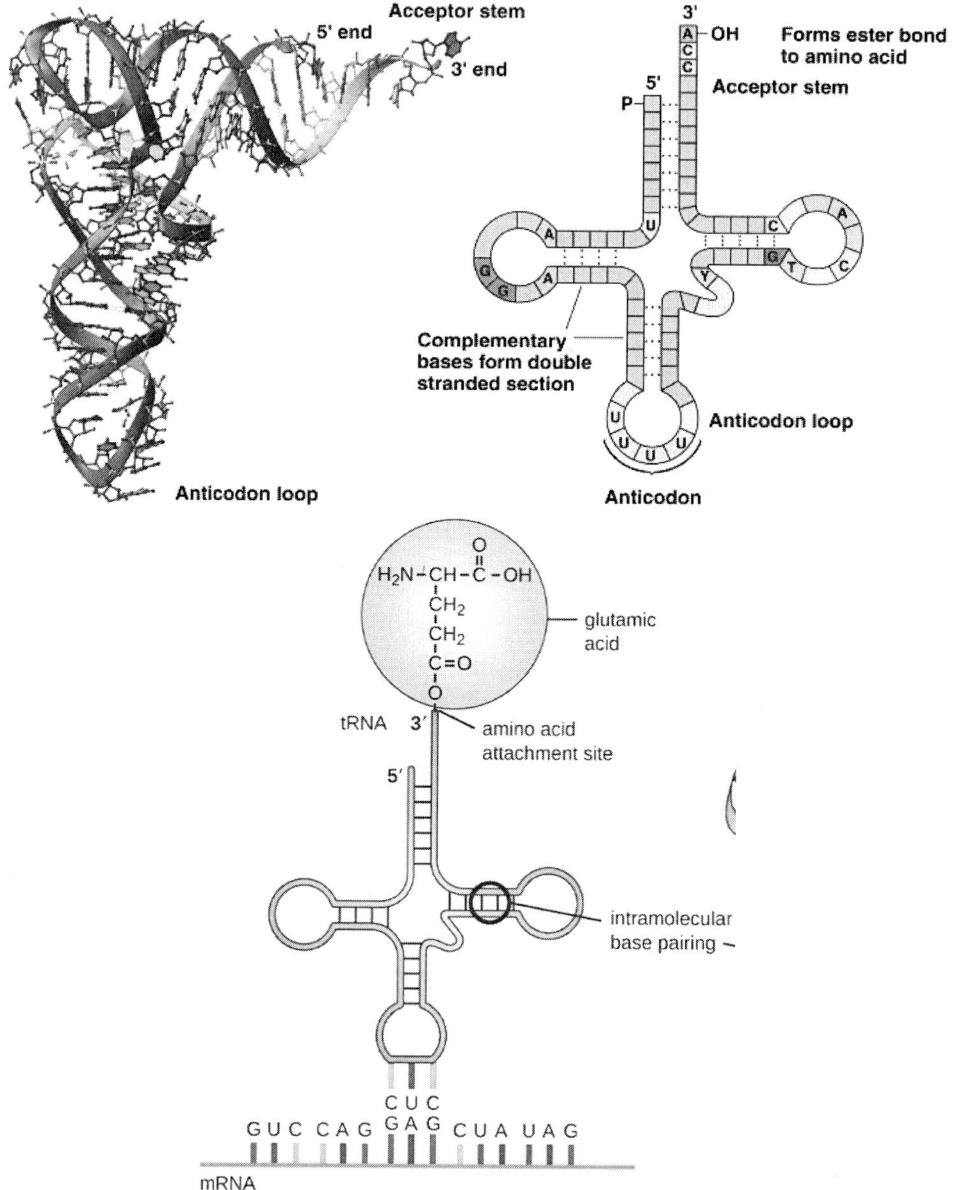

Figure 12.12. Conformation of tRNA (Transfer RNA).

Globular Conformation of tRNA (Transfer RNA)

Characteristics

1. All tRNA's have unusual bases such as methyladenine, methylcytosine, Ribothynine *etc.* due to methylation of normal bases.
2. It passes DNA like double helical stricture by A:U and C:G near unity.
3. All tRNA's require Mg for stabilization.
4. All tRNA's have Guanine base at the 5th terminal end. The single stranded portion contains CCA at 3' end. Amino acid is attached at this 3' end.
5. Amino acids are attracted at the terminal and with adenine (CCA end)
6. It attracts on a place on mRNA during translation process.
7. It will liberate the amino acid in favour of other amino acid by forming peptide bond in the presence of the enzyme peptidyl transferase.

Table 12.2. Difference between DNA and RNA

Parameters	*DNA*	*RNA*
Full Name	Deoxyribonucleic acid	Ribonucleic acid
Structure	Double stranded helix	Single stranded
Sugar	Deoxyribose	Ribose
Nitrogenous Bases	Adenine Thymine Guanine Cytosine	Adenine Uracil Guanine Cytosine
Base pairing	Adenine – Thymine Guanine – Cytosine	Adenine – Uracil Guanine - Cytosine
Propagation	Self-replicating	Synthesized from DNA

Functions of RNA

- RNA is a nucleic acid messenger between DNA and ribosomes.
- It serves as the genetic material in some organisms (viruses).
- Some RNA molecules play an active role within cells by catalyzing biological reactions, controlling gene expression, or sensing and communicating responses to cellular signals.
- Messenger RNA (mRNA) copies DNA in the nucleus and carries the info to the ribosomes (in cytoplasm).
- Ribosomal RNA (rRNA) makes up a large part of the ribosome; reads and decodes mRNA.

- Transfer RNA (tRNA) carries amino acids to the ribosome where they are joined to form proteins.
- Certain RNAs are able to catalyse chemical reactions such as cutting and ligating other RNA molecules, and the catalysis of peptide bond formation in the ribosome; these are known as ribozymes.

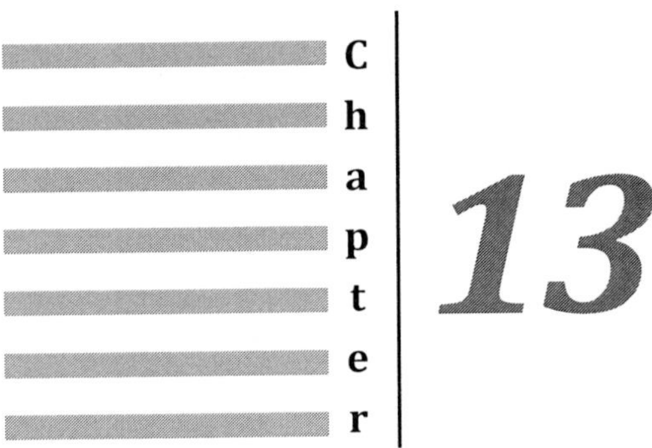

DNA Replication

The mechanisms that make life possible depend on the structure of the double-stranded DNA molecule. **DNA replication is the process in which, each strand of the existing DNA molecule acts as a template for the production of new strand, and the sequence of nucleotides of the synthesized (growing) strand is determined by base complementarity.** This mechanism of DNA replication is called **semiconservative replication**, because each of the strands of the parental double helix is conserved (or the double helix is half-conserved) during the process.

Small chromosomes, such as those of bacteria and viruses, replicate as single units called **replicons**. Replication begins from a unique site, the origin of replication. Large eukaryotic chromosomes contain multiple replicons, each with its own origin, which fuse as they replicate. All origins contain AT-rich sequences where the strands initially separate. AT-rich regions are more easily opened than GC-rich regions. The genome is actively protected molecular machines continually scan DNA, comparing the complementary strands to find copying errors and looking for damage caused by UV radiation and chemical mutagens. When errors are found, they are cut out and corrected.

Each sugar is linked to the next via the phosphate group, creating a polymer chain composed of a repetitive sugar-phosphate backbone with a series of bases protruding from it. The DNA polymer is extended by adding monomers **at one end normally its 3' end** because 3' end is having free OH group, it is necessary for the addition of the new nucleotide. The bases protruding from the existing strand bind to bases of the strand being synthesized, according to a strict rule defined by the complementary structures of the bases: **A binds to T and C binds to G**. This base-pairing holds fresh monomers in place and thereby controls the selection of which one of the four monomers shall be added to the growing strand next. In this way, a double-stranded structure is created, consisting of two exactly complementary sequences of As, Cs, Ts, and Gs. The two strands twist around each other, forming a double helix. The bonds between the base pairs are weak compared with the sugar-phosphate links, and this allows the two DNA strands to be pulled apart without breakage of their backbones. At the time of cell division each strand can serve as a template, to synthesis a fresh complementary DNA strand, in this way the hereditary information is multiplied and transferred from single parent cell to two daughter cells. In different types of cells, this process of DNA replication occurs at different rates.

Replication of DNA

1. Conservative method
2. Dispersive method
3. Semi conservative method.

1. Conservative Method

According to conservative model, during DNA replication two parental DNA strand act as template and directs synthesis of an entirely new double-stranded DNA molecule. After completion of replication, that parental *DNA* remains together and newly-formed daughter strands are together.

2. Dispersive Method

Old molecule disintegrates in the process of replication and two molecules are synthesised. The method suggests that replication involves the fragmentation of DNA molecule in such a way that new daughter molecule consists of sections of an old and new along with each strand. Both methods are not proved scientifically.

3. Semi-conservative Method

In the first stage, the two strands of DNA begins to uncoil at one end. The strands separate by breaking of 'H' bonds, between the bases. The two uncoiled strands act as a template for synthesizing new strands by adding appropriate complementary bases from the cytoplasmic pool of nucleotides. After completion of replication one double strand molecule is converted in to two, each double strand is consist of one parental strand and one daughter strand. This method of replication is called Semi-conservative method. This method is most accepted and supported by many experiments among one is Meselson and Stahl's experiment (Figure 13.1).

DNA Replication – Semi-Conservative Mechanism

It is the process of producing two identical replicas from one original DNA molecule. This biological process occurs in all living organisms and is the basis for biological inheritance. The key to the mechanism of DNA replication is the fact that each strand of the DNA double helix carries the same information because their base sequences are complementary. Thus, during replication, the two parental strands separate and each acts as a template to direct the enzyme-catalyzed synthesis of a new complementary daughter strand following the normal base pairing rules (A with T; G with C).

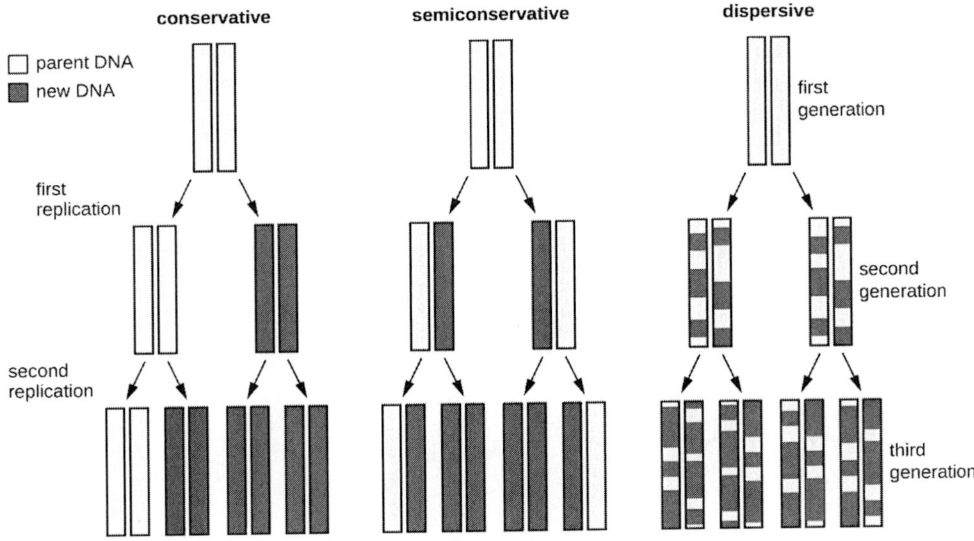

Figure 13.1. Semi-Conservative Mechanism of DNA Replication.

The two new double-stranded molecules then pass to the two daughter cells at cell division. The point at which separation of the strands and synthesis of new DNA takes place is known as the replication fork. **This semi-conservative mechanism was demonstrated experimentally in 1958 by Meselson and Stahl.**

Meselson and Stahl Experiment of DNA Replication

Three concepts were put forward to explain the replication process *i.e.*, Conservative, Semiconservative and Dispersive. But experimental evidence shown that DNA replication occurs based on semiconservative concept in living organisms. This was explained by Mathew Meselson and Franklin Stahl in the year 1958. Meselson and Stahl grew *Escherichia coli* cells for many generations in a medium in which ^{15}N (heavier) had been substituted for the normal ^{14}N (lighter). This made the bacterial DNA denser than normal because atoms of ^{15}N were used instead of the normal lighter ^{14}N atoms in all the nitrogenous bases of DNA. They then transferred the multiplying cells to fresh growth medium containing normal ^{14}N.

Semi-conservative Mechanism

During the cultivation period, they harvested bacteria at regular intervals for analysis. They assumed for each round of bacterial reproduction the DNA would be duplicated. They predicted that the DNA of cells grown on medium containing ^{15}N would have a greater density than the DNA of cells grown on medium containing ^{14}N.

These heavier and lighter molecules can be separated by Cesium Chloride Equilibrium Density Gradient Centrifugation. Meselson and Stahl observed that the DNA of the parental bacteria (grown on ^{15}N containing medium) was heavier. When these bacteria were transferred to ^{14}N containing medium, the DNA harvested from them was lighter than the DNA of the bacteria from ^{15}N containing medium. Subsequent culture of the first generation bacteria on ^{14}N containing medium and the analysis of DNA from them indicated that there were two types of DNA molecules-one having the density similar to the first generation bacteria and the other lighter than the DNA of both parental and first generation bacteria. The following table summarises the results of Meselson and Stahl experiment conducted for establishing that the DNA replication is semiconservative (Figure 13.2).

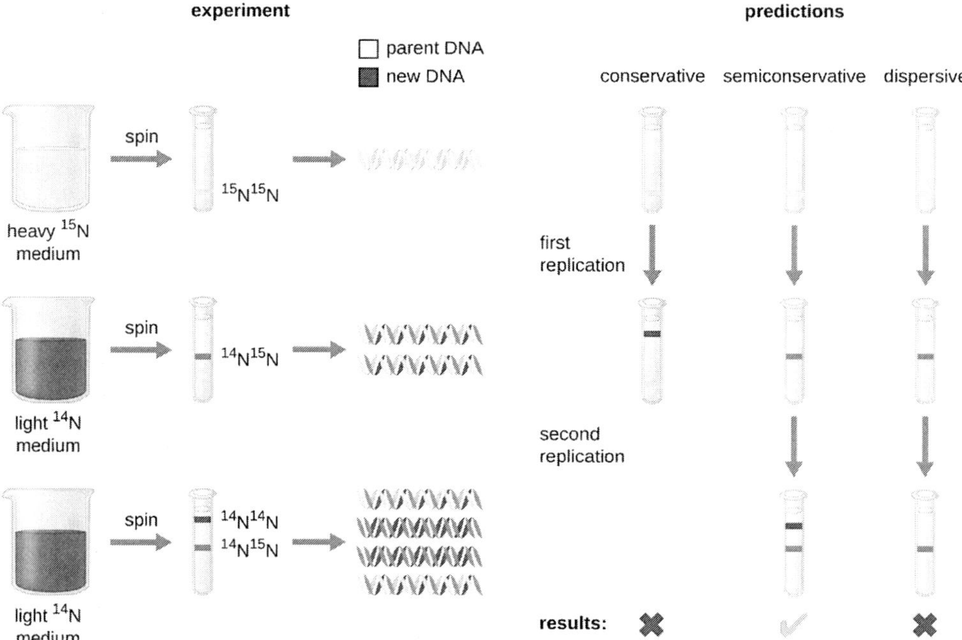

Figure 13.2. Semi-Conservative Mechanism Experiment.

From the above experiment, Meselson and Stahl concluded that during the replication of the DNA each parent DNA strand was serving as a template for a new, complementary DNA strand, which thencombined with the parent DNA strand to form a double helix. The method of DNA replication determined by Meselson and Stahl has been termed semisconservative because one strand of the original DNA (semi) is brought over (conserved) to each new double helix.

1. Topoisomerases

Topoisomerases are groups of enzymes concerned with breaking and resealing of DNA strand. These can be of two types: (i) Type I which makes break in only one strand of DNA and (ii) Type II which makes the break in both strands of DNA. In prokaryotes, type I enzyme was originally called omega protein and it relaxes only negatively super coiled strand of DNA but in eukaryotes, it can relax both negative as well as positive super coils. Type II isomerases have similar mode of action both in prokaryotes and eukaryotes.

Table 13.1. Enzymes Involved in DNA Replication

Sl.No.	*Enzyme*	*Function*
1	**Topoisomerase**	Changing the super helical nature of DNA
2	**Helicase**	Unwinding and separating of parental strands
3	**Single Strand Binding proteins**	Stabilize the unwound template or parental DNA
4	**DNA Polymerase**	Catalyzing the connection of nucleotides to form new DNA strand in 5' to 3' direction
5	**Primase**	Synthesis of the RNA primer
6	**DNA Ligase**	Joining the Okazaki fragments
7	**RNAse H**	Destruction of the used RNA primer

2. Helicase

Unwinding and separating of parental strands of DNA in to two separate strands and make the way for DNA replication

3. Single Strand Binding Proteins (Unwinding and single strand binding proteins)

SSB protein stabilizes single stranded structure of DNA. M.W.=74,000. SS DNA is found in bacteriophages. During binding reactions, it extends rapidly covering the SS DNA for stabilization.

4. DNA Polymerase

DNA polymerases are a group of enzymes that are used to make copies of DNA templates, essentially used in DNA replication mechanisms. These enzymes make new copies of DNA from existing templates and also function by repairing the synthesized DNA to prevent mutations. **DNA polymerase catalyzes the formation of the phosphodiester bond which makes up the backbone of DNA molecules.** It uses a magnesium ion in catalytic activity to balance the charge from the phosphate group. The enzyme is found and used in the DNA replication of both prokaryotic and eukaryotic cells. Several types of DNA polymerase enzymes have been discovered with the first one to be discovered named **DNA polymerase I**. Each of these types plays a major role in replication and DNA repair mechanisms. However, DNA polymerases are not used for initiating the synthesis of new strands, but in the extension of already existing DNA or RNA strands which are paired with a template strand. DNA polymerase starts its mechanism after a short RNA fragment is known as a primer is created and paired with a template DNA strand.

DNA polymerase acts by synthesizing the new DNA strand by adding new nucleotides that match those of the template, extending towards the 3' end. Each nucleotide is linked with a phosphodiester bond. DNA polymerases are very accurate in their mechanism with minimal errors of less than one error for every 10^7 nucleotides. Some types of DNA polymerase have the ability to proofread and remove unmatched bases of nucleotides and correct them. Prokaryotes containing three major type of DNA polymerase those are DNA polymerase I II III. Where as the eukaryotic cell contains five DNA polymerase α, β, γ, δ, and ε. Polymerase γ is found in the cell mitochondria and it actively replicates the mitochondrial DNA, while polymerase α, β, δ are found in the cell nucleus hence are involved in the nuclear DNA replication.Polymerase α and δ are majorly applied and active in dividing cells hence involved in replication while polymerase β is active in both dividing and nondividing cells hence it is involved in the repair of DNA damage.

DNA Polymerase's Polymerization Activity

The enzyme requires the 5'- triphosphates of each of the four nucleotides (dATP, dTTP, dGTP and dCTP), Mg^{2+} and pre-existing DNA. This DNA should provide two essential components, one serving a primer function and the other a template function. The primer provides a terminus with a free 3'-OH to which nucleotides are added during DNA synthesis. DNA polymerase cannot initiate the synthesis of DNA *de novo*. It has an absolute requirement for 3'-hydroxyl on preexisting DNA chain. DNA polymerase catalyses the formation of a phophodiester bonds between the 3'-OH at the end of the primer DNA chain and the 5'phospahte of incoming deoxyribonucleotide. DNA polymerase requires a DNA template and short primer sequence to synthesize the new sreand. The template DNA provides the nucleotide sequence that specifies the complementary sequence of the new DNA chain.

DNA Polymerase's Exonuclease Activity

The main enzymatic activity of DNA polymerases is the **5' ⇒ 3'** synthetic activity. However, DNA polymerases possess two additional activities of importance for both replication and repair. These additional activities include a 5' ⇒ 3' exonuclease function and a 3' ⇒ 5' exonuclease function. The 5' ⇒ 3' exonuclease activity allows the removal of ribonucleotides of the RNA primer, utilized to initiate DNA synthesis, along with their simultaneous replacement with deoxyribonucleotides by the 5' ⇒ 3' polymerase activity. The 5' ⇒ 3' exonuclease activity is also utilized during the repair of damaged DNA. The 3' ⇒ 5' exonuclease function is utilized during replication to allow DNA polymerase to remove mismatched bases. It is possible (but rare) for DNA polymerases to incorporate an incorrect base during replication. These mismatched bases are recognized by the polymerase immediately due to the lack of Watson-Crick base-pairing. The mismatched base is then removed by the 3' ⇒ 5' exonuclease activity and the correct base inserted prior to progression of replication. **This process is called proof reading** of the DNA, necessary for conservation and maintaining of genetic purity from one generation to next generation.

Table 13.2. Different Types of DNA Polymerase Enzyme and its Property

Properties	*DNA Polymerase I*	*DNA Polymerase II*	*DNA Polymerase III*
Polymerase activity	Synthesizing short DNA strands in the place of RNA primer to fill the gap between Okazaki fragments in lagging strand during DNA replication.	Restart replication and synthesizing DNA strand after replication stops due to DNA strand damages.	It is responsible for the synthesis of new strands by adding nucleotides to the 32 -OH during replication
Exonuclease 5' -3'	Yes	No	No
Exonuclease 3' -5'	Yes	Yes	Yes (proof reading activity)

5. Primase

DNA polymerase need short neucleotide strand for initiating polymerization activity so this enzyme synthesis the short strand of RNA it act as a primer for starting replication

6. DNA Ligase

This enzyme is specifically used in joining the Okazaki fragments synthesised in a discontinuous DNA synthesis.

7. RNAse H

It is used to destruct the used RNA primer present in the DNA strand after completion of replication

Steps Involved in DNA Replication

Transient Breaking of DNA by Topoisomerases

During the unwinding of the DNA molecule (*E.coli* DNA spins around 3000 revolutions per minute to allow the unwinding) there is every possibility to form DNA supercoils. The formation of supercoils is prevented by the required axes of rotation (swivel) provided by enzymes called DNA topoisomerases. The topoisomerases catalyse the transient breaks in DNA molecules but use covalent linkages to themselves to hold on to the cleaved molecules.

Unwinding of DNA with Helicases

Semiconservative replication of DNA requires that the two strand of a parental DNA molecule be separated during the synthesis of new complementary strands. This separation needs an unwinding mechanism. The unwinding process is catalysed by enzymes called DNA helicases. DNA helicases unwind DNA molecules using energy derived ATP.

Binding of SSB Proteins

Once the DNA strands are unwound by DNA helicase, they must be kept in an extended single stranded form for replication. The binding of SSB proteins to single stranded DNA is cooperative; that is, the binding of the first SSB monomer stimulates the binding of additional monomers at contiguous sites on the DNA chain. Without the SSB protein binding, the complementary strands could renature of form intrastrand hairpin lops by hydrogen bonding between short segments of complementary nucleotide sequences.

RNA Priming and Formation of Primosomes

Once the replication fork has formed, the synthesis of new DNA strands is initiated by RNA primers synthesise by DNA primase. A single RNA primer is sufficient for the continuous replication of the leading strand, but the discontinous replication of the lagging strand requires an RNA primer to start the synthesis of each Okazaki fragment. The initiation of Okazaki fragments on the lagging strand is carried out by the primosome, a protein complex containing DNA primase and DNA helicase.

Formation of Replisomes

The complete replication apparatus that move along the replication fork is called replisome. The replisome contains the DNA polymerase III holoenzyme, one catalytic correreplicates the leading strand, the second catalytic core replicates the lagging strand, and the primosome unwinds the parental DNA molecule and synthesises the RNA primers needed for the discontinuous synthesis of the lagging strand.

Covalent Closure of Nicks by DNA Ligase

During the replication of the lagging strand, RNA primers are used. The DNA polymerase I replaces these RNA primers, and the **single strand breaks left by polymerase are sealed by DNA ligase.**

Mechanisms of DNA Replication

The process of DNA replication begins at specific sites in the chromosomes termed origins of replication, requires a primer bearing a free 3'-OH, proceeds specifically in the 5' ⇒ 3' direction on both strands of DNA concurrently and results in the copying of the template strands in a semiconservative manner. The semiconservative nature of DNA replication means that the newly synthesized daughter strands remain associated with their respective parental template strands. The large size of eukaryotic chromosomes and the limits of nucleotide incorporation during DNA synthesis, make it necessary for multiple origins of replication to exist in order to complete replication in a reasonable period of time. The precise nature of origins of replication in higher eukaryotic organisms is unclear. However, it is clear that at a replication origin the strands of DNA must dissociate and unwind in order to allow access to DNA polymerase. Unwinding of the duplex at the origin as well as along the strands as the replication process proceeds is carried out by helicases. The resultant regions of single-stranded DNA are stabilized by the binding of single-strand binding proteins. The stabilized single-stranded regions are then accessible to the enzymatic activities required for replication to proceed. The site of the unwound template strands is termed the replication fork.

Synthesis of DNA proceeds in the 5' ⇒ 3' direction through the attachment of the 5'-phosphate of an incoming dNTP to the existing 3'-OH in the elongating DNA strands with the concomitant release of pyrophosphate. Initiation of synthesis, at origins of replication, occurs simultaneously on both strands of DNA. Synthesis then proceeds bidirectionally, with one strand in each direction being copied continuously and one strand in each direction being copied discontinuously. During the process of DNA polymerases incorporating dNTPs into DNA in the 5' ⇒ 3' direction they are moving in the 3' ⇒ 5' direction with respect to the template strand. In order for DNA synthesis to occur simultaneously on both template strands as well as bidirectionally one strand appears to be synthesized in the 3' ⇒ 5' direction. In actuality one strand of newly synthesized DNA is produced discontinuously.

The strand of DNA synthesized continuously is termed the **leading strand** and the discontinuous strand is termed the **lagging strand**. The lagging strand of DNA is composed of short stretches of RNA primer plus newly synthesized DNA approximately 1000-2000 bases long (the approximate distance between adjacent nucleosomes). **The lagging strands of 1-2 kb long DNA are also called Okazaki fragments.** The concept of continuous strand synthesis is somewhat of a misnomer since DNA polymerases do not remain associated with a template strand indefinitely. The ability of a particular polymerase to remain associated with the template strand is termed its' processivity. The longer it associates the higher the processivity of the enzyme. DNA polymerase processivity is enhanced by additional protein activities of the replisome identified as processivity accessory proteins.

A model has been proposed where **DNA polymerases exist as dimers associated with the other necessary proteins at the replication fork and identified as the replisome.** The template for the lagging strand is temporarily looped through the replisome such that the DNA polymerases are moving along both strands in the 3' ⇒ 5' direction simultaneously for short distances, the distance of an Okazaki fragment. As the replication forks progress along the template strands the newly synthesized daughter strands and parental template strands reform a DNA double helix. The means that only a small stretch of the template duplex is single-stranded at any given time.

The progression of the replication fork requires that the DNA ahead of the fork be continuously unwound. Due to the fact that eukaryotic chromosomal DNA is attached to a protein scaffold the progressive movement of the replication fork introduces severe torsional stress into the duplex ahead of the fork. This torsional stress is relieved by DNA topoisomerases. Topoisomerases relieve torsional stresses in duplexes of DNA by introducing either double- (topoisomerases II) or single-stranded (topoisomerases I) breaks into the backbone of the DNA. These breaks allow unwinding of the duplex and removal of the replication-induced torsional strain. The nicks are then resealed by the topoisomerases.

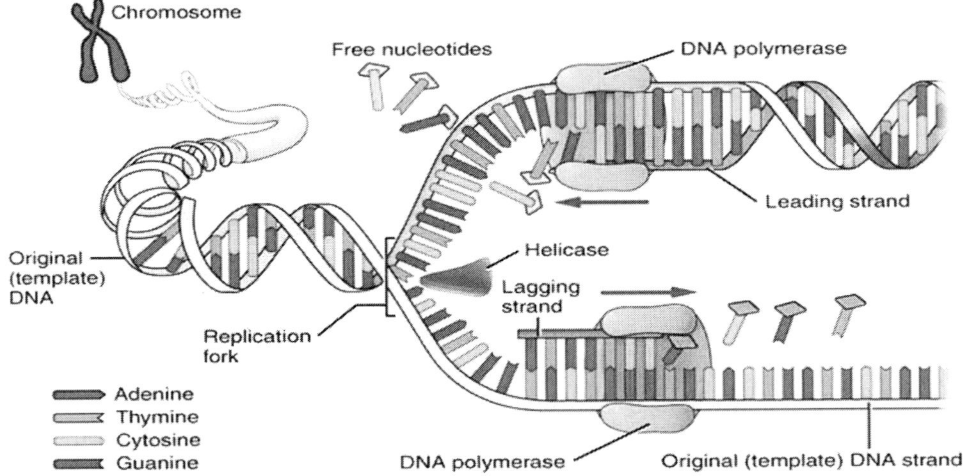

Figure 13.3. Process of DNA Replication.

The RNA primers of the leading strands and Okazaki fragments are removed by the repair DNA polymerases simultaneously replacing the ribonucleotides with deoxyribonucleotides. The gaps that exist between the 3'-OH of one leading strand and the 5'-phosphate of another as well as between one Okazaki fragment and another are repaired by DNA ligases thereby, completing the process of replication (Figure 13.3).

Amino Acids and their Classification and Genetic Codes, Transcription

Amino Acids and their Classification

Amino acids, the tiny building blocks of proteins occupies a prominent position among all the other nutrients and are reported as the molecule of source of life. More than 300 amino acids are found in nature but only **20 amino acids** are standard and present in protein because they are coded by genes. Other amino acids are modified amino acids and called non-protein amino acids. Some are residues modified after a protein has been synthesized by posttranslational modifications; others are amino acids present in living organisms but not as constituents of proteins. Out of 20 naturally occurring amino acids, **Asparagine** was the first discovered amino acid in the year 1806 followed by **Cysteine, Leucine** and **Glycine**. All the 20 amino acids involved in the construction of proteins were identified in the year 1935 and this discovery marked phenomenal significance in understanding the proteins, its structure and functions. Amino acid, as the name implies has amine ($-NH_2$) group and carboxylic acid (-COOH) with additional functional R group which acts as a side chain. Thus amino acids possess molecules of carbon, nitrogen, oxygen and hydrogen. The R group alone varies from one amino acid to the other thus contributing to 20 different natural amino acids.

Structure of Amino Acid

All 20 of the common amino acids are alpha-amino acids. They contain a carboxyl group, an amino group, and a side chain (R group), all attached to the α-carbon (Figure 14.1). The 20 amino acids involved in the construction of proteins are Glycine, Valine, Leucine, Isoleucine, Arginine, Cysteine, Lysine, Proline, Threonine, Methionine, Histidine, Tyrosine, Serine, Alanine, Phenylalanine, Glutamine, Glutamate, Asparagine, Aspartic acid and Tryptophan.

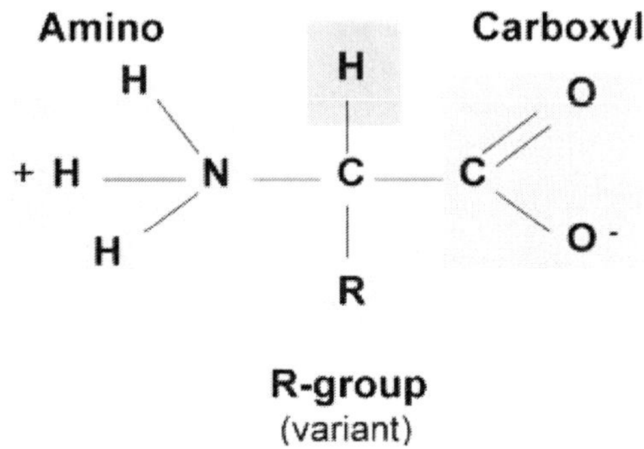

Figure 14.1. Common Structure of Amino Acid.

Classification

Based on the characteristic of the functional group amino acids are classified as polar, non-polar, acidic and basic amino acids. Based on their mode of availability (on the basis of nutrition) amino acids are divided into essential (dietary intake), non-essential amino acids (synthesized in the body through metabolic process) and conditionally non-essential and also amino acid is classified on the basis of the metabolic fate (Table 14.1, 2 and 3).

Classification of Amino Acids on the Basis of R-group (Figure 14.2 and Table 14.1)

1. Nonpolar, Aliphatic Amino Acids

The R groups in this class of amino acids are nonpolar and hydrophobic *e.g.* Glycine, Alanine, Valine, Leucine, Isoleucine and Methionine.

2. Aromatic Amino Acids

Phenylalanine, Tyrosine and Tryptophan, with their aromatic side chains, are relatively nonpolar (hydrophobic). All can participate in hydrophobic interactions.

3. Polar, Uncharged Amino Acids

The R groups of these amino acids are more soluble in water, or more hydrophilic, because they contain functional groups that form hydrogen bonds with water. This class of amino acids includes serine, threonine, cysteine, proline, asparagine and glutamine.

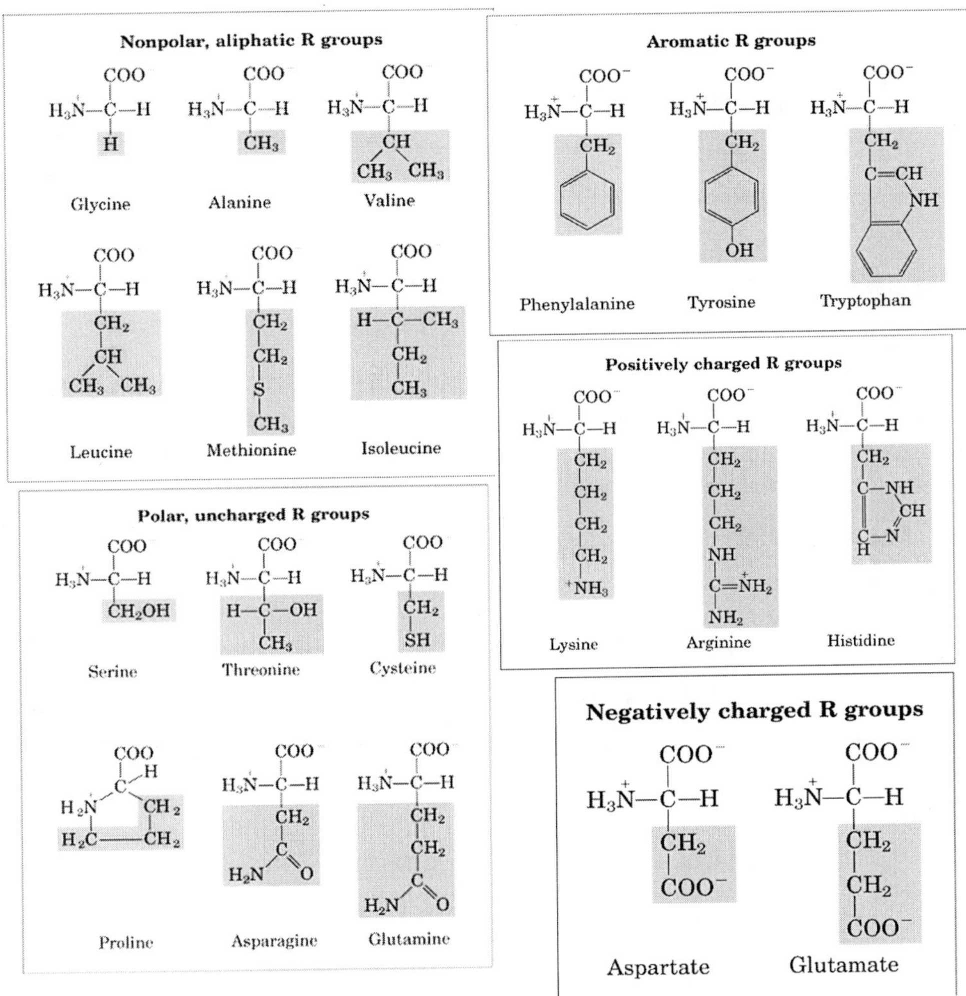

Figure 14.2. Classification of Amino Acids on the R Group.

Table 14. 1. Classification of Amino Acids on the Basis of R-group

Nonpolar, Aliphatic Amino Acids	*Aromatic Amino Acids*	*Polar, Uncharged Amino Acids*	*Acidic Amino Acids*	*Basic Amino Acids*
Glycine	Phenylalanine	Serine	Glutamic acid	Lysine
Alanine	Tyrosine	Threonine	Aspartic acid	Arginine
Valine	Tryptophan	Cysteine		Histidine
Leucine		Proline		
Isoleucine		Asparagine		
Methionine		Glutamine		

4. Acidic Amino Acids

Amino acids in which R-group is acidic or negatively charged *e.g.* Glutamic acid and Aspartic acid.

5. Basic Amino Acids

Amino acids in which R-group is basic or positively charged *e.g.* Lysine, Arginine and Histidine

Classification of Amino Acids on the Basis of Nutrition

1. Essential Amino Acids

Nine amino acids cannot be synthesized in the body. Therefore, these amino acids must be obtained from the diet in order for protein synthesis to occur. These essential amino acids are histidine, isoleucine, leucine, lysine, methionine, phenylalanine, threonine, tryptophan and valine.

2. Non-essential Amino Acids

These amino acids can be synthesized in the body itself and hence not necessarily need to be acquired through diet *e.g.,* Arginine, glutamine, tyrosine, cysteine, glycine, proline, serine, ornithine, alanine, asparagine and aspartate.

3. Conditionally Non-essential Amino Acids

Conditional amino acids are usually not essential, except in times of illness and stress. Conditional amino acids include: Glycine, Arginine, Cysteine, Glutamine, Proline and Tyrosine.

Table 14.2.Classification of Amino Acids on the Basis Nutrition

Essential Amino Acids (Nine)	*Non-essential Amino Acids (Eleven)*	*Conditionally Non-essential Amino Acids*
Histidine, Isoleucine, Leucine, Lysine, Methionine, Phenylalanine, Threonine, Tryptophan, Valine.	Arginine, Glutamine, Tyrosine, Cysteine, Glycine, Proline, Serine, Ornithine, Alanine, Asparagine, Aspartate.	Glycine, Arginine, Cysteine, Glutamine, Proline, Tyrosine

Classification of Amino Acids on the Basis of the Metabolic Rate

1. Glucogenic Amino Acids

These amino acids serve as precursors for glucose formation in gluconeogenesis. For example Glycine, alanine, serine, aspartic acid, asparagine, glutamic acid, glutamine, proline, valine, methionine, cysteine, histidine, and arginine.

2. Ketogenic Amino Acids

Amino acids Leucine and Lysine are breakdown to form ketone bodies.

3. Both Glucogenic and Ketogenic Amino Acids

These amino acids breakdown to form precursors for both ketone bodies and glucose formation for example Isoleucine, Phenylalanine, Tryptophan, and tyrosine.

Table 14.3. Based on Metabolic Fate

Glucogenic Amino Acids	*Ketogenic Amino Acids*	*Glucogenic and Ketogenic Amino Acids*
Glycine, alanine, serine, aspartic acid, asparagine, glutamic acid, glutamine, proline, valine, methionine, cysteine, histidine, and arginine	Leucine and Lysine	Isoleucine, Phenylalanine, Tryptophan, and tyrosine

Genetic Code

There are 20 amino acids involved in protein synthesis and there are only 4 bases in the DNA coding for all the amino acids. **Nirenberg** who has found that three bases code for one amino acid and thus it is possible to code for all the amino acids. The number and the sequence of bases in mRNA specifying an amino acid is known as a codon. While the set of bases in **tRNA which base pair with a codon of mRNA is known as anti-codon**. The sequence of bases in an anti-codon is exactly the opposite of that present in the codon. Since the codon and anticodon segments run anti-parallel to each other when they base pair, Codons are written in 5' - 3' direction, where as anticodons are usually written in 3'- 5' direction. The set of all the codons that specify the 20 amino acids is termed as the genetic code.

It is clear from various experiments that a sequence of three nucleotides in mRNA code for an amino acid and hence the genetic code is called the triplet code. **Three codons UAA, UAG and UGA do not code for any amino acid and hence they are called nonsense codons or stop codons or termination codons** as they provide stop signal for termination. The codon *i.e.* **AUG is known as start codon or initiation codon as it starts the synthesis of polypeptide chain**. This codon also codes for amino acid methionine. In eukaryotes, the starting amino acid is **methionine**, while in prokaryotes it is N-formyl methionine (Figure 14.3).

Nature/Properties of Genetic code; There are several important features or properties of a genetic code.

1. **The code is triplet:** The triplet code was first suggested by **Gammow in 1954**. In a triplet code, three RNA bases code for one amino acid.
2. **The code is universal**: The same genetic code is applicable to all forms of organisms from microbes to human beings.
3. **The code is comma less:** The genetic code is without a comma or break. The codons are continuous and there are no breaks between the codons.

A change or deletion of a single base in the code will alter the entire sequence of amino acid to be synthesized.

1st base

2nd base	U		C		A		G		3rd base
U	UUU	Phenylalanine	UCU	Serine	UAU	Tyrosine	UGU	Cysteine	U
	UUC	Phenylalanine	UCC	Serine	UAC	Tyrosine	UGC	Cysteine	C
	UUA	Leucine	UCA	Serine	UAA	Stop	UGA	Stop	A
	UUG	Leucine	UCG	Serine	UAG	Stop	UGG	Tryptophan	G
C	CUU	Leucine	CCU	Proline	CAU	Histidine	CGU	Arginine	U
	CUC	Leucine	CCC	Proline	CAC	Histidine	CGC	Arginine	C
	CUA	Leucine	CCA	Proline	CAA	Glutamine	CGA	Arginine	A
	CUG	Leucine	CCG	Proline	CAG	Glutamine	CGG	Arginine	G
A	AUU	Isoleucine	ACU	Threonine	AAU	Asparagine	AGU	Serine	U
	AUC	Isoleucine	ACC	Threonine	AAC	Asparagine	AGC	Serine	C
	AUA	Isoleucine	ACA	Threonine	AAA	Lysine	AGA	Arginine	A
	AUG	Methionine (Start)	ACG	Threonine	AAG	Lysine	AGG	Arginine	G
G	GUU	Valine	GCU	Alanine	GAU	Aspartic Acid	GGU	Glycine	U
	GUC	Valine	GCC	Alanine	GAC	Aspartic Acid	GGC	Glycine	C
	GUA	Valine	GCA	Alanine	GAA	Glutamic Acid	GGA	Glycine	A
	GUG	Valine	GCG	Alanine	GAG	Glutamic Acid	GGG	Glycine	G

Nonpolar, aliphatic Polar, uncharged Aromatic Positively charged Negatively charged

Figure 14.3. Genetic Code.

4. **The code is non-overlapping:** Three nucleotides or bases code for one amino acid and six bases will code for two amino acids. In a non – overlapping code, one base or letter is read only once.
5. **The code is non – ambiguous:** Out of the 64 codons, **61 code for 20 different amino acid, while 3 are nonsense codons**. None of the codons code for more than one amino acid.
6. **The code is degenerate:** In most cases, several codons code for the same amino acid. Only two amino acids, *viz.* **tryptophan and methionine** are coded by one codon each. Nine amino acids are coded by two codons each, one amino acid (isoleucine) by three codons each, five amino acids by four codons each and three amino acids by six codons each. This type of redundancy of genetic code is called degeneracy of genetic code. Such a system provides protection to the organisms against many harmful mutations. If one base of codon is mutated, there are other codons, which will code for the same amino acid and thus there will be no alteration in polypeptide chain.
7. **The code has polarity:** The code has a definite direction for reading of message, which is referred to as polarity. Reading of code in opposite direction will naturally specify for another amino acid example: GUC codes for valine, if reversed, CUG codes for Leucine. Crick postulated the wobble hypothesis in 1966 to account for the degeneracy of genetic code.

Wobble Hypothesis

The **first two bases on the codon and last two bases of anti codon** are usually the important ones, the third base of codon and first base of anticodon may be in some cases one of the four bases and the triplet would still code for the same amino acid as long as the first two bases are the same and have the same sequence. **This concept is known as the Wobble hypothesis.**

Transcription – mRNA Synthesis

Transcription is the process by which the information contained in a section of DNA is transferred to a newly assembled piece of messenger RNA (mRNA). During this process, one strand of the DNA double helix is used as a template to synthesize a mRNA mediated by the enzyme **RNA polymerase**. The mRNA, that produced after transcription is called as **primary transcript.** The primary transcripts of prokaryotes are different from the eukaryotes and this difference is due to the differences in genome organization of prokaryotes and eukaryotes. During the process of transcription a single strand of RNA is synthesized using a double stranded DNA molecule as a template. At a time out of two DNA strand only one strand is actively used as a template in the transcription process, this is known as the **template strand, otherwise called as antisense strandor noncoding strand. The sense strand or coding strand or nontemplate strand is complementary to the antisense strand, and is not transcribed**. The RNA sequence that is made is a complementary copy of the nitrogenous bases of the anti-sense strand and exactely similar to the sense strand. The only difference between sense strand and mRNA molecule is thymine (T) is substituted with uracil (U). If guanine (G) base is part of the sequence on the sense DNA strand, then the RNA molecule has a cytosine (C) base added to its sequence at that point (Figure 14.4)

The process of transcription is catalyzed by a multi subunit enzyme called RNA polymerase, which needs as substrates double stranded DNA, and the ribonucleotides ATP, UTP, CTP and GTP. One at a time, this enzyme adds ribonucleotides to a growing RNA strand by joining incoming ribonucleotide triphosphates to the ribose sugar molecule of the last nucleotide of the growing RNA strand. Two of the phosphate groups are removed from the triphosphate and a covalent bond is formed between the remaining phosphate and the third carbon atom of the ribose sugar at the end of the RNA strand. Transcription process begins with binding of the RNA polymerase enzyme to the DNA molecule at a region known as the **promoter site**. The RNA synthesis takes place within locally unwound segment of DNA, this site is right in front of a gene where transcription will begin. Left side from the site of transcription starts is **called upstream sequencs nucleotides present this side are indicated with – symbol like -1,-2,-3,-4 *etc....* and right side of the transcription initiation site is called as down stream sequences.** Nucleotides which are present in down stream indicated with + symbol as +1,+2,+3,+4 *etc....*(Figure 14.5). In bacteria, this region contains two short sequences of bases that appear to be the same in all, or most promoters. The RNA polymerase enzyme does not copy the promoter into the

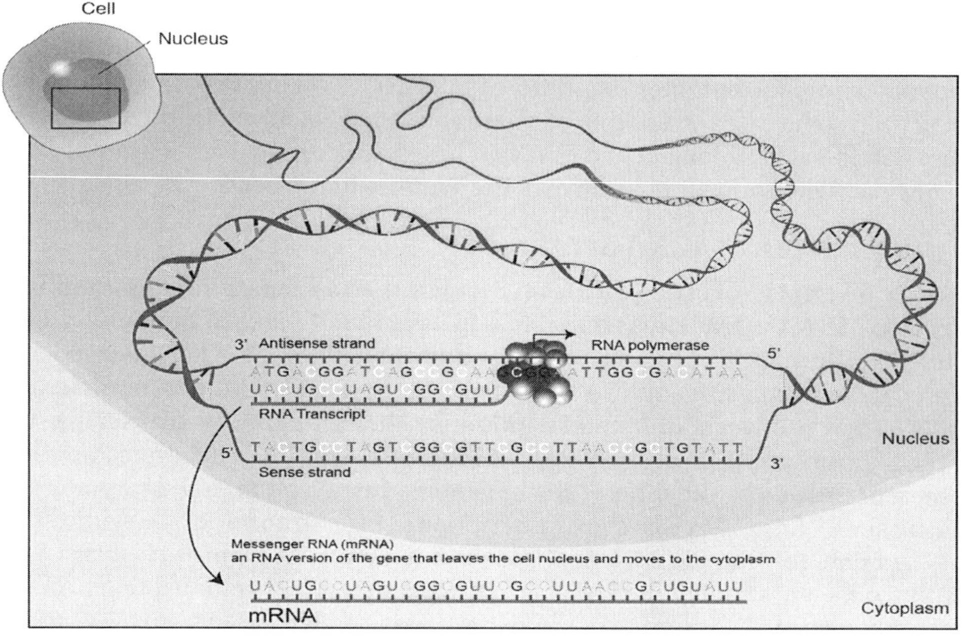

Figure 14.4. Process of Transcription.

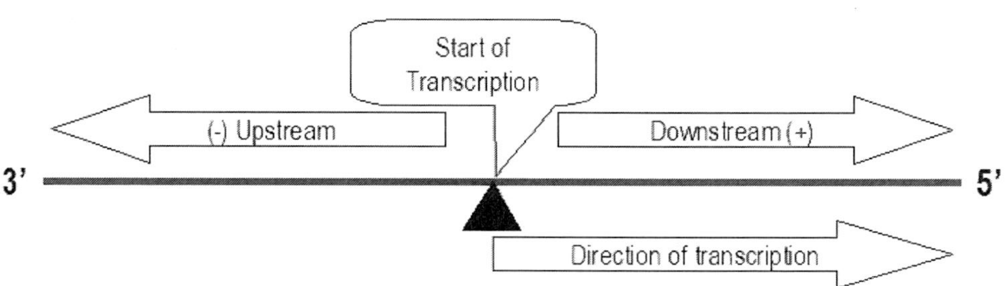

Figure 14.5. Transcription Initiation Site of the Gene.

RNA, but begins the synthesis of the RNA at a specific nucleotide sequence called the **start signal or initiation site** which is often the bases GTA on the DNA (which then become the bases CAU on the RNA molecule).

Transcription

Transcription of mRNA from DNA is catalyzed by a single RNA polymerase on the template DNA strand in the presence of substrate Ribonucleotide triphosphates (NTPs): ATP, CTP, GTP, UTP. Transcription containing three three distinct stage *i.e.*, initiation, elongation and termination (Figure 14.6).

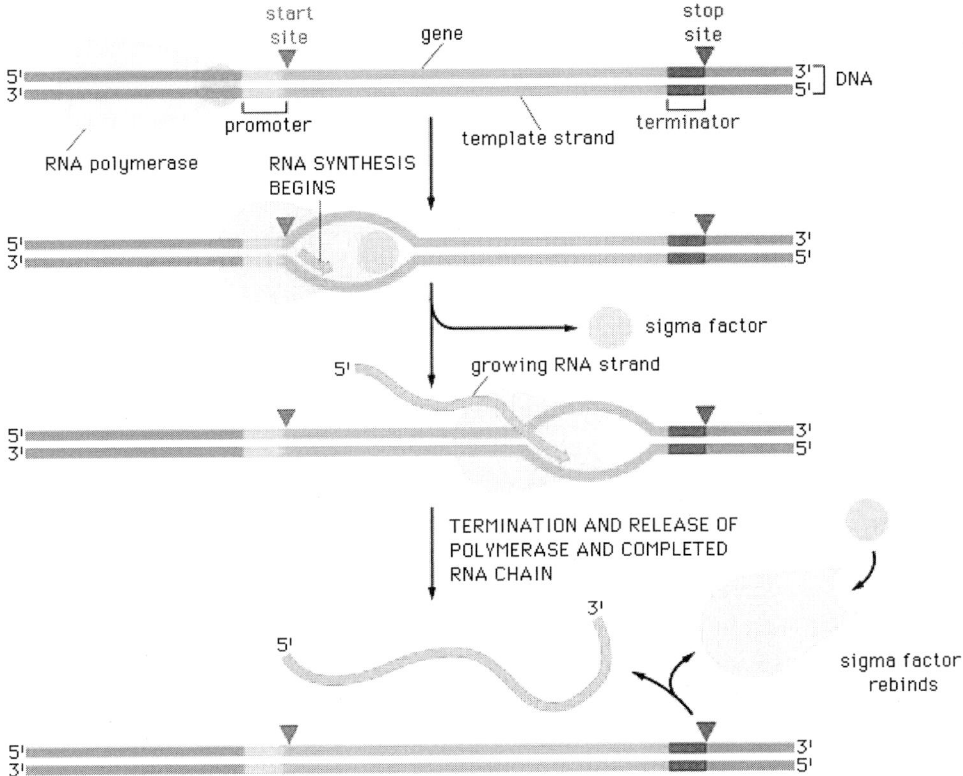

Figure 14.6. Whole Process of Transcription.

RNA Polymerase

RNA polymerase that catalyzes prokaryotic transcription is complex, multimeric protein. The *E. coli* RNA polymerase has a molecular weight of about 4,80,000 and consists of five polypeptides. Two of these polypeptides are identical; thus the enzyme contains four distinct polypeptides. **The complete RNA polymerase molecule, the holoenzyme, has the composition of α2, β, β' and σ. The α subunits are involved in the assembly of the tetrameric core ($\alpha 2\beta\beta'$) of RNA polymerase.** The β subunit contains the ribonucleotide triphosphate binding site and the β' subunit harbours the DNA template binding site. One subunit of σ factor, is involved only in the initiation of transcription, it plays no role in chain elongation. After RNA chain initiation has occurred, the σ factor is released, and chain elongation is catalyzed by the **core enzyme ($\alpha 2\beta\beta'$).** The function of σ factor is to recognize and bind RNA polymerase to the transcription intiation or promoter sites in DNA.

Prokaryote Transcription

Initiation Phase

- ☆ During initiation, RNA polymerase recognizes a specific site on the DNA, upstream from the gene that will be transcribed, called a **promoter site** and then unwinds the DNA locally.
- ☆ The holoenzyme binds to a promoter region about 40–60 bp in size and then initiates transcription. The first nucleotide transcribed sequence is mentioned as +1.
- ☆ Within the promoter two six base pair sequences that are particularly important for promoter function and they are highly conserved between species.
- ☆ These two promoter elements lie at positions –10 and –35, that is about 10 and 35 bp, respectively, upstream of where transcription will begin.
- ☆ **The –10 sequence has the consensus TATAAT bases known as the Pribnow box**, because this element was discovered by Pribnow. It is an important recognition site that interacts with the σ factor of RNA polymerase.
- ☆ The **–35 sequence has the consensus TTGACA bases** and is important in DNA unwinding during transcriptional initiation.
- ☆ RNA polymerase does not need a primer to begin transcription; having bound to the romoter site, the RNA polymerase begins transcription directly (Figure 14.7).

Elongation Phase

- ☆ After transcription initiation, the σ factor is released from the transcriptional complex to leave the core enzyme (α2 ββω) which continues elongation of the RNA transcript.
- ☆ The core enzyme contains the catalytic site for polymerization, probably within the β subunit.
- ☆ The RNA polymerase then synthesizes RNA in the 5' →3' direction, using the four ribonucleoside 5-triphosphates (ATP, CTP, GTP, UTP) as precursors.
- ☆ The 3-OH at the end of the growing RNA chain attacks the α phosphate group of the incoming ribonucleoside 5-triphosphate to form a 3'- 5' phosphodiester bond.
- ☆ The complex of RNA polymerase, DNA template and new RNA transcript is called a **ternary complex** (*i.e.* three components) and the region of unwound DNA that is undergoing transcription is called the transcription bubble.

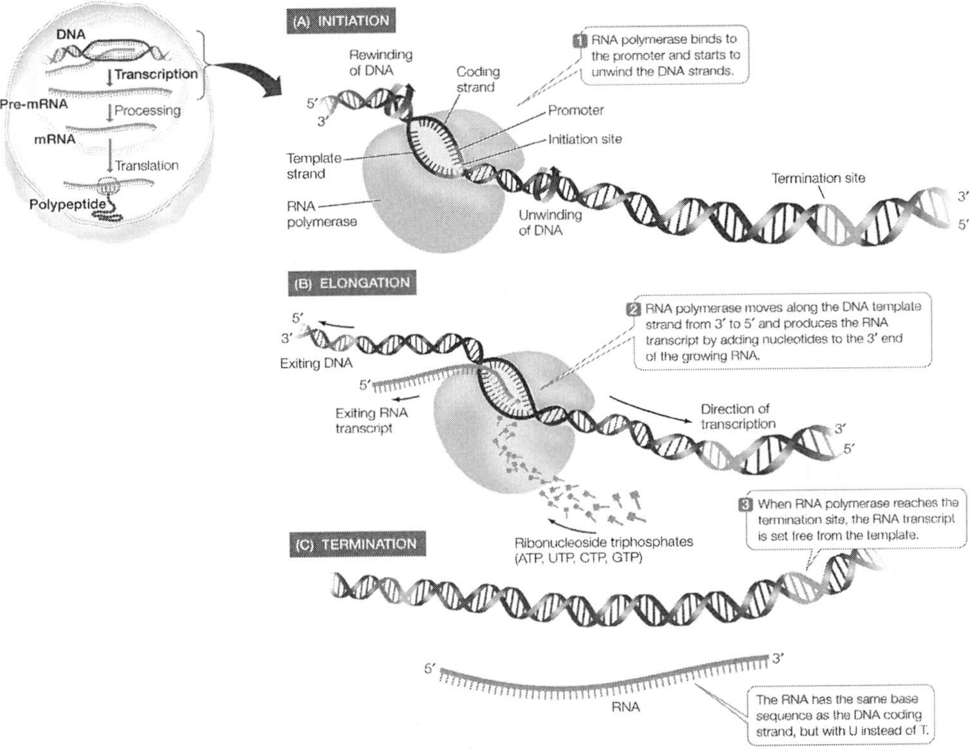

Figure 14.7. Different Phase of Prokaryote Transcription.

- ☆ The RNA transcript forms a transient RNA–DNA hybrid helix with its template strand but then peels away from the DNA as transcription proceeds.
- ☆ The DNA is unwound ahead of the transcription bubble and after the transcription complex has passed, the DNA rewinds.
- ☆ Thus, during the elongation, the RNA polymerase uses the antisense (-) strand of DNA as template and synthesizes a complementary RNA molecule.
- ☆ The RNA produced has the same sequence as the non-template strand, called the sense (+) strand (or coding strand) except that the RNA contains U instead of T.
- ☆ In the bacterial chromosome, sometimes one strand is used as template, sometimes the other strand can act as a template, it is depending up on the DNA strand which code the gene need to be expressed at that specific time. Any one of the both strand can act as a template based on the need,but both strand will not act as a gene at the same time.

- The correct strand to be used as template is identified for the RNA polymerase by the presence of the promoter site (Figure 14.7).

Termination Phase

- Transcription continues until a termination sequence is reached.
- The most common termination signal is a GC-rich region that is a palindrome, followed by an AT-rich sequence.
- The RNA made from the DNA palindrome is self- complementary and so base pairs internally to form a hairpin structure rich in GC base pairs followed by four or more U residues (**rho independent termination**).
- However, not all termination sites have this hairpin structure. Those that lack such a structure require an additional protein, called **rho**, to help recognize the termination site and stop transcription (**rho dependent termination**).
- Thus the RNA polymerase encounters a termination signal and ceases transcription, releasing the RNA transcript and dissociating from the DNA (Figure 14.7).

Transcription in Eukaryotes

- Although the overall process of RNA synthesis is similar in prokaryotes and eukaryotes, the process is considerably more complex in eukaryotes. In eukaryotes, RNA is synthesized in the nucleus and RNAs that encode proteins must be transported to the cytoplasm for translation on ribosomes.
- The complexity of eukaryotic transcription is evident from the involvement of three different RNA polymerases in the process of RNA synthesis.
- Eukaryotic transcription process is catalyzed by three different types of RNA polymerases and designated as RNA polymerases I, II and III. These enzymes are more complex, with 10 or more subunits, than the *E. coli* RNA polymerase (Table 14.4).
- Moreover, unlike the *E. coli* RNA polymerase, all the three enzymes require the assistance of other proteins called transcription factors, in order to initiate the synthesis of RNA chains.

Table 14.4. Types and Function of different RNA Polymerase Enzyme in Eukaryotes

Enzyme	Location	Function	Products
RNA polymerase I	Nucleolus	Catalyzes the synthesis of ribosomal RNAs except the small 5S RNA	Ribosomal RNA excluding 5S rRNA
RNA polymerase II	Nucleus	Transcribes nuclear genes that encode proteins and perhaps other genes specifying hnRNA	Nuclear pre mRNA
RNA polymerase III	Nucleus	Catalyzes the synthesis of transfer RNA molecules, the 5S rRNA molecules and small nuclear RNA	tRNA, 5S rRNA, and other small nuclear RNA

RNA Processing

In prokaryotes, RNA transcribed from protein-coding genes (messenger RNA, mRNA), requires little or no modification prior to translation. Because prokaryotes are not having any introns in the protein coding gene. Mostly translation is started before finishing the transcription of mRNA in cytoplasm itself. So mRNA no need travel and wait for long time for translation. But in the eukaryotic pre-mRNA undergoes extensive processing before it is ready to be translated. The additional steps involved in eukaryotic mRNA maturation create a molecule with a much longer half-life than a prokaryotic mRNA. Eukaryotic mRNAs last for several hours, whereas the typical *E. coli* mRNA lasts no more than five seconds. Pre-mRNAs are first coated in RNA-stabilizing proteins; these protect the pre-mRNA from degradation while it is processed and exported out of the nucleus. The three most important steps of pre-mRNA processing are the addition of stabilizing and signaling factors at the 5' and 3' ends of the molecule, and the removal of intervening sequences (introns) thatdo not specify the amino acids occur in between the exons.

mRNA Processing

The Pre-mRNA (Primary transcripts) molecules are processed to mature mRNA by 5'-capping, 3'-cleavage and polyadenylation and splicing in Eukaryotes. **Eukaryotic pre mRNA, is converted in to mature mRNA after necessary modification is called mRNA processing** (Figure 14.8).

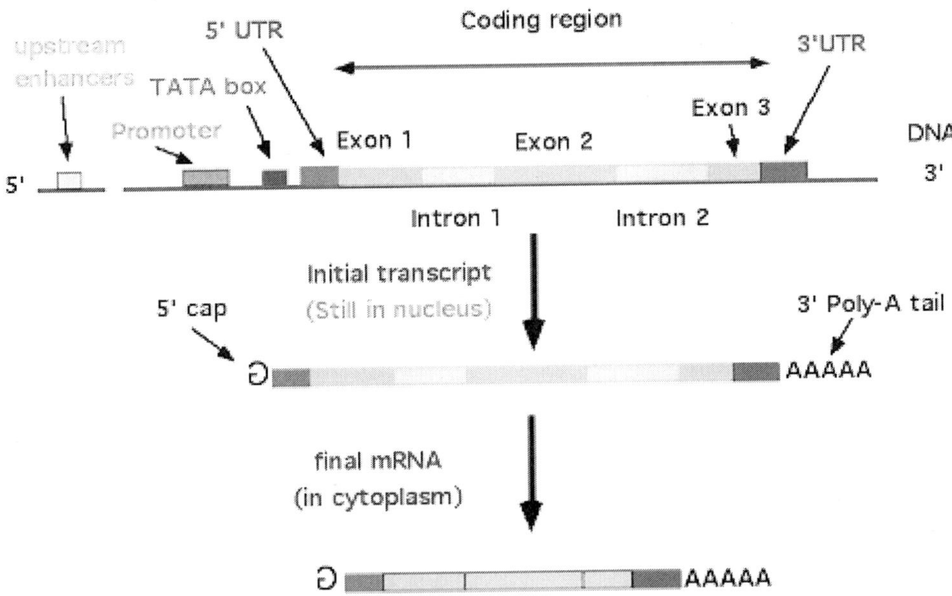

Figure 14.8. Processing of Eukaryotic mRNA.

Table 14.5. Difference between Prokaryotic and Eukaryotic Transcription

	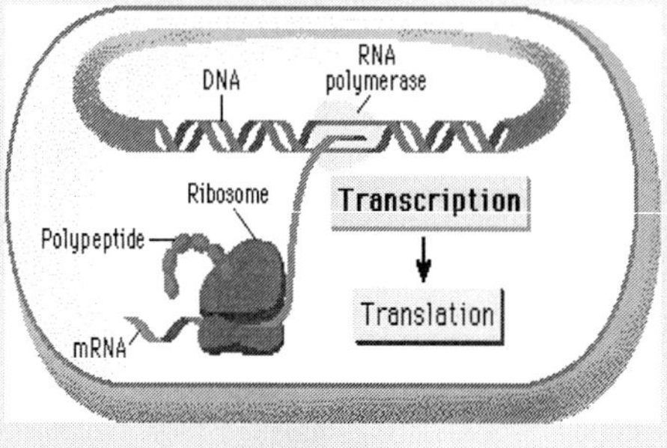 *Prokaryotic Transcription*	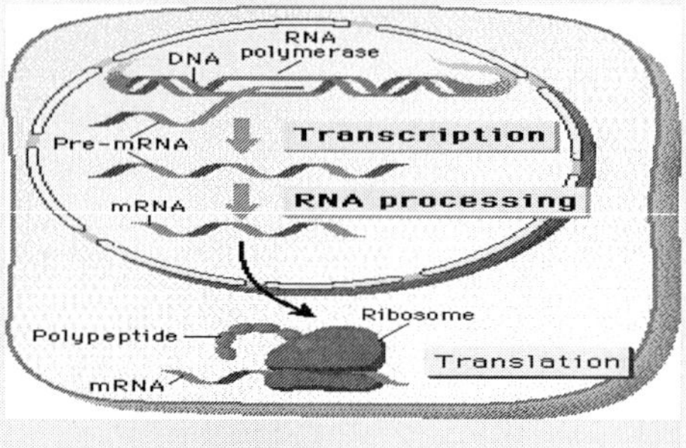 *Eukaryotic Transcription*
1	Coupled transcription-translation is the rule.	Coupled transcription translation is not possible.
2	Occurs in the cytoplasm.	Occurs in the nucleus.
3	There is no definite phase for its occurrence.	Take place in the G1 and G2 phases of cell cycle.
4	A single RNA polymerase synthesises all the three types of RNA (mRNA, tRNA, rRNA).	The RNA polymerases I, II and III synthesizes rRNA, mRNA and tRNA respectively.
5	RNAs are released and processed in the cytoplasm.	RNAs are released and processes in the nucleus.
6	Initiation of transcription does not need any proteins or initiation factors.	Initiation of transcription requires proteins called transcription factors. These are TFIIA, TFIIB, TFIID, TFIIE, TFIIF AND TFIIH. These recognise TATA BOX.
7	Pre RNA molecules are released and processed in the cytoplasm.	Pre RNA are released and processed in the nucleus.
8	RNA polymerases are complexes of five polypeptides.	RNA polymerases are complexes of 10-15 polypeptides.
9	The mRNA primary transcript has fewer surplus nucleotides.	The mRNA primary transcript has a large number of surplus nucleotides.
10	Transcriptional unit has one or more genes (Polycistronic).	Transcriptional unit has only one gene (Monocistronic).
11	Transcription and translation nearly simultaneous. Little process of mRNA	Processing of hnRNA includes:· Addition of 5'cap(7 methylguanosine)· Addition of 3'poly A tail.
12	The 23S, 16S and 5S rRNAs are formed from a single primary transcript.	The 28S, 18S, 5.8S and 5S rRNAS are formed from two primary transcripts.
13	Inhibitors:**Rifampicin:** RNA polymerase binds to β subunit.**Actinomycin**-Intercalates to interrupt transcription.	Inhibitors:α **amanitin**: Inhibits RNA polymerase 2 most srongly

5'-capping

The 5'-end is chemically modified by the addition of a **7-methylguanosine** residue.

3'-cleavage and polyadenylation

In most pre-mRNAs, the mature 3'-end of the molecule is generated by cleavage followed by the addition of a tail of A residues (polyadenylation) which is called the poly(A) tail.

Splicing

The process of cutting the pre-mRNA to remove the introns and joining together of the exons is called **splicing**.

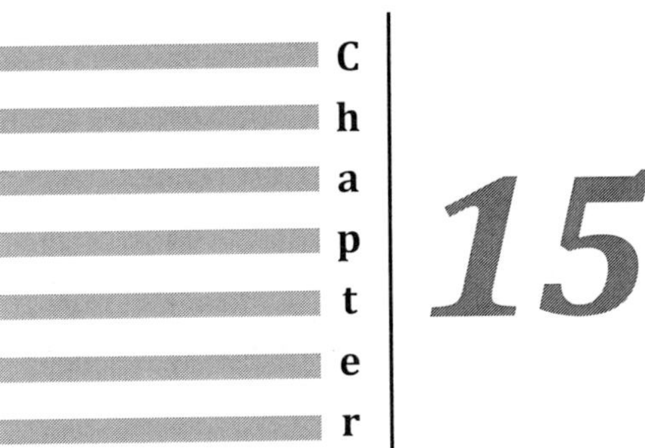

Translation and Protein Synthesis

Protein Synthesis

The translation is a process of synthesizing proteins in a chain of amino acids known as polypeptides. It takes place in the ribosomes found in the cytosol or those attached to the rough endoplasmic reticulum. The functions of the ribosome are to read the sequence of the codons in mRNA and the tRNA molecules that transfer or transport or bring the amino acids to the ribosomes in the correct sequence. The translation process involves reading the genetic code in mRNA to make proteins. The entire translation has three phases: Initiation, elongation, and termination.

- During initiation, the mRNA–ribosome complex is formed and the first codon (always AUG) binds the first aminoacyl tRNA (called initiator tRNA).
- During the elongation phase, the other codons are read sequentially and the polypeptide grows by addition of amino acids to its C-terminal end.
- This process continues until a termination codon (Stop codon), which does not have a corresponding aminoacyl-tRNA with which to base pair, is reached.
- At this point, protein synthesis ceases (termination phase) and the finished polypeptide is released from the ribosome

Translation Machinery

The translation process is aided by translation machinery composed of,

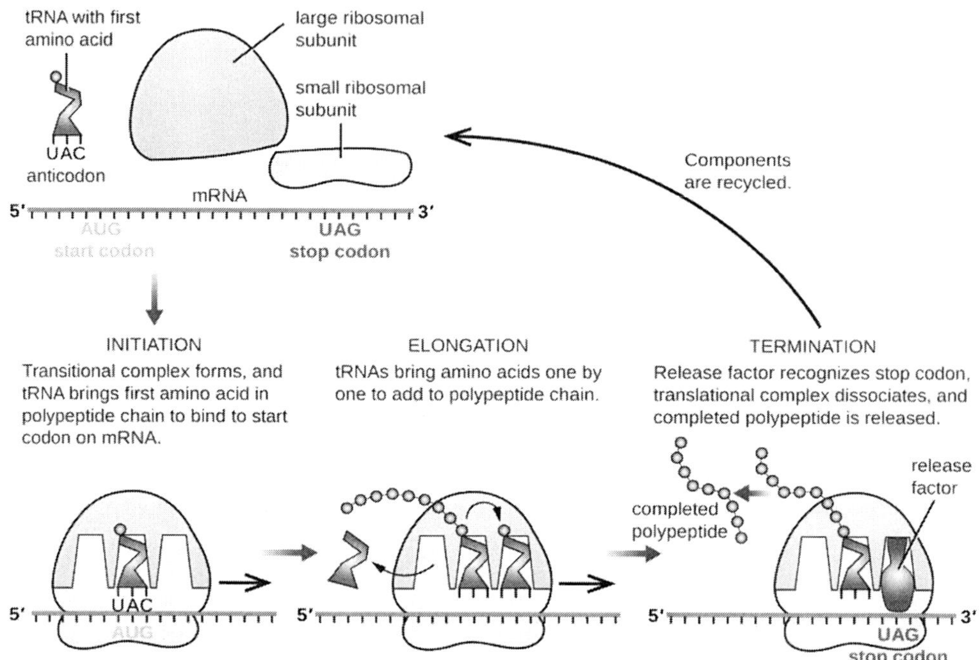

Figure 15.1. The Process of Protein Synthesis (Translation).

Ribosomes

- Ribosomes are made of ribosomal RNA (rRNA) and proteins, and therefore they are also names ribozymes because the rRNA has enzymatic activity. the rRNA has the peptidyl transferase activity that bonds the amino acids.
- The ribosomes have two subunits of rRNA and proteins, **a large subunit with three active sites (E, P, A)** which are critical for the catalytic activity of ribosomes (Fig15.2).

Transfer RNA (tRNA)

- Each tRNA has an anticodon which is complementary to the codon code for amino acid present in the mRNA. For example; Phenylaline is coded by 5'UUC 3', therefore the anticodon that carried by tRNA will be 3'AAG 5', therefore when the codon 5'UUC 3' appears, an anticodon 3'AAG 5' of tRNA will bind to it temporarily.
- When tRNA is bound to mRNA, then tRNA releases its amino acid. rRNA then helps to form peptide bonds between the amino acids as they are transported to the ribosomes one by one, thus creating a polypeptide chain. The polypeptide chain keeps growing until it reaches a stop codon (Figure 15.2).

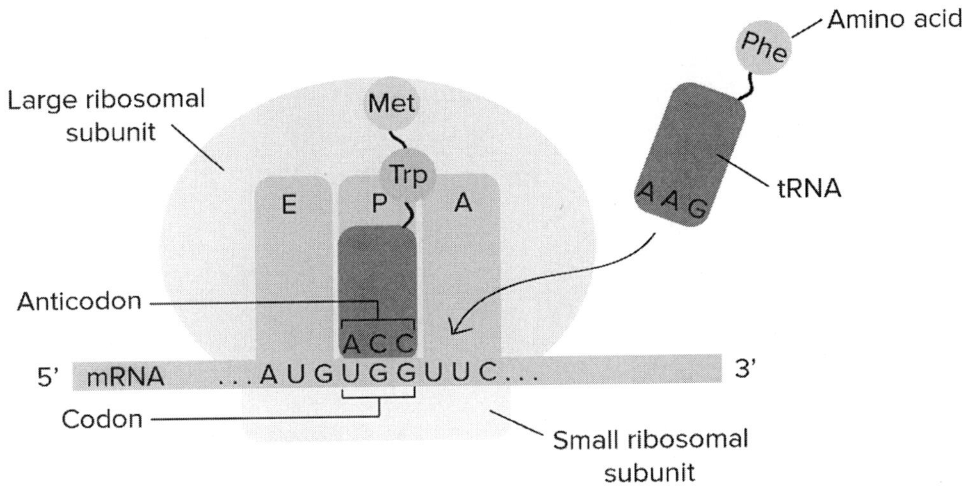

Figure 15.2. Components are Involved in Translation.

Synthesis of Aminoacyl-tRNA

- Each tRNA molecule has a cloverleaf secondary structure with the anticodon accessible at the end of the anticodon stem loop.
- During synthesis of the aminoacyl-tRNA, the amino acid is covalently bound to the A residue of the CCA sequence at the 3' end.
- Each tRNA molecule carries only a single amino acid.
- Synthesis of aminoacyl-tRNAs is crucially important for two reasons:
  1. Each amino acid must be covalently linked to a tRNA molecule in order to take part in protein synthesis, which depends upon the 'adaptor' function of tRNA to ensure that the correct amino acids are incorporated.
  2. The covalent bond that is formed between the amino acid and the tRNA is a high energy bond that enables the amino acid to react with the end of the growing polypeptide chain to form a new peptide bond.
- For this reason, the synthesis of aminoacyl-tRNA is also referred to as **amino acid activation.**
- The attachment of an amino acid to a tRNA is catalyzed by an enzyme called **aminoacyl-tRNA synthetase.**
- A separate aminoacyl-tRNA synthetase exists for every amino acid, making 20 synthetases in total.
- The synthesis reaction occurs in two steps.
  1. The first step is the reaction of an amino acid and ATP to form an aminoacyl-adenylate (also known as aminoacyl-AMP).

2. In the second step, without leaving the enzyme, the aminoacyl group of aminoacyl-AMP is transferred to the 3' end of the tRNA molecule to form aminoacyl-tRNA (Figure 15.3)

The overall reaction is:

Amino acid + ATP + tRNA → aminoacyl-tRNA + AMP + PP$_i$

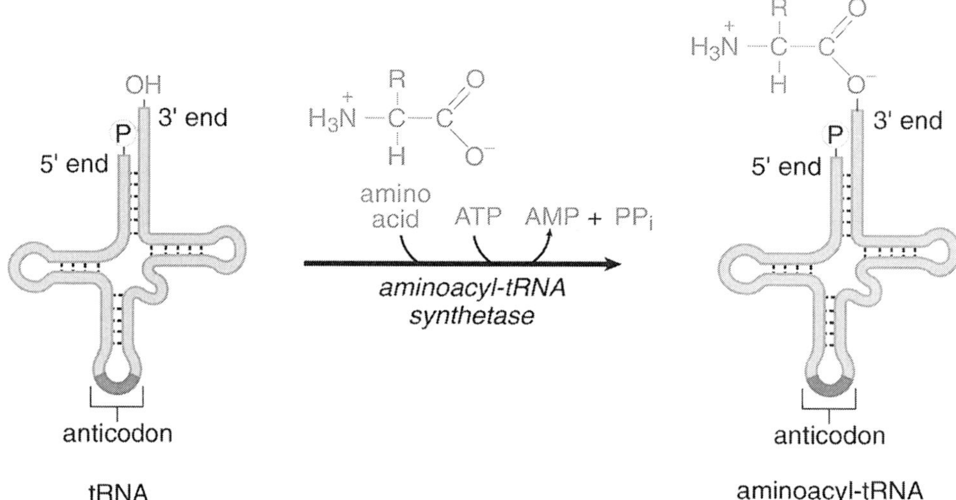

Figure 15.3. Synthesis of Aminoacyl-tRNA.

Enzymes Involved in Translation

- Peptidyl transferase is the main enzyme used in Translation. It is found in the ribosomes with an enzymatic activity that catalyzes the formation of a covalent peptide bond between the adjacent amino acids.
- The enzyme's activity is to form peptide bonds between adjacent amino acids using tRNAs during translation.
- It is located in the large subunit of the ribosomes and therefore, the primary function of peptidyl transferase is to catalyze the addition of amino acid residues allowing the polypeptide chain to grow.
- The peptidyl transferase enzyme is entirely made up of RNA and its mechanism is mediated by ribosomal RNA (rRNA), which is a ribozyme, made up of ribonucleotides.
- In prokaryotes, the **23S subunit contains the peptidyl transferase in eukaryotes, it is found in the 28S subunit** (Figure 15.3).

Translation Process in Prokaryotes

Translation involves translating the sequence of a messenger **RNA** (mRNA) molecule to a sequence of amino acids during protein synthesis. The messenger RNA (mRNA), the product of transcription and splicing, carries the code for the order of insertion of amino acids. This genetic code is a triplet code without punctuation. The mRNA also contains signals for initiation and termination of a polypeptide chain. The initiation signals are near its 5' end, while the termination signals are near its 3' end. Thus, the translation process has three steps *viz.* 1) polypeptide chain initiation, 2) chain elongation and 3) chain termination. A variety of protein factors, usually loosely bound to ribosomes, are also required. Many are needed for proper initiation of polypeptide chain synthesis, while others are required for binding incoming aminoacyl tRNAs to the ribosome and moving the ribosome relative to the mRNA (translocation) after each addition step.

Initiation

The initiation of translation includes all events that precede the formation of a peptide between the first two amino acids of the new polypeptide chain. The initiation process involves the 30S subunit of the ribosme, a special initiator tRNA, an mRNA molecule, three soluble proteins initiation factors: IF-1, IF-2 and IF-3 and one molecule of GTP. In the first stage of the initiation of translation, a free 30S subunit interacts with an mRNA molecule and initiation factors. The 50S subunit joins the complex to form the 70S ribosome in the final step of the initiation process. The addition of 50S subunit results in the release of all the initiation factors and the addition of 50S ribosomal subunit positions the initiator tRNA, methionyl tRNAfMet, in the peptidyl site (P site) with the anticodon of the tRNA aligned with the AUG initiation codon of the mRNA. The synthesis of polypeptides is initiated by a special tRNA, designated tRNAfMet. This means that all polypeptides begin with methionine during synthesis. **Methionyl tRNAfMet is the only aminoacyl-tRNA that can enter the P-site directly, without first passing through the aminoacyl site (A site).** With the initiator AUG positioned in the P site, the second codon in the mRNA is in the A site, dictating the amino-acyl tRNA binding specificity at that site and setting the stage for the second phase in polypeptide synthesis, chain elongation (Figure 15.4).

Generally, there are three steps in the initiation process of translation;

1. Initiation of the binding of mRNA to the small ribosome subunit (the 30S) with the help initiator factor IF3. This dissociates the ribosomal subunits into two.
2. The initiator factor IF2 then binds to the Guanine-triphosphate (GTP) and to the initiator fMet-tRNA to the P-site of the ribosomes.
3. A ribosomal protein splits the GTP that is bound to IF2 thus helping in driving the assembly of the two ribosomal subunits. The IF3 and IF2 are released.

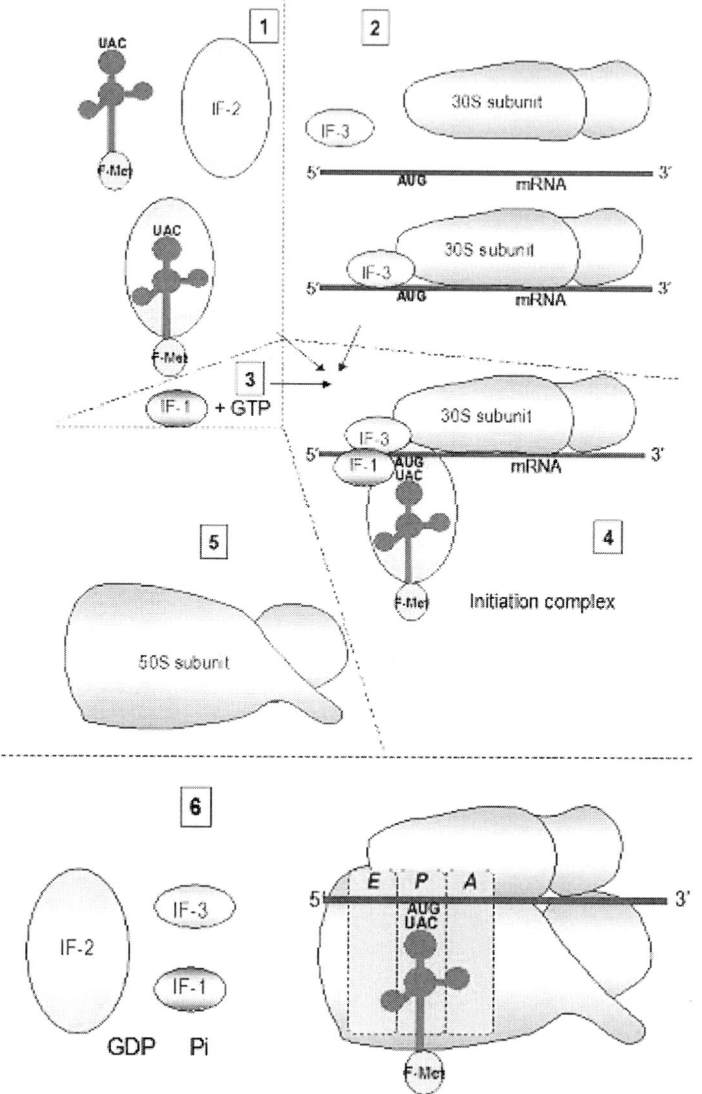

Figure 15.4. Various Steps in Translation Initiation.
1-3: Formation of IF-2/tRNAtMet and IF-3/mRNA/30S subunit complex; 4: The complexes formed in step 1 combine with each other, IF-1 and GTP to form the 30S initiation complex; 5-6: After IF-3 is released, the 50S subunit joins the initiation complex; GTP is cleaved and IF-1 and If-2 are released.

Elongation

The elongation of protein synthesis is aided by three protein factors *i.e.* **EF-Tu, EF-Ts**, and **EF-G**. The process of polypeptide chain elongation involves addition of amino acid to the growing polypeptide and has three steps: 1) binding of an aminoacyl-tRNA to the A site of the ribosome, 2) transfer of the growing polypeptide chain from the tRNA in the P site to the tRNA in the A site by the formation of a new polypeptide bond and 3) translocation of the ribosome along the mRNA to position the next codon in the A site. During step 3, the charged tRNA is translocated from A site to P site and the uncharged tRNA is moved from P site to E site. These three steps are repeated in a cyclic manner throughout the elongation process. The binding of an aminoacyl-tRNA to the A site of the ribosome requires an elongation factor EF-Tu and a molecule of GTP (EF-Tu-GTP). The second step of polypeptide bond formation between the amino acids in P site and A site is catalyzed by peptidyl transferase, an enyzymatic activity built into the 50S subunit of the ribosome. During the third step in chain elongation, the peptidyl-tRNA in the A site of the ribosome is translocated to the P site, and the uncharged tRNA in the P site is translocated to the E site, as the ribosome moves three nucleotides toward the 3' end of the mRNA molecule. The translocation step requires GTP and elongation factor G (EF-G). The translocation of peptidyl-tRNA from the A site to the P site leaves the A site unoccupied and the ribosome ready to begin the next cycle of chain elongation.

Therefore, three distinct steps are involved in translation, and these are;

1. The mediation of elongation Factor-Tu (EF-Tu) in the entry of amino-acyl-tRNAs to the A site. This entails the binding of EF-Tu to GTP, which activates the EF-Tu-GTP complex to bind to tRNA. The GTP then hydrolyses to GDP releasing an energy-giving phosphate molecule, thus driving the binding of aminoacyl-tRNA to the A site. At this point the EF-Tu is released, leaving the tRNA in the A-site.
2. Elongation factor EF-Ts then mediates the releasing of EF-Tu-GDP complex from the ribosomes and the formation of the EF-Tu-GTP.
3. During this translocation process, the polypeptide chain on the peptidyl-tRNA is transferred to the aminoacyl-tRNA on the A-site during a reaction that is catalyzed by a peptidyl transferase. The ribosomes then move one codon further along the mRNA in the 5' to 3' direction mediated by the elongation factor EF-G. This step draws its energy from the splitting of GTP to GDP. Uncharged tRNA is released from the P-site, transferring newly formed peptidyl-tRNA from the A-site to the P-site.

Termination

Termination of the translation process is triggered by an encounter of any of the three stop codons (UAA, UAG, UGA). These triplet stop codons, however, are not recognized by the tRNA but by protein factors known as the **release factors, (RF1 and RF2)** found in the ribosomes. The RF1 recognizes the triplet UAA and UAG while RF2 recognizes UAA and UGA. A third factor also assists in catalyzing the termination process and it's known as **Release factor 3 (RF3).** When the peptidyl-tRNA from the elongation step arrives at the P site, the release factor of the stop codon binds to the A site. These releases the polypeptide from the P site allowing the ribosomes to dissociate into two subunits by the energy derived from GTP, leaving the mRNA. After many ribosomes have completed the translation process, the mRNA is degraded allowing its nucleotides to be reused in other transcription reactions. Termination is completed by the release of the mRNA molecule from the ribosome and the dissociation of the ribosome into its subunits. The ribosomal subunits are then ready to initiate another round of protein synthesis (Figure 15.5).

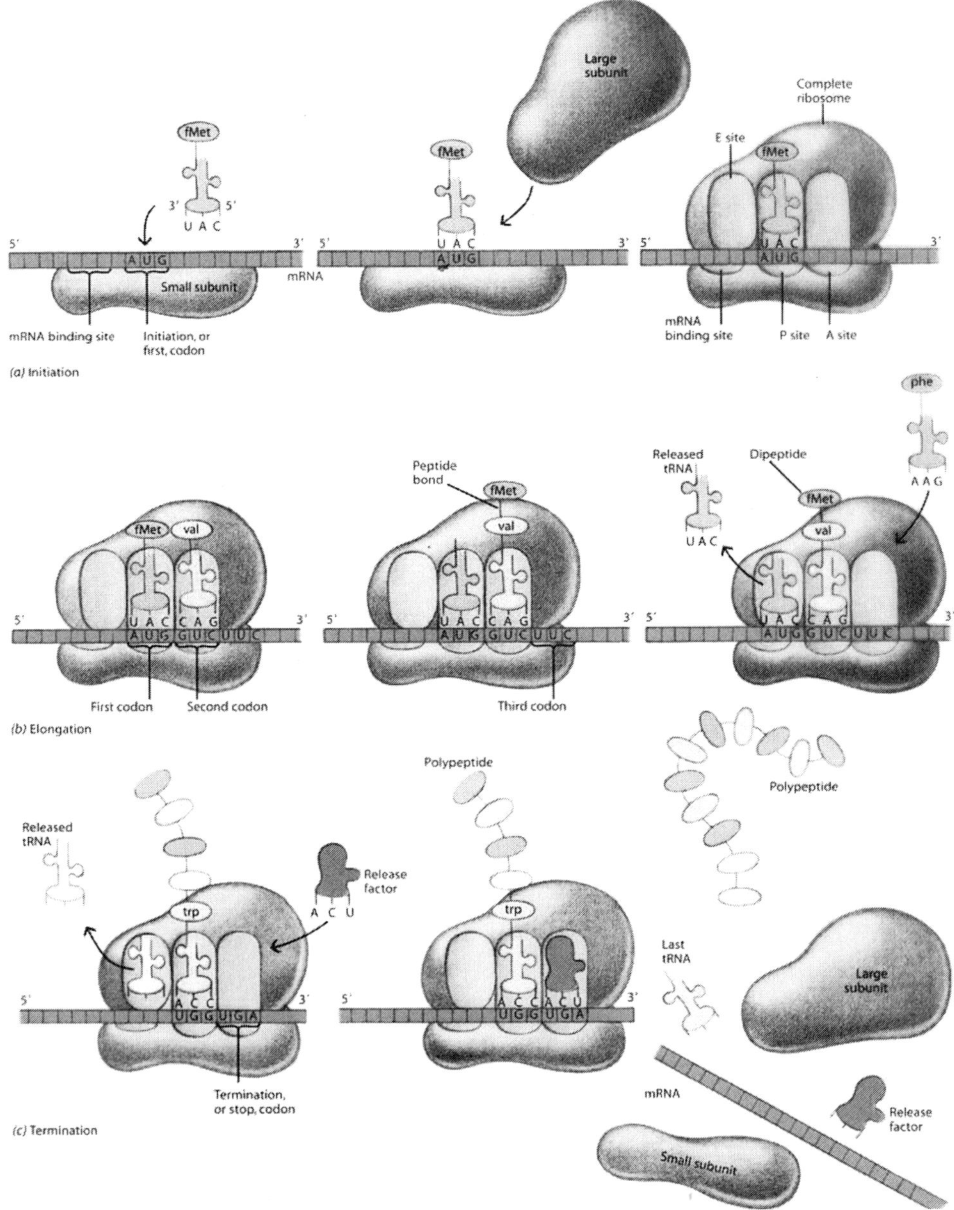

Figure 15.5. Protein Synthesis.

Table 15.1. Comparison between Eukaryotic and Prokaryotic Translation

Sl.No.	*Eukaryotes*	*Prokaryotes*
1.	The mRNA for translation is monocistronic, coding for a single gene of polypeptides	The mRNA for translation is polycistronic, thus coding for several genes of polypeptides
2.	The three types of RNA polymerase are used for the synthesis of cellular RNA.	A single type of RNA polymerase is used to control the synthesis of the types of RNA molecules
3.	It involves both subunits of the 80S ribosomes *i.e.* 40S and 60S subunits.	It involves 70S ribosomes of 30S and 50S subunits.
4.	Transcription and translation take place separately hence they do not overlap.	Transcription and translation can overlap or happen simultaneously
5.	The pre mRNA or an mRNA undergoes modification before they are translated.	The mRNA doesn't undergo any modification before translation.
6.	They do have a special initiator complex of tRNA.	A special initiator tRNA Met-tRNA$_f$ or Met – tRNA is used.
7.	The starting amino acid is methionine.	The starting amino acid is N-formyl methionine
8.	They have a single initiation and termination site.	They have several initiation and termination sites.
9.	The Ribosomal Binding Site is Kozak sequence that is centered around the start codon	The ribosomal binding site (RBS) on mRNA is the Shine-Dalgarno sequence that lies -10 nucleotides ahead of the initiation codon.
10.	Several initiation factors are involved in initiating the synthesise of the polypetide chain *i.e.* eIF-2 (eIF-2, eIF-2al, eIF-a2, eIF-a)	It involves three initiation factors IF-1, IF-2, and IF-3.
11.	There are two chain elongation factors, EF-1 and EF-2	There are three chain elongation factors, EF-Tu, EF-Ts, and EP-G.
12.	There is a single release factor eRF for recognition of three termination codons (UAA, UAG, and UGA).	There are three release factors (RF-1 or RF-2 and RF-3) for recognition of termination codons.
13.	The genetic code may differ in mitochondria and chloroplast.	The genetic code is the same in every prokaryotic organism.

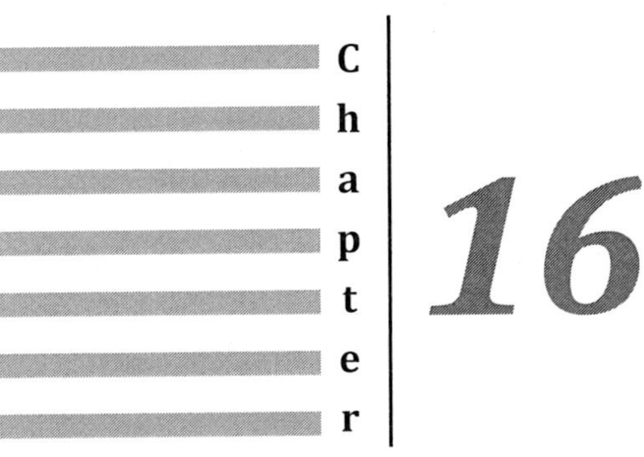

Structure of a Gene

Gene Structure

A gene is the basic physical and functional unit of heredity. Each gene has a specific sequence of DNA containing genetic information required to make a specific protein or RNA. **A gene may exist in alternative forms called alleles.** Understanding gene structure is the foundation of understanding gene annotation, expression, and function. Much of gene structure is broadly similar between eukaryotes and prokaryotes. These common elements largely result from the shared ancestry of cellular life in organisms over 2 billion years ago. Key differences in gene structure between eukaryotes and prokaryotes reflect their divergent transcription and translation machinery.

History of Genes

The classical principles of genetics were deduced by Gregor Mendel in 1865 on the basis of breeding experiments with peas. He assumed that each trait is determined by a pair of inherited 'factors' which are now called gene. Mendel's work was rediscovered in 1900 by Hugo de Vries, Correns and Tschermak. **Wilhelm Johannsen coined the term 'GENE' in 1909. William Bateson in 1905 coined the term genetics.** In 1972, Walter Fiers and his team determined the sequence of a gene in bacteriophage MS2 coat protein.

Common Gene Structure Features

The structures of both eukaryotic and prokaryotic genes involve several nested sequence elements. Each element has a specific function in the multistep process of gene expression. The sequences and lengths of these elements vary, but the same general functions are present in most genes. Although DNA is a double-stranded molecule, typically only one of the strands encodes information that the RNA polymerase reads to produce protein coding mRNA or non-coding RNA (tRNA and rRNA). This 'sense' or 'coding' strand, runs in the 5' to 3' direction where the numbers refer to the carbon atoms of the backbone's ribose sugar. The promoter is located at the 5' end of the gene (3' end of non coding strand or template strand or antisense DNA strand) and is composed of a core promoter sequence and a proximal promoter sequence. The core promoter marks the start site for transcription by binding RNA polymerase and other proteins necessary for copying DNA to RNA. The proximal promoter region binds transcription factors that modify the affinity of the core promoter for RNA polymerase. The structures of genes are intimately linked to their functions. Genes are often thought of as only the protein coding regions of DNA. However, coding sequences are only a minority component of the overall gene. Multiple untranscribed and untranslated DNA regions are necessary for proper gene function in all organisms. All regions of gene structure are important for determining phenotype, and so mutations in any of these sections have the potential to alter function (Figure 16.1).

Prokaryotes

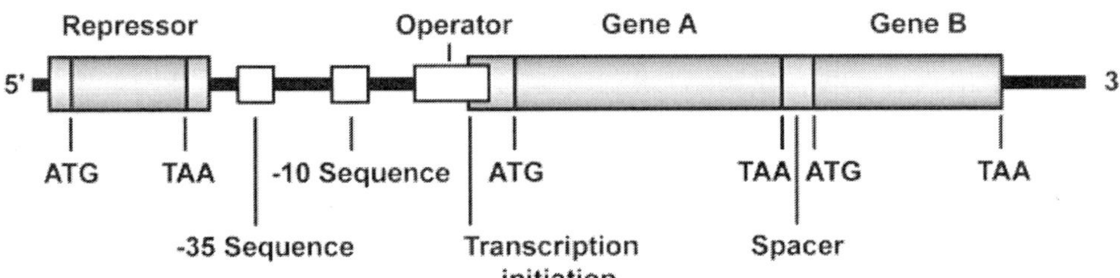

Eukaryotes

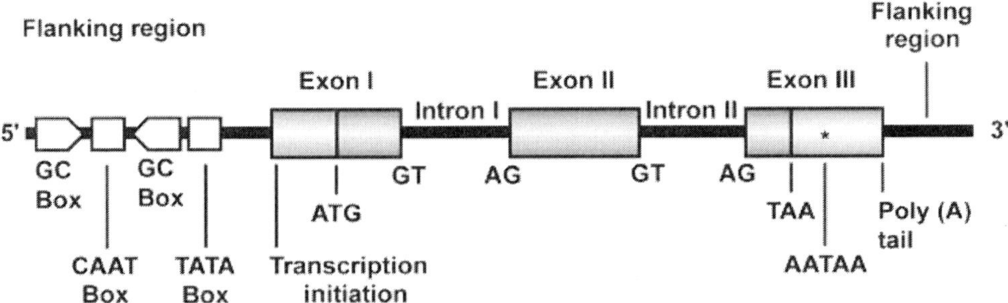

Figure 16.1. Gene Structure of Prokaryotes and Eukaryotes.

Eukaryotic Gene Structure

- ☆ Exons
- ☆ Introns
- ☆ Promoter sequences
- ☆ Terminator sequences
- ☆ Upstream sequences
- ☆ Downstream sequences
- ☆ Enhancers and silencers (upstream or downstream)
- ☆ Signals (Upstream sequence signal for addition of cap. Downstream sequences signal for addition of poly A tail)

Exons: coding sequence, transcribed and translated. Coding for amino acids in the polypeptide chain. Vary in number, sequence and length. A gene starts and ends with exons (5' to 3'). Some exon includes untranslated (UTR) region.

Introns: coding sequences are separated by non- coding sequences called introns. Any nucleotide sequence that are removed when the primary transcript is processed to give the mature RNA are called introns. All introns share the base sequence GT in the 5'end and AG in the 3'end. Introns were 1st discovered in 1977 independently by Phillip Sharp and Richard Roberts.

Promoters: A promoter is a regulatory region of DNA located in the upstream region of DNA which controlling gene expression.

1. **Core promoter** – transcription start site (-34), it is a binding site for RNA polymerase. General transcription factor binding sites.
2. **Proximal promoter**-contain primary regulatory element Approx. -250, specific transcription factor binding sites. **TATA box or hogness box (-30 to -80) and CAAT (upstream TATA) are two distinct sequences.** These together are responsible for binding of RNA polymerase II which is responsible for transcription

Upstream (5'end): 5'UTR serve several functions including mRNA transport and initiation of translation. Signal for addition of cap (7 methyl guanisine) to the 5'end of the mRNA. The cap facilitates the initiation of translation stabilization of mRNA.

Downstream (3'end): 3'UTR serves to add mRNA stability and attachment site for poly-A-tail. The translation termination codon TAA. AATAA sequence signal for addition of poly A tail.

Terminator:Recognized by RNA polymerase as a signal to stop transcription.

Enhancer: Enhances the transcription of a gene. Upto few thousand bp upstream.

Silencers: Reduce or shut off the expression of a nearby gene.

The structure of eukaryotic genes includes features not found in prokaryotes (Figure 16.2). Most of these relate to post transcriptional modification of pre-mRNAs to produce mature mRNA ready for translation into protein. Eukaryotic genes typically have more regulatory elements to control gene expression compared to prokaryotes. A key feature of the structure of eukaryotic genes is that their transcripts are typically subdivided into exon and intron regions. Exon regions are retained in the final mature mRNA molecule, while intron regions are spliced out (excised) during post-transcriptional processing. Indeed, the intron regions of a gene can be considerably longer than the exon regions. Once spliced together, the exons form a single continuous protein-coding regions, and the splice boundaries are not detectable. Eukaryotic post-transcriptional processing also adds a 5' cap to the start of the mRNA and a polyadenosine tail to the end of the mRNA. These additions stabilise the mRNA and direct its transport from the nucleus to the cytoplasm, although neither of these features are directly encoded in the structure of a gene. Regulatory sequence controls when and where expression occurs for the protein coding region. Promoter and enhancer regions regulate the transcription of the gene into a pre-mRNA which is modified to remove introns (spiliced mRNA) and add a 5' cap and poly-A tail (processed mRNA). The mRNA 5' and 3' untranslated regions (mature mRNA) regulate translation into the final protein product.

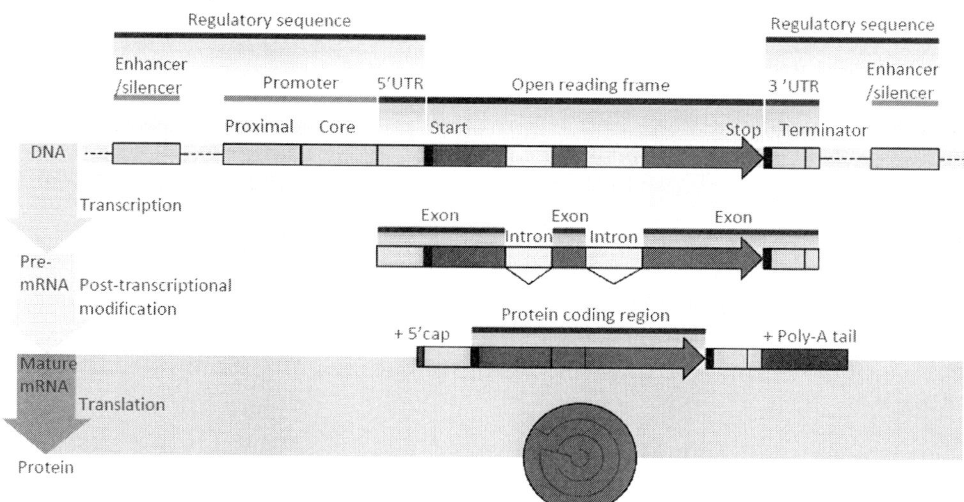

Figure 16.2. The Structure of a Eukaryotic Protein-Coding Gene.

Prokaryotic Gene Structure

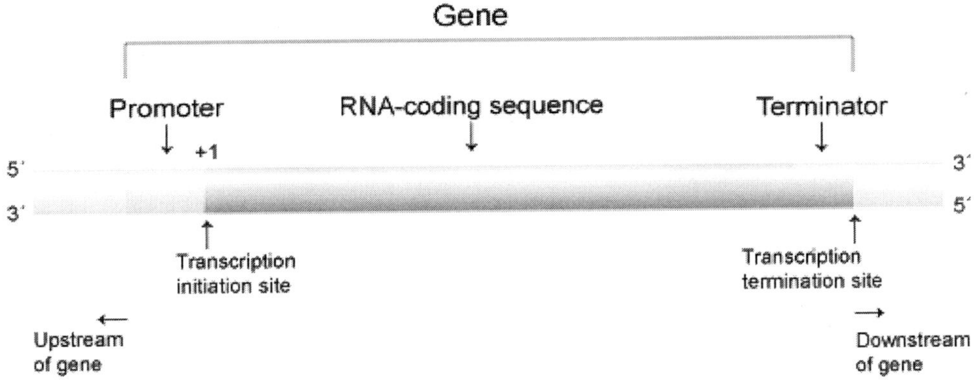

Figure 16.3. Monocistronic Gene (Single Gene) Structure in Prokaryotes.

Structural Features of Gene

Small genomes are about 0.5 to 10 million bp. Prokaryotic genes are collinear with their proteins. It consists of a) promoter elements b) Coding region c) terminal region or terminator (Figure 16.3).

a) Promoter Elements

The upstream elements from the start of the coding region include promoter sequences. 50 to 100 nucleotides upstream of the start codon- transcriptional initiation site or START site. (Any nucleotide present on the left is denoted by (-) symbol and the region is called upstream element. *e.g.* -10, -20,-35 *etc.* Start site symbolized by +1. Any sequence to the right of the start is downstream elements and numbered as +10, +35 *etc.*)

At -65 to -60 of promoter contains activator elements. They are involved in activation of the polymerase. At -200 to -1000 enhancer sequence to enhances transcription by 100 to 200 folds. At -10 there is a sequence TATAAT or PRIBNOW BOX. At -35 another consensus sequence TTGACA. These two are the most important promoter elements recognized by transcription factors.

b) Coding Region

Starts with an initiator codon and ends with termination codon. No introns (uninterrupted) in between coding regions and collinear to its mRNA.

c) Terminal Region of the Gene

Sequences for the termination of transcription. It takes place by Rho dependent mode or Rho independent mode.

Most of the genes have following conserved structural features in general.

- The coding region starts with an initiator codon (ATG) and the reading frame ends in a terminator codon (TAA, TGA, TAG). The upstream elements from the start of the coding region include **promoter elements**.
- Nearly 50 to 100 nucleotides upstream of the start codon, is the first nucleotide at which transcription initiates, it means, it is at this site the first nucleotide is incorporated into the transcribed RNA. **The site is called transcriptional initiation site or START**.
- Any nucleotide present on the left of the start is denoted by **(-) symbol** and the region is called **upstream element**. The numbers are written as -10, -20, -35 *etc.*
- Nearly -10 nucleotides upstream of the start, there is a sequence called **TATAAT or Pribnow** box. **The start site is the first nucleotide and symbolized by +1,** any sequence to the right of the start is called downstream elements and numbered as +10, +35 and so on. **At –35 there is another consensus sequence TTGACA**. These two sequences are the most important promoter elements, for if there is any change in their sequence and position, transcriptional initiation suffers.

The meaning of a promoter essentially is a distinct sequence module recognized by transcription factors that recruits RNA polymerase (as a holozyme) and bind to the sequence tightly and initiate transcription by unwinding the helically coiled DNA into **transcriptional bubble**. In addition to -10 and -35 sequences one finds up Stream sequences such as activator and enhancer elements. One also finds another sequence called **Operator elements** to which Repressors/Activators bind.

Prokaryotes (Polycistronic Gene)

The overall organisation of prokaryotic genes is markedly different from that of the eukaryotes (Figure 16.4). The most obvious difference is that prokaryotic ORFs are often grouped into a polycistronic operon under the control of a shared set of regulatory sequences. These ORFs are all transcribed onto the same mRNA and so are coregulated and often serve related functions (*e.g.* 3 structural genes in *lac* Operon, 5 structural genes in *trp* operon) Each ORF typically has its own ribosome binding site (RBS) so that ribosomes simultaneously translate ORFs on the same mRNA. Having multiple ORFs on a single mRNA is only possible in prokaryotes because their transcription and translation take place at the same time and in the same sub cellular location. The operator sequence next to the promoter is the main regulatory element in prokaryotes. Repressor proteins bound to the operator sequence physically obstructs the RNA polymerase enzyme, preventing transcription.

According to the **Benzer's** (1955) **modern concept of gene**, it may be subdivided into different units such as Recon, Muton, Cistron and Operon.

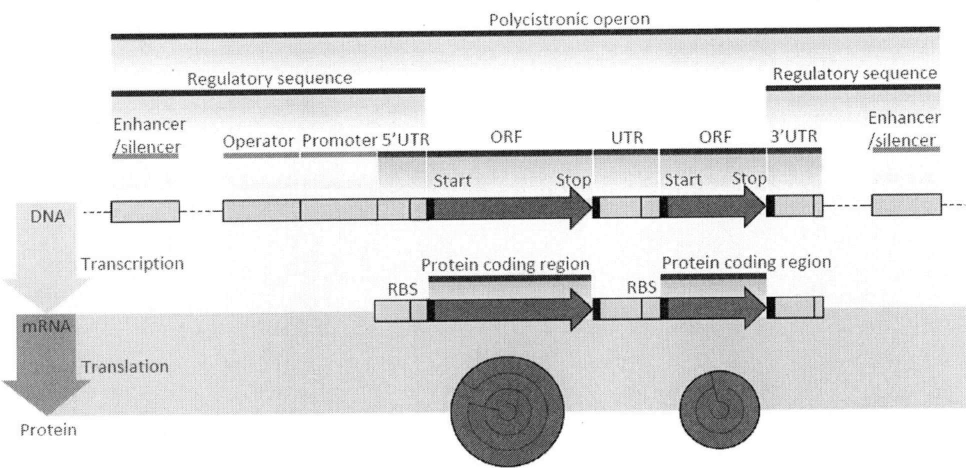

Figure 16.4. The Structure of a Prokaryotic Operon of Protein Coding Genes.

Recon

It is that smallest portion of a gene which can undergo crossing over and recombination and may be as small as a single nuclecotide pair.

Muton

It is the smallest unit of a gene that can undergo mutation and can involve a pair of nucleotides.

Cistron

It is the functional unit which can synthesize one polypeptide.

Operon

It is a group of genes having an operator a structural gene and other genes in sequence which all function as a unit.

Regulation of Gene Expression, Operon Concept

The basic mechanism for the control of gene expression was discovered in 1961 by **Francois Jacob** and **Jacques Monod** at the Pasteur Institute in Paris. Their findings became known as the **Operon concept** of Prokaryotic gene regulation. Regulation of gene expression is the mechanism which control the gene expression *i.e.*, whether the information coded by the gene is transcribed into mRNA and inturn translated in to a functional protein or not under particular environment. The fluctuation in the immediate environment of the organism is coped with by such regulation. An ***E.coli*** bacterial cell, for instance, is dependent for its nutrients on the eating habit of its human host. If the bacterium does not get the amino acid tryptophan from the host's food, it activates a pathway to make its own tryptophan (as it needs this amino acid in order to survive) from another compound. Like this, the bacteria tune their gene expression according to changing environments.

Regulation of Gene Expression

Genes contain the information necessary for living cells to survive and reproduce. In most organisms, genes are made of DNA, where the particular DNA sequence determines the function of the gene. A gene is transcribed (copied) from DNA into RNA, which can either be non-coding (ncRNA) with a direct function, or an intermediate messenger (mRNA) that is then translated into protein. Each of these steps is controlled by specific sequence elements, or regions, within the gene. Every gene, therefore, requires multiple sequence elements to be functional. This includes the sequence that actually encodes the functional protein or ncRNA, as well as multiple regulatory sequence regions. These regions may be as short as a few base pairs, up to many thousands of base pairs long.

The structures of both eukaryotic and prokaryotic genes involve several nested sequence elements. Each element has a specific function in the multistep process of gene expression. Although DNA is a double-stranded molecule, typically only one of the strands encodes information that the RNA polymerase reads to produce protein coding mRNA or non-coding RNA. This 'sense' or 'coding' strand, runs in the 5' to 3' direction where the numbers refer to the carbon atoms of the backbone's ribose sugar. The open reading frame (ORF) of a gene is therefore usually represented sense strand and it is always read 5' to 3' direction. Regulatory sequences are located at the extremities of genes. These sequence regions can either be just prior to the transcribed region (the promoter) or separated by many kilobases (enhancers and silencers). The core promoter marks the start site for transcription by binding RNA polymerase and other proteins necessary for copying DNA to RNA. Genes may be regulated by multiple enhancer and silencer sequences that further modify the activity of promoters by binding activator or repressor proteins. Enhancers and silencers may be distantly located from the gene, many thousands of base pairs away. The binding of different transcription factors, therefore, regulates the rate of transcription initiation at different times and in different cells. Regulation occurs in the process of transcriptional stage of gene expression (either synthesizing of mRNA strand or not) is called transcriptional level gene regulation. Control of gene expression that occurs during the post transcriptional phase when transcripts are processed by splicing, clipping, and modification is called as Post transcriptional control of gene expression.

The core promoter of eukaryotic genes typically requires additional activation by promoter elements for expression to occur. The core promoter of prokaryotic genes, conversely, is sufficient for strong expression and is regulated by repressors. Ribo-switches are another important regulatory sequence commonly present in prokaryotic UTRs. These sequences switch between alternative secondary structures in the RNA depending on the concentration of key metabolites. The secondary structures then either block or reveal important sequence regions such as RBSs. Introns are extremely rare in prokaryotes and therefore introns, do not play a significant role in prokaryotic gene regulation.

An additional layer of regulation occurs for protein coding genes after the mRNA has been processed to prepare it for translation to protein. Only the region between the start and stop codons encodes the final protein product. **The flanking untranslated regions (UTRs) contain further regulatory sequences.** The 3' UTR contains a terminator sequence, which marks the end point for transcription and releases the RNA polymerase. The 5' UTR binds the ribosome, which translates the protein coding region into a string of amino acids that fold to form the final protein product. Regulation occur in the translational stage whether gene encoded protein is synthesized from mRNA or not is called traslational level gene regulation. Some times gene is transcribed in to mRNA and mRNA translated in the encoded protein but that protein may not be functional because of improper protein folding. Protein folding pattern and interaction between polypeptides is the deciding factor for that particular protein become either functional or non functional. If regulation occur in the protein folding stage that regulation is called post translational gene regulation.

Operon Concept of Prokaryotic Gene Regulation

An operon is a functioning unit of DNA containing a cluster of genes under the control of a single promoter. The genes are transcribed together into a mRNA strand, either translated together in the cytoplasm (polycistronic mRNAs) or undergo splicing to create monocistronic mRNAs that are translated separately, *i.e.* several strands of mRNA that each encode a single gene product.

An **Operon** consists of a group of structural genes whose transcription is regulated by the same set of genes *viz.*, regulator gene, promoter and operator sequences.

(or)

An operon is a unit of prokaryotic gene expression and regulation, comprising structural genes and control elements (promoter and operator sequence) in DNA which is recognized by the regulatory proteins.

Operon Structure

Operons are regions of DNA that contain clusters of related genes. They are made up of a promoter region, an operator, and multiple related genes. The operator can be located either within the promoter or between the promoter and the genes. RNA polymerase initiates transcription by binding to the promoter region. The location of the operator is important as its regulation either allows or prevents transcription of the genes into mRNA (Figure 17.1).

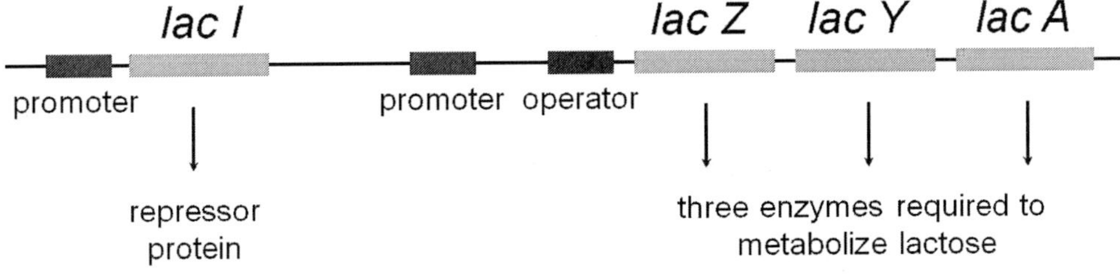

Figure 17.1. Structure of Lac Operon.

- ☆ **Structural Genes:** Genes that code for proteins required by the cell (for functioning as an enzyme or to be structural proteins) are called **Structural genes**. The three structural genes are transcribed to give a single mRNA molecule that codes for all the three proteins. A mRNA molecule coding for more than one protein is known as **Polygenic** (or **Polycistronic**) transcript.

☆ **Regulatory Genes:** Genes that code for proteins which, in turn, regulate the expression of other genes, are called **Regulatory genes (*lac I* in *Lac* operon).**

Operon Function

An operon is a complete package for gene expression and synthesis of polypeptides. By combining the related genes, all polypeptides required for a specific function are synthesized in response to a single stimulus. For example, the bacterium *Escherichia coli* contains a number of genes clustered into operons and regulons: the Lac operon which is involved in lactose degradation, and the Trp operon which is involved in tryptophan biosynthesis. These operons are turned on when the gene products are needed. **Operons can be under negative or positive control**. Negative control involves turning off the operon in the presence of a repressor; this can be either inducible or repressible. **An inducible operon** is one that is usually off. In the absence of an inducer the operator is blocked by a repressor molecule. When the inducer is present it interacts with the repressor protein, releasing it from the operator and allowing transcription to proceed (*Lac* operon). **A repressible operon** is one that is usually on but which can be repressed in the presence of a repressor molecule it needs co repressor for its binding to the operotor. The repressor binds to the operator presence of co repressor in such a way that the movement or binding of RNA polymerase is blocked and transcription cannot proceed (*Trp* operon).

(i) Inducible System:

Active Repressor + Operator → System OFF

Active Repressor + Inducer → Inactive Repressor → System ON

(ii) Repressible System:

Repressor = Inactive Repressor → System ON

Repressor and co-repressor complex →Active repressor → System OFF

Inducible operons are generally involved in catabolic pathways, or the breakdown of a nutrient while repressible operons are generally involved in anabolic pathways, or the synthesis of an essential component. Positive control of an operon is when gene expression is stimulated by the presence of a regulatory protein.

The Lac Operon

Jacob and Monod proposed the lac operon model to explain the regulation of the synthesis of an enzyme, **β-galactosidase**. The lac operon in *E.coli*, only expressed when lactose is available as a substrate and glucose is not available. The Lac operon is an inducible operon; in the absence of lactose the operator is blocked by a repressor protein. This was the first study of metabolic regulation based on genetic analysis of the lac system.

Structural Genes of Lac Operon

Bacterial structural genes are mostly organized as clusters, consisting of genes coding for proteins whose functions are related or involved in single pathway. There are three structural genes clustered together in Lac operon. The Lac operon is the classic operon example, and is responsible for the degradation of the milk protein lactose. The operon is made up of a promoter with operator, and **three genes (*lacZ, lacY*, and *lacA*) which encode β-galactosidase, permease, and transacetylase**. The regulator gene and regulatory sequences for this cluster of three genes are the ***lacI***gene, the **lac O** operator, and the **Lac P** promoter respectively. The entire system, comprising the structural genes and the regulatory (=control) elements, forms a common unit called the Lac Operon (Figures 17.2 and 17.3).

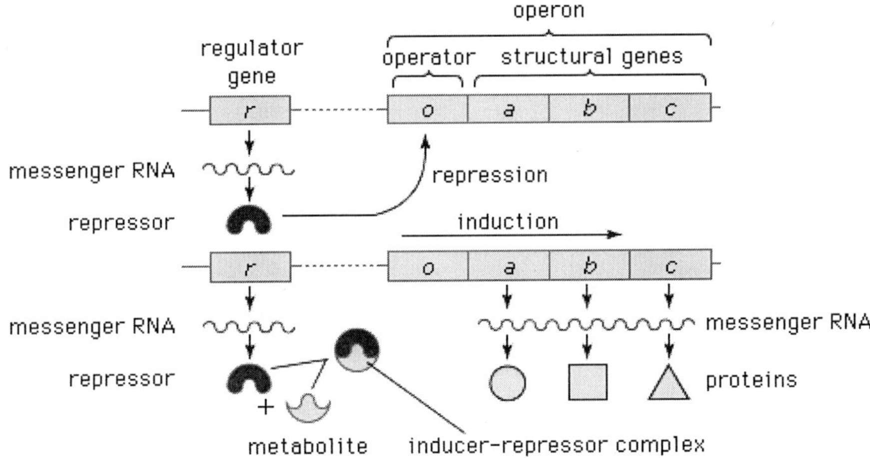

Figure 17.2. Lac Operon of *E. coli*.

lacZ Gene

The *lacZ* gene codes for the enzyme **β-galactosidase**; the enzyme breaks the β-galactoside into its components Sugar *e.g.* Lactose is cleaved into glucose and galactose for further metabolism and formation of **allolactose (isomer of lactose)**.

Lactose $\xrightarrow[\beta\text{-Galactosidase}]{H_2O}$ Glucose + Galactose

lacY Gene

lacY gene codes for the **β-galactoside Permease**; this transports the β-galactosides into the cell.

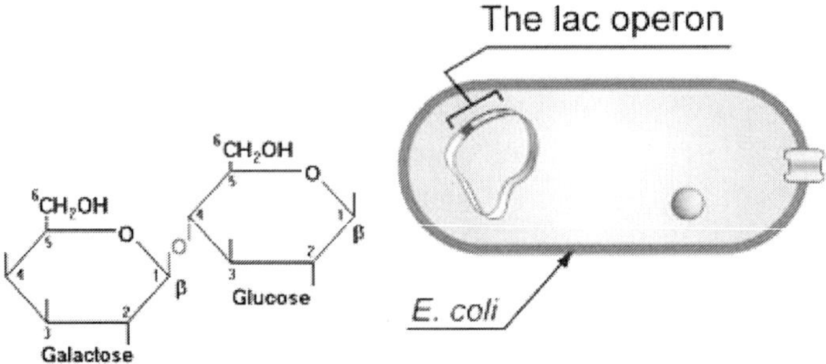

lacA Gene

lacA genes codes for **β-galactoside transacetylase**, an enzyme that transfers an acetyl group from acetyl~CoA to β-Galactosides.

The expression of the *Lac* operon is controlled by the regulatory gene *LacI*, located prior to the promoter region. *LacI* encodes an allosteric repressor protein that keep the Lac operon "off". In order for the Lac operon to be turned on, an inducer molecule must inactivate the repressor protein. The inducer molecule in this system is **allolactose, an isomer of lactose**. When lactose and its isomer are present in the cell, allolactose will bind to allosteric sites on the repressor protein, changing its conformation and rendering it inactive. As the repressor protein detaches from the operator, RNA polymerase can bind to the promoter, transcription can occur, and the three lactose degradation genes can be synthesized.

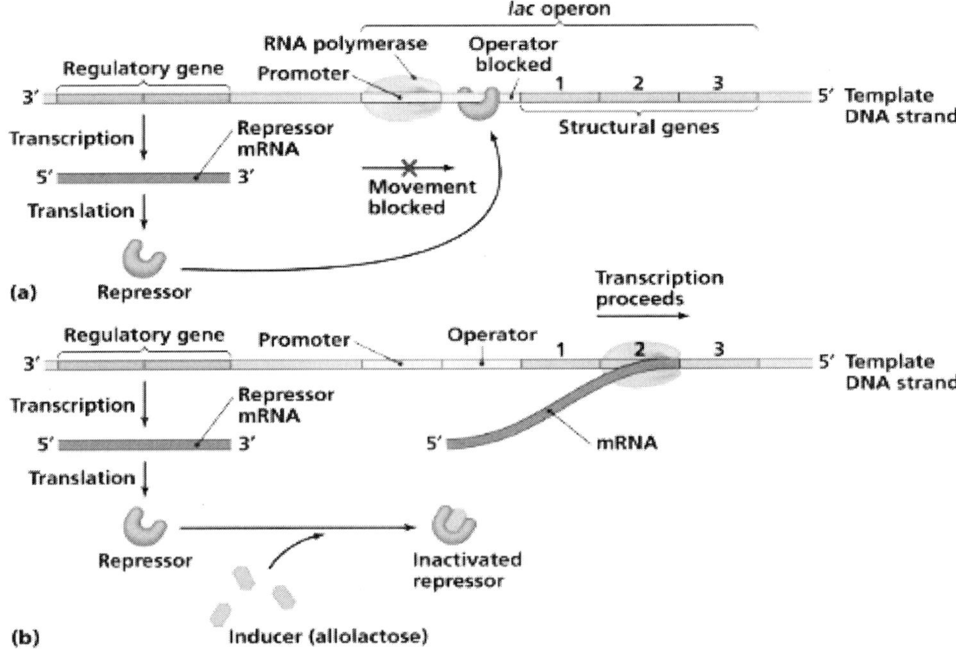

Figure 17.3. Structure of the Lac Operon and the Adjacent *lacI* Repressor Gene.

Trp Operon

The Trp operon is responsible for synthesis of the amino acid trytophan when it is not available in the environment. The Trp operon is made up of a promoter with an operator, and five genes that encode enzymes for tryptophan synthesis. The Trp operon is regulated by the regulatory gene *trpR*, a gene that is located at a distance from the Trp operon. The Trp operon is an example of a repressible operon; it is on unless turned off by a repressor protein. The repressor protein is synthesized by *trpR*. While the repressor protein is always present in the cell, it is synthesized in an inactive form. **When a corepressor is present, in this case tryptophan**, it binds to the repressor protein in an allosteric site. This changes the conformation of the protein such that it can bind to the operator and block transcription by preventing the binding of RNA polymerase to the promoter. In this way the cell saves energy by not producing tryptophan when it is already present Figure 17.4.

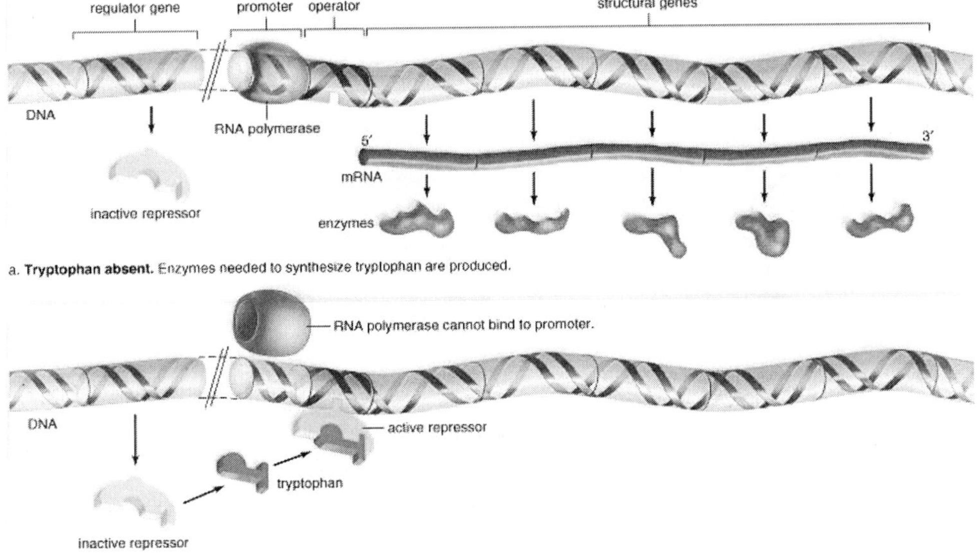

Figure 17.4. Structure of the Trp Operon and the Regulatory Region.

Positive Gene Regulation

The Lac operon is also under positive gene regulation. While the removal of the repressor protein in the presence of lactose is required for synthesis of the *lacZ*, *lacY*, and *lacA* genes. The level of gene expression is controlled by the amount of the preferred energy source, glucose, available in the cell. This control is regulated by an allosteric regulatory protein, catabolite activator protein (CAP). When glucose levels in the cell are low, the organic molecule cyclic AMP is in high concentration. Cyclic AMP activates CAP by binding to the allosteric sites, causing CAP to attach to the Lac operon promoter. Unlike the repressor proteins, binding of CAP to the *Lac* operon stimulates gene expression. When the cell glucose levels increase, the cyclic AMP levels in the cell decrease, and the activator protein will disassociate from the promoter. Transcription will return to low levels, or will turn off if the repressor protein reattaches (Figure 17.5).

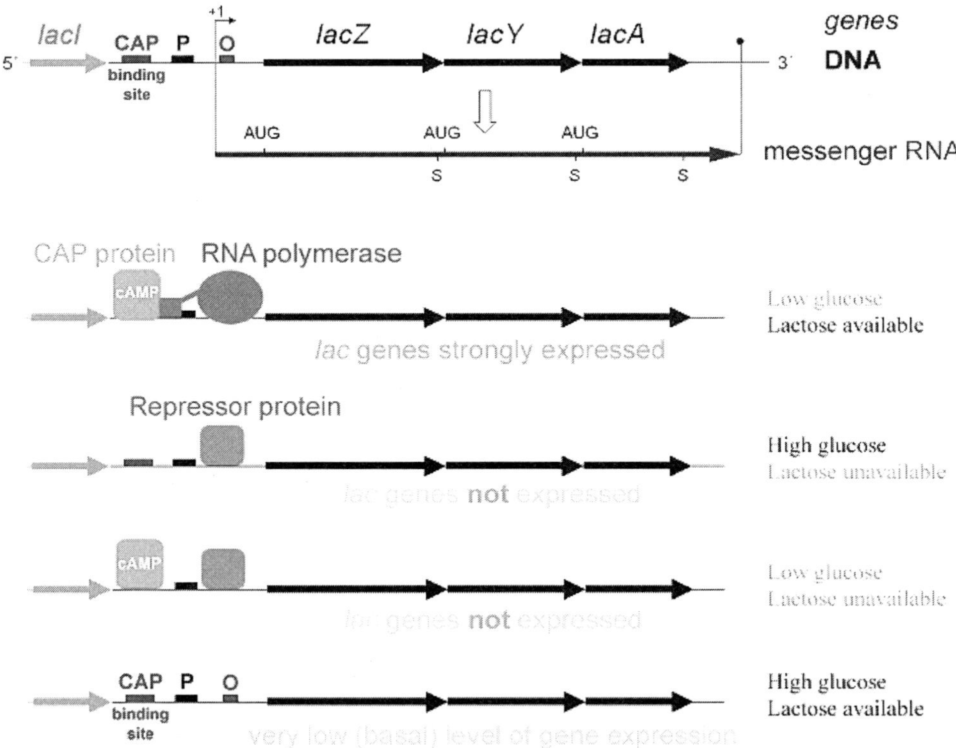

Figure 17.5. *Lac* Operon and its Control Elements (Positive regulation).

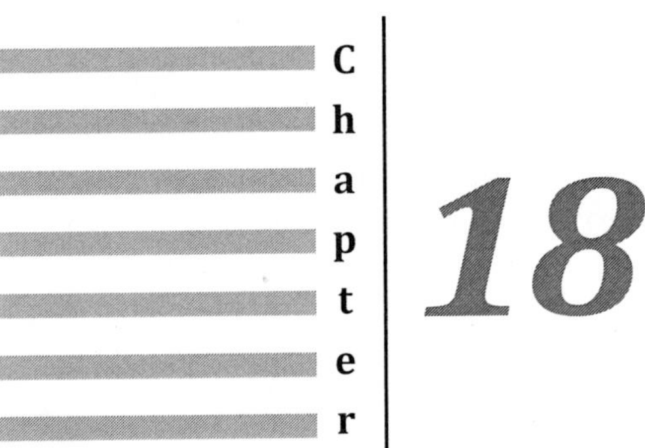

Blotting Techniques and Polymerase Chain Reaction

Blotting Techniques

The transfer of nucleic acid/protein molecule from an electrophoretic gel to any membrane (nitrocellulose filter or nylon membrane or PVDF membrane) by capillary action is known as **blotting.**

Southern Blotting

Southern Blot is the analytical technique used in molecular biology, immunogenetics and other molecular methods to detect or identify DNA of interest from a mixture of DNA sample or a specific base sequence within a strand of DNA. The technique was developed by a molecular biologist **E.M. Southern in 1975**; so named as Southern blotting in his honour. The transfer of DNA fragment from an electrophoretic gel to the nitrocellulose filter or nylon membrane by capillary action is known as **Southern blotting** (Figure 18.1). It involves DNA-DNA hybridization and the basic steps in southern blotting are:

1. DNA is first separated from target cells following standard methods of genomic DNA extraction and then purified.
2. Restriction endonucleases are used to cut high-molecular-weight DNA strands into smaller fragments. One or more restriction enzymes can be used to achieve such fragments.
3. The separation may be done by agarose gel electrophoresis in which the negatively charged DNA fragments move towards the positively charged

anode, the distance moved depending upon the size of DNA fragments. Larger fragment will move slowly whereas smaller fragment will move fast in the agarose gel.

4. Partial depurination is done by the use of dilute HCl which promotes higher efficient transfer of DNA fragments by breaking it down into smaller pieces.
5. DNA is then denatured with a mild alkali such as an alkaline solution of NaOH. This causes the double stranded DNA to become single-stranded, making them suitable for hybridization. DNA is then neutralized with NaCl to prevent re-hybridization before addition of the probe.
6. The denatured fragments are then transferred onto a **nylon or nitrocellulose filter membrane** which is done by placing the gel on top of a buffer saturated filter paper, then laying nitrocellulose filter membrane on the top of gel. Finally some dry filter papers are placed on top of the membrane. Fragments are pulled towards the nitrocellulose filter membrane by capillary action and result in the exact print of the gel in membrane.
7. The nitrocellulose membrane is removed from the blotting stack, and the membrane with single stranded DNA bands attached on to it is baked in a vacuum or regular oven at 80 °C for 2-3 hours or exposed to ultraviolet radiation to permanently attach the transferred DNA onto the membrane (UV crosslinking).
8. The baked membrane is treated with a solution containing 0.2 per cent each of Ficoll, polyvinyl pyrolidone, and Bovine serum albumin, to prevent the non specific binding of the radio-active probe (pre treatment).
9. The membrane is then exposed to a hybridization probe which is a single DNA fragment with a specific sequence whose presence in the target DNA is to be determined.
10. The probe DNA is labeled so that it can be detected, usually by incorporating radioactivity or tagging the molecule with a fluorescent or chromogenic dye. This probe hybridizes with complimentary DNA on the membrane resulting in DNA-DNA hybridization.
11. After hybridization, the membrane is thoroughly washed with a buffer to remove the probe that is bound nonspecifically or any unbound probes present.
12. The hybridized regions are detected autoradiographically by placing the nitrocellulose membrane in contact with a photographic film which shows the hybridized DNA molecules. The pattern of hybridization is visualized on X-ray film by autoradiography in case of a radioactive or fluorescent probe is used or by the development of color on the membrane if a chromogenic detection method is used.

Applications of Southern blotting

- Identifying specific DNA in a DNA sample.
- Detection of mutations, deletions or gene rearrangements in DNA
- It can be used to map the restriction site around a single copy gene sequence in any genome.
- It is used for DNA finger printing preparation of RFLP maps, detection and identification of transferred genes in the transgenic individuals *etc.*
- It is used to detect the size of the gene fragment from a genome and that how many copies of the gene are present in the genome.

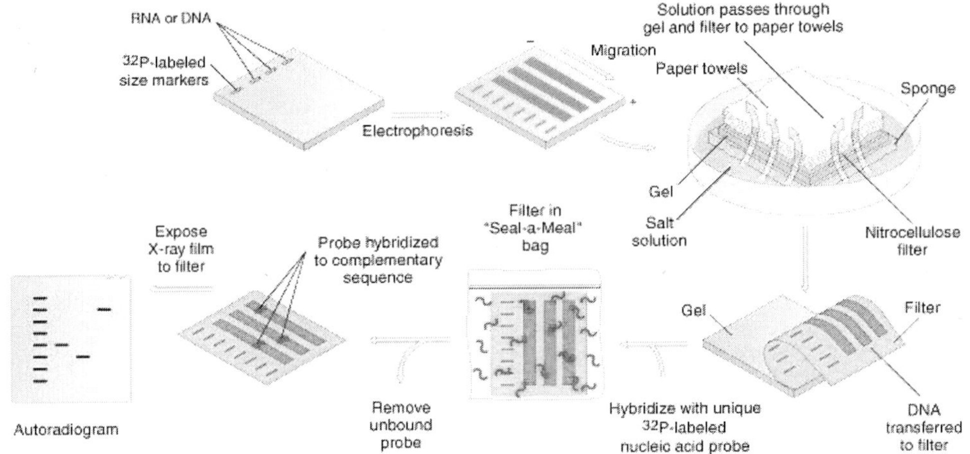

Figure 18.1. Southern Blotting Technique.

Northern Blotting

Northern blotting, the name was extrapolated from Southern blotting. The Northern blot is a technique used to study gene expression by **detection of RNA** (or isolated mRNA) in a sample. The procedure for the Northern blotting is same as that of the Southern blotting technique, except for the alkali denaturation step before transfer. Since RNA is single stranded, in Northern blotting, depurination is not necessary as alkali would hydrolyze the RNA molecules. Once transferred, the procedure for Southern and Northern blotting is identical.

Applications of Northern Blotting

- Northern blots give information about the size of the mRNA.
- Northern blots can help to identify whether a genomic clone has regions that are transcribed and, if the RNA on the blot is made from different tissues, where these transcripts are made.

☆ With northern blotting it is possible to observe cellular control of particular gene expression levels during differentiation, morphogenesis, as well as abnormal or diseased conditions.

Western Blotting

Identification of a specific protein in a complex mixture of proteins can be done by a technique known as **western blotting**. Western blotting (also called immunoblotting because an antibody is used to specifically detect its antigen) was introduced by **Towbin and co-workers** in 1979 and is now a routine technique for protein analysis.

In this method, known antigens of well-defined molecular weight are separated by SDS-PAGE and blotted onto **nitrocellulose or PVDF membrane**. The separated bands of known antigens are then probed with the sample suspected of containing antibody specific for one or more of these antigens. Reaction of an antibody with a band is detected by using either radio labeled or enzyme-linked secondary antibody that is specific for the species of the antibodies in the test sample (Figure 18.2).

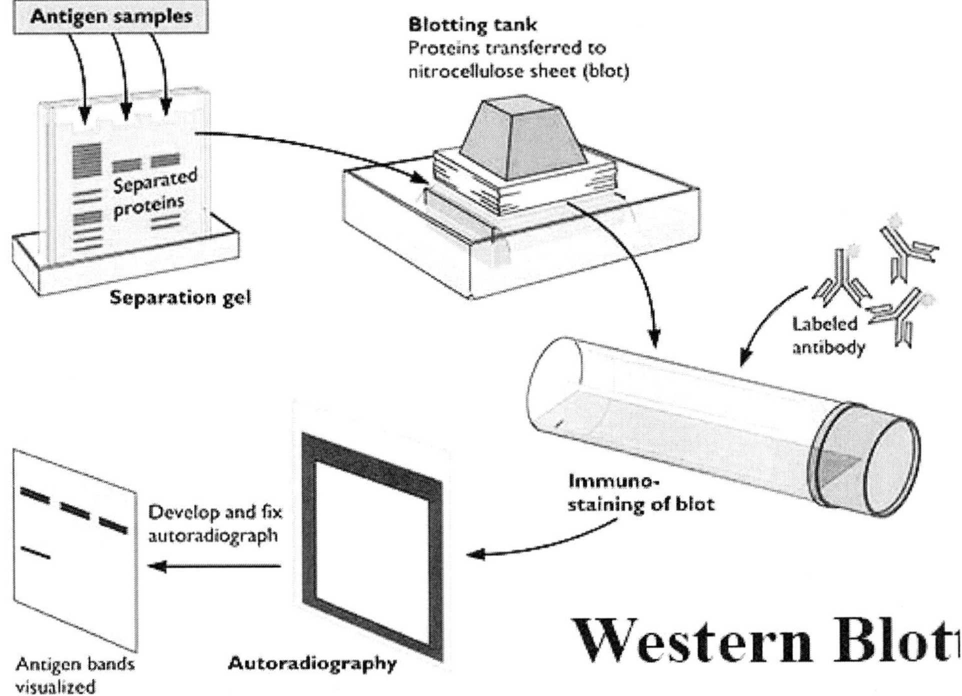

Figure 18.2. Steps in Western Blotting Technique.

This technique consists of three major processes:

1. Separation of proteins by size (Electrophoresis).

2. Transfer to a solid support (Blotting)
3. Marking target protein using a proper primary and secondary antibody to visualize (Detection).

- Western blotting is usually done on a tissue homogenate or extract.
- **SDS-PAGE (Sodium dodecyl sulphate polyacrylamide gel electrophoresis)**, a type of gel electrophoresis is used to separate various proteins in a mixture according to their electrophoretic mobility which depends on charge, size of protein molecule and structure of the proteins.
- Proteins present in the tissue homogenate are moved within the gel produce various size bands, that should be transferred in to a Nitrocellulose (NC) or Polyvinylidene difluoride (PVDF) membrane.
- Proteins transferring in to membrane can be achieved in number of ways, but most common are electrophoretic transfer (Elecroblotting) and microfiltration (Dot blotting).
- In general electrophoretic transfer is used to transfer proteins following electrophoretic separation by native or **SDS-PAGE and** microfiltration is used to transfer proteins that are in solution with out doing any electrophoresis.
- During blotting, proteins combine with nitrocellulose membrane based on hydrophobic interaction. Pre-activation of membrane is not needed.
- Then blotted membrane is treated with a Bovine serum albumin (BSA) solution, to prevent the non specific binding of the antibodies in the membrane **(Blocking)** since membrane has high affinity to the protein and antibody molecules.
- The membrane is then incubated with antibodies specific to the protein of interest. For detection of the proteins primary antibody and secondary antibody conjugated with enzyme is used.
- After hybridization of antigen and antibody, the unbound antibody is washed off using wash buffer leaving only the bound antibody to the protein of interest.
- After binding of the enzyme–antibody conjugate, addition of a chromogenic substrate, specific to the enzyme conjugated with secondary body,a substrate reacts with the enzyme and produces a highly colored and insoluble product causes the appearance of a colored band at the site of the target antigen.
- The thickness of the band corresponds to the amount of protein present; thus doing a standard can indicate the amount of protein present.
- The antigen–antibody complexes (protein recognized by the antibody) that form in membrane can be visualized in a variety of ways.

- ☆ If the protein of interest is bound by a radioactive antibody, its position on the blotted membrane can be determined by exposing the membrane to a sheet of X-ray film, a procedure called **autoradiography**.
- ☆ However, the most generally used detection procedures employ enzyme-linked antibodies against the protein.
- ☆ The site of the protein of interest can be determined with much higher sensitivity if a chemiluminescent compound along with suitable enhancing agents is used to produce light at the antigen site.

Application of Western Blotting

1. Identification of a specific protein in a complex mixture of proteins.
2. Estimation of the size of the protein as well as the amount of protein present in the mixture.
3. It is most widely used as a confirmatory test for diagnosis of many diseases like HIV,Herps, Hepatitis *etc.*, where this procedure is used to determine whether the patient has antibodies that react with one or more viral proteins or not.
4. It can be used to identify the nature of protein or epitope effectively

Polymerase Chain Reaction (PCR)

The polymerase chain reaction (PCR) was originally developed in 1983 by the American biochemist **Kary Mullis**. He was awarded the Nobel Prize in Chemistry in 1993 for his pioneering work. **Polymerase chain reaction** (**PCR**) is a common laboratory technique used to make millions of copies of a particular region of DNA or gene. Using PCR it is possible to generate thousands to millions of copies of a particular section of DNA from a very small amount of template DNA with in a few hours of time. Typically, the goal of PCR is to make enough of the target DNA region that can be analyzed or used for visualization by gel electrophoresis or sent for sequencing or cloned into a plasmid for further experiments.

Taq polymerase

Like DNA replication in an organism, PCR requires a DNA polymerase enzyme that makes new strands of DNA, using existing strands as templates. The DNA polymerase typically used in PCR is called ***Taq* polymerase**, after the heat-tolerant bacterium *Thermus* ***aquaticus*** from which it was isolated. *T. aquaticus* lives in hot springs and hydrothermal vents. Its DNA polymerase is highly heat-stable and is most active around 70°C (a temperature at which a human or *E. coli* DNA polymerase would be nonfunctional). This heat-stability makes Taq polymerase ideal for PCR.

PCR Primers

Like other DNA polymerases, *Taq* polymerase can only make DNA if it's given a short of oligo nucleotidesequence called as a **primer,** that provides a starting point for DNA synthesis. PCR primers are short pieces of single-stranded DNA, usually around 20-30 bp (nucleotides) in length. Two primers are used in each PCR reaction (forward and reverse primer), and they are designed in such a way that they flank the target region (region that should be copied). The primers bind to the template by complementary base pairing (Figure 18.3).

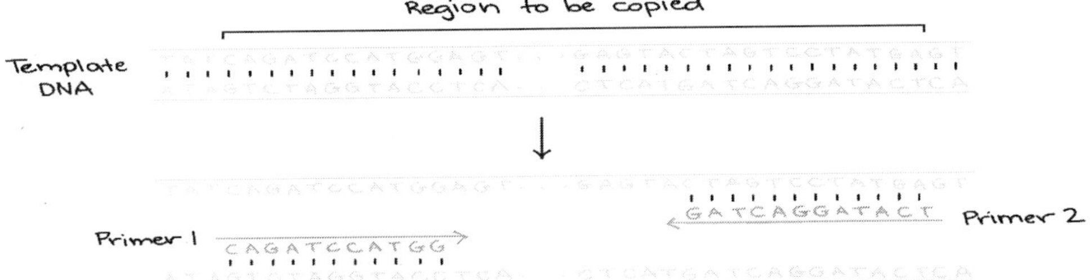

Figure 18.3. Primers Binds Respective Template by Complementary Base Pairing.

Template DNA Containing Target Region Need to be Amplified

5' TATCAGATCCATGGAGT.GAGTACTAGTCCTATGAGT 3' (Sence Strand)

3' ATAGTCTAGGTACCTCA.CTCATGATCAGGATACTCA 5' (Antisence Strand)

Primer 1: 5' CAGATCCATGG 3' (Forward primer)

Primer 2: 5' TCATAGGACTAG 3'(Reverse primer)

When the primers are bound to the template, they can be extended by the polymerase, and the region that lies between them will get copied. Both the primers, synthesis the new strand 5' to 3' direction towards the region to be copied. New strand always needed free OH group in the 3rd position of ribose sugar (3' end) for the addition of new nucleotide, so growing chain always will be 5' to 3' direction not in 3' to 5' direction. Like other DNA polymerases, *Taq* polymerase can only synthesize DNA in the 5' to 3' direction. When the primers are extended, the region that lies between them will be copied (Figure 18.4).

Basic Requirement of PCR

PCR involves a process of continuous heating and cooling is called thermal cycling which is carried out by thermal cycler machine. Whatever the template DNA may be, principle behind the PCR is same. Five core 'ingredients' are required to set up a PCR. These are:

- ✰ The DNA template containing target region need to be amplified
- ✰ Primers (Forward and reverse primer),short stretches of DNA that initiate the PCR reaction, designed to bind to either side of the section of DNA need to be copied

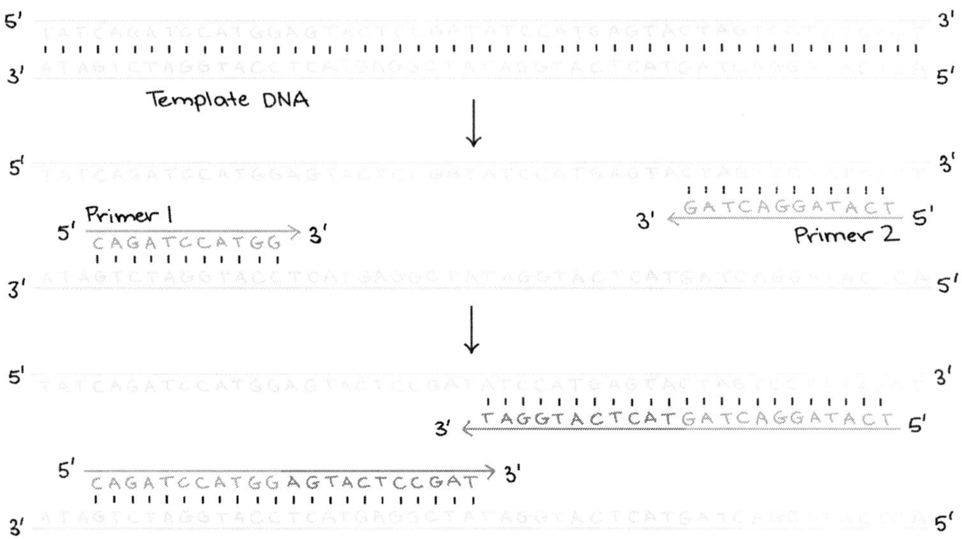

Figure 18.4. Extension of Primer and Synthesizing of New Strand.

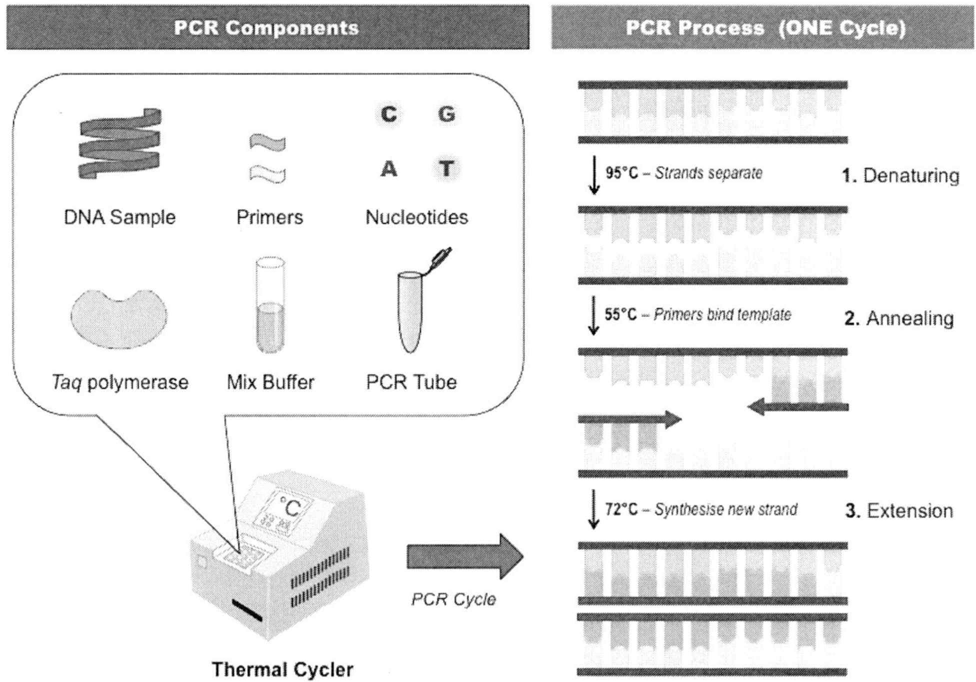

Figure 18.5. PCR Components and Steps in PCR Reaction.

- ☆ DNA bases (A, C, G and T) (also known as dNTPs) are the building blocks of DNA needed to add the growing are newly synthesizing DNA strand
- ☆ Taq polymerase enzyme for polymerization of new strand
- ☆ Taq buffer with Mg ions to ensure the right conditions for the polymerization reaction (Figure 18.5).

There are three stages **Denaturation, annealing and extension** will be repeated up to 25-35 times, in each time the number of DNA copies will be increased in **2^n times, here 'n' represents** the number of cycle (Figure 18.5. and Figure 18.6).

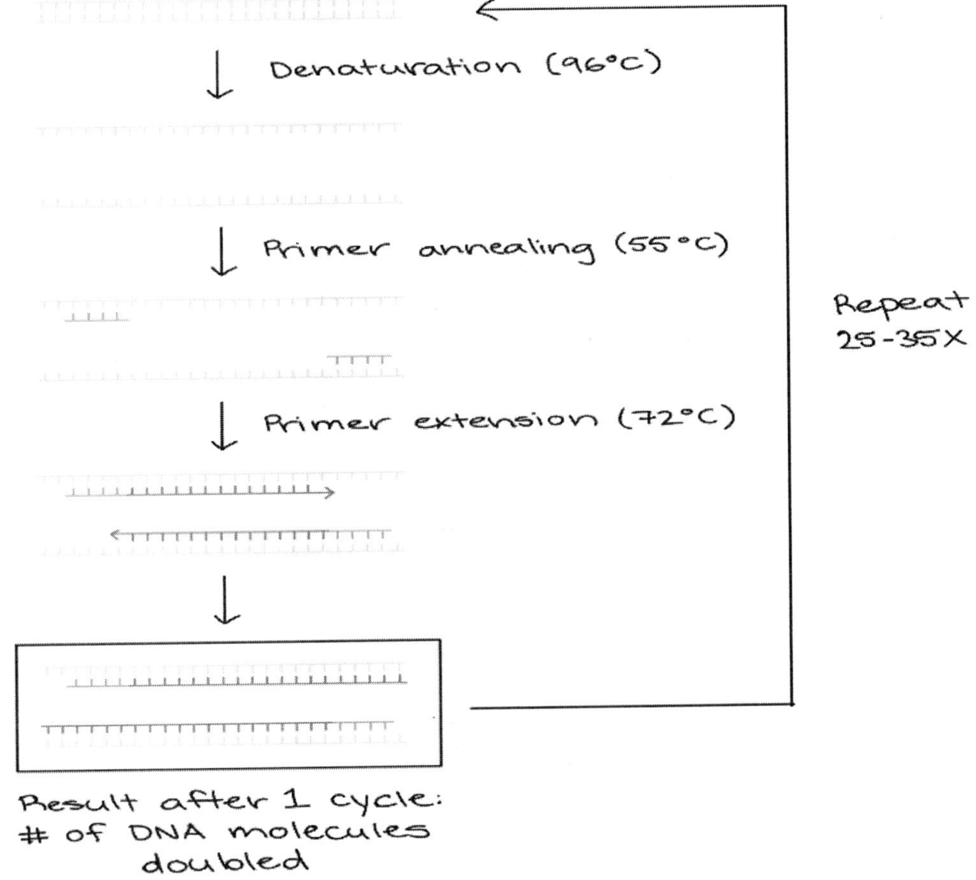

Figure 18.6. Complete Cycle of PCR

Different Stage of PCR

1. Initial Denaturation

This is the first step of PCR. In this double stranded DNA will be denatured in to single stranded. Since more amount of DNA present in the initial sample, it require **3-5 min at 94-95°C**for getting complete denaturation. This step is only once in the whole PCR reaction.

2. Denaturing Stage

- ☆ During this stage the cocktail containing the template DNA and all the other core ingredients is heated to 94-95°C.
- ☆ The high temperature causes the hydrogen bonds between the bases in two strands of template DNA to break and the two strands to separate.
- ☆ This results in two single strands of DNA, which will act as templates for the production of the new strands of DNA.
- ☆ It is important that the temperature is maintained at this stage for long enough to ensure that the DNA strands have separated completely.
- ☆ This usually takes between 45-60 seconds.

3. Annealing Stage

- ☆ During this stage the reaction is cooled to 50-60°C. This enables the primers to attach the specific location on the single-stranded template DNA, where it finds complementary base sequence by forming hydrogen bonding (the exact melting temperature is not uniform, It varied depends up on the primers used).
- ☆ Primers are single strands of DNA or RNA sequence that are around 20 to 30 bases in length.
- ☆ The primers are designed to be complementary in sequence to short sections of DNA on each end of the sequence to be copied.
- ☆ Primers served as the starting point to Taq DNA polymerase enzyme for DNA synthesis.
- ☆ The two separated strands of DNA are complementary and run in opposite directions in which forward primer and reverse primer will bind in respective strand.
- ☆ This step usually takes about 30-45 seconds (Figure 18.7).

4. Extending Stage (Extension)

- ☆ During this final step, the heat is increased to 72°C to enable the new DNA to be made by a special Taq DNA polymerase enzyme which adds DNA bases.
- ☆ Taq DNA polymerase is an enzyme taken from the heat-loving bacteria *Thermus aquaticus*.
- ☆ This bacteria normally lives in hot springs so can tolerate temperatures above 80°C.
- ☆ The bacteria's DNA polymerase is very stable at high temperatures, which means it can withstand the temperatures needed to break the strands of DNA apart in the denaturing stage of PCR.

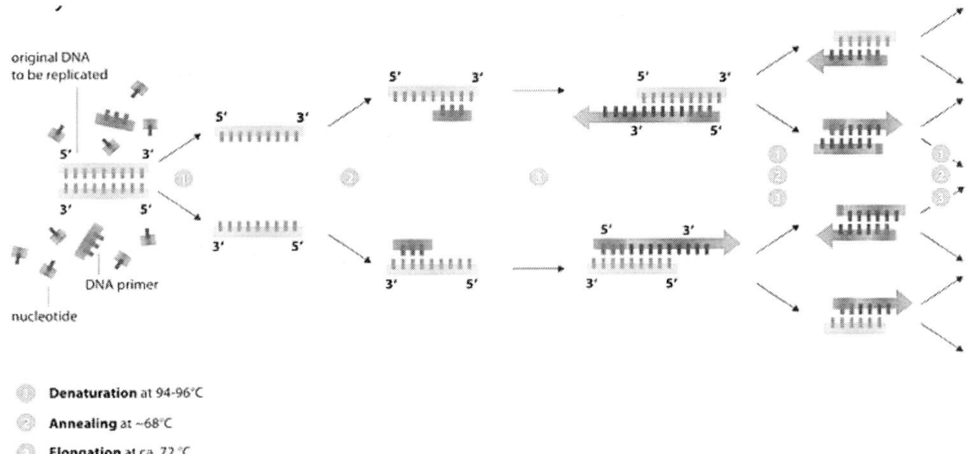

Figure 18.7. Exponential Amplification of PCR.

- DNA polymerase from most other organisms would not be able to withstand these high temperatures, for example, human polymerase works ideally at 37°C (body temperature).
- 72°C is the optimum temperature for the Taq polymerase to build the complementary strand. It attaches to the primer and then adds DNA bases to the single strand one-by-one in the 5' to 3' direction.
- The duration of this step depends on the length of DNA sequence being amplified but usually takes around one minute to copy 1,000 DNA bases (1Kb).
- These three processes of thermal cycling are repeated 20-40 times to produce lots of copies of the DNA sequence of interest.
- During this cycling first cycle product will act as a tempelate for the next
- The result is a huge number of copies of the specific DNA segment is produced in a relatively short period of time.

5. Final Extension

- This is the lost step of PCR and this also conducted only once in whole PCR reaction used to keep for 5-10 min at 72°C.
- This step helps to finish the incomplete reactions occurred during 25-35 times repetition of 2, 3 and 4th step of PCR. After this step product analysis should be done with amplified PCR product. In product analysis The amplified DNA (PCR product) is electrophoretically migrated according to their molecular size by performing agarose gel electrophoresis. The amplified DNA forms clear bands in agarose gel which can be visualized under ultra-violet (UV) light in Gel DOC instrument. Amplified product

with positive result will be stored at 4°C for short term or it can be stored for long time at -20°C for future analysis.

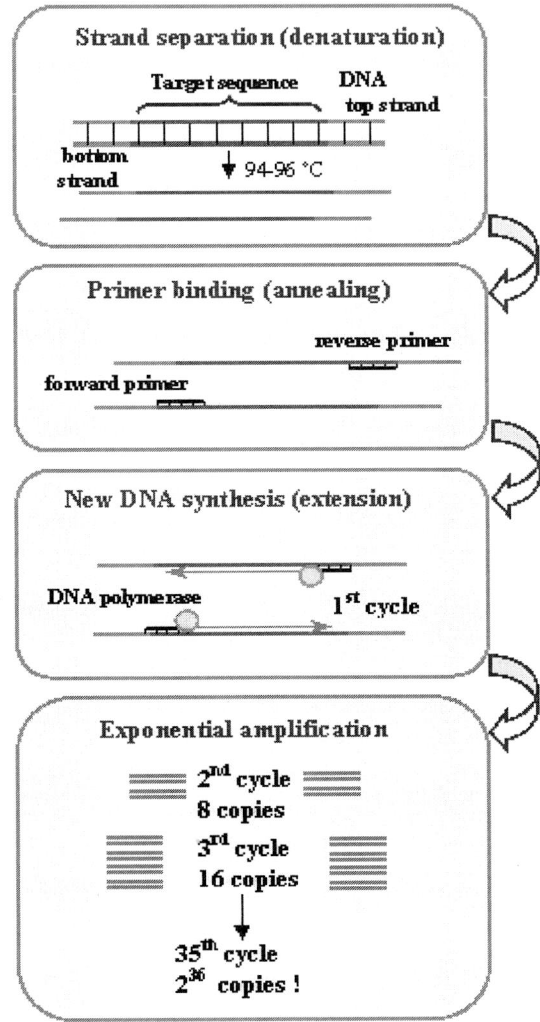

Figure 18.8. Overall Process of the Polymerase Chain Reaction (PCR).

Application

- PCR for Site Directed Mutagenesis -This technique is used for introduction of mutations at the desired place in a DNA sequence by altering the sequences of primers.
- Detection of recombinant DNA from transgenic crop.
- DNA sequencing and cloning

- DNA based phylogenetic studies.
- Functional analysis of genes
- Diagnosis of hereditary diseases
- Identification of genetic finger prints used in forensics and paternity studies
- The detection and Diagnosis of infectious diseases
- It can be used to determine the sex of embryos.

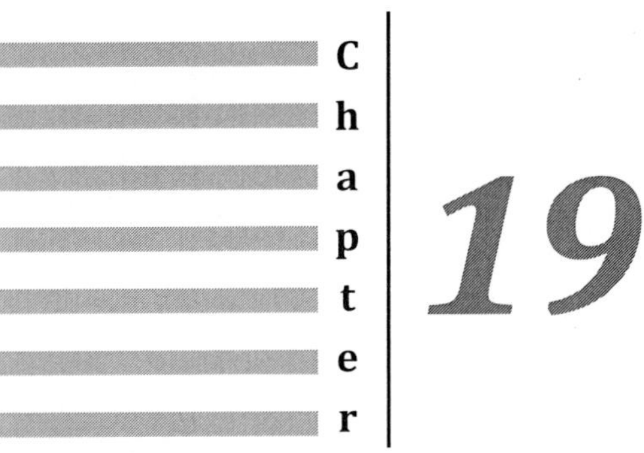

DNA Sequencing Methods

Determination of the precise order of nucleotides within a DNA molecule is popularly known as **DNA sequencing**. The development of DNA sequencing techniques with enhanced speed, sensitivity and throughput are of utmost importance for the study of biological systems. About four decades ago in the year **1977, Sanger and Maxam–Gilbert** made a breakthrough that revolutionized the world of biological sciences by sequencing the **5,386-base bacteriophage** φ **X174**. From the year 1977 to till date DNA sequencing came across much advancement in terms of sequencing tools and techniques. The modern era DNA sequencing are dealing with next generation sequencing and many other advancement are available to the researchers, practitioners, and academicians at a very reasonable cost with highest accuracy. The biological databases are being flooded with a huge flow of sequences coming out from various organisms across the world. Today the researchers and scientists across the various fields are utilizing these data for a variety of applications including food security by developing better crops and crop yields, livestock, improved diagnostics, prognostics and therapies for many complex diseases.

Maxam–Gilbert Method

Allan Maxam and Walter Gilbert developed a method for sequencing single-stranded DNA by a two-step catalytic process involving **piperidine and two chemicals *i.e.* dimethyl sulfate and hydrazine that selectively attack purines and pyrimidines.** Purines react with dimethyl sulfate and pyrimidines react with hydrazine in such a way these chemicals modified the bases by adding the methyl group (methylation) and break the glycoside bond between the ribose sugar and the base, later the modified base got displaced from the DNA strand. Piperidine catalyzes cleavage of phosphodiester bonds where the base has been displaced. Moreover, dimethyl sulfate and piperidine selectively cleave guanine nucleotides (G) but dimethyl sulfate and piper idine in presence of formic acid cleave both **guanine and adenine nucleotides(G and C).** Similarly, hydrazine and piperidine cleave both thymine and cytosine nucleotides (C and T), whereas hydrazine and piperidine in presence of 1.5 M NaCl only cleave cytosine **nucleotides (C)**. The concentration of the modifying chemicals is controlled to introduce on average one modification per DNA molecule.z

Maxam-Gilbert sequencing requires denaturation of DNA fragment to be sequenced in to single strand and radioactive labeling at one 5' end of the single strand. This labeled single strand DNA is subjected to four separate cleavage reactions, each of which creates a population of labeled cleavage products ending in known nucleotides. The reactions are loaded on high percentage polyacrylamide gels and the fragments are resolved by electrophoresis. The gel then is transferred to a light-proof X-ray film cassette, a piece of X-ray film placed over the gel, and the cassette placed in a freezer for several days. Wherever a labeled fragment stopped on the gel, the radioactive tag would expose the film due to particle decay (autoradiography). The dark autoradiography bands on the film represent the 5' to 3' DNA sequence when read from bottom to top. The process of base calling involves interpreting the banding pattern relative to the four chemical reactions. For example, a band in the lanes corresponding to the C reaction and also the C+T reactions called a C. If the band present in the C+T reaction lane but not in the C reaction lane it is called as T. The same decision process can be obtained for the G only and the G+A reaction lanes. Sequences can be confirmed by running replicate reactions on the same gel and comparing the autoradiographic patterns between replicates (Figure 19.1).

Sanger's Sequencing

Frederick Sanger and his colleagues developed the method of sequencing known as **chain termination method or dideoxy method.** This method soon became popular and common method of sequencing used by molecular biologists because of its ease to use and reliability. In this there is less use of toxic chemicals and also less amount of radioactivity is used when compared to Maxam method. Sanger's method was automated and it became the commonly used method of DNA sequencing. Some of next generation sequencing methods are followed the principle and working based on Sanger sequencing method. DNA is synthesized from four deoxynucleotide triphosphates. Each new nucleotide is added to the 3' – OH group of the last nucleotide of that strand. So new nucleotide can be added to the any growing or newly synthesizing DNA strand only in the presence of free OH, at the 3' end, in the absence of free OH the new nucleotide will not be added, so growing chain will get terminated. The dideoxy method gets its name from the critical role played by synthetic nucleotides (dideoxy nucleotides) that lack the -OH at the 3' carbon atom in ribose sugar (Figure 19.2). A dideoxynucleotide can

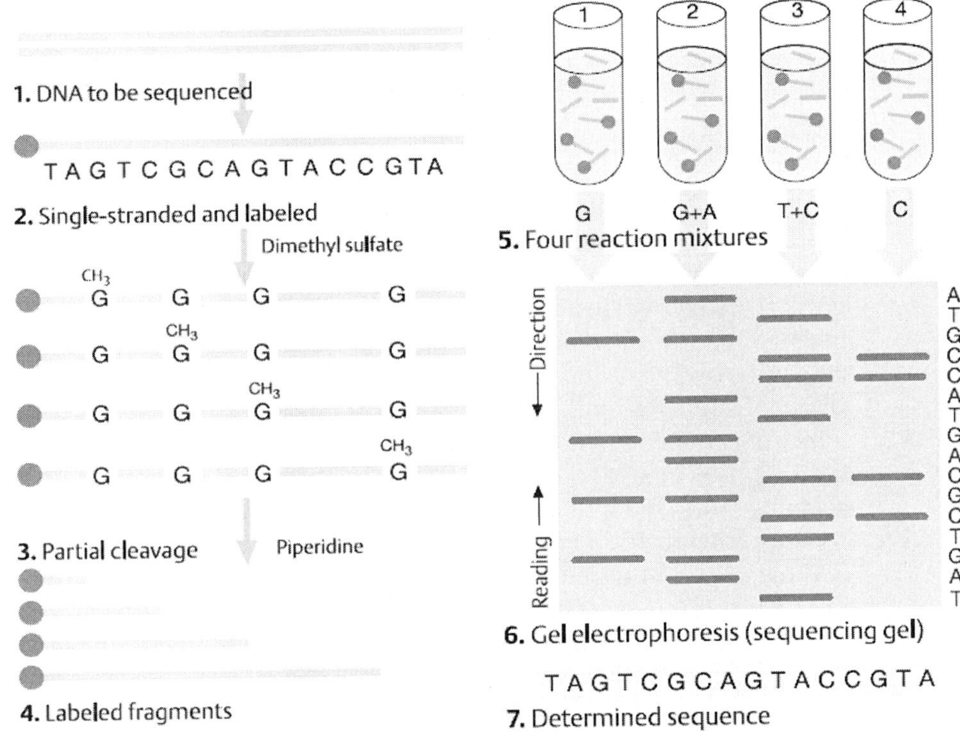

Figure 19.1. Maxam–Gilbert Sequencing Method.

be added to the growing DNA strand. When it is added it stops chain elongation because there is no 3' -OH for the next nucleotide to be attached. For this reason, the dideoxy method is also called the **chain termination method.**

P—P—P—C 5'
O
Thymine
C4'
1' C
Deoxythymidine triphosphate (dTTP)
3' 2'
C—C
OH H

P—P—P—C 5'
O
Thymine
C4'
1' C
Dideoxythymidine triphosphate (ddTTP)
3' 2'
C—C
H H

Figure 19.2. Structure of Deoxy and Dideoxynucleotide (dTTP).

Various steps involved in the Sanger sequencing methods :

1. The region of DNA to be sequenced is amplified in some way and then denatured to produce single stranded DNA.
2. A sequencing primer is annealed to the single stranded DNA.
3. DNA sequencing takes advantage of the fact that a growing chain of nucleotides, extending in the 5' to 3' direction. Because all four normal nucleotides are present, chain elongation proceeds normally until, by chance, DNA polymerase inserts a dideoxy nucleotide instead of the normal deoxynucleotide. ddNTPs differs from conventional dNTPs because of the absence of a hydroxyl residue at the 3'position of deoxyribose. These ddNTPs can be incorporated in to the DNA chain by DNA polymerases by their 5'triphosphate groups but the absence of a 3'hydroxyl residue in ddNTP will not allow to form the phosphodiester bond to the next dNTP. It leads to prevention of extension of the growing DNA chain. In such a way dideoxy nucleotide is added to the **normal nucleotide (1:100 ratio)**, allow DNA strands will succeed in adding several hundred nucleotides before insertion of the dideoxy by performing four separate reactions, each containing a DNA polymerase and a small amount of one of the four dideoxynucleotides in addition to all four deoxynucleotides, four separate sets of chain-terminated fragments can be produced (Figure 19.3. shows the reaction tube of ddATP in The dideoxy sequencing method and Autoradiography of polyacrylmide gel electrophoresis).
4. Following the replication/termination step, these chain terminated fragments will remain bound to the single stranded DNA molecule which has acted as a template. By heating these partially double stranded molecules and adding a denaturing agent such as formamide, the single stranded chain termination molecules can be released from their template and separated using high resolution denaturing gel electrophoresis.
5. The sequence of the original region of DNA is then finally deduced by examining the relative positions of the dideoxynucleotide chain termination products in the four lanes of the denaturing gel like in Maxam–Gilbert sequencing method

Automated DNA Sequencing

With the many advancements in technology that has been achieved since 1974, it is no surprise that the Sanger method has become outdated. However, the new technology that has emerged to replace this method is based on the same principles of Sanger's method. Automated sequencing has been developed so that more DNA can be sequenced in a shorter period of time. Instead of using radiolabeled primer in the automated procedures fluorescent labelling is used. So in the automated sequencing the reactions are performed in a single tube containing all four ddNTP's,

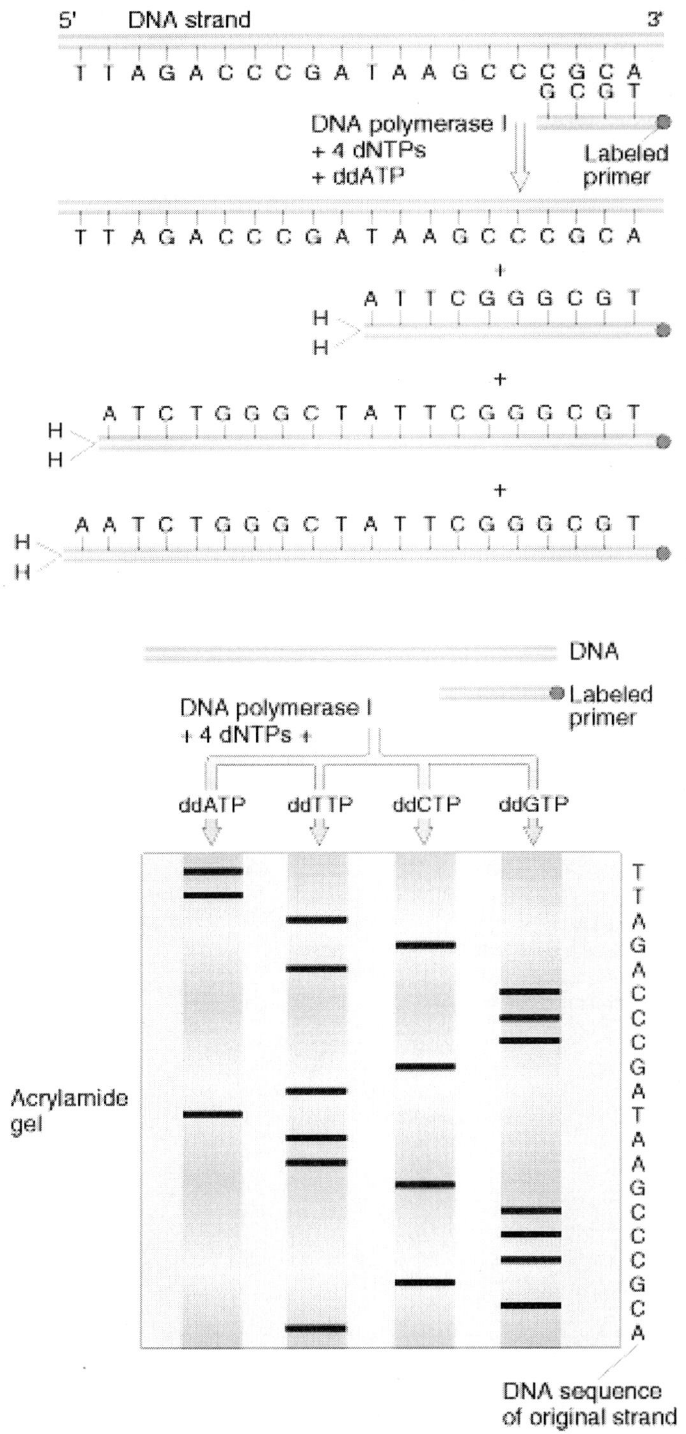

Figure 19.3. Dideoxy Sequencing Method (Sanger sequencing).

each labeled with a different color dye *i.e.* ddATP (orange), ddGTP (green), ddCTP (blue) and ddTTP (red). Since the four dyes fluoresce at different wavelengths, a laser then reads the gel to determine the identity of each band according to the wavelengths at which it fluoresces. The results are then depicted in the form of a chromatogram, which is a diagram of colored peaks that correspond to the nucleotide in that location in the sequence (Figure 19.4).

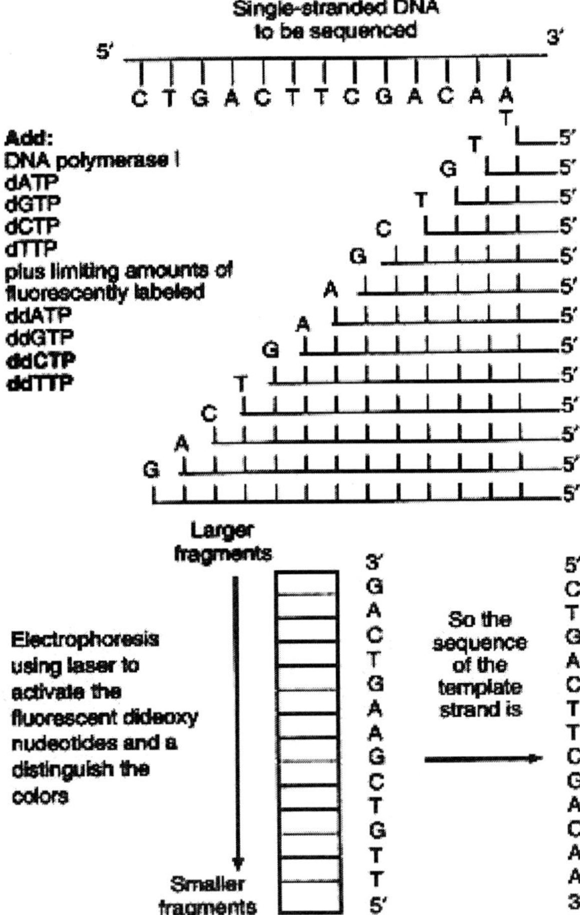

Figure 19.4. Automated DNA Sequencing.

Pyrosequencing

In 1996, Pal Nyren's group reported that natural nucleotide can be used to obtain efficient incorporation during a sequencing-by-synthesis protocol. The detection was based on the pyrophosphate (inorganic biphosphate) released during the DNA polymerase reaction, the quantitative conversion of pyrophosphate to ATP by sulfurylase and the subsequent production of visible light by firefly luciferase.

In a cascade of enzymatic reaction, visible light is generated that is proportional to the number of incorporated nucleotides. The cascade starts with a nucleic acid polymerization reaction in which inorganic biphosphate (PPi) is released as a result of nucleotide incorporation by polymerase. The released PPi is subsequently converted to ATP by ATP sulfurylase, which provides the energy to luciferase to oxidize luciferin and generate light. The light so generated is captured by a CCD camera and recorded in the form of peaks known as pyrogram (compared with electropherograms in Sanger's method). Apyrase, a nucleotide degrading enzyme, degrades unincorporated nucleotides, and ATP. After degradation another nucleotide is added. Sequencing is achieved by sequentially introducing each of the four dNTPs into the flow cell. Presence or absence of light burst of each picotiter well indicates the incorporation of corresponding nucleotide, therefore, added nucleotide is known. It reveals the identity of complementary base on the template DNA in that well.

Shotgun Sequencing

Shotgun sequencing is a sequencing method designed for analysis of DNA sequences longer than 1000 base pairs, up to and including entire chromosomes. This method requires the target DNA to be broken into random fragments. After sequencing individual fragments, the sequences can be reassembled on the basis of their overlapping regions.

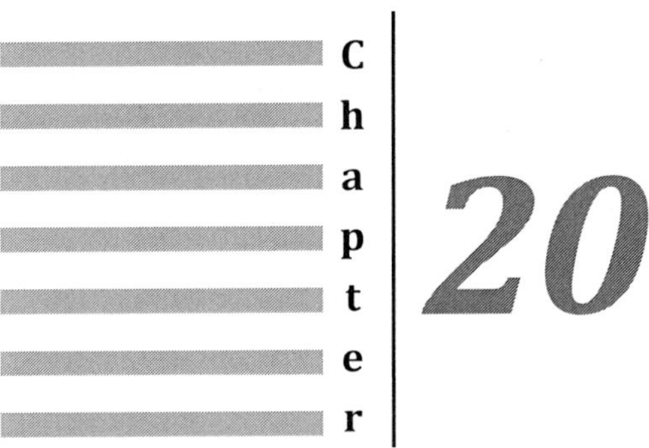

DNA Manipulation Enzymes: Polymerase, Restriction Endonucleases and Ligases

The process of DNA cloning involves placing a relatively short fragment of a genome, which might contain the gene or other sequence of interest, in an autonomously replicating piece of DNA, known as a vector, forming recombinant DNA, which can be replicated independently of the original genome, in host species. **Propagation of the host organism containing the recombinant DNA forms a set of genetically identical organisms, or a clone this process is called cloning.**

The essential steps involved in DNA cloning are:

1. Generating DNA fragments,
2. Cutting and joining the DNA fragments to vector DNA molecules,
3. Introducing the vectors carrying the foreign DNA into host cells where they can replicate
4. Selecting or identifying the clone(s) of recipient cells that have acquired the recombinant DNA molecules

Many enzymes are used in DNA cloning and analysis such as DNA polymerases, restriction endonucleases, ligases, reverse transcriptase, phosphatase, kinase, *etc.*

DNA Polymerase: Tool for Polymerization

A DNA polymerase is an enzyme that synthesizes DNA molecules from their nucleotide building blocks. DNA polymerases are essential for DNA synthesis.

DNA polymerases are widely used in molecular biology laboratories, notably for the polymerase chain reaction (PCR), DNA sequencing, and molecular cloning. **In 1956, Arthur Kornberg and colleagues** discovered the enzyme **DNA polymerase I, also known as Pol I, in *Escherichia coli*.** They described the DNA replication process by which DNA polymerase copies the base sequence of a template DNA strand. Subsequently in 1959, Kornberg was awarded the Nobel Prize in Physiology or Medicine for this work. DNA polymerase can add free nucleotides only to the 3' end of the newly forming strand. This results in elongation of the newly forming **strand in a 5'-3' direction** (Figure 20.1).

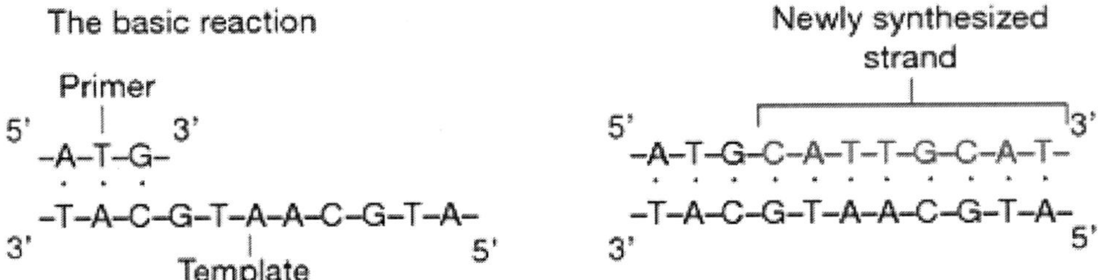

Figure 20.1. Polymerization of Short Strand by DNA Polymerase.

Four types of DNA polymerase are used routinely in genetic engineering.

i. DNA Polymerase I

DNA polymerase I is usually prepared from *E. coli*. **This enzyme attaches to a short single-stranded region (or nick) in a mainly double-stranded DNA molecule**, and then synthesizes a completely new strand, degrading the existing strand as it proceeds. DNA polymerase I is therefore an example of an enzyme with a **dual activity-DNA polymerization and DNA degradation (nuclease activity)** (Figure 20.2).

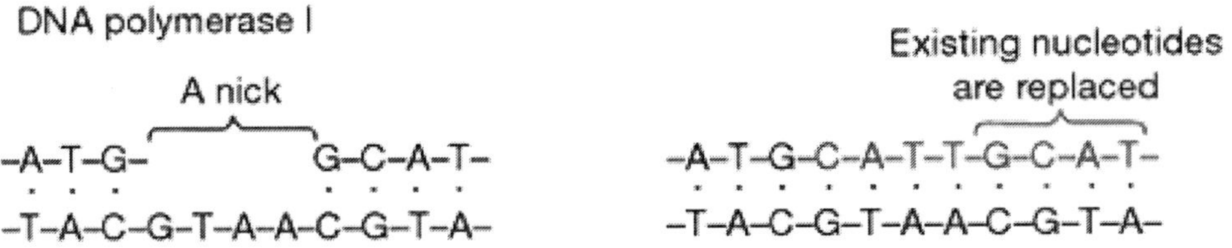

Figure 20.2. Polymerization and Exonuclease Activity of DNA Polymerase.

ii. Klenow Fragment

It is obtained by modifying the DNA polymerase I. The modification is the **removal of the nuclease activity** segment of DNA polymerase I, which leaves a modified enzyme that retains the polymerase function but is unable to degrade DNA. This modified enzyme can still synthesize a complementary DNA strand on a single-stranded template, but as it has no nuclease activity it cannot continue the synthesis once the gap or nick is filled in (Figure 20.3).

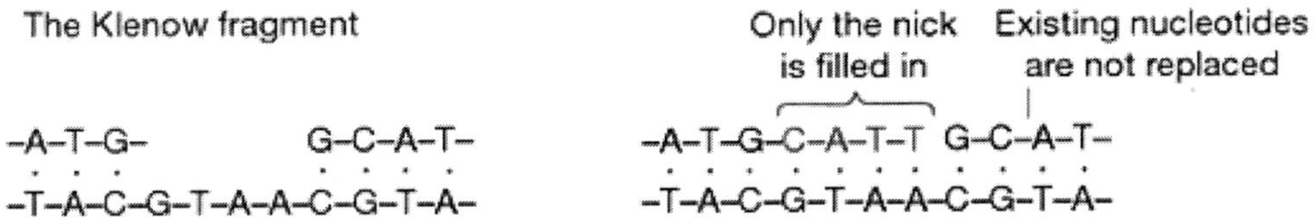

The Klenow fragment

-A-T-G- G-C-A-T-
-T-A-C-G-T-A-A-C-G-T-A-

Only the nick is filled in

Existing nucleotides are not replaced

-A-T-G-C-A-T-T G-C-A-T-
-T-A-C-G-T-A-A-C-G-T-A-

Figure 20.3. Polymerization Activity of Klenow Fragment.

iii. *Taq* Polymerase

The *Taq* DNA polymerase used in the polymerase chain reaction (PCR) is the DNA polymerase I enzyme of the bacterium ***Thermus aquaticus***. This organism lives in hot springs, and many of its enzymes, including the Taq DNA polymerase, are thermostable, meaning that they are resistant to denaturation by heat treatment. This is the special feature of ***Taq* DNA polymerase that makes it suitable for PCR,** because if it was not thermostable it would be inactivated when the temperature of the reaction is raised to 94°C to denature the DNA.

iv. Reverse Transcriptase

Reverse transcriptase is an enzyme involved in the replication of several kinds of virus. **Reverse transcriptase is unique in that it uses as a template not DNA but RNA**. The ability of this enzyme to synthesize a DNA strand complementary to an RNA template is central to the technique called complementary DNA (cDNA) cloning (Figure 20.4).

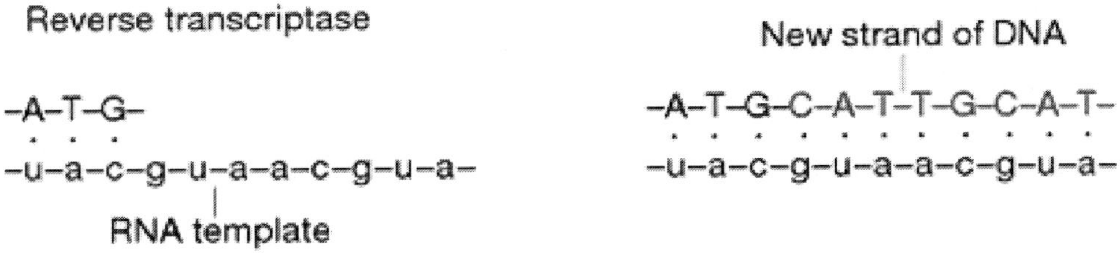

Reverse transcriptase

-A-T-G-
-u-a-c-g-u-a-a-c-g-u-a-

RNA template

New strand of DNA

-A-T-G-C-A-T-T-G-C-A-T-
-u-a-c-g-u-a-a-c-g-u-a-

Figure 20.4. DNA Synthesized from RNA Template by Reverse Transcriptase.

Restriction Endonucleases: Tool for Cutting DNA Molecules

In 1970 the first restriction endonuclease enzyme **HindII** was isolated. For the subsequent discovery and characterization of numerous restriction endonucleases, in **1978 Daniel Nathans, Werner Arber, and Hamilton O. Smith awarded for**

Nobel Prize for Physiology or Medicine. Since then, restriction enzymes have been used as an essential tool in recombinant DNA technology

A restriction enzyme is a protein that recognizes a specific, short nucleotide sequence and cuts the DNA only at that specific site, which is known as restriction site or target sequence. More than 400 restriction enzymes have been isolated from the bacteria. In live bacteria, restriction enzymes function to defend the cell against invading viral bacteriophages. Restrictions sites in the viral genome are cleaved by the bacterium's restriction enzymes, fragmenting and destroying the DNA of invading bacteriophages before it can incorporate into the host's genome and take over the cell. A bacterium is immune to its own restriction enzymes, even if it has the target sequences ordinarily targeted by them. This is because the bacterial restriction sites are **highly methylated**, making them unrecognizable to the restriction enzyme(Figure 20.5).

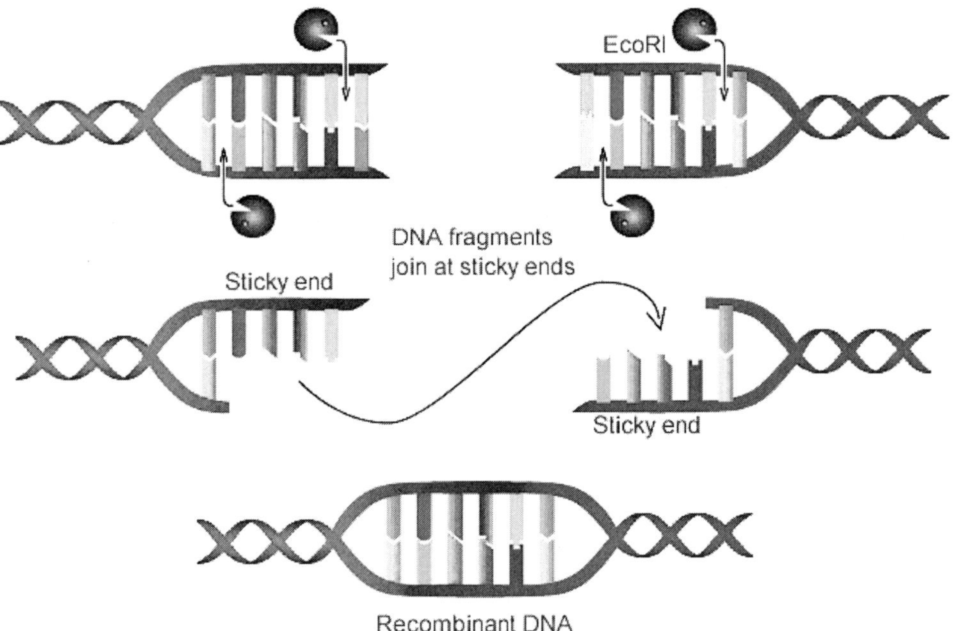

Figure 20.5. Restriction Endonuclease Activity.

When a restriction enzyme cleaves a restriction site present in the recognition sequence, the reaction creates highly reactive "sticky ends" on the broken DNA. By cutting open vector DNA with the same restriction enzymes used to cleave the target DNA, complementary "sticky ends" are created. This fosters the insertion of the target DNA into the vector. **The fragment is "glued in" with DNA ligase**, which creates the phosphodiester bonds necessary to complete the sugar-phosphate backbone of the newly transgenic DNA. Some restriction enzymes also cut DNA to form "blunt" ends (without single-stranded tails), which also can be inserted into target DNA via the action of DNA ligase (Figure 20.6).

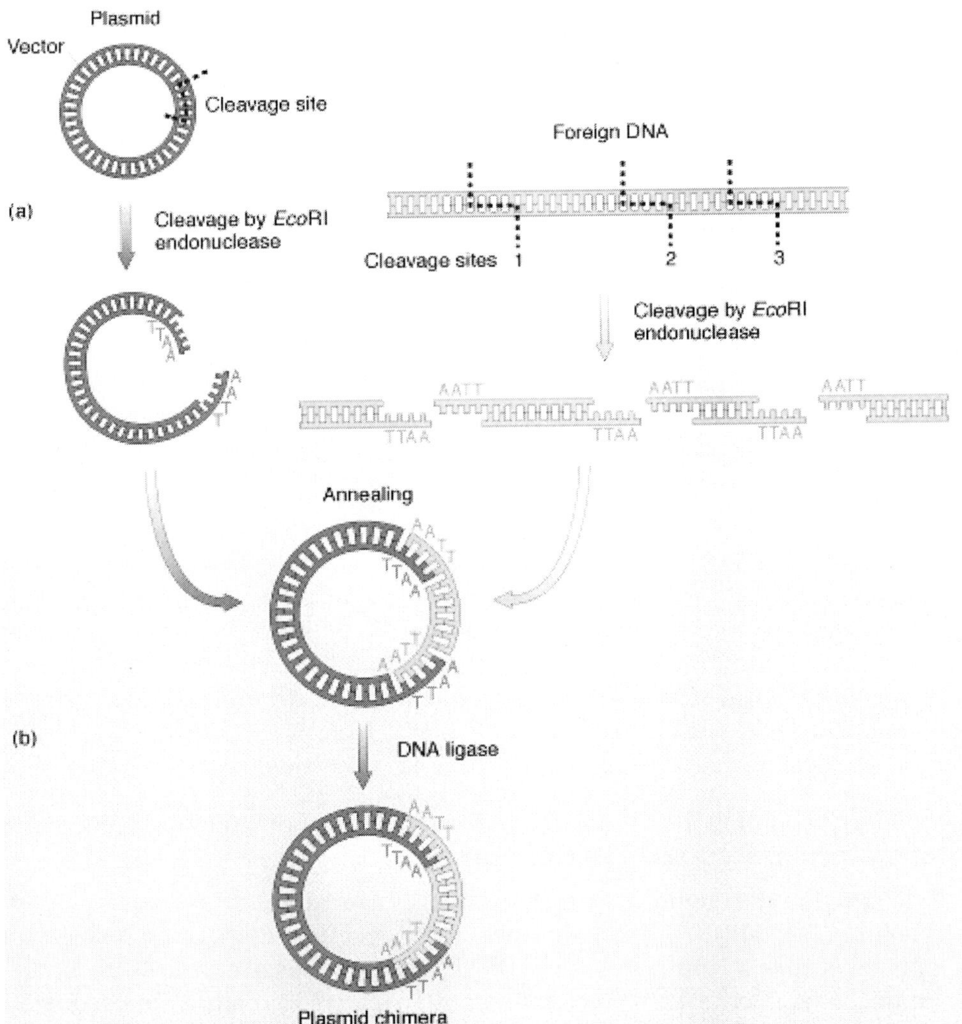

Figure 20.6. Restriction and Ligation of DNA Molecule in to Recombinant DNA (rDNA).

Identification of Restriction Enzymes

Restriction enzymes are named for the organism from which they were first isolated. For example. *Eco*RI is isolated from *E. coli* strain RY13. *Eco* refers to the genus and species (1st letter of genus; 1st two letters of specific epithet), R is the strain of *E. coli*, I (Roman numeral) indicates it was the first enzyme of that type isolated from *E. coli* RY13. *Bam*HI is isolated from *Bacillus amyloliquefaciens* strain

H. *Sau3A* is isolated from *Staphylococcus aureas* strain 3A. Another example, *HindIII* was discovered in *Haemophilus influenza* (strain d). The Roman numerals are used to identify specific enzymes from bacteria that contain multiple restriction enzymes indicating the order in which restriction enzymes were discovered in a particular strain (Figure 20.7).

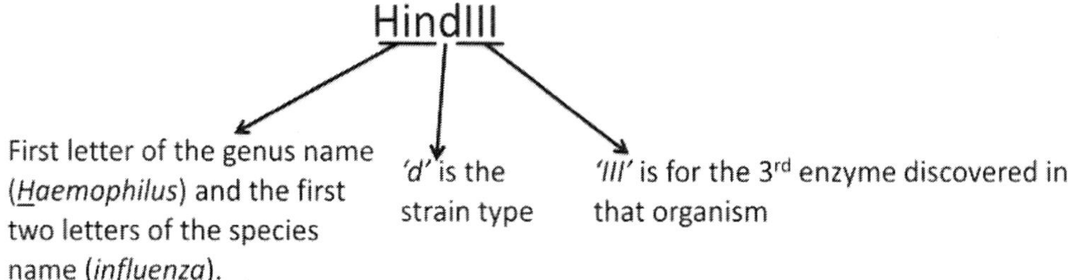

Figure 20.7. Nomenclature of Restriction Endonucleases.

Types of Restriction Endonucleases

The restriction endonucleases can be divided into three groups as type I, II and III. Types I and III are rather complex and have only a limited role in genetic engineering. Type II restriction endonucleases, on the other hand, are the cutting enzymes that are so important in gene cloning. Type II restriction enzymes has a specific recognition sequence at which it cuts a DNA molecule. A particular enzyme cleaves DNA at the recognition sequence and nowhere else. For example, the restriction endonuclease called *Pvu*I (isolated from *Proteus vulgaris*) cuts DNA only at the hexanucleotide CGATCG. In contrast, a second enzyme from the same bacterium, called *Pvu*II, cuts at a different hexanucleotide, in this case CAGCTG.

Characters of Restriction Enzymes

Restriction and modification are mediated by separate enzymes so it is possible to cleave bacterial DNA in the absence of modification. Cleavage of nucleotide sequence occurs at the restriction site. These enzymes are used to recognize rotationally symmetrical sequence which is often referred as palindromic sequence. **They require only Mg^{2+} as a cofactor and ATP is** not needed for their activity. Type II endonucleases are widely used for mapping and reconstructing DNA *in vitro* (recombinant DNA technology) because they recognize specific sites and cleave just with in that sites.

Blunt Ends and Sticky Ends

The exact nature of the cut produced by a restriction endonuclease is of considerable importance in the design of a gene cloning experiment. Many restriction endonucleases make a simple double-stranded cut in the middle of the recognition sequence resulting in a **blunt end or flush end. *Pvu*II and *Alu*I**

are examples of blunt end cutters. Other restriction endonucleases cut DNA in a slightly different way. With these enzymes the two DNA strands are not cut at exactly the same position instead restrict each strand in different position but with in the recognition site. These type of cleavage is staggered, usually by two or four nucleotides, so that the resulting DNA fragments have short single-stranded overhangs at each end. These are called **sticky or cohesive ends** (Figure 20.8).

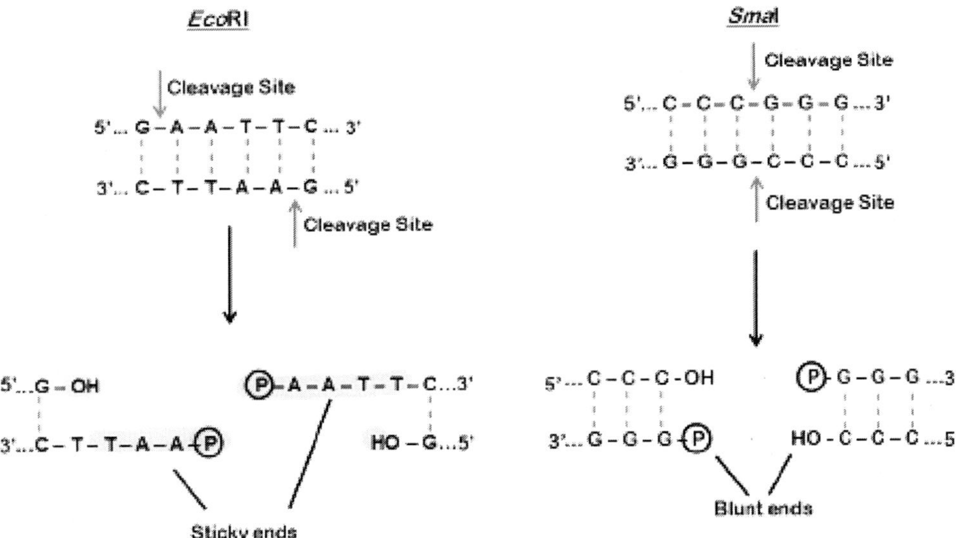

Figure 20.8. Production of Sticky and Blunt End by Restriction Endonuclease.

Table 20.1. Recognition Sequence of some Frequently Used Restriction Enzymes

ENZYME	ORGANISM	RECOGNITION SEQUENCE*	BLUNT OR STICKY END
*Eco*RI	*Escherichia coli*	GAATTC	Sticky
*Bam*HI	*Bacillus amyloliquefaciens*	GGATCC	Sticky
*Bgl*II	*Bacillus globigii*	AGATCT	Sticky
*Pvu*I	*Proteus vulgaris*	CGATCG	Sticky
*Pvu*II	*Proteus vulgaris*	CAGCTG	Blunt
*Hind*III	*Haemophilus influenzae* R_d	AAGCTT	Sticky
*Hin*fI	*Haemophilus influenzae* R_f	GANTC	Sticky
*Sau*3A	*Staphylococcus aureus*	GATC	Sticky
*Alu*I	*Arthrobacter luteus*	AGCT	Blunt
*Taq*I	*Thermus aquaticus*	TCGA	Sticky
*Hae*III	*Haemophilus aegyptius*	GGCC	Blunt
*Not*I	*Nocardia otitidis-caviarum*	GCGGCCGC	Sticky
*Sfi*I	*Streptomyces fimbriatus*	GGCCNNNNNGGCC	Sticky

Table 20.2. The Properties of Three Types of Restriction Endonucleases

Property	*Type I*	*Type II*	*Type III*
Structure	Enzyme complex of 500-600 k dal composed of thre eseparate subunits	Normally homodimers of 20-70 k dal	Heterodimers with subunits of 70 and 100 k dal
Aboundance	Less commen than Type II	Most common	Rare
Composition	Multi enzyme complex with R (endonuclease), M (methylase) and S (specificity) subunits	Separate enzymes; endonuclease is a homodimer, methylase is a monomer	M subunit provides specificity on its own; functions as methylase; as heterodimer with R subunit; functions as methylase endonuclease
Cofactors	Mg^{2+}, ATP, S-adenosyl-methionine (SAM)	Mg^{2+} only	Mg^{2+} and ATTeP
Recognition sites	15 bp length	Commonly Hexanucleotides but also tetra/penta and octanucleotides	Asymmetric recognition sites.
Cleavage	Non-specific, variable distance (100-1000 nucleotides) from recognition site	Precise cleavage within recognition site at defined distance	Precise cleavage at a fixed distance; 25-27 nucleotides from recognition site
DNA cleavage requirements	Two recognition sites in any orientation	Single recognition site	Two recognition sites in ahead-to-head orientation
Restriction and modification	Single multifunctional enzyme	Separate nuclease and methylase	Separate enzymes sharing a common subunit
Example	*Eco*K	*Eco*RI	*Mbo*II

Cleavage Patterns of Some Common Restriction Endonucleases

The recognition and cleavage sites and cleavage patterns of *HindIII, SmaI, EcoRI,* and *BamHI* are shown. Cleavage by an endonuclease creates DNA sequence with either a sticky end or blunt end. The blunt ended fragments can be joined to any other DNA fragment with blunt ends using linkers/adapters, making these enzymes useful for certain types of DNA cloning experiments (Figure 20.9).

Ligases: Tool for joining DNA fragments

Joining DNA fragments by forming **phosphodiester bonds** is yet another fundamental step in rDNA technology. This process is called as **ligation and is achieved by the catalytic reaction of enzymes called ligases.** These enzymes catalyses the formation of phosphodiester bonds between DNA molecules and facilitate the joining the nicked strand. The ligase enzymes of *E. coli* and phage T_4

have the ability to seal the single stranded nicks between nucleotides in a duplex DNA.

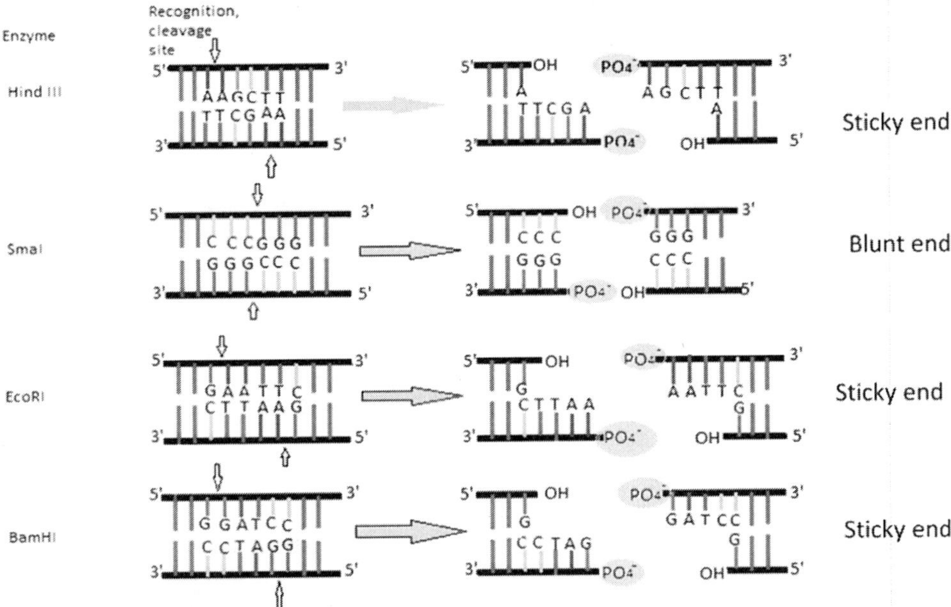

Figure 20.9. Cleavage Patterns of Restriction Enzyme.

Ligation Reaction

Although the reactions catalyzed by the ligases enzymes of *E. coli* and T_4 are similar, they differ in their cofactor requirements. The T_4 enzyme requires ATP, while the *E. coli* enzymes requires NAD^+. In each case the cofactor is split to form an enzyme-AMP complex. The complex binds to the nick, which must expose a 5'- phosphate and 3'-OH group, and makes a covalent bond in the phosphodiester chain (Figure 20.10).

DNA Modifying Enzymes

There are numerous enzymes that modify DNA molecules by addition or removal of specific chemical groups.

1. Alkaline Phosphatase

Enzyme alkaline phosphatase extracted from *E. coli* or calf intestine removes the phosphate group present in the 3' end of the DNA molecule.

2. Polynucleotide Kinase

Polynucleotide kinase enzyme extracted from *E. coli* infected with bacteriophage has the capacity to add phosphate group to the 5' end of the DNA molecule.

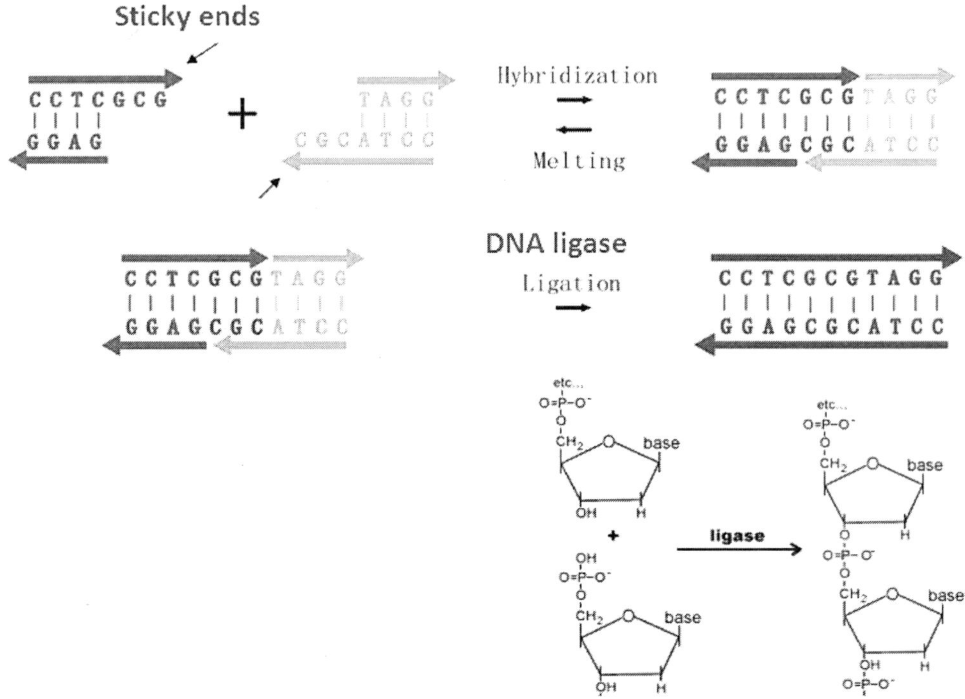

Figure 20.10. Joining of Nicks through DNA Ligase.

3. Terminal Deoxynucleotidyl Transferase

Terminal deoxynucleotidyl transferase enzyme is extracted from calf thymus tissue, which has the capacity to add one or more number of nucleotide to the 3' terminus of the DNA molecule. Action of this enzyme in the presence of just one deoxyribonucleotide, results in a homopolymer tail, and the reaction is called homopolymer tailing.

4. Exonuclease III

E. coli exonuclease III cleave from the ends of linear DNA. Exonuclease III digested DNA from the 3' terminus of the DNA molecule.

5. Nuclease S1

S1 endonuclease (from the fungus *Aspergillus oryzae*) only cleaves single strands including single-stranded nicks in the double-stranded molecules. It also changes the cohesive ends to blunt ends.

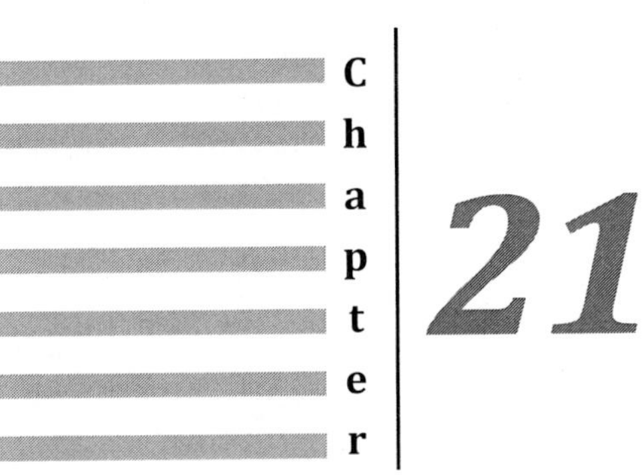

Different Type of Vectors: Plasmids, Phagemids, Cosmids and BAC

A prime requisite for a gene cloning experiment is the selection of a suitable cloning vector, *i.e.,* a DNA molecule that acts as a vehicle for carrying a foreign DNA fragment when inserted into it and transports it into a host cell, which is usually a bacterium, or other types of living cells. A wide variety of natural replicons exhibit the properties that allow them to act as cloning vectors, however, vectors may also be designed to possess certain minimum qualification to function as an efficient agent for transfer, maintenance, and amplification of target DNA.

In 1970s, when recombinant DNA technology was being first developed, only a limited number of vectors were available based on either high copy number plasmids or λ phage. Later phage M13 was developed as a specialist vector to facilitate DNA sequencing; over a time a series of specialist vectors were constructed for specific purpose like vectors based on *Escherichia coli* plasmids (***e.g.* pBR 322, pUC, pGEM**), bacteriophages (***e.g.* λ, M13, P1**), chimeric plasmids (***e.g.* cosmid, phagemid, phasmid, and fosmid**) viruses (***e.g.* cauliflower mosaic virus, potato virus X, Gemini virus, *etc.*)** and artificial chromosomes (***e.g.* YAC, BAC, PAC**) and *Agrobacterium tumefaciens* based vectors.

Properties of an Ideal Vector

1. It should be low-molecular weight, easy to isolate and purify.
2. It should be easily introduced into the host cells.
3. The vector should have suitable marker genes that allow easy detection or/and selection of the transformed the host cell. *e.g.* Genes for ampicillin and Tetracycline resistance.

4. The cells transform with recombination DNA should be indentifiable (or) selectable from those transformed by the unaltered vector.
5. Single sites for a large number of restriction endonucleases, preferably in genes with a scorable phenotype.
6. It should be able to replicate autonomously that is independent of the replication of host chromosome.
7. When expression of the DNA insert is desired, the vector should contain suitable regulatory elements like promoter, operator, and ribosome binding sites.

Based upon utilization the vectors classified as two types.

1. Cloning Vectors

Vectors used for propagation of DNA inserts in a suitable host are called cloning vectors. These are mostly used in construction of gene libraries. A number of organisms can be used as sources for cloning vectors. Some are created synthetically, as in the case of yeast artificial chromosomes and bacterial artificial chromosomes, while others are taken from bacteria and bacteriophages. In all cases, the vector needs to be genetically modified in order to accommodate the foreign DNA by creating an insertion site where the new DNA will be inserted. Example: PUC cloning vectors, pBR322 cloning vectors, BAC, YAC, phage vectors *etc.*

2. Expression Vectors or Expression Construct

Vector is designed for the expression of gene of insert *i.e.*, production of the protein specified by the DNA insert is called as expression vector. Apart from the three DNA sequences (origin of replication, selectable markers and multiple cloning sites), the expression vectors have promoter sequences and some additional sequences to facilitate the gene expression.

Plasmid Vectors

These are the most common vectors for the prokaryotic host cells. Plasmids are small, circular, double- stranded DNA molecules exists in the cytoplasm of many strains of bacteria. Plasmids are independent of the chromosome of bacterial cell and range in size from 1,000 to 2,00,000 base pairs. Some of the examples of naturally occurring plasmids are Ti plasmids, F-factors, R- factors, ColE1 plasmid, *etc.* (Figure 21.1).

The bacterial cells benefit from the presence of plasmids, which often carry genes that express proteins able to confer antibiotic resistance. These also protect bacteria by carrying genes for resistance to toxic heavy metals, such as mercury, lead, and cadmium; and plasmids are responsible for conjugation. It is very important to note that naturally occurring plasmids do not have all necessary sequences which are required by a DNA molecule to act as a profitable vector. Due to this, natural plasmids are extracted and modified by inserting suitable DNA segments and a complete vector DNA molecule is made. Plasmid-cloning vectors are derived from bacterial plasmids and are the most widely used, versatile, and easily manipulated ones.

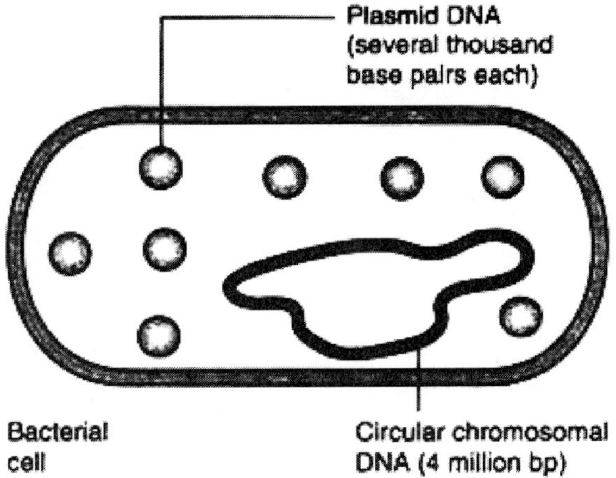

Figure 21.1. Plasmids in Bacterial Cells.

The following are different types of plasmid vectors:

I. pBR322

This was the first widely used, purpose built plasmid vector. pBR322 has a relatively small size of 4,363 bp. In pBR322 an insert of at least six kbp can be cloned. Also this vector has a reasonably high copy number (~15 copies per cell), which can be increased 200-fold by treatment with a protein-synthesis inhibitor-chloramphenicol amplification (Figure 21.2).

The nomenclature of pBR 322:

1. 'p' indicates as a plasmid.
2. **'BR' identifies Boliver and Rodriguez, the two researchers who developed it.**
3. '322' distinguishes those plasmids from others (like pBR 325, pBR 327 *etc.*) developed in the same laboratory.

The Construction of pBR322

1. Origin of Replication

It carries a fragment of plasmid pMB1 that acts as an origin for DNA replication and thus ensures multiplication of the vector.

2. Selectable Marker

It carries two antibiotic resistance genes, ampicillin and tetracycline.

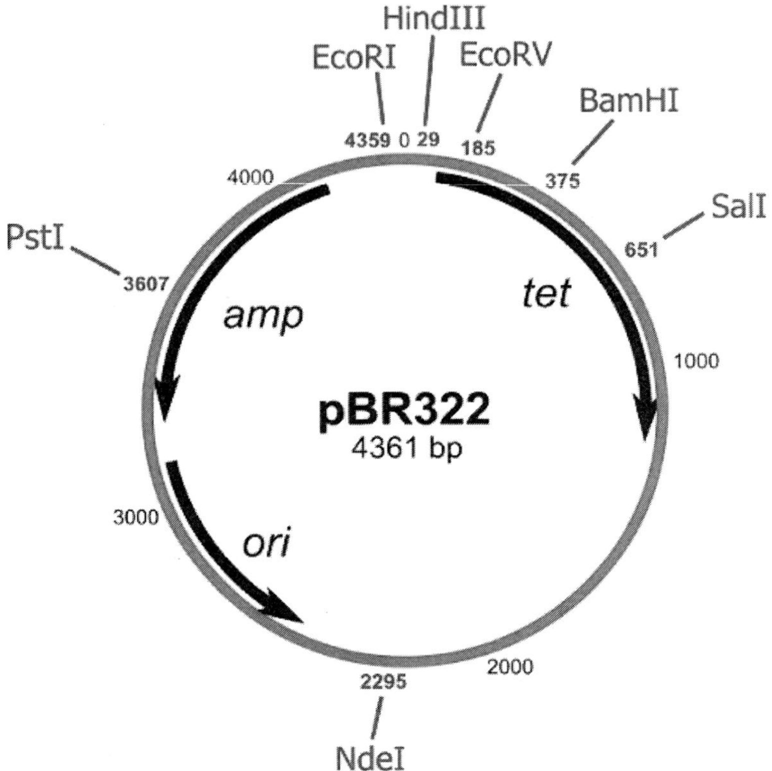

Figure 21.2. Structure of pBR322.

3. *Cloning Sites*

It carries a number of unique restriction sites. Some of these are located in one of the antibiotic resistance genes (*e.g.* sites for Pst I, Pvu I, and Sac I are found in Amp resistance gene and BamHI and Hind III in Tet resistance gene). Cloning into one of these sites inactivates that antibiotic gene, this allowing recombinants to be differentiated from non-recombinants. Inactivating the functional gene in the vector molecule by inserting a foreign gene or DNA fragment is known **insertional inactivation.** Host cells that takes up the foreign DNA from the surrounding environment those cells are called transformed cells and this process is called **transformation**. Transformed cells have two possibilities 1. Host cells transformed with recombinant DNA **(vector + gene of interest)** 2. Host cells transformed with **self ligated vector (with out gene of interest).** Every vector has some mechanism associated for screening of transformed cells with recombinant DNA (vector + gene of interest) from the transformed with non-recombinant DNA(self ligated vector).

pBR322 has several unique restriction sites that can be used to open up the vector for insertion of a new DNA fragment. For example, restriction enzyme BamHl, cuts pBR322 at just one position, within the cluster of genes that code for resistance to tetracycline. A recombinant pBR322 molecule, one that carries an extra piece of DNA in the BamHl site is no longer able to confer tetracycline resistance on its host, as one of the necessary genes is now disrupted by the inserted DNA. Cells containing this recombinant pBR322 molecule are still resistant to ampicillin, but sensitive to tetracycline (amp^R tef^s).

Screening for pBR322 recombinants is performed in the following way. After transformation the cells are plated onto ampicillin medium and incubated until colonies appear. All of these colonies are transformants (remember, untransformed cells are amp^s and so do not produce colonies on the selective medium), but only a few contain recombinant pBR322 molecules: most contain the normal, self-ligated plasmid. To identify the recombinants the colonies are replica plated into agar medium that contains tetracycline. After incubation, some of the colonies grow, but others do not. Those colonies growing in the tetracycline containing agar medium consist the normal pBR322 without DNA insert so tetracycline resistance gene still functional (amp^R tet^R). The colonies that do not grow on tetracycline agar are recombinants (amp^R tef^s); once their positions are known, samples for further study can be recovered from the original ampicillin agar plate. **This type of screening of recombinants is called as replica plate technique** (Figure 21.3).

Uses of pBR322

It is widely used as a cloning vector. In addition to this, it has been widely used as a model system for study of prokaryotic transcription and translation.

Advantages of pBR322

1. Small size (~ 4.4 kb) enables easy purification and manipulation.
2. Two selectable markers (amp and tet) allow easy selection of recombinant DNA.
3. It can be amplified up to 1000-3000 copies per cell when protein synthesis is blocked by the application of chloramphenicol.

Disadvantages of pBR322

1. It has very high mobility i. e; it can move to another cell in the presence of a conjugative plasmid like F-factor. The nic-bom (bom=basis of mobility) region of pBR322 is responsible for this feature. Due to this, the vector may get lost in a population of mixed host cells.
2. There is a limitation in the size of the gene of interest that it can accommodate.
3. Not a very high copy number is present as is expected from a good vector.
4. Although insertional inactivation of an antibiotic resistance gene provides an effective means of recombinant identification, the method is made inconvenient by the need to carry out two screenings, one with

the antibiotic that selects for transformants, followed by the second screen, after replica plating, with the antibiotic which distinguishes recombinants. This makes the screening process time- consuming and laborious.

(a) Colonies on ampicillin medium

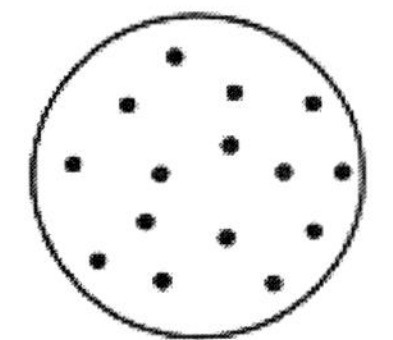

(b) Replica plating

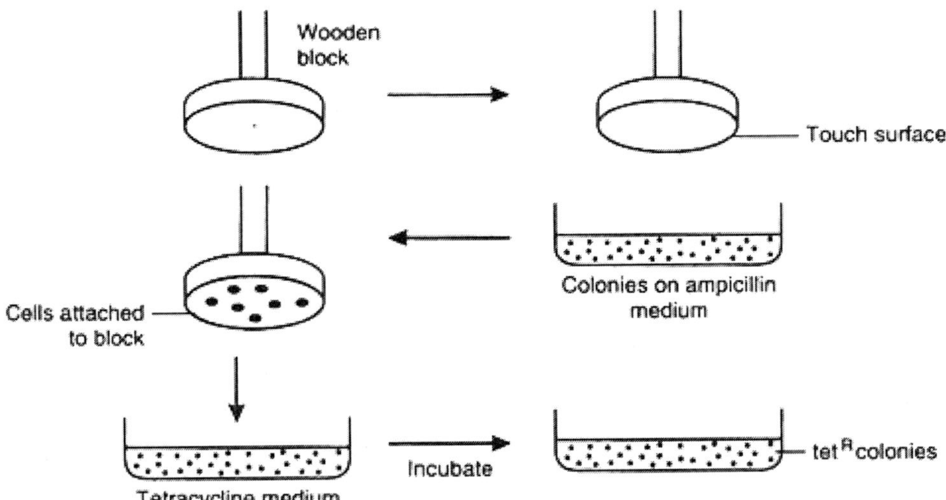

(c) amp R tet R colonies grew on tetracycline medium

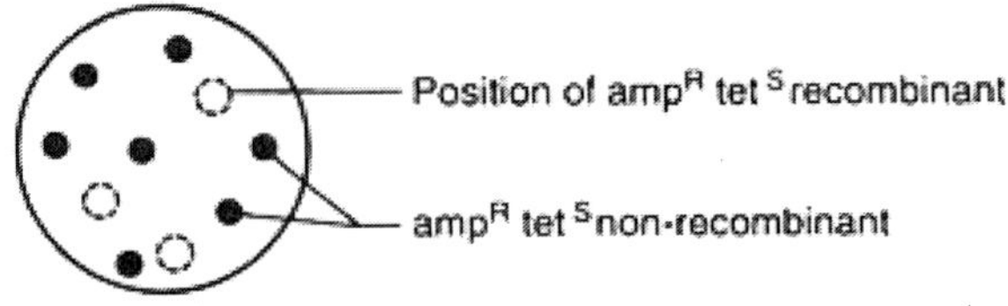

Figure 21.3. Screening of pBR322 through Replica Plate Method.

II. pBR327

Another vector **pBR327** was derived from pBR322, by deletion of nucleotides between 1,427 to 2,516. These nucleotides are deleted to reduce the size of the vector and to eliminate sequences that were known to interfere with the expression of cloned DNA in eukaryotic cells. pBR327 still contains genes for resistance against two antibiotics (tetracycline and ampicillin).

pBR327 has following two advantages over pBR322:

1. pBR327 has high copy number (30-45 copies per cell).
2. It lacks mobility.

III. pUC Vectors

pUC are obtained by modifying the pBR322 vector. pUC vectors are smaller than pBR322 of being only ~2.7 kb. But comparatively they have a high copy number. A mutation within the origin of replication produces 500 to 600 copies of the plasmid per cell without amplification (Figure 21.4).

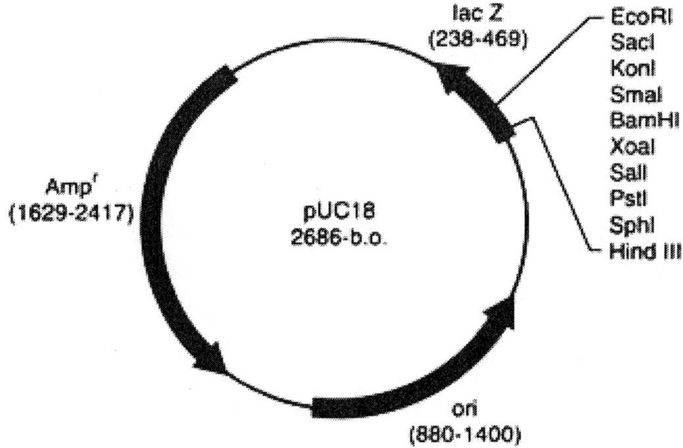

Figure 21.4. Structure of pUC18 Vectors.

The Nomenclature of pUC Vectors

The nomenclature of 'pUC' can be understood with the following explanation:

1. 'p' indicates the plasmid.
2. **'UC' stands for university of California where it was first developed by J. Messing *et al.***

Many pUC type vectors developed and numbered as pUC8, pUC18, pUC19 and so on. They are just the series of pUC and have been named just to differentiate from each other.

The Construction of pUC Vectors

1. Origin of Replication: It is derived from the origin of replication of pBR322. The ColE1origin of replication of pBR322 has been modified by carrying out a chance mutation so that each transformed *E. coli* cell has 500-600 copies of the plasmid.
2. Selectable Marker: It has an ampicillin resistant gene. The transformed host cells can grow on media having ampicillin whereas non-transformed cells die.
3. *lac Z'* gene having Multiple Cloning Site (MCS).
4. The *lac Z'* is incorporated into this vector codes for the enzyme beta-galactosidase which acts on a chromogenic substrate called X-gal (present in bacterial culture media). Beta-Galactosidase is one of the series of enzymes involved in breakdown of lactose to glucose and galactose. It is normally coded by the gene *lac Z*, which resides on *E. coli* chromosome. Some strains of *E. coli* JM103, JM109 used as a host of pUC series vectors have a modified *lacZ* gene, *i.e.,* deleted segment of lacZα gene coding for the α-peptide portion of beta-galactosidase. These mutants can synthesize the enzyme only when they harbour a plasmid, such as pUC, that carries the missing *lacZ*α gene segment of the *lacZ* gene. When pUC8 vector enters in to *E. coli* host cell, the host genome and plasmid encode for different parts of the β-galactosidase enzyme, which interact each other and produce active enzme enable to hydrolase lactose. **This process is called as α- complementation.** The expression of *lac Z'* gene is induced by another compound present in the same media called Iso-propyl-thiogalactoside (IPTG). When the enzyme substrate reaction takes place, then the X- gal is converted from white to a blue compound. The *lac Z'* gene itself has MCS in pUC vector. Hence, when the gene of interest is introduced into the *lac Z'* gene, it fails to code for functional beta-galactosidase and the substrate (X-gal) is never converted to coloured substances. So transformed cells with the gene of interest will be in white colour because of non-functional *lacZ* gene and cells with self ligated vector (with out gene of interest) will appear in blue colour in the agar media. This type of screening is called as **blue-white screening** (Figure 21.5).

Uses of pUC Vectors

pUC vectors can be used both as cloning vector and expression vector. When used as an expression vector its sequences are slightly modified to meet necessary requirements.

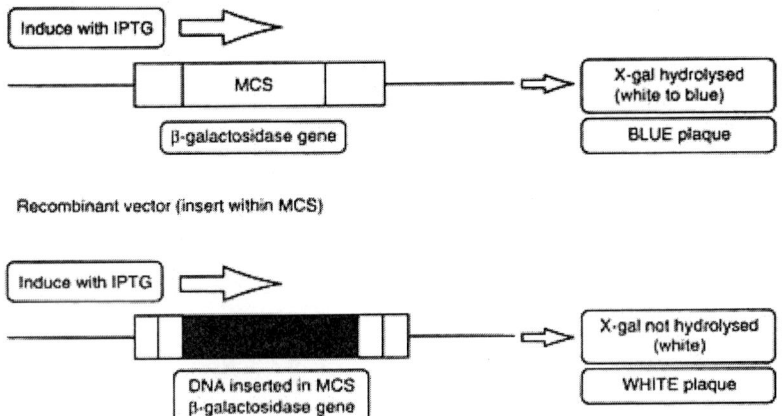

Figure 21.5. Selection of Recombinant Vectors through Blue White Colony Screening Method

Advantages of pUC Vectors

The pUC vectors offer following major advantages over pBR322 vectors:

(a) High copy number of 500-600 copies per cell.

(b) Easy and single step selection.

(c) The unique restriction sites used for cloning are clustered within the MCS. This allows cloning of a DNA fragment having two different sticky ends.

Disadvantages of pUC

It cannot accommodate a gene of interest larger than 15kb.

Table 21.1. Insert DNA Size of different Vectors

Types of Vector	*Insert DNA Size (in kb)*
Plasmid	0.5 to 8
Bacteriophage Lambda	9 to 25
Cosmid	30 to 45
BAC	50 to 300
YAC	250 to 2000

Bacteriophage Derived Vectors

Bacteriophages, or phages as they are commonly known, are viruses that specifically infect bacteria. Like all viruses, phages are very simple in structure, consisting merely of a DNA (or occasionally ribonucleic acid (RNA)) molecule carrying a number of genes, including several for replication of the phage, surrounded by protective coat or capsid made up of protein molecules.

The general pattern of infection, which is the same for all types of phage, is a three-step process:

1. The phage particle attaches to the outside of bacterium and injects its DNA chromosome into the cell.
2. The phage DNA molecule is replicated, usually by specific phage enzymes coded by genes on the phage chromosome.
3. Other phage genes direct synthesis of protein components of capsid, and new phage particles are assembled and released from the bacterium.

With some phage types the entire infection cycle is completed very quickly, possibly in less than 20min. This type of rapid infection is called a lytic cycle, as release of the new phage particles is associated with lysis of the bacterial cell. The characteristic feature of a lytic infection cycle is that phage DNA replication is immediately followed by synthesis of capsid proteins, and the phage DNA molecule is never maintained in a stable condition in the host cell. In contrast to a lytic cycle, lysogenic infection is characterized by retention of the phage DNA molecule in the host bacterium, possibly for many thousands of cell divisions. Fred Blatter and his colleagues were the first to develop a bacteriophage as vector.

The following are different types of phage vectors:

I. Bacteriophage M13 Vectors

General Biology

The M13 family of vectors is derived from bacteriophage M13. This is a male specific (infects *E. coli* having f. pili), lysogenic filamentous phage with a **circular single-stranded DNA genome about 6,407 bp (6.4 kb) in length.** Once inside the host-cell the single-stranded DNA of M13 phage acts as the template for synthesis of a complementary strand, resulting in normal double-stranded DNA.

The Attraction of M13 as a Cloning Vector

Several features of M13 make this phage attractive as the basis for a cloning vector. The genome is less than 10 kb in size, well within the range desirable for a potential vector. In addition, the double-stranded replicative form (RF) of the M13 genome behaves very much like a plasmid, and can be treated as such for experimental purposes.

It is easily prepared from a culture of infected *E. coli* cells and can be reintroduced by transfection. Most importantly, **genes cloned with an M13-based vector can be obtained in the form of single- stranded DNA. Single-stranded version of cloned genes are useful for several techniques, notably DNA sequencing and *in vitro* mutagenesis.** Using an M13 vector is an easy and reliable way of obtaining single-stranded DNA for this type of work (Figure 21.6).

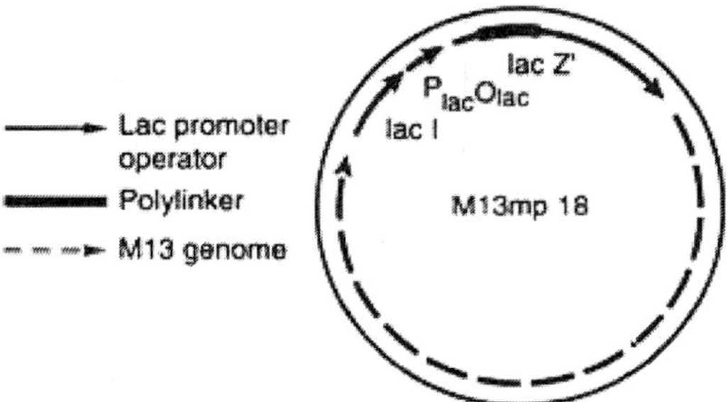

Figure 21.6. Structure M13 Vector.

Advantages of Bacteriophage M13 Vector

1. *Advantages over Lambda Phage Vector*

M13 is an example of a filamentous phage and is completely different in structure from lambda. Furthermore, the M13 DNA molecule is much smaller than the lambda genome, being only 6407 nucleotides in length. It is circular and is unusual in that it consists entirely of single- stranded DNA. The smaller size of the M13 DNA molecule means that it has room for fewer genes than the lambda genome. This is possible because the M13 capsid is constructed from multiple copies of just three proteins (requiring only three genes), whereas synthesis of the lambda head- and-tail structure involves over 15 different proteins. In addition, M13 follows a simpler infection cycle than lambda and does not need genes for insertion into the host genome. Injection of an M13 DNA molecule into an *E. coli* cell occurs via the pilus, the structure that connects two cells during sexual conjugation.

2. *Other Advantages*

M13-based vectors are that they contain the same poly-linker and alpha-peptide fragments as the pUC series and recombinants can be selected by the blue and white colour test. Also the size of the genome is below 10 kb and so is easy to handle (Figure 21.7).

Disadvantages of Bacteriophage M13 Vectors

The following are the disadvantages of bacteriophage M13 vectors:

1. Gene of interest more than 2kb cannot be cloned.
2. It has low yield of DNA.
3. The phage produce many toxins in high concentration.

II. Lamda Phage Vectors

Cloning vectors derived from λ bacteriophage are commonly used as it provides an approximately 16-fold advantage in cloning efficiency in comparison with the most efficient plasmid cloning vectors. Phage λ is a linear double-stranded phage approximately 49 kb in length. It infects *E. coli* with great efficiency by injecting its DNA through the cell membrane.

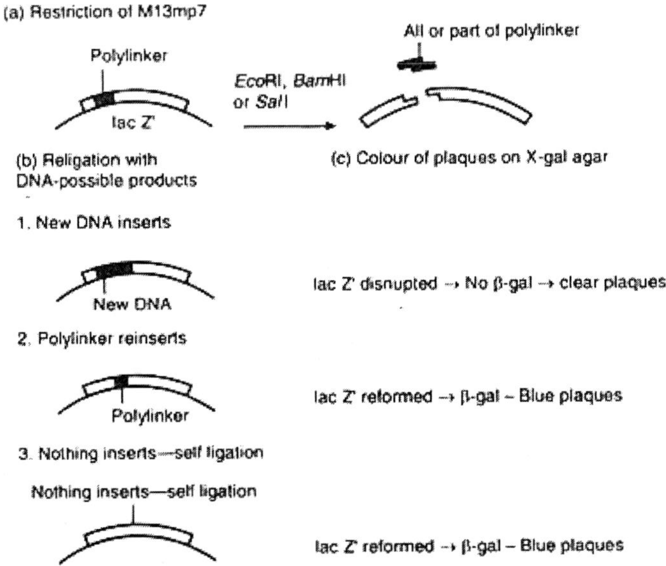

Figure 21.7. Cloning with Bacteriophage M13 Vectors.

Types of Lambda Vectors

There are two types of lambda cloning vectors.

(a) Lambda Insertion Vectors

In this case a large segment of the non-essential region has been deleted, and the two arms ligated together. An insertion vector possesses at least one unique restriction site into which new DNA can be inserted. The size of the DNA fragment that an individual vector can carry depends on the extent to which the non-essential region has been deleted, *e.g.* λ gtl0, λZAP11(Figure 21.8).

(b) Lambda Replacement Vectors

These vectors have two recognition sites for the restriction endonucleases. These sites flank a segment of DNA that is replaced by the DNA to be cloned. Often the replaceable fragment (or stuffer fragment) carries additional restriction sites that can be used to cut it up into small pieces so that its own reinsertion during a cloning experiment is very unlikely. Replacement vectors are generally designed to carry large pieces of DNA than insertion vectors can handle *e.g.* λEMBL, λ GEMll (Figure 21.9).

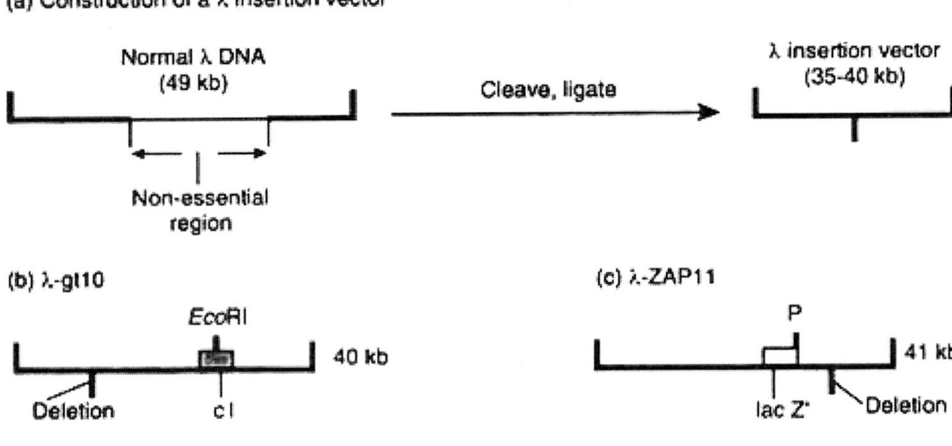

Figure 21.8. Lambda Phage Insertion Vectors

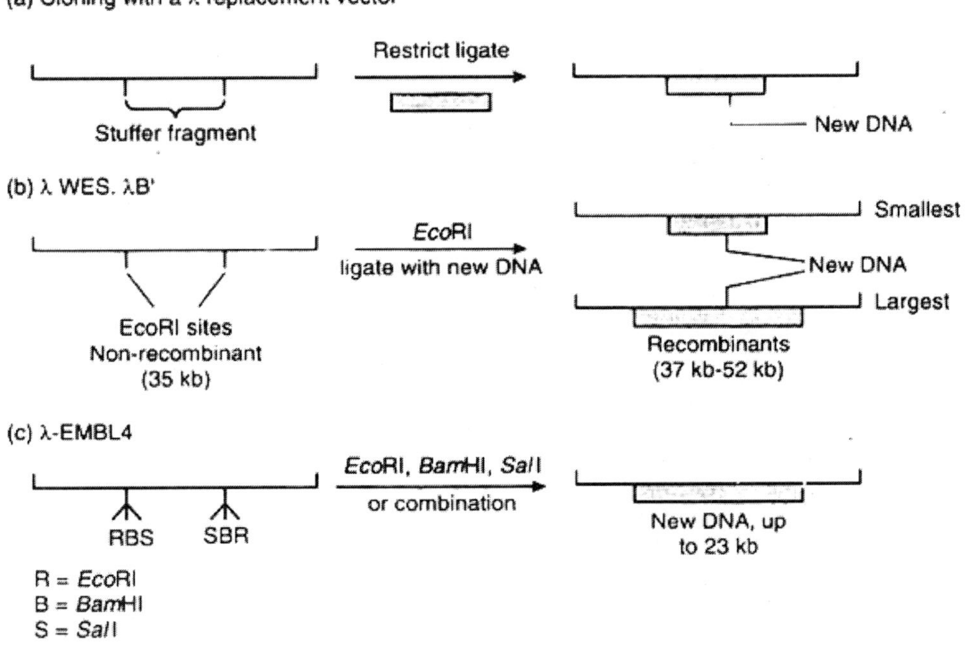

Figure 21.9. Lambda Phage Replacement Vectors.

The Phagemid Vectors

Although M13 vectors are very useful for the production of single-stranded versions of cloned genes they do have one disadvantage. There is a limit to the size of DNA fragment that can be cloned with an M13 vector, with 1500bp generally being looked on as the maximum capacity. To get around this problem a number of novel vectors have been constructed which are the hybrids of plasmids and M13 vectors. We call them phagemids (**'phage' from M13 bacteriophage and 'mid' from plasmid**).

Construction of Phagemid Vector

A typical phagemid has following parts:

1. Phage M13 origin of replication.
2. A portion of lac Z' gene driven by lac promoter.
3. A multiple cloning site (MCS) with lac Z' gene.
4. Phage T7 and T3 promoter sequences flanking the MCS sequences.
5. ColE1 origin of replication.
6. amp^R resistant gene.

Plasmids that carry the M13 replication origin in addition to a conventional origin of dsDNA synthesis can be replicated either as dsDNA from the latter or as single-stranded DNA from the M13 origin. Replication from the M13 origin requires the appropriate proteins (such as gene II protein) to be provided from a helper phage also replicating within the cell.

Replication generates single-stranded DNA which can then be packaged into phage coats. Examples of phagemids are the vectors pUC118, 119 and 120.

They are replicated as plasmids until the cell containing them is co-infected with a helper phage, such as M13K07, which provides the proteins for single-stranded DNA synthesis and packaging. M13K07 is an M13 phage that has been modified, most importantly by the incorporation of a plasmid replication origin.

Replication from this origin allows the helper phage to be present in a high copy number per cell and, therefore, to provide the larger quantities of the proteins that are required to replicate and package the phagemid molecule.

M13K07 also contains a kanamycin resistance gene to allow for selection for the presence of the helper phage. (Of course, it is possible that the M13K07 helper phage may be packaged too, but in practice the packaged phagemid molecules are found to be in a 100-fold excess over the helper phage)

Another example of these vectors is the pBluescript series, such as pBluescriptIIKSÞ. This series of plasmids contains, in addition to features already described, promoters from the *E. coli* bacteriophages T3 or T7, which are useful for expressing cloned sequences (Figure 21.10).

Uses of Phagemid Vectors

This vector is a multipurpose vector as it can serve as following:

1. A cloning vector.

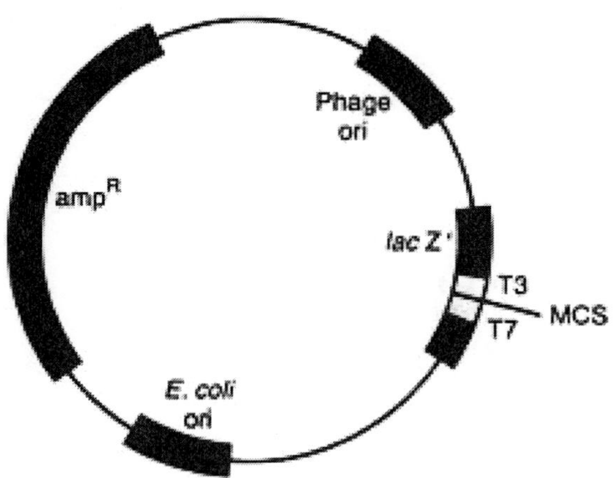

Figure 21.10. Structure pBluescript Phagemid Vector.

2. An expression vector
3. A sequencing vector.

Advantages of Phagemid Vectors

The main advantage of the phagemid system is that it can be used to provide single-or double-stranded material without any re-cloning.

Cosmid Vectors

Cosmids are hybrids between a phage DNA molecule and a bacterial plasmid or are basically a plasmid that carries a cos site, the substrate for **enzymes that package φ λDNA molecule into phage coat proteins.** The *in vitro* packaging reaction works not only with phage genome but also with any DNA molecule that carries cos site separated by **37–52 kb of** DNA. It also needs a selectable marker, such as ampicillin resistance gene, and a plasmid origin of replication. As cosmids lack all the λ genes, they are not able to produce plaques. Instead colonies are formed on selective media, just as with a plasmid vector. The loading capacity of cosmids varies depending on the size of the vector itself but usually lies around 40–45 kb much more than a phage λ vector can accommodate. After packaging *in vitro*, the particle is used to infect suitable host. The recombinant cosmid DNA is injected into the cell where it circularizes like phage DNA but replicates as a normal plasmid without the expression of any phage functions. Transformed cells are selected on the basis of a vector antibiotic resistance marker. Cosmids provide an efficient means of cloning large pieces of DNA. Because of their capacity to carry large fragments of DNA, cosmids are particularly attractive for constructing libraries of eukaryotic genome fragments (Figure 21.11).

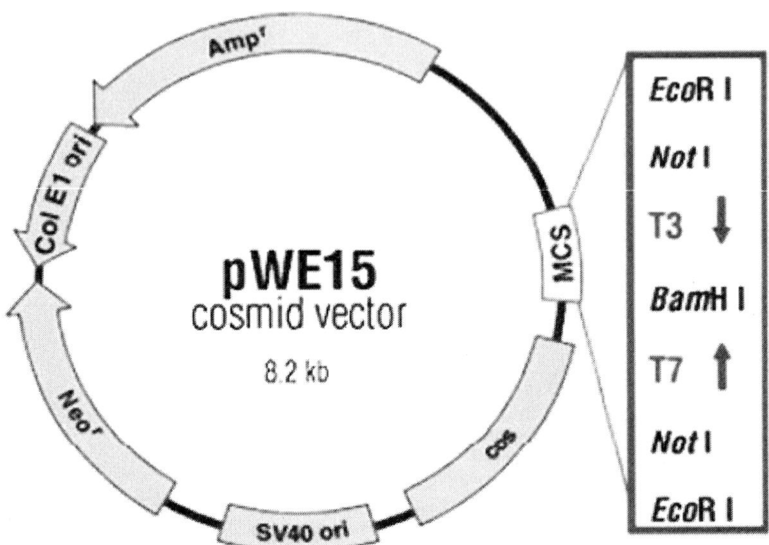

Figure 21.11. Cosmid Vectors.

Uses of Cosmid Vectors

Cosmids are used for construction of genomic libraries of eukaryotes since these can be used for cloning large fragments of DNA.

Advantages of Cosmids

Followings are advantages of cosmid vectors:

1. These can be used to clone gene of interest up to 40 kb.
2. As the lambda phage will insert the recombinant DNA into the host cell, an extra step of inserting the recombinant DNA into the host cell is not performed.
3. Easy screening method is found.

Shuttle Vectors

Shuttle vectors are those which can multiply into two different unrelated species. Shuttle reactors are designed to replicate in the cells of two species, as they contain two origins of replication, one appropriate for each species as well as genes that are required for replication and not supplied by the host cell, *i.e.*, it is self-sufficient with the process of its replication (Figure 21.12).

Disadvantage

The presence of two replication origins sometimes poses special problems, one portion of replication origin of one species is totally unrelated to another and interferes with the replication of other host. Hence, in a shuttle vector various types of replication origins are to be inserted and checked before experimenting.

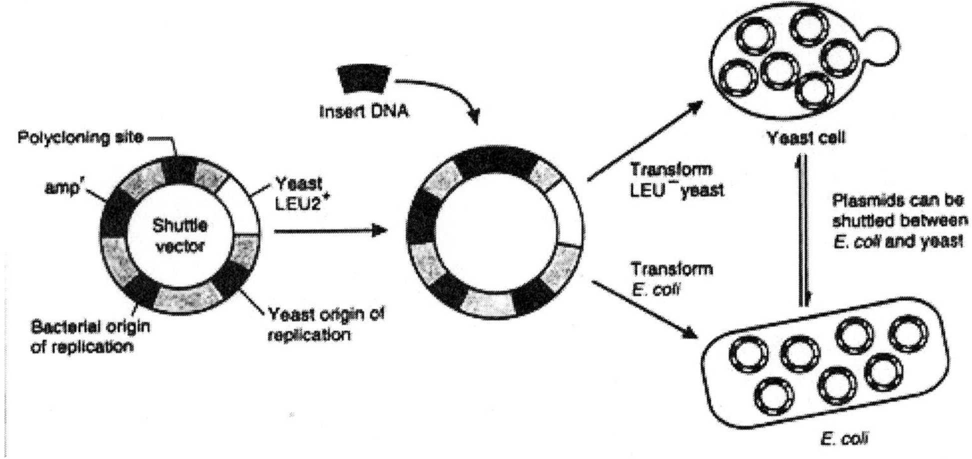

Figure 21.12. An Yeast/Bacteria Shuttle Vector.

Artificial Chromosomes

Artificial chromosomes are synthetically designed DNA molecules of known structure, which are assembled in vitro (in the laboratory) from specific DNA sequences that acts like a natural chromosome. Artificial chromosomes are circular or linear vectors that are stably maintained in, usually, 1-2 copies per cell.

They are huge in size in comparison to other vectors but can clone very large segments of chromosomes (even an entire chromosome). Before seeing different types of artificial chromosomes the three key components of an eukaryotic chromosomes can be seen which are necessary for its stable maintenance inside a cell.

1. The centromere, which is required for the chromosome to be distributed correctly to daughter cells during cell division.
2. Two telomeres, the structures at the ends of a chromosome, which are needed for the ends to be replicated correctly in order and which also prevent the chromosome from being nibbled away by exonucleases.
3. The origin of replication, which are the positions along the chromosome at which DNA replication initiates, similar to the origin of replication of a plasmid.

Once we have defined the chromosomal structure of an eukaryotic organism (like humans and yeast), then we can isolate the key components of their chromosomes and join them together to form an artificial chromosome. Then into this artificial chromosome we can insert our gene of interest which can be subsequently cloned in its respective cell.

2. Bacterial Artificial Chromosomes (BAC)

Bacterial Artificial Chromosomes (BACs) are cloning vectors based on the extra-chromosomal plasmids of *E.coli*, called F factor or fertility factor, used for transforming and cloning in bacteria, usually *E. coli*. F-plasmids play a crucial role because they contain partition genes that promote the even distribution of plasmids after bacterial cell division. This vector is useful for cloning DNA fragments up to 350 kb, but can be handled like regular bacterial plasmid vectors, and is very useful for sequencing large stretches of chromosomal DNA. The replication of F factor is strictly controlled by the regulatory functions of *E. coli*; as a result F factor is maintained as a low-copy number (*i.e.*, one or two copies per cell). This allows stable maintenance of large DNA inserts and reduces the potential for recombination between DNA fragments carried by the vector, which was a limitation observed with cosmid-cloning system. In addition to stable maintenance, the structural stability of F factors allows complex genomic DNA inserts to be maintained with a great degree of structural stability in the *E. coli* host. The structure of a typical BAC is given in Figure 21.13.

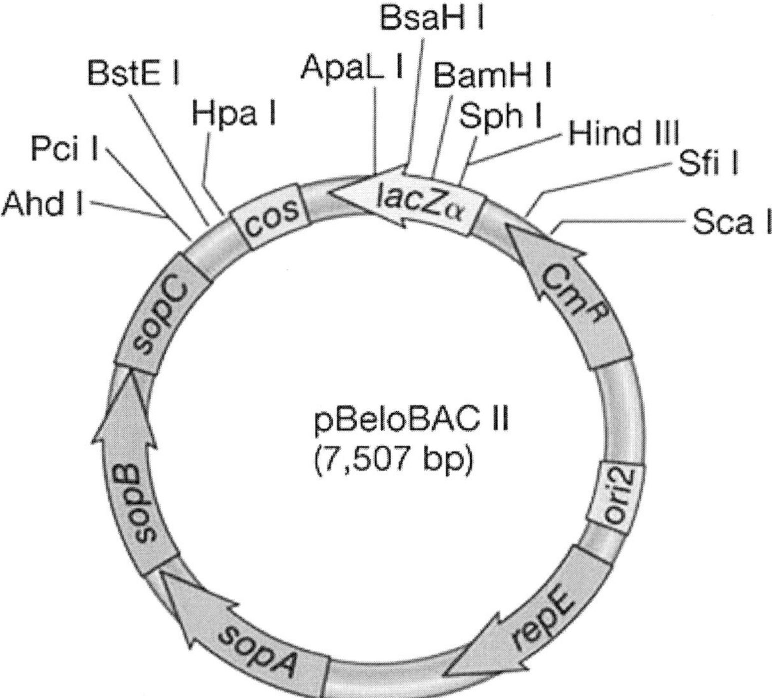

Figure 21.13. Different Components of Bacterial Artificial Chromosomes (BAC).

BAC Vector Cloning Site

The cloning segment of BAC vector includes (1) two bacteriophage markers lambda cosN and P1 loxP, (2) three restriction enzyme sites (EcoRI, HindIII, and BamHI) for cloning, and (3) a GC- rich NotI restriction enzyme site for potential excision of inserts. The cosN site provides a fixed position for cleavage by bacteriophage lambda enzyme terminase, which allows the convenient generation of a linear form of the BAC DNA. The cosN site is also used to package approximately 50 kb DNA into bacteriophage lambda head as a particle. The method known as Fosmid for F-based cosmid system is extremely efficient, thus very useful when DNA is precious or available in small amounts. The P1 loxP site allows the retro fitting of additional components to BAC vector at a later stage. The loxP site is also utilized to linearize BACs through the P1 phage protein Cre, which catalyses strand exchange between two DNA strands at the loxP sites. Examples of BAC are pBACe3.6, pBeloBAC11 *etc.*

DNA Library

Gene sequence are arranged in genome in a random fashion and without knowing genomic sequences selecting or isolating a gene is very difficult. Hence, there are two ways to represent a genomic sequence information into the multiple small fragments in the form of a library:

(1) Genomic library; (2) cDNA library.

1. Genomic Library

A genomic library is an organism specific collection of DNA covering the entiregenome of an organism. It contains all DNA sequences such as expressed genes, non expressed genes, exons, introns, promoter, terminator regions and other DNA sequences. Construction of a genomic DNA library involves isolation, purification and fragmentation of genomic DNA followed by cloning of the fragmented DNA using suitable vectors. Vectors with DNA fragments (organism's entire genome fragment) will be transferred in to specific host cells. Those cells covering entire genome and will be maintained as a genomic library. The library created contains representative copies of all the DNA fragments of that particular organism. An outline of the construction of genomic library is given in Figure 21.14.

Steps in Genomic Library Construction

1. Isolation of genomic DNA

Total genomic DNA is isolated and purified from which organism genomic library need to be constructed. The eukaryotic cell nuclei are purified by digestion with protease and organic (phenol-chloroform) extraction.

2. Generation of Suitable Size F3ragments

Next step generation of genomic DNA into suitable small size fragments. The derived genomic DNA is too large to incorporate into a vector and needs to be broken up into desirable fragment sizes. Fragmentation of DNA can be achieved by physical method and enzymatic method, most preferably enzymatic method of re**striction digestion followed by with** mechanical shearing**.**

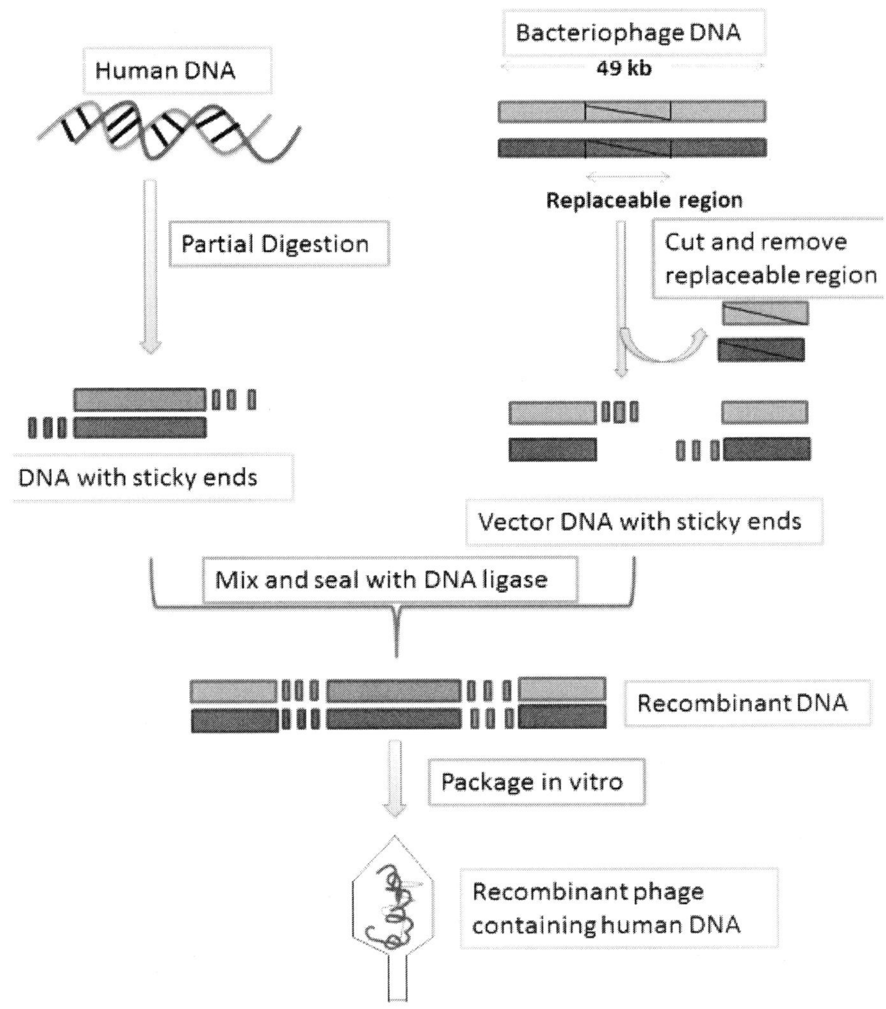

Figure 21.14. Construction of Genomic Library.

Restriction Digestion

Genomic DNA can be digested with a frequent DNA cutting enzyme such as EcoR-I, BamH-I or Sau3A to generate the random sizes of DNA fragments. The criteria to choose the restriction enzyme or pair of enzymes in such a way so that a reasonable size DNA fragment will be generated. As fragments are randomly generated and are relatively big enough, it is likely that each and every genomic sequence is presented in the pool. As size of the DNA fragment is large, complete genome will be presented in very few number of clones. In addition, genomic DNA can be fragmented using a mechanical shearing. If a organism has a genome size of $2x10^7$ kb and an average size of the fragment is 20kb, then no. of fragment, n= 10^6. In reality, this is the minimum number to represent a given fragment in the library where as the actual number is much larger.

3. *Cloning into the Suitable Vector*

Depending upon organism and size of genome, this library is either prepared in a bacterial vector(Phage vector) or in yeast artificial chromosome (YAC). The suitable vector to prepare the genomic library can be selected based on size of the fragment of genomic DNA and carrying capacity of the vector (Table 21.2). In the case of fragment generated by restriction enzyme, vector can be digested with the same enzyme and put for ligation to get clone.

Cloning of Genomic DNA

Various vectors are available for cloning large DNA fragments. λ phage, yeast artificial chromosome, bacterial artificial chromosome *etc.* are considered as suitable vectors for larger DNA and λ replacement vectors like λDASH and EMBL3 are preferred for construction of genomic DNA library. T_4 DNA ligase is used to ligate the selected DNA sequence into the vector.

(i) λ replacement vectors: The λEMBL series of vectors are widely used for genomic library construction. The multiple cloning sites of these vectors flanking the stuffer fragment contain promoters for the $T_3$and T_7 RNA polymerases. The restriction digestion of the recombinant vector generates short fragments of insert DNA left attached to these promoters.

(ii) High-capacity vectors: The high capacity cloning vectors used for the construction of genomic libraries are cosmids, bacterial artificial chromosomes (BACs), P1-derived artificial chromosomes (PACs) and yeast artificial chromosomes (YACs). They are designed to handle longer DNA inserts, much larger than for λ replacement vectors. So they require lower number of recombinants to be screened for identification of a particular gene of interest.

4. *Transformation to get Colonies*

Post ligation, clones are transformed in a suitable host to get colonies. A suitable host can be a bacterial strain or yeast. Those population will be maintained as a genomic library of the organism and any gene of that particular organism at any time can be isolated by screening from that particular population.

Advantages of Genomic Libraries

- ☆ Identification of a clone encoding a particular gene of interest.
- ☆ It is useful for prokaryotic organisms having relatively small genomes.

- Genomic libraries from eukaryotic organisms are very important to study the genome sequence of a particular gene, including its regulatory sequences and its pattern of introns and exons.

Disadvantages of Genomic Library

- Genome libraries from eukaryotes having very large genomes contain a lot of DNA which does not code for proteins and also contain non-coding DNA such as repetitive DNA and regulatory regions which makes them less than ideal.
- Genomic library from a eukaryotic organism will not work if the screening method requires the expression of a gene.

Applications

- To determine the complete genome sequence of a given organism.
- To study and generate transgenic animals through genetic engineering, serving as a source of genomic sequence.
- To study the function of regulatory sequences *in vitro.*
- To study the genetic mutations.
- Used for genome mapping, sequencing and the assembly of clone contigs.

Table 21.2. DNA Carrying Capacity of the Vector

Vector	*Insert size*	*Features*
λ phages	9 to 20-30 kb	Genome size-47 kb, efficient packaging system,replacement vectors usually employed, used to study individual genes.
Cosmids	30 to 45 kb	Contains cos site of λ phage to allow packaging,propagate in *E. coli* as plasmids, useful for sub-cloning of DNA inserts from YAC, BAC, PAC *etc.*
Fosmids	35-45 kb	Contains F plasmid origin of replication and λ cos site, low copy number, stable.
Bacterial artificial chromosomes (BAC)	50 to 300kb	Based on F- plasmid, relatively large and high capacity vectors.
P1 artificial chromosomes (PACs)	50 to 300 kb	Derived from DNA of P1 bacteriophage, combines the features of P1 and BACs, used to clone larger genes and in physical mapping, chromosome walking as well as shotgun sequencing of complex genomes.
Yeast artificial chromosomes (YAC)	250 to 2000kb	Allow identification of successful transformants (BAC clones are highly stable and highly efficient)

cDNA Library

A cDNA library represents total mRNA present at a particular stage of an organism into multiple clones containing small DNA fragments. cDNA library preparation same as a genomic library preparation, but the difference here is mRNA is isolated from organism instead of DNA and from that mRNA, complementary DNA (cDNA) is synthesized. Then those cDNA is integrated in to specific vector followed by transferred in to the host cell. So the cDNA library is having only coding sequence and devoid of all other sequence such as introns, promoter, terminator regions *etc.*

Construction of cDNA Library

1. Isolation of mRNA
2. Preparation of complementary DNA fragments
3. Cloning in suitable vector system
4. Transformation in suitable host (Figure 21.15).

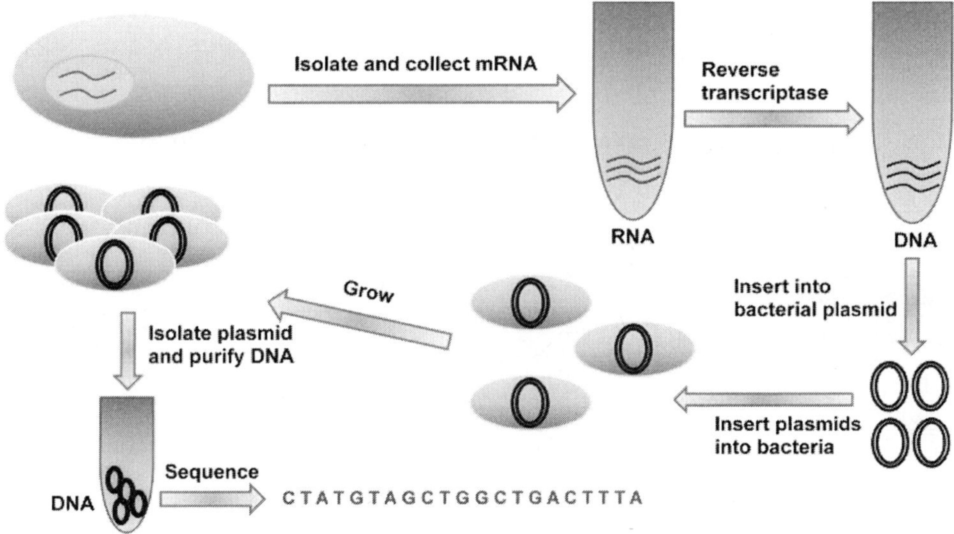

Figure 21.15. Construction of cDNA Library.

1. Isolation of mRNA

Total mRNA isolated from the specific tissue at particular organisam, which cDNA library need to be constructed by following standard mRNA isolation method.

2. Preparation of Complementary DNA (cDNA)

1. First DNA strand (cDNA) is synthesized from mRNA as a template with a reverse transcriptase enzyme using oligo dT as a primer.
2. Presence of poly A tail on mRNA 3' end it is easy to synthesize first DNA strand followed by degradation of RNA template from DNA : RNA hybrid by treating with RNase H.
3. Second DNA strand is synthesized using existing first DNA strand as a template with DNA polymerase enzyme.

3. Cloning of cDNA into the Vector

The cDNA is ligated into the suitable vector to generate clone.

4. Transformation to get Colonies

Post ligation, clones are transformed in a suitable host to get colonies. A suitable host can be bacterial strain or yeast.

Comparison of Genomic and cDNA Libraries

cDNA library has revolutionized the field of molecular genetics and recombinant DNA technology. It consists of a population of bacterial transformants or phage lysates in which each mRNA isolated from an organism is represented as its cDNA insertion in a vector. cDNA libraries are used to express eukaryotic genes in prokaryotes. In addition, cDNAs are used to generate expressed sequence tags (ESTs) and splices variant analysis. Some of the differences of cDNA library with genomic library are presented in Table 21.3.

Table 21.3. Differences of cDNA Library with Genomic Library

Features	*Genomic Library*	*cDNA Library*
Sequences present	Ideally, all genomic sequences	Only structural genes that are transcribed
Contents affected by		
(a) Developmental stage	No	Yes
(b) Cell type	No	Yes
Features of DNA insert(s)representing a gene:		
(a) Size	As present in genome	Ordinarily, much smaller
(b) Introns	Present	Absent
(c) 5′- and 3′- regulatory sequences	Present	Absent
As compared to the genome		
(a) Enrichment of sequences	In amplified genomic libraries	For abundant mRNAs
(b) Redundancy in frequency	In amplified libraries	For rare mRNA species
(c) Variant forms of agene	Not possible	For such genes, whose RNA transcripts are alternatively spliced

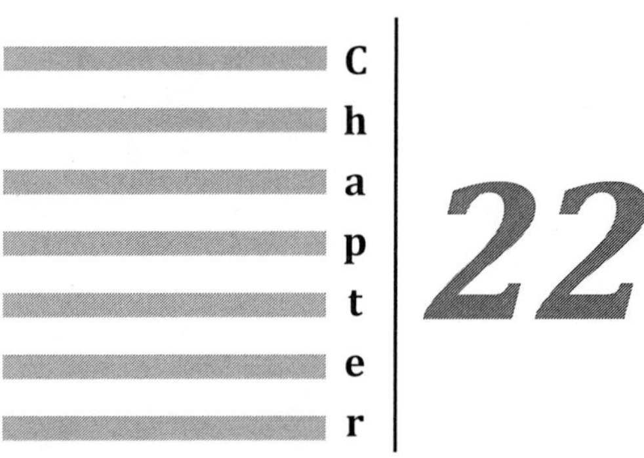

Construction of Recombinant DNA Molecules and Bacterial Transformation

Recombinant DNA refers to the **creation of new combinations of DNA** segments that are not found together in nature. The isolation and manipulation of genes allows for more precise genetic analysis as well as practical applications in medicine, agriculture and industry. **Molecular cloning (i.e. gene cloning) involves creating recombinant DNA and introducing it into a host cell to be replicated.** One of the basic strategies of molecular cloning is to move desired genes from a large, complex genome to a small, simple one. The process of *in vitro* recombination makes it possible to cut different strands of DNA, with a restriction enzyme and join the DNA molecules together via complementary base pairing.

Construction of the Recombinant DNA (rDNA) Molecule

Overview of making recombinant DNA as follows: Isolate DNA →Cut with restriction enzymes →Ligate into cloning vector →transform recombinant DNA molecule into host cell →each transformed cell will divide many, many times to form a colony of millions of cells, each of which carries the recombinant DNA molecule (DNA clone) (Figure 22.1). Recombinant DNA in a living organism was first achieved in **1973 by Herbert Boyer, of the University of California at San Francisco, and Stanley Cohen, at Stanford University**, who used *E. coli* restriction enzymes to insert foreign DNA into plasmids.

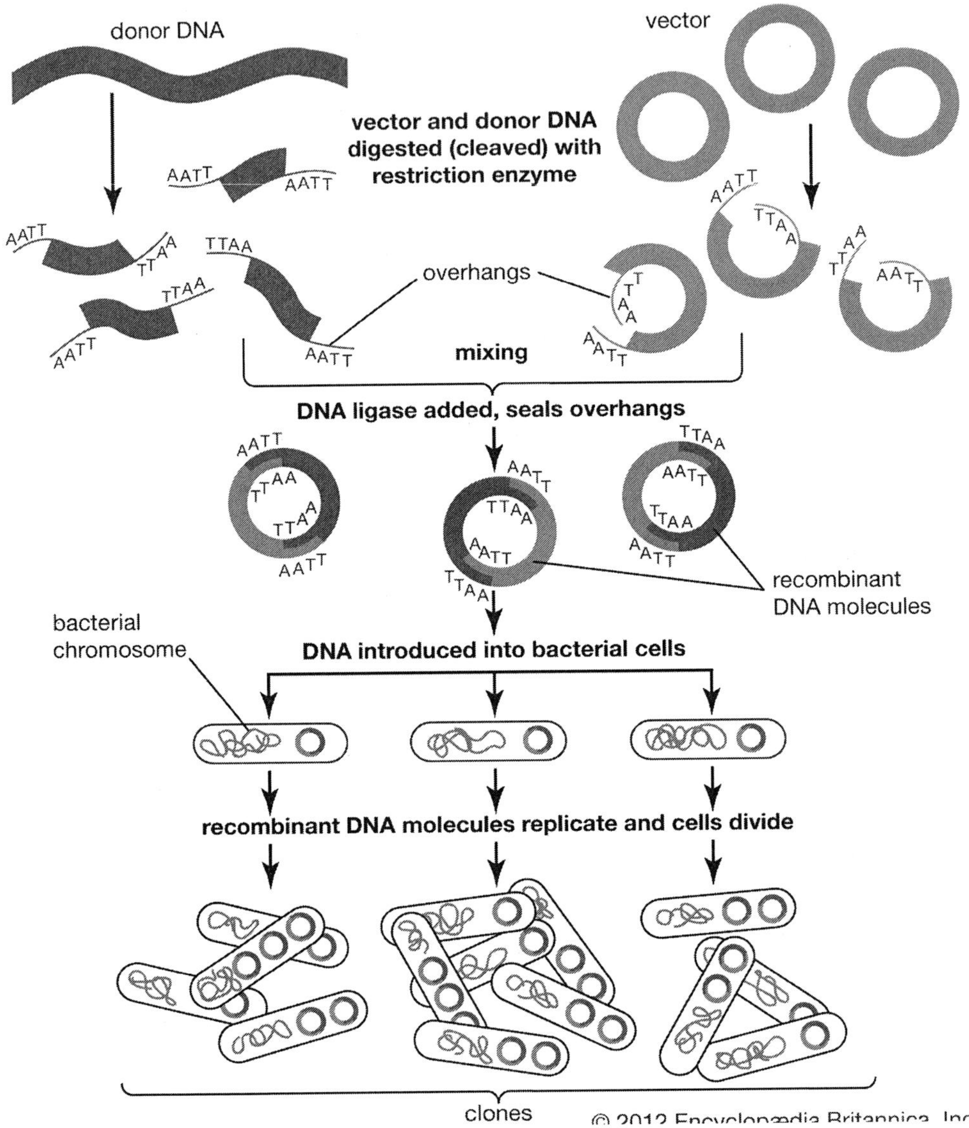

Figure 22.1. Overview of rDNA Molecule Construction and Cloning.

Step 1

To construct the recombinant DNA, first the total cell DNA consisting the gene of interest and the plasmid vector DNA has to be prepared. Total cell DNA may be from a culture of bacteria or a plant or animal cells, or from any other type of organism that is being studied. It consists of either the genomic DNA or extra chromosomal DNA molecules, such as plasmids. The second type of DNA (vector) that should be pure plasmid DNA. Preparation of plasmid DNA from a culture of bacteria follows the same basic steps as purification of total cell DNA, with the crucial difference that at some stage the plasmid DNA must be separated from the chromosomal DNA present in the cell.

Step 2

Restriction enzymes act as molecular scissors that cut DNA at specific locations. These reactions are called **restriction enzyme digestions**. The vector molecule must be cleaved at a single position, to open up the circle so that new DNA can be inserted. If the vector is cut more than once then it will be broken into two or more separate fragments and will be of no use as a cloning vector. Furthermore, each vector molecule must be cut at exactly the same position on the circle, as random cleavage is not satisfactory. The technique agarose gel electrophoresis reveals the progress of the restriction enzyme digestion. This technique involves running out the DNA on an agarose gel. On the application of current, the negatively charged DNA travels to the positive electrode and is separated out based on size. This allows separating and cutting out the digested DNA fragments (Figure 22.2).

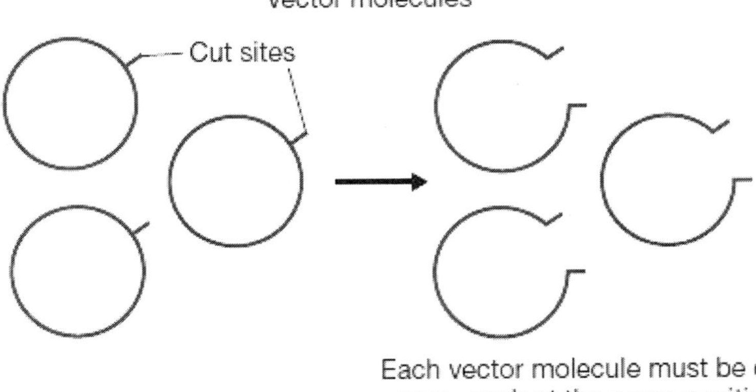

Figure 22.2. Vector Restricted with Restriction Endonuclease Enzyme.

Step 3

It is also necessary to cleave the DNA that is to be cloned. There are two reasons for this. First, if the aim is to clone a single gene, which may consist of only 2 or 3 kb of DNA, then that gene will have to be cut out of the large DNA molecules. Second, large DNA molecules may have to be broken down simply to produce fragments small enough to be carried by the vector. Most cloning vectors exhibit a preference for DNA fragments that fall into a particular size range. Restriction endonucleases allow us to cut DNA molecules in the precise, reproducible manner required for gene cloning. Both vector DNA and gene need to be cloned should be restricted with same restriction endonuclease enzyme (Figure 22.3).

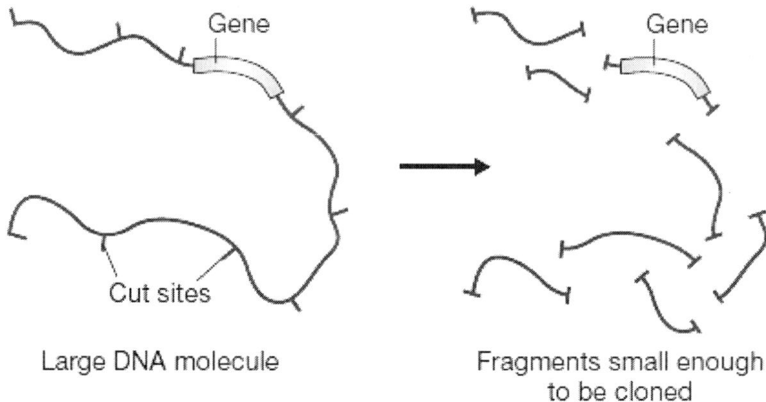

Figure 22.3. Gene of Interest is Restricted with same Restriction Endonuclease Enzyme.

Step 4

- The final step in construction of a recombinant DNA molecule is the joining together of the vector molecule and the DNA to be cloned. The purified DNA and the vector of interest, both are cut with the same restriction enzyme gives the restricted fragment of DNA and the clevead vector, The cut ends of vector and foreign DNA both sharing complementary bases and join together by ligation process and the enzyme that catalyzes the reaction is called **DNA ligase.**
- The resulting DNA molecule is a hybrid of two DNA molecules – the DNA of interest and the vector. In the terminology of genetics this intermixing of different DNA strands is called **recombination**. Hence, this new hybrid DNA molecule is also called a **recombinant DNA** molecule and the technology is referred to as the **Recombinant DNA Technology** (Figure 22.4).

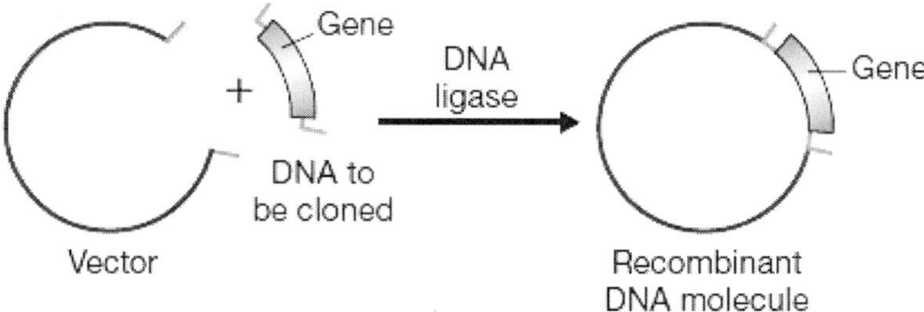

Figure 22.4. Gene of Interest and Vector both Ligated with DNA Ligase Enzyme.

Applications of Recombinant DNA Technology

- Recombinant DNA is used to identify, map and sequence genes, and to determine their function.
- Recombinant proteins are widely used as reagents in laboratory experiments and to generate antibody probes for examining protein synthesis within cells and organisms.
- Many additional practical applications of recombinant DNA are found in industry, food production, human and veterinary medicine, agriculture, and bioengineering.
    1. **Application in Agriculture:** Transgenic crops development *e.g.* Bt-Cotton to protect the plant against boll worms.
    2. **Application of medicines:** Insulin production in genetically modified *E.coli*.
    3. **Gene Therapy:** It is used as an attempt to correct the gene defects which give rise to heredity diseases.

Limitations of Recombinant DNA Technology

- Destruction of native species in the environment the genetically modified species are introduced in.
- Resilient plants can theoretically give rise to resilient weeds which can be difficult to control.
- Cross contamination and migration of proprietary DNA between organisms.
- Recombinant organisms contaminating the natural environment.
- The recombinant organisms are population of clones, vulnerable in exact same ways. A single disease or pest can wipe out the entire population quickly.
- Creation of superbug is hypothesized.
- Ethical concern about humans trying to play God and mess with the nature's way of selection. It is exaggerated by the fear of unknown of what all can be created using the technology and how is it going to impact the civilization.
- Many people worry about the safety of modifying food and medicines using recombinant DNA technology.

Linkers and Adopters in rDNA Technology

For construction of an rDNA, compatible sticky ends are desirable on the DNA molecules to be ligated together. Often these sticky ends can be provided by digesting both the vector and the DNA to be cloned with the same restriction endonuclease, or with different enzymes that produce the same sticky end, but it is not always possible to do this. A common problematic situation occurs where the vector molecule has sticky ends, but the DNA fragments to be cloned are blunt-ended. Under these circumstances either linkers or adapters can be used to put the correct sticky ends onto the DNA fragments.

Linkers

They are short pieces of double stranded DNA, of known nucleotide sequence, that are synthesized artificially. A typical linker can be a blunt-ended molecule, but contains a restriction site. DNA ligase can attach linkers to the ends of larger blunt ended DNA molecules. The digestion with the specific restriction enzyme cleaves the attached linkers at the recognition sequences, producing a cleaved linker attached to the original DNA fragment, now carrying the sticky ends. This modified fragment is ready for ligation into a cloning vector having a complementary sticky end.

Adaptors

Another method of attaching sticky ends to a blunt-ended molecule is by using the Adaptors. **Adaptors, like linkers, are short synthetic oligonucleotides**. But unlike linkers, an adaptor is synthesized so that it already has one sticky end. The idea is to ligate the blunt end of the adaptor to the blunt ends of the DNA fragment, to produce a new molecule with sticky ends.

Transformation: The Uptake of DNA by Bacterial Cells

In nature, transformation is one of the processes by which bacteria obtains free DNA from their close environment. Close study of these organisms has revealed that they possess sophisticated mechanisms for DNA binding and uptake. **In 1928, Frederick Griffith** reported what is now known as Griffith's Experiment, the first widely accepted demonstrations of bacterial transformation. Most species of bacteria, including *E. coli*, take up only limited amounts of DNA under normal circumstances. In order to transform these species efficiently, the bacteria have to undergo some form of physical and/or chemical treatment that enhances their ability to take up DNA. Cells that have undergone this treatment are said to be competent.

Preparation of Competent *E. coli* Cells and Transformation

In the early 1970s, it was observed that *E. coli* cells that had been soaked in an ice cold salt solution were more efficient at DNA uptake than unsoaked cells. A solution of **50 mM calcium chloride ($CaCl_2$)** is traditionally used, although other salts, notably rubidium chloride, are also effective. $CaCl_2$ causes the DNA to precipitate onto the outside of the cells, or perhaps the salt is responsible for some kind of change in the cell wall that improves DNA binding. In any case, soaking in $CaCl_2$ affects only DNA binding, and not the actual uptake into the cell. When DNA is added to treated cells, it remains attached to the cell exterior, and is not at this stage transported into the cytoplasm. The actual movement of DNA into competent cells is stimulated by heat shock cells by **42°C for 90 sec or by electrophoration** (Figure 22.5).

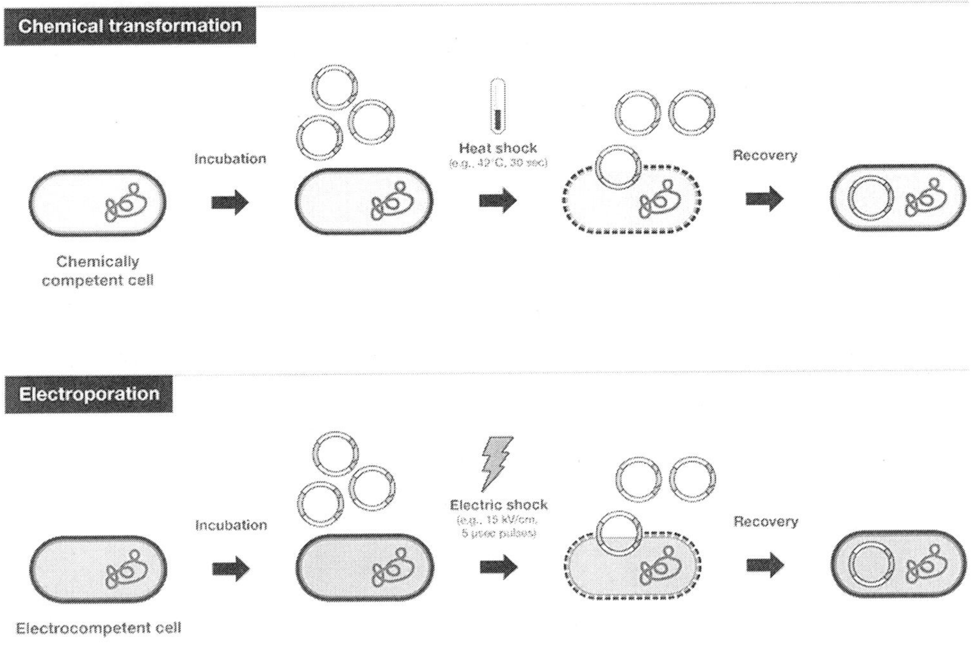

Figure 22.5. Bacterial Transformation through Heat Chock and Electrophoration Method.

Selection for Transformed Cells

Generally during the transformation of competent cells, 1 ng of the plasmid vector can yield 1000–10,000 transformants, this represents the uptake of only 0.01 per cent of all the available molecules. Furthermore, 10,000 transformants is only a very small proportion of the total number of cells that are present in a competent culture. This means that some way must be found to distinguish a cell that has taken up a plasmid from the many thousands that have not been transformed. Uptake and stable retention of a plasmid is usually detected by looking for expression of the genes carried by the plasmid. For example, *E. coli* cells are normally sensitive to the growth inhibitory effects of the antibiotics ampicillin and tetracycline. However, cells that contain the plasmid pBR322 are resistant to these antibiotics. This is because pBR322 carries two sets of antibiotic resistance genes, *amp*^{R} *and tet*^{R}. After a transformation experiment with pBR322, only those *E. coli* cells that have taken up a plasmid are resistant to ampicillin and tetracycline and able to form colonies on an agar medium that contains ampicillin or tetracycline; non-transformants, which are still susceptible to these antibiotics, do not produce colonies on the selective

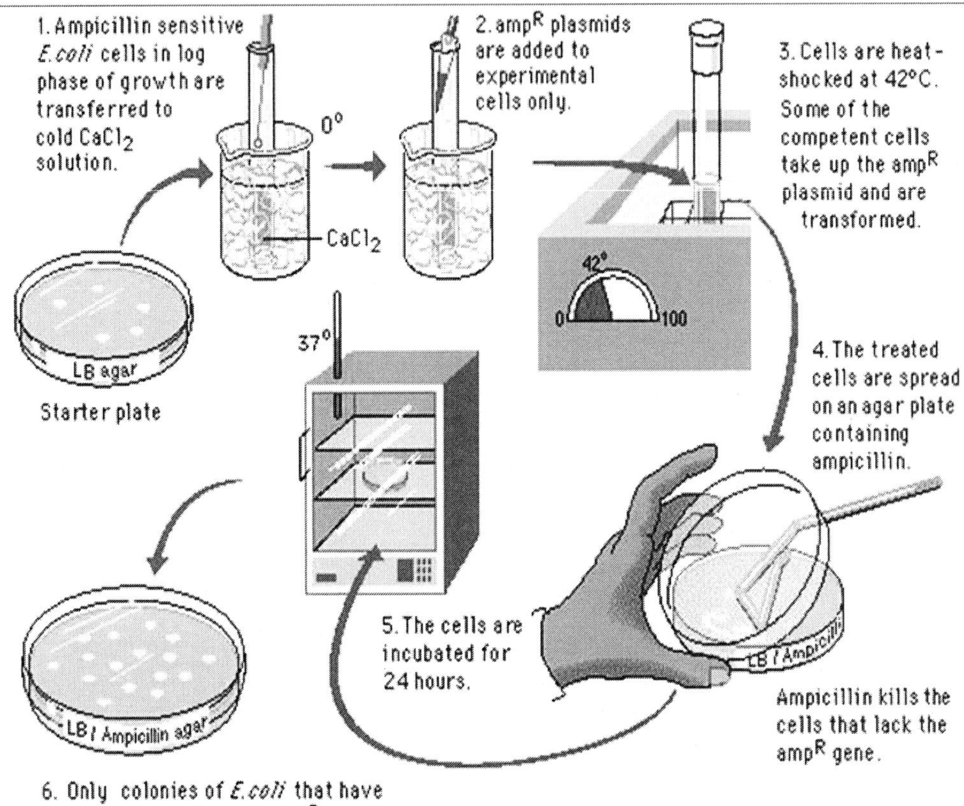

Figure 22.6. Screening of Bacterial Transformation through Antibiotic Resistance Marker.

medium. Transformants and non-transformants are therefore easily distinguished (Figure 22.6). Another method of selection is based upon the functional *lacZ* gene present in the transformed cells. After transformation of bacterial cells either electrophoration or heat shock method with pUC type vectors, transformed bacterial cells in special agar medium (with X gal) produce blue and white colour colonies. Blue colour colonies are having functional lacZ gene in their MCS region. White colour colony bacteria containing gene of interest in their MCS site of pUC vectors. So the lacZ gene is not functional in white colour cells thats why those not able to produce any colour. Blue colour cell is transformed with self ligated vector where as white colour bacterial colonies are transformed with recombinant DNA. This type of screening is called as blue white screening (Figure 22.7).

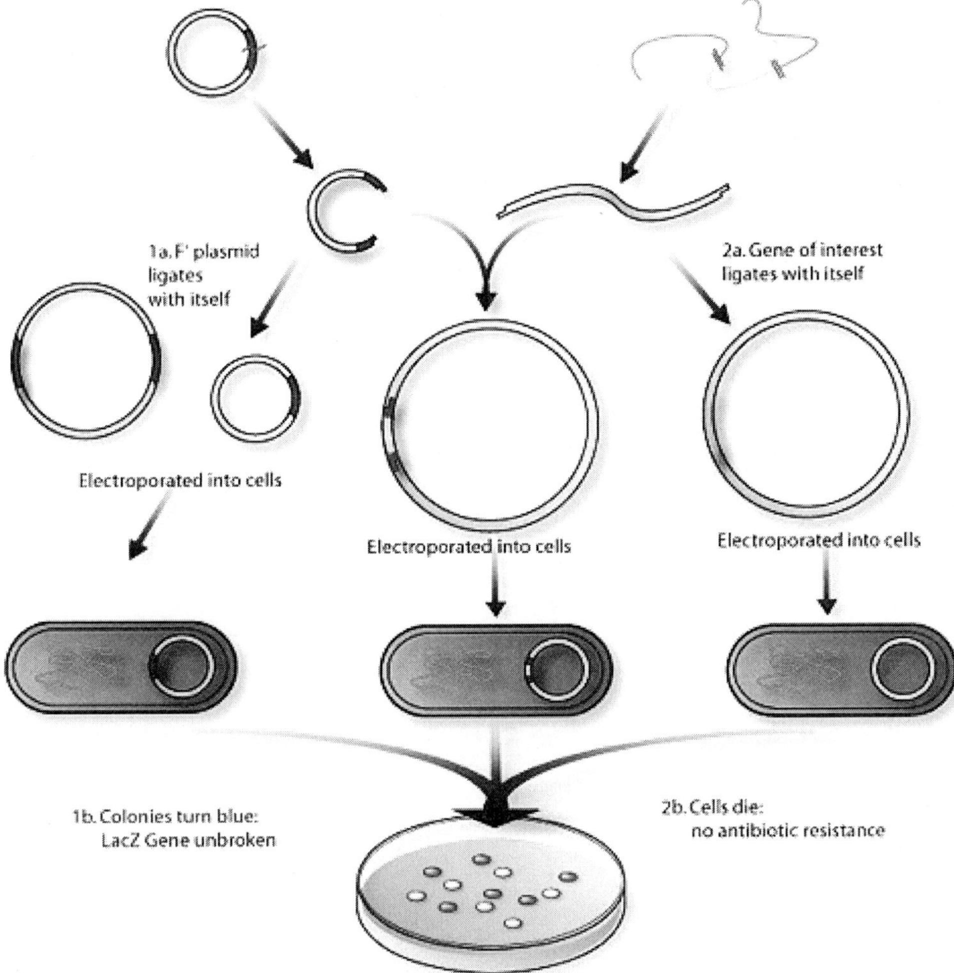

Figure 22.7. Screening of Bacterial transformation through Blue white screening method

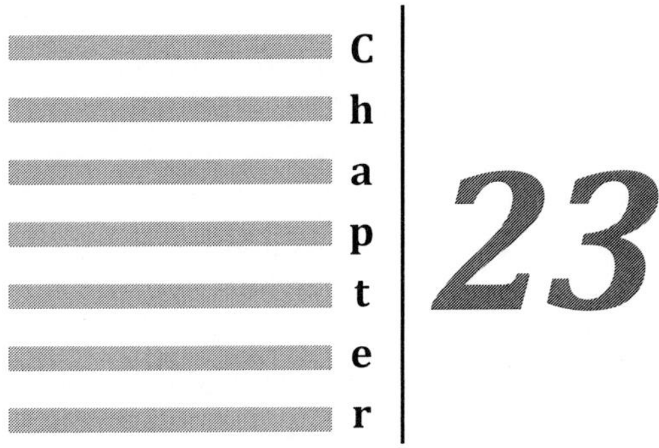

Direct and Indirect Gene Transfer Methods in Plants: Microinjection, Electrophoration, Particle Bombardment, *Agrobacterium* Mediated Method

Biotechnology has provided several unique opportunities that include: access to novel molecules, ability to change the level of gene expression, capability to change the expression pattern of genes and develop transgenic plants with novel genes. As a result of advancement in genetic engineering and controlling of gene expression pattern, there has been a rapid progress in genetic transformation method and it act as a inevitable tool for crop improvement. To achieve genetic transformation in plants, we need to construct a vector (genetic vehicle) which transports the genes of interest, flanked by the necessary controlling sequences *i.e.* promoter and terminator, and deliver the genes into the host plant. The two kinds of gene transfer methods in plants are:

I. Direct or vector less DNA transfer
II. Indirect or vector-mediated gene transfer

I. Direct or Vector-less DNA Transfer

The term direct or vector less transfer of DNA is used when the foreign DNA is directly introduced into the plant genome without the help of a vector. Direct DNA transfer methods rely on the delivery of naked DNA into the plant cells. This is in contrast to the *Agrobacterium* or vector-mediated DNA transfer which may be regarded as indirect methods. *Agrobacterium* has not been used successfully to transform all plant species that have been tested. Many important agronomic crops cannot be transformed using this method. There are two major reasons for the failure of *Agrobacterium* to be used with all species: i) inability of the bacterium to transfer DNA into these plants as all plant species are not susceptible to infection by *Agrobacterium* and ii) failure to regenerate plants after transformation. Since *Agrobacterium* transformation is not successful with some plant species, a variety of other methods have been developed. These all use physical methods to deliver DNA into plant cells. Majority of the direct DNA transfer methods are simple and effective. The major disadvantage of direct gene transfer is that the frequency of transgene rearrangements is high. This results in higher transgene copy number, and high frequencies of gene silencing. And in fact, several transgenic plants have been developed by this approach. The methods used for direct gene transfer in plants are:

1. Microinjection

Microinjection is a direct physical method involving the mechanical insertion of the desirable DNA into a target cell. The target cell may be the one identified from intact cells, protoplasts, callus, embryos, meristems, *etc.* Microinjection is used for the transfer of cellular organelles for the manipulation of chromosomes (Figure 23.1).

The technique of microinjection involves the transfer of the gene through a micropipette **(0.5-10.0 pm tip)** into the cytoplasm/nucleus of a plant cell or protoplast. While the gene transfer is done, the recipient cells are kept immobilized in agarose embedding, and held by a suction holding pipette (on the left of the photograph). As the process of microinjection is complete, the transformed cell is cultured and grown to develop into a transgenic plant. In fact, transgenic tobacco and *Brassica napus* have been developed by this approach. The major limitations of microinjection are that it is slow, expensive, and has to be performed by trained and skilled personnel.

2. Electrophoration

Electrophoration basically involves the use of high field strength electrical impulses to reversibly permeabilize the cell membranes for the uptake of DNA. This technique can be used for the delivery of DNA into intact plant cells and protoplasts. The plant material is incubated in a buffer solution containing the desired foreign/ target DNA, and subjected to high voltage electrical impulses. This results in the formation of pores in the plasma membrane through which DNA enters and gets integrated into the host cell genome. In the initial days, only protoplasts were used for gene transfer by electrophoration. Now a days, intact cells, callus cultures

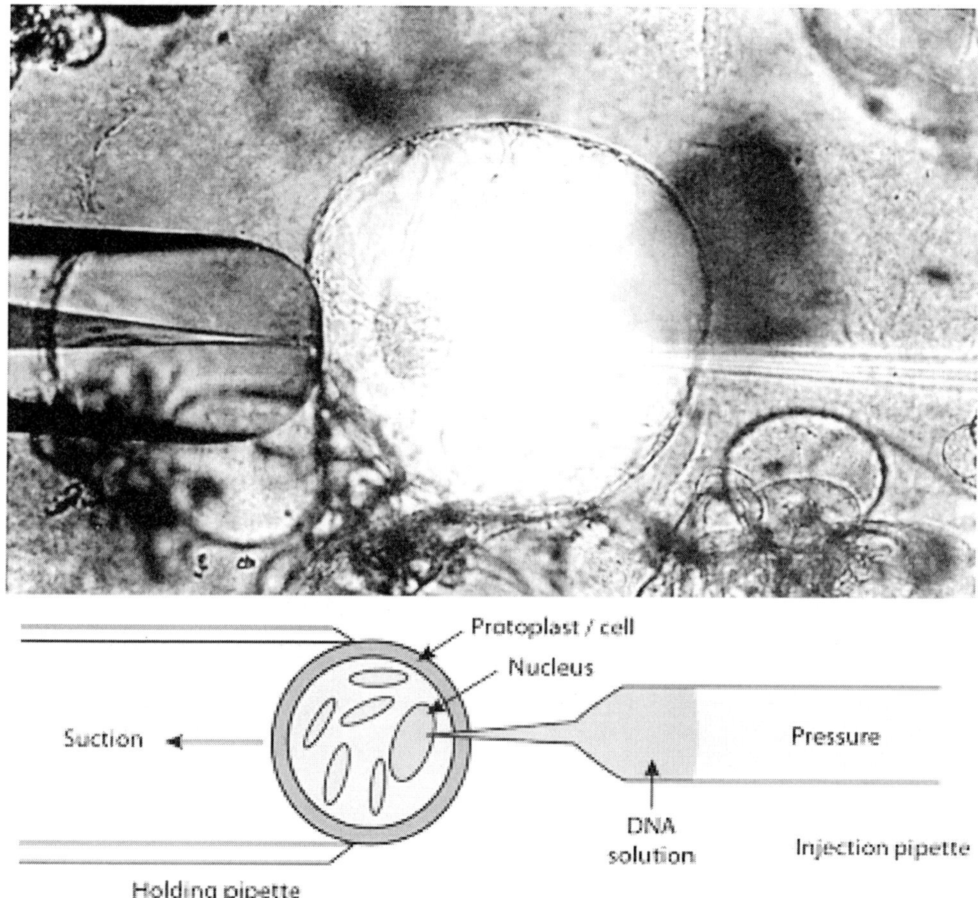

Figure 23.1. Microinjection of DNA by Holding Pipette Method.

and immature embryos can be used with suitable pre- and post-electrophoration treatments. Electrophoration has been successfully used for the production of transgenic plants of many cereals *e.g.* rice, wheat, maize (Figure 23.2).

Advantages of Electrophoration

i. This technique is simple, convenient and rapid, besides being cost-effective.

ii. The transformed cells are at the same physiological state after electrophoration.

iii. Efficiency of transformation can be improved by optimising the electrical field strength, and addition of spermidine.

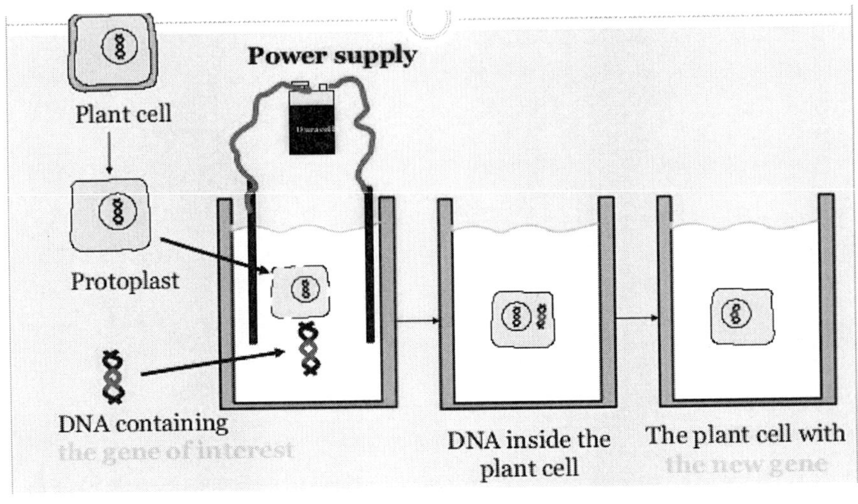

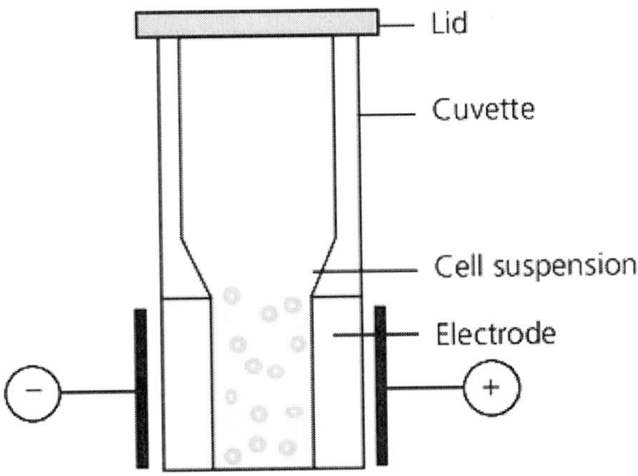

Figure 23.2. Electrophoration Unit for DNA Transformation.

Limitations of Electrophoration

i. Under normal conditions, the amount of DNA delivered into plant cells is very low.

ii. Efficiency of electrophoration is highly variable depending on the plant material and the treatment conditions.

iii. Regeneration of plants is not very easy, particularly when protoplasts are used.

3. Particle Bombardment (Biolistics)

Prerequisite for Particle Bombardment System of gene transfer

Macro and Micro carriers

- ☆ Micro carriers (micro projectiles), the tungsten or gold particles coated with DNA, are carried by macro carriers (macro projectiles). These macro-carriers are inserted into the apparatus and pushed downward by rupturing the disc.
- ☆ The stopping plate does not permit the movement of macro carrier while the micro carriers (with DNA) are propelled at a high speed into the plant material. Here the DNA segments are released which enter the plant cells and integrate with the genome.

Plant Material Used in Bombardment

Two types of plant tissue are commonly used for particle bombardment:

1. Primary explants which can be subjected to bombardment that are subsequently induced to become embryogenic and regenerate.
2. Proliferating embryonic tissues that can be bombarded in cultures and then allowed to proliferate and regenerate.

In order to protect plant tissues from being damaged by bombardment, cultures are maintained on high osmoticum media or subjected to limited plasmolysis.

Transgene Integration in Bombardment

It is believed (based on the gene transfer in rice by biolistics) that the gene transfer in particle bombardment is a two stage process.

1. In the pre-integration phase, the vector DNA molecules are spliced together. This results in fragments carrying multiple gene copies.
2. Integrative phase is characterized by the insertion of gene copies into the host plant genome.

The integrative phase facilitates further transgene integration which may occur at the same point or a point close to it. The net result is that particle bombardment is frequently associated with high copy number at a single locus. This type of single locus may be beneficial for regeneration of plants.

a) Particle Bombardment Mediated Transformation

Particle (or micro projectile) bombardment is the most effective method for gene transfer, and creation of transgenic plants. This is the most widely used method of direct DNA delivery method and a main alternative to *Agrobacterium*-mediated transformation method. This method has received the most attention for cereal crop transformation. It has been successfully used for the transformation of many cereals, *e.g.* rice, wheat, maize. In fact, the first commercial genetically modified crops such as maize containing Bt-toxin gene were developed by this approach.

The micro projectile bombardment method was initially named as biolistics by its inventor Sanford (1988). Biolistics is a combination of biological and ballistics. There are other names for this technique- particle gun, gene gun, bio blaster. The aims are to penetrate cells or tissues with accelerated metal micro-projectile (Also known as microcarriers), which are coated with DNA (containing gene of interest). **Such micro-projectile, of tungsten or gold** (used because of their high densities), have been shown to penetrate cells when accelerated at high velocities, and the DNA can be released and expressed transiently or can be stably integrated into chromosomes. A diagrammatic representation of micro projectile bombardment system for the transfer of genes in plants is depicted in Figure 23.3, and briefly described below.

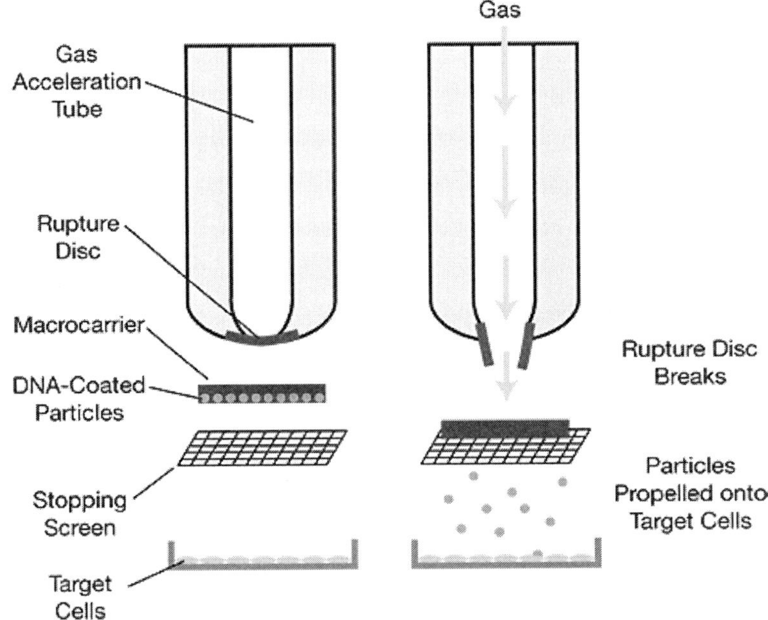

Figure 23.3. A diagrammatic representation of micro projectile bombardment system for the transfer of genes in plants

b) The Biolistic PDS-1000/He device

This device is the most widely used particle delivery system for gene transfer. DNA is delivered in cells in association with microscopic metal particles called microcarriers that are propelled at high velocity towards target tissues.

The microcarriers (gold or tungsten) are accelerated on a plastic sheet, called macrocarrier, which is driven by shock wave of helium gas. A small high pressure chamber within the gas acceleration tube is filled with helium gas to a selected pressure. The chamber has been temporarily sealed by rupture disc. **Helium gas** is supplied by a high pressure helium tank. When critical pressure for the rupture disc is reached; it bursts and releases powerful gas shock wave. In the path of the gas shock is the micro-carrier launch assembly where shock wave energy is transferred to microcarriers. The macrocarriers are positioned under a steel ring and is held in place by a thin lip around its perimeter. Upon firing the macrocarrier separates from its holder and flies unimpeded downwards until it impacts against rigid stopping screen. It is retained by the stopping screen. The microcarriers, however, are launched and continue downwards until they impact and penetrate target cells. During operation of the device, as much of the air in the main chamber is removed with a vacuum pump.

Factors Affecting Bombardment

Several attempts are made to study the various factors, and optimize the system of particle bombardment for its most efficient use. Some of the important parameters are described.

1. Nature of Micro Particles

Inert metals such as tungsten, gold and platinum are used as micro particles to carry DNA. These particles with relatively higher mass will have a better chance to move fast when bombarded and penetrate the tissues.

2. Nature of Tissues/Cells

The target cells that are capable of undergoing division are suitable for transformation.

3. Amount of DNA

The transformation may be low when too little DNA is used. On the other hand, too much DNA may result is high copy number and rearrangement of transgenes. Therefore, the quantity of DNA used should be balanced. Recently, some workers have started using the chemical aminosiloxane to coat the micro particles with low quantities of DNA adequate enough to achieve high efficiency of transformation.

4. Environmental Parameters

Many environmental variables are known to influence particle bombardment. These factors (temperature, humidity, photoperiod *etc.*) influence the physiology of the plant material, and consequently the gene transfer. It is also observed that some explants, after bombardment may require special regimes of light, humidity, temperature *etc.*

The technology of particle bombardment has been improved in recent years, particularly with regard to the use of equipment. A commercially produced particle bombardment apparatus namely PDS-1000/HC is widely used these days.

Advantages of Particle Bombardment

i. Gene transfer can be efficiently done in organized tissues.

ii. Different species of plants can be used to develop transgenic plants.

Limitations of Particle Bombardment

i. The major complication is the production of high transgene copy number. This may result in instability of transgene expression due to gene silencing.

ii. The target tissue may often get damaged due to lack of control of bombardment velocity.

iii Sometimes, undesirable chimeric plants may be regenerated.

4. Liposome-Mediated Transformation

Liposomes are artificially created lipid vesicles containing a phospholipid membrane. They are successfully used in mammalian cells for the delivery of proteins, drugs *etc.* Liposomes carrying genes can be employed to fuse with protoplasts and transfer the genes. The efficiency of transformation increases when the process is carried out in conjunction with polyethylene glycol (PEG). Liposome-mediated transformation involves adhesion of liposomes to the protoplast surface, its fusion at the site of attachment and release of plasmids inside the cell (Figure 23.4).

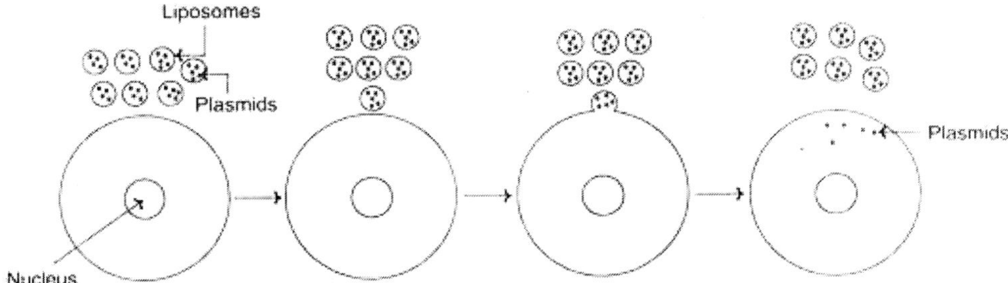

Figure 23.4. Fusion of Plasmid-Filled Liposomes with Protoplasts.

Advantages of Liposome Fusion

i. Being present in an encapsulated form of liposomes, DNA is protected from environmental insults and damage.

ii. DNA is stable and can be stored for some time in liposomes prior to transfer.

iii. Applicable to a wide range of plant cells.

iv. There is good reproducibility in the technique.

Limitations of Liposome Fusion

The major problem with liposome-mediated transformation is the difficulty associated with the regeneration of plants from transformed protoplasts.

5. Polyethylene Glycol (PEG)-Mediated Transfer

Polyethylene glycol (PEG), in the presence of divalent cations (using Ca^{2+}), destabilizes the plasma membrane of protoplasts and renders it permeable to naked DNA. In this way, the DNA enters nucleus of the protoplasts and gets integrated with the genome. The procedure involves the isolation of protoplasts and their suspension, addition of plasmid DNA, followed by a slow addition of **40 per cent PEG-4000 (w/v)** dissolved in mannitol and calcium nitrate solution. As this mixture is incubated, protoplasts get transformed.

Advantages of PEG-Mediated Transformation

i. A large number of protoplasts can be simultaneously transformed.

ii. This technique can be successfully used for a wide range of plant species.

Limitations of PEG-Mediated Transformation

i. The DNA is susceptible for degradation and rearrangement.

ii. Random integration of foreign DNA into genome may result in undesirable traits.

iii. Regeneration of plants from transformed protoplasts is a difficult task.

II. Indirect or Vector-Mediated Gene Transfer Method

Indirect gene transfer (also known as **vector-mediated gene transfer**) involves the introduction of exogenous **DNA** into the plant genome via biological **vector** bacteria and virus. Among the various vectors used in plant transformation, the Ti plasmid of ***Agrobacterium tumefaciens*** has been widely used. *Agrobacterium tumefaciens* is a soil-borne, Gram-negative phytopathogenic bacterium. It is rod shaped and motile, and belongs to the bacterial family of Rhizobiaceae. This bacteria is known as "**natural genetic engineer**" of plants because these bacteria have natural ability to transfer T-DNA of their plasmids into plant genome upon infection of cells at the wound site and cause an unorganized growth of a cell mass known as crown gall. This bacterium is considerd as the natural expert of inter-kingdom gene transfer. In fact, the major credit for the development of plant transformation techniques goes to the natural unique capability of *A. tumefaciens.* This bacteria contains Ti plasmids (approximate size 200 kb) exist as independent replicating circular DNA molecules. Ti plasmids contain T-DNA (transferred DNA) region having the genes for the biosynthesis of auxin (aux), cytokinin (cyt) and opine (ocs), and is flanked by left and right borders. These three genes-aux, cyto and ocs are referred to as oncogenes, as they are the determinants of the tumor phenotype. T-DNA borders, a set of 24 bp sequences present on either side (right and left) of T-DNA are also transferred to the plant cells. these 24 bp sequences of right and left border is most important in transfering T-DNA from Ti plasmid without these region transfer of the T-DNA region is not occur. Other then T-DNA region it also contain the genes responsible for the transfer of T-DNA into the host plant are located outside T-DNA and the region is referred to as vir or virulence region. Vir region codes for proteins involved in T-DNA transfer. At least nine vir-gene operons have been identified. These include vir A, vir G, vir B1, vir C1, vir D1, D2 and D4, and vir E1, and E2 (Figure 23.5).

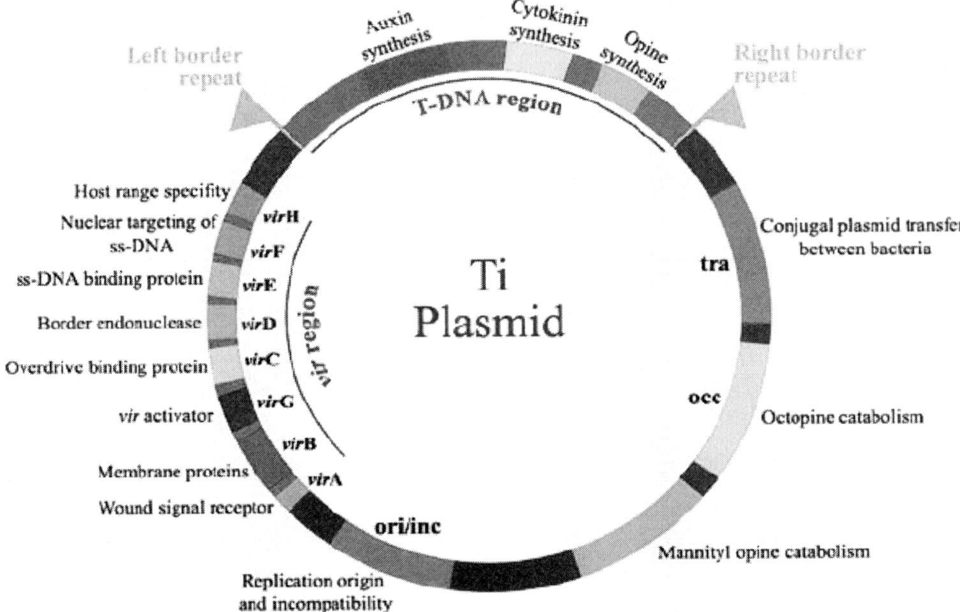

Figure 23.5. Structure of Ti Plasmid.

Ti Plasmid-Derived Vector Systems

It is possible to insert a desired DNA sequence (gene) into the T-DNA region (of Ti plasmid), and then use *A. tumefaciens* to deliver this gene(s) into the genome of plant cell. In this process, Ti plasmids serve as natural vectors. However, there are several limitations to use Ti plasmids directly as cloning vectors:

i. Ti plasmids are large in size (200-800 kb). Smaller vectors are preferred for recombinant experiments. For this reason, large segments of DNA of Ti plasmid, not essential for cloning, must be removed.

ii. Absence of unique restriction enzyme sites on Ti plasmids.

iii. The phytohormones (auxin, cytokinin) produced prevent the plant cells being regenerated into plants. Therefore auxin and cytokinin genes must be removed.

iv. Opine production in transformed plant cells lowers the plant yield. Therefore opine synthesizing genes which are of no use to plants should be removed.

v. Ti plasmids cannot replicate in *E. coli*. This limits their utility as *E. coli* is widely used in recombinant experiments. An alternate arrangement is to add an origin of replication to Ti plasmid that allows the plasmid to replicate in *E. coli*.

Considering the above limitations, Ti plasmid- based vectors with suitable modifications have been constructed.

These vectors are mainly composed of the following components:

1. The right border sequence of T-DNA which is absolutely required for T-DNA integration into plant cell DNA.
2. A multiple cloning site (poly-linker DNA) that promotes the insertion of cloned gene into the region between T-DNA borders.
3. An origin of DNA replication that allows the plasmids to multiply in *E. coli*.
4. A selectable marker gene (*e.g.* neomycin phosphotransferase) for appropriate selection of the transformed cells.

Two types of Ti plasmid-derived vectors are used for genetic transformation of plants 1. Co-integrate vectors; 2. Binary vectors.

Co-integrate Vector

Co-integrate vector system, containing the disarmed and modified Ti plasmid containing foreign gene (intermediate cloning vector) and recepter Ti plasmid containing T-DNA region. The desired foreign gene (target-gene) is first cloned in the multiple cloning site of the intermediate vector. The cloning process is carried out in *E. coli*, the bacterium where the cloning is most efficient. The intermediate vector is mated with *Agrobacterium* so that the foreign gene is mobilised into the *Agrobacterium*. This transformed *Agrobacterium* cells containing both receptor Ti plasmid and intermediate vector are selectively isolated when grown on a minimal medium containing spectinomycin. The selection process becomes easy since *E. coli* does not grow on a minimal medium in which *Agrobacterium* grows. Within the *Agrobacterium* cells, intermediate plasmid gets integrated into the receptor Ti plasmid to produce co-integrate plasmid. This plasmid containing plant transformation marker (*e.g.* npt II) gene and cloned target gene between T-DNA borders is transferred to plant cells. The transformed plant cells can be selected on a medium containing kanamycin when the plant and *Agrobacterium* cells are incubated together (Figures 23.6 and 23.8).

Binary Vector

The binary vector system consists of an *Agrobacterium* strain along with a disarmed Ti plasmid called **vir helper plasmid** (the entire T-DNA region including borders deleted while virulance region is retained). It may be noted that both of them are not physically linked (or integrated). A binary vector with T-DNA can

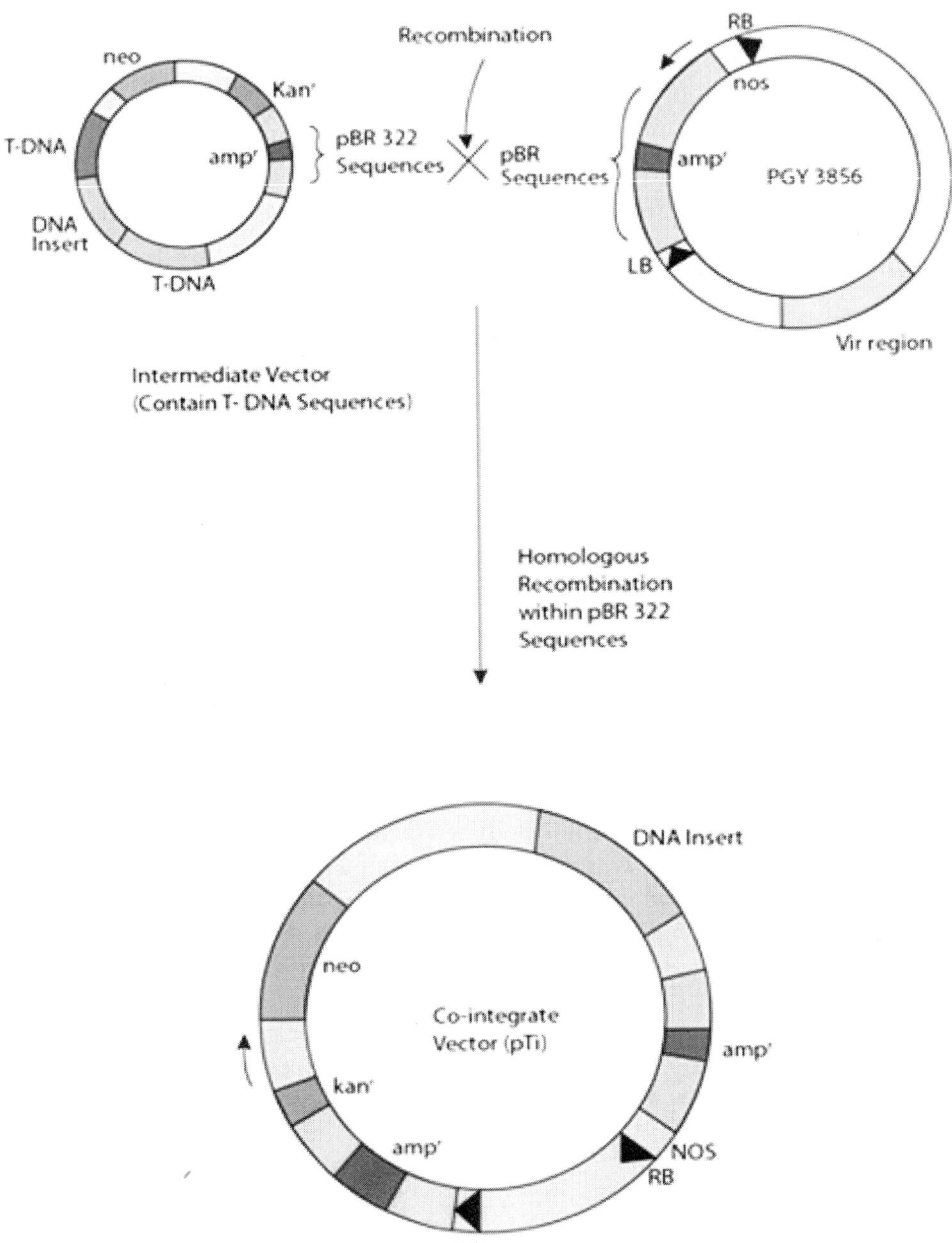

Figure 23.6. Co-integrate Vector System.

replicate in *E. coli* and *Agrobacterium*. The target (foreign) gene of interest is inserted into the multiple cloning site of the binary vector. In this way, the- target gene is placed between the right and left border repeats and cloned in *E. coli*. By a mating process, the binary vector is mobilised from *E. coli* to *Agrobacterium*. Now, the virulence gene proteins of T-DNA present in the helper plasmid facilitate the transfer of T-DNA of the vector into plant cells (Figures 23.7 and 23.8).

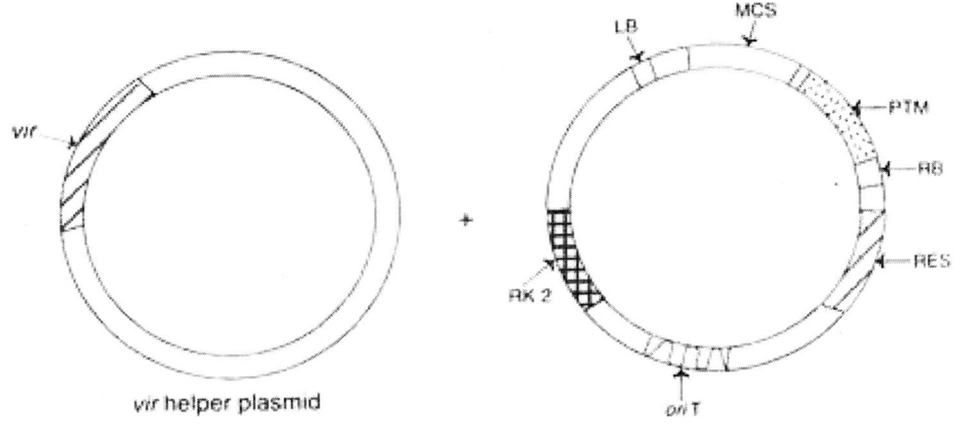

Figure 23.7. Binary Vector System.

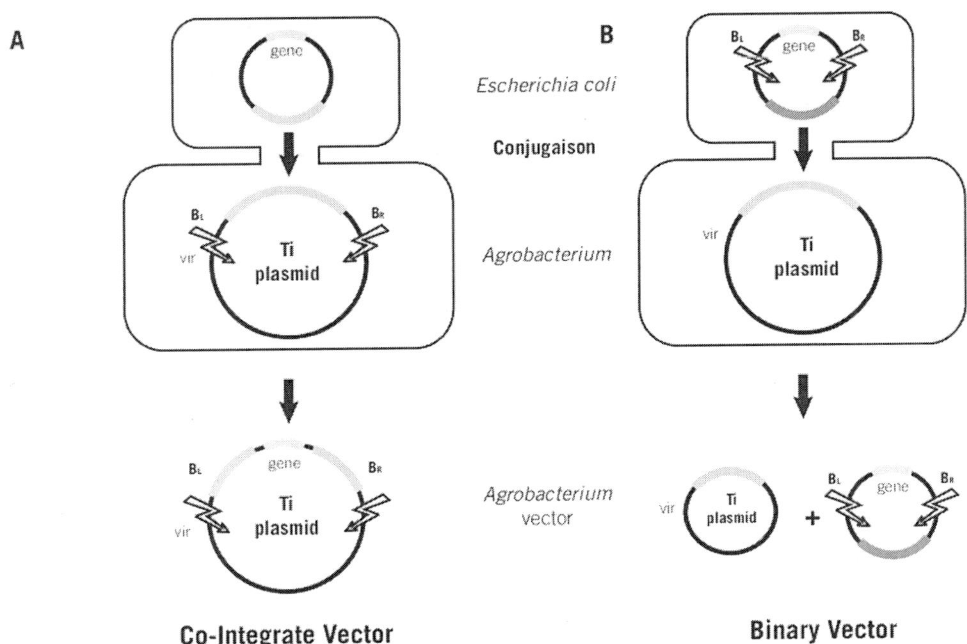

Figure 23.8. Comparison of Co-integrate and Binary Vector System.

Whole Process of Transfer of T-DNA and Integration into Plant Cell

The process of T-DNA transfer from Ti Plasmid and it integration into the host plant genome is briefly described (Figure 23.9).

1. Signal Induction to *Agrobacterium*

The wounded plant cells release certain chemicals- phenolic compounds and sugars which are recognized as signals by *Agrobacterium*.

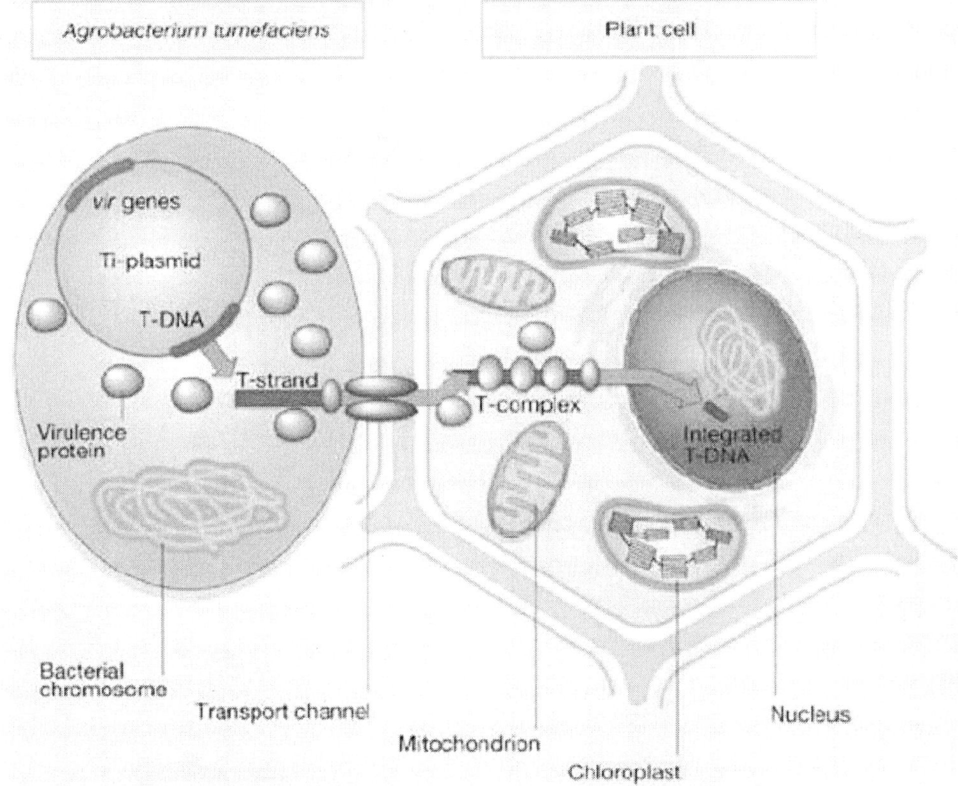

Figure 23.9. T-DNA Transfer and Integration into Plant Cell.

2. Attachment of *Agrobacterium* to Plant Cells

The *Agrobacterium* attaches to plant cells through polysaccharides, particularly cellulose fibres produced by the bacterium.

3. Production of Virulence Proteins

As the signal induction occurs in the *Agrobacterium* cells attached to plant cells, a series of events take place that result in the production of virulence proteins. To start with, signal induction by phenolics stimulates vir A which in turn activates (by phosphorylation) vir C. This induces expression of virulence genes of Ti plasmid to produce the corresponding virulence proteins (D1, D2, E2, B *etc.*).

4. Production of T-DNA Strand

The right and left borders of T-DNA are recognized by vir D1/vir D2 proteins. These proteins are involved in the production single-stranded T-DNA (ss DNA), its protection and export to plant cells. The ss T-DNA gets attached to vir D2.

5. Transfer of T-DNA out of *Agrobacterium*

The ss T-DNA - vir D2 complex in association with vir G is exported from the bacterial cell.

6. Transfer of T-DNA into Plant Cells and Integration

The T-DNA-vir D2 complex crosses the plant plasma membrane. In the plant cells, T-DNA gets covered with vir E2. This covering protects the T-DNA from degradation by nucleases; vir D2 and vir E2 interact with a variety of plant proteins which influences T-DNA transport and integration. The T-DNA-vir D2-vir E2 - plant protein complex enters the nucleus through nuclear pore complex. Within the nucleus, the T-DNA gets integrated into the plant chromosome through a process referred to illegitimate recombination. This is different from the homologous recombination, as it does not depend on the sequence similarity.

Agrobacterium-Mediated Gene Transfer Method in Plants

Agrobacterium-mediated technique is the most widely used for the transformation of plants and generation of transgenic plants. Transformation Technique consists of following steps:

1. Development of *Agrobacterium* carrying the co-integrate or binary vector with the desired gene.
2. Identification of a suitable explant *e.g.* cells, protoplasts, tissues, calluses, organs.
3. Co-culture of explants with *Agrobacterium.*
4. Killing of *Agrobacterium* with a suitable antibiotic (Rifampicin) without harming the plant tissue.
5. Selection of transformed plant cells from non transformed plant cells (Kanamycin).
6. Regeneration of whole plants.

The important requirements for gene transfer in higher plants through *Agrobacterium* mediation are, i. The explants of the plant must produce phenolic compounds **(*e.g.* autosyringone)** for activation of virulence genes ii. Transformed cells/tissues should be capable to regenerate into whole plants.

Disarmed Ti plasmids (oncogenic genes, which is involved producing galls removed from the T-DNA region without affecting the right and left border) are used as gene vectors for delivering useful foreign genes into target plant cells and tissues. It is possible to insert a desired DNA sequence (gene) or foreign gene into the T-DNA region (of Disarmed Ti plasmid), then use *A. tumefaciens* to deliver this gene(s) into the genome of plant cell. In this process, Ti plasmids serve as natural vectors. However, there are several limitations to use Ti plasmids directly as cloning vectors. So for artificially constructed Ti plasmid-derived vector systems *i.e.*, 1. cointegrate vector and 2. Binary vector are used for plant transformation.

To transform plants, leaf discs (in case of dicots) or embryogenic callus (in case of monocots) are collected and infected with ***Agrobacterium*** carrying recombinant disarmed Ti-plasmid vector (either cointegrate vector or Binary vector system). The infected tissue is then cultured (co-cultivation) on shoot regeneration medium for 2-3 days during which time the transfer of T-DNA along with foreign genes takes place. After this, the transformed tissues (leaf discs/calli) are transferred onto selection cum plant regeneration medium supplemented with usually lethal concentration of an antibiotic to selectively eliminate non-transformed tissues. After 3-5 weeks, the regenerated shoots (from leaf discs) are transferred to root-inducing medium, and after another 3-4 weeks, complete plants are transferred to soil following the hardening (acclimatization) of regenerated plants. The molecular techniques like PCR and southern hybridization are used to detect the presence of foreign genes and its expression in the transgenic plants (Figure 23.10).

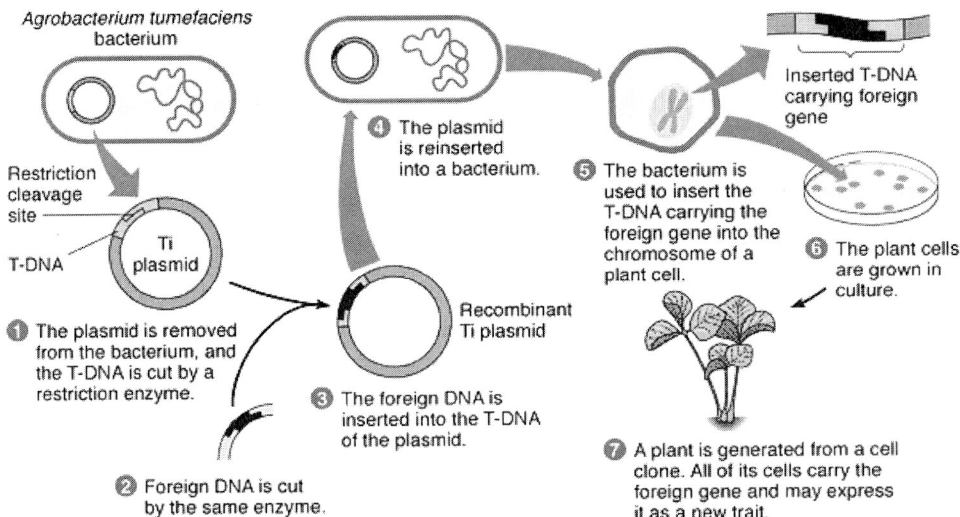

Figure 23.10. *Agrobacterium*-Mediated Gene Transfer Method.

Advantages of *Agrobacterium*-Mediated Transformation

i. This is a natural method of gene transfer.

ii. Agrobacterium can conveniently infect any explant (cells/tissues/organs).

iii. Even large fragments of DNA can be efficiently transferred.
iv. Stability of transferred DNA is reasonably good.
v. Transformed plants can be regenerated effectively.

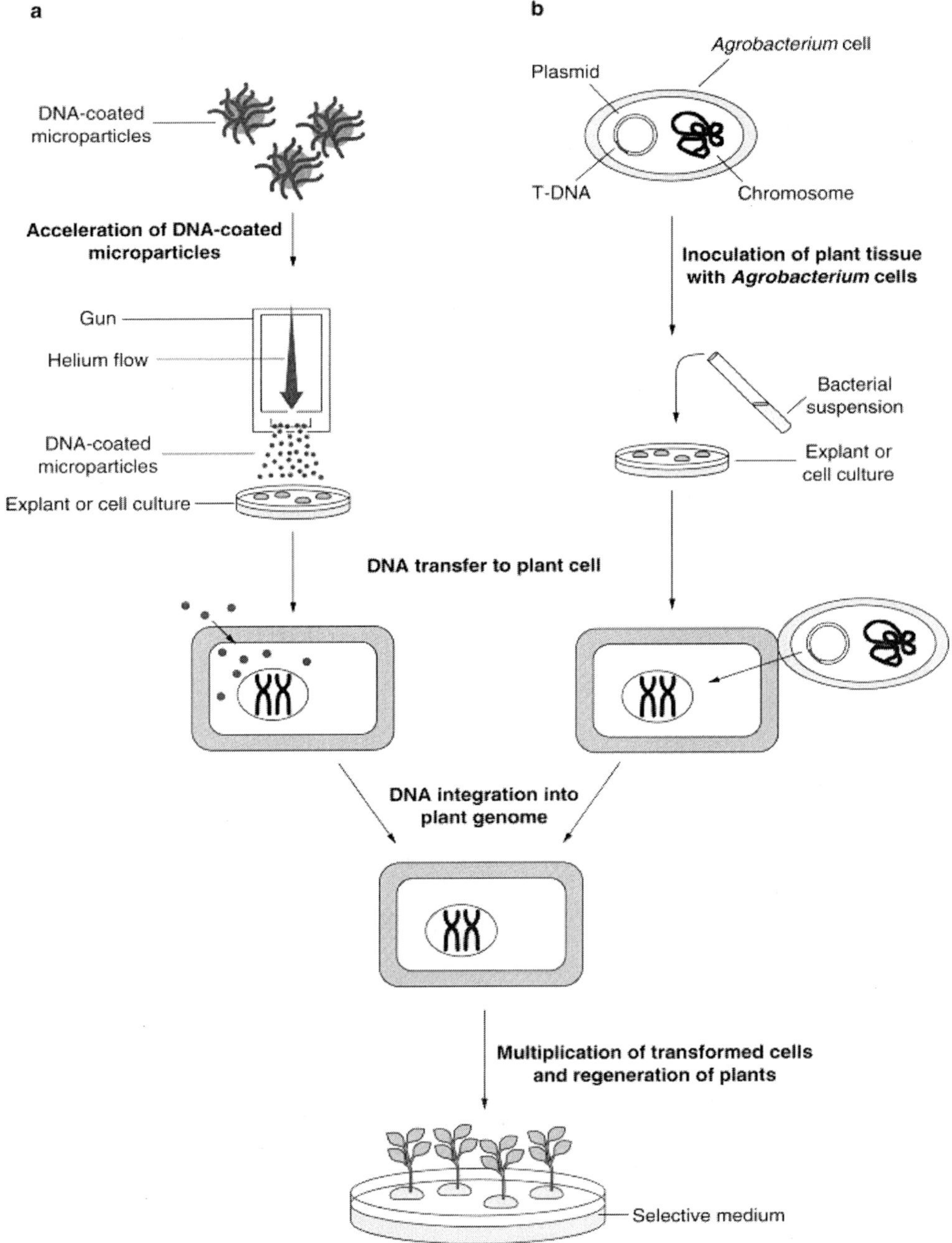

Figure 23.11. Direct and Indirect DNA Transformation Method.

Limitations of *Agrobacterium*-Mediated Transformation

i. There is a limitation of host plants for *Agrobacterium*, since many crop plants (monocotyledons *e.g.* cereals) are not infected by it. In recent years, virulent strains of *Agrobacterium* that can infect a wide range of plants have been developed.

ii. The cells that regenerate more efficiently are often difficult to transform, *e.g.* embryonic cells lie in deep layers which are not easy targets for Agrobacterium.

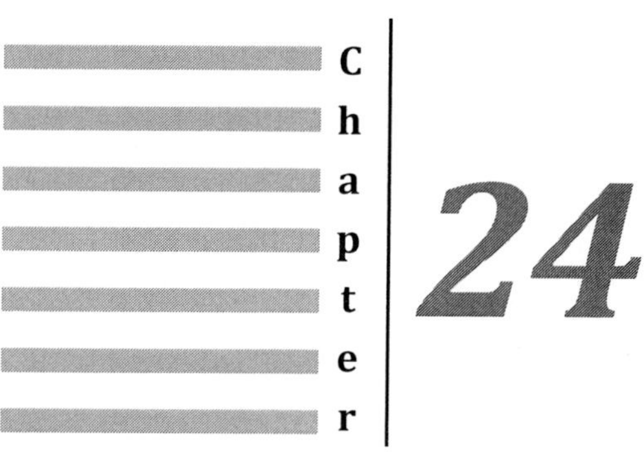

Tissue Specific Promoters, Selectable and Scorable Markers, Reporter Genes and Molecular Analysis of Transgenic Plants

Plant transformation vectors are special vectors which are used in genetic transformation of plants or production of transgenic plants. Generally the plant transformation vectors have the gene of interest, a promoter sequence, a reporter gene and a selectable marker.

Promoters

The promoter acts as the regulator for the level of gene expression *i.e.* when, where and how much of the gene product (protein) is produced. Factors that bind to promoters react to signals from the organism or/and the surrounding environment. The source and type of signal determines the type of promoters that are activated. In genetic engineering, there are three major types of promoters used, depending on the level of gene expression and specificity required:

1. Constitutive Promoters

They facilitate expression of the gene in all tissues regardless of the surrounding environment and development stage of the organism. Such promoters can turn on the gene in every living cell of the organism, all the time, throughout the organism's lifetime. *e.g.* - Cauliflower mosaic virus (CaMV) 35S, opine promoters, plant ubiquitin (Ubi), rice actin 1 (Act-1) and maize alcohol dehydrogenase 1 (Adh-1). CaMV 35S is the most commonly used constitutive promoter for high levels of gene expression in dicot plants. Maize Ubi and rice Act-1 are the currently the most commonly used constitutive promoters for monocots.

2. Tissue-Specific or Development-Stage-Specific Promoters

They facilitate expression of a gene in specific tissue(s) or at certain stages of development while leaving the rest of the organism unmodified. In the case of plants, such promoters might specifically influence expression of genes in the roots, fruits, or seeds, or during the vegetative, flowering, or seed-setting stage. *e.g.* Barley hordein gene promoters (for seed gene expression), tomato pz7 and pz130 gene promoters (for ovary gene expression), tobacco RD2 gene promoter (for root gene expression), banana TRX promoter and melon actin promoter (for fruit gene expression).

3. Inducible Promoters

They are activated by external factors. External factors may be abiotic such as heat, water, salinity, chemical, or biotic like pathogen or insect attack. Promoters that react to abiotic factors are the most commonly used in plant genetic engineering because these can easily be manipulated. Such promoters respond to chemical compounds such as antibiotics, herbicides or changes in temperature or light. *e.g.* Ethanol inducible promoter.

Marker Genes

Monitoring and detection of plant transformation systems in order to know whether the **'gene of interest'** has been successfully transferred into the plant cells, is done with the help of marker gene(s). The marker gene(s) is/are introduced into the plant transformation vector along with the gene of interest.

Types of Marker Genes

1. Reporter/Scoreable/Screenable genes
2. Selectable marker genes

Reporter Genes

These marker genes can show immediate expression of transgenes in the cells/ tissue. A reporter gene is useful in the analysis of transgenic expression and for standardization of the parameters for successful gene transfer protocol. An ideal reporter gene should have the following features:

- Detection with high sensitivity.
- Low endogenous background.
- Assayed by an easy, non-destructive and quantitative assay.

Common Reporter Genes

- β-**glucuronidase (GUS)** – The bacterial gene ***uidA*** encoding β-**glucuronidase (GUS)** is the most frequently used reporter gene isolated from *E.coli*. In transgenic plant β-glucuronidase enzyme will be synthesized upon the expression of *uidA* gene, which breaks down substrate **X-Gluc (5 bromo-4 chloro-3 indol beta D glucuronide)** to give a coloured reaction (blue colour), so that its presence can be detected *in situ*. The detection is a non-radioactive assay using X-Gluc. This reporter gene does not require DNA extraction, electrophoresis or autoradiography (Figure 24.1).

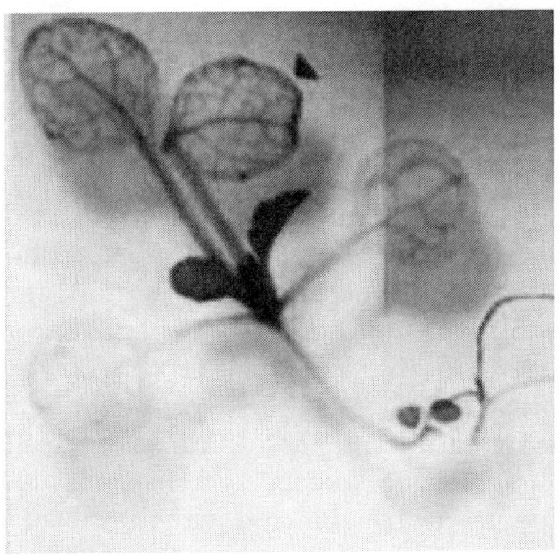

Figure 24.1. Gene Expression in Transgenic Young Plants.

- β-**galactosidase (*lacZ*)**- The bacterial gene *lacZ* is encoding the enzyme β-**galactosidase** which acts on a chromogenic substrate called X-gal, when the enzyme substrate reaction takes place, the **X- gal** is converted from white to a blue compound. The expression of *lacZ* gene is induced by **Iso-propyl-thiogalactoside (IPTG)**. When the transformed bacterial cells with gene of interest fails to code for beta-galactosidase and in this case the substrate (X-gal) is never converted to the blue colour but transformed cells without gene of interest produce blue colour colonies. Insertional inactivation takes place in *lacZ* gene when gene of interest is integrated in to the MCS present in the *lacZ* gene, so gene is not able to produce functional protein. This type of screening is called **blue-white screening** (Figure 24.2).

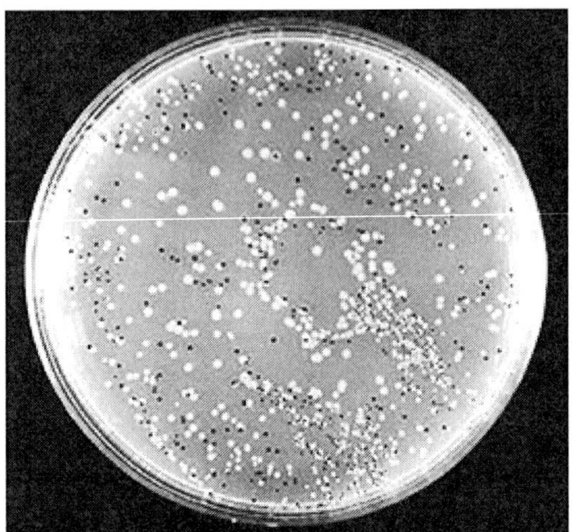

Figure 24.2. Blue White Screening.

☆ **Green Fluorescent Protein (GFP)** – The green fluorescent protein gene is an ideal reporter and selectable marker for gene expression analysis and plant transformation. Gene for GFP has been obtained from **jellyfish *Aequorea victoria***. GFP is a small protein surrounding a fluorescent chromophore. It emits green fluorescent light in the blue to ultraviolet range. The formation of green fluorescence can be detected under fluorescent microscope. Visual detection is possible at any time in living cells without any destruction and without the addition of any cofactor or external substrate. In addition blue-white screening product does not adversely affect cell growth, regeneration and fertility of transformed plants (Figure 24.3).

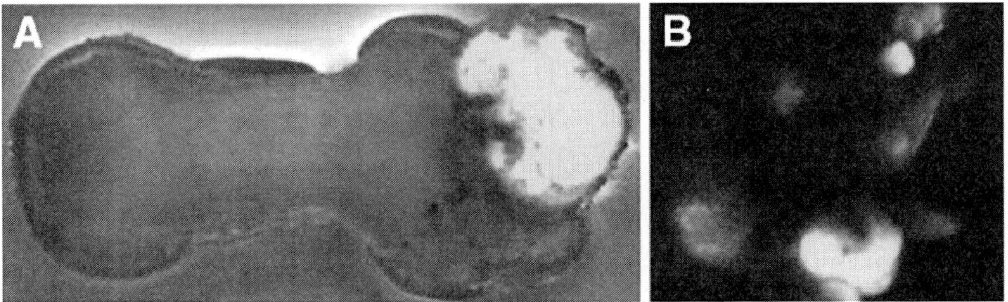

Figure 24.3. Transformed Cells Emits Green Colour Fluorescence.

☆ **The Firefly Luciferase (Luc)**- Luciferase gene **(*luc+*)** isolated from the **North American firefly, *Photinus pyralis*** catalyzes the oxidative decarboxylation of luciferin, to oxyluciferin in the presence of ATP, oxygen and magnesium ions. Luminescense in terms of light production can be recorded in a luminometer (Figure 24.4).

$$\text{Luciferin} + O_2 + \text{ATP} \longrightarrow \text{Oxyluciferin} + CO_2 + H_2O + \text{AMP} + \text{light}$$

$$\left[\begin{array}{l} E + LH_2 + \text{ATP} \longrightarrow E \cdot LH_2\text{–AMP} + PP_i \\ E \cdot LH_2\text{–AMP} + O_2 \longrightarrow E \cdot P\ (\text{oxyluciferin}) + CO_2 + \text{AMP} + \text{light} \end{array}\right]$$

Figure 24.4. Transformed Cells Emits Light (Luminescense).

Selectable Marker Genes

Selection of transformed cells is a key factor in developing successful methods for genetic transformation. This is done by certain selectable marker genes which are present in the vector along with the gene of interest. Selectable markers are an integral part of plant transformation strategies. The selectable marker genes enable the transformed cells to survive on media containing toxic levels of selection agent while non-transformed cells get killed. A large number of such selectable marker genes have become available *viz.,* antibiotic, antimetabolite and herbicide resistance genes, hormone biosynthetic genes and genes conferring resistance to toxic levels of amino acids or amino acid analogs.

I. Antibiotic Resistance Markers

1. Neomycin Phosphotransferase II

Neomycin Phosphotransferase II enzyme is the most widely used selectable marker and it is encoded by the ***npt*II** gene from Tn5 transposon. The commonly used selection agents are **kanamycin, neomycin, geneticin**. The NPT II enzyme inactivates these antibiotics, thus allowing the transformed tissues containing this gene to survive.

2. Aminoglycoside 3 Phosphotransferae II

Aminoglycoside 3 phosphotransferae II enzyme is the commonly used selectable marker and it is encoded by the ***kan*** gene from bacteria. The commonly used selection agent is **kanamycin**.

3. Hygromycin Phosphotransferase

Hygromycin Phosphotransferase gene (*hpt*) is derived from *E.coli.* The selective agent used is **Hygromycin B** antibiotic which interferes with protein synthesis and kills the non-transformed cells quickly (Figure 24.5).

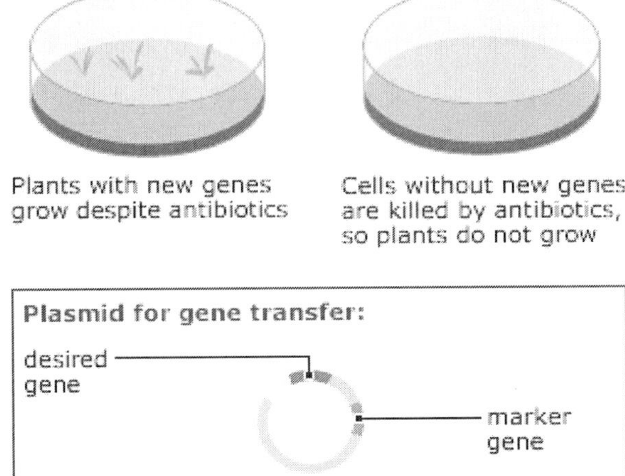

Figure 24.5. Transformed Cells Exhibits Antibiotic Resistance.

II. Herbicide Resistance Markers

1. *Bar Gene*

The ***bar*** gene encodes **for phosphinothricin acetyl transferase (PAT)** enzyme. The PAT enzyme converts the **Bialophos/Phosphinothricin** herbicides (selection agent) into a non-herbicidal form thus allowing the transformed tissues to survive in the presence of these herbicides. This gene is derived from ***Streptomyces hygroscopicus*** **or** ***Streptomyces viridochromogenes***.

2. *aro A Gene*

The *aro A* gene encodes for a *mutant Enol pyruvyl shikimate synthase* (*EPSPS*) enzyme which has the resistance to glyphosate herbicide (selection agent). This gene was isolated from ***Agrobacterium*** **spp.**

3. *gox Gene*

The ***gox*** **gene** isolated from ***Achromobacter*** **LBAA** encodes for **Glyposate oxidoreductase (GOX)** enzyme which degrade glyphosate herbicide (selection agent). The organism containing this gene has the resistance glyphosate herbicide

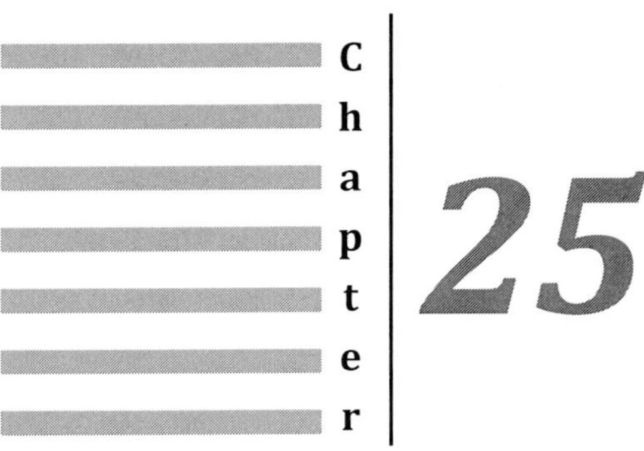

Transgenic Plants: Herbicide, Pest and Disease Resistant, Abiotic Stress Resistant

Transgenic Plants with Beneficial Traits

During the last decades, a tremendous progress has been made in the development of transgenic plants using the various techniques of genetic engineering. The plants, in which a functional foreign gene has been incorporated by any biotechnological methods that generally are not present in the plant, are called transgenic plants. Transgenic plants have many beneficial traits like insect resistance, herbicide tolerance, delayed fruit ripening, improved oil quality, *etc.*

Some of the commercially grown transgenic plants in developed countries are: **"Roundup Ready" soybean, 'Freedom II squash, 'High- lauric' rapeseed (canola), 'Flavr Savr' and 'Endless Summer' tomatoes. During 1995, full registration was granted to genetically engineered Bt gene containing insect resistant 'New Leaf' (potato), 'Maximizer' (corn), 'BollGard' (cotton) in USA.**

Herbicide Tolerance

Weeds are unwanted plants which decrease the crop yields and by competing with crop plants for light, water and nutrients. Many method are adopted to control weeds sucessfully in crop plants, among one of the important method is controlling weeds by applying herbicides *i.e.*, Glyphosate, Phosphinothricin, Bromoxynil *etc.*, Application of herbicide not only kill the weeds but also kill the plants, so development of herbicide tolerant crops is one of the important strategy to control weeds upon applying herbicides. Glyphosate is a glycine derivative and is a herbicide which is found to be effective against the 76 of the world's worst 78 weeds.

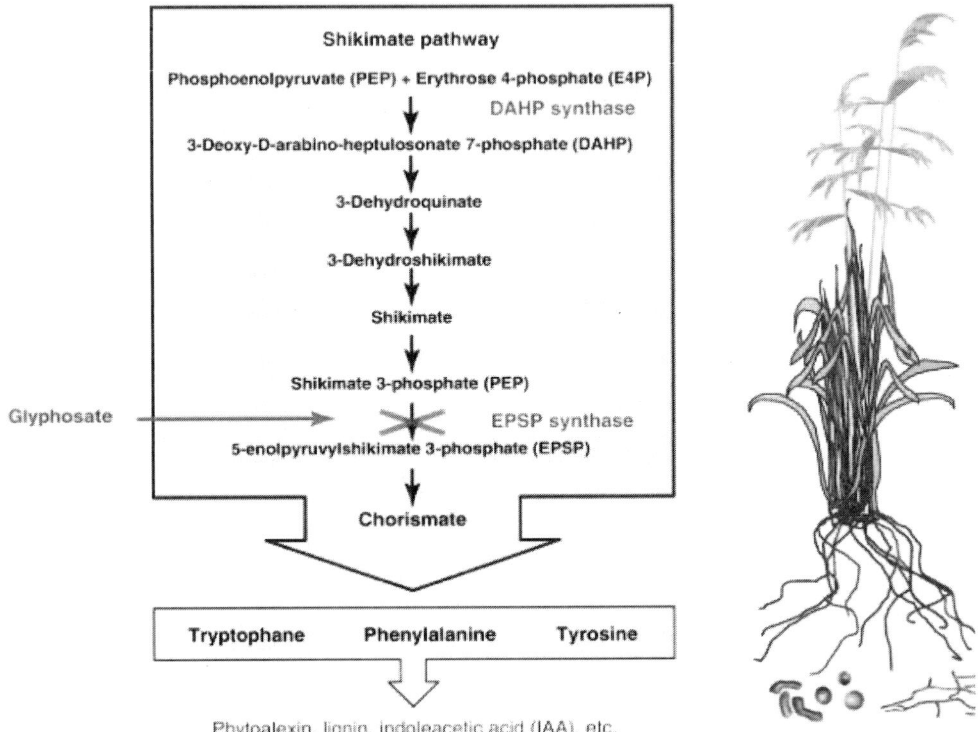

Figure 25.1. Glyphosate Inhibition Action on Plants Aromatic Amino Acid Synthesis Pathway.

It kills the plant by being the **competitive inhibitor of the enzyme 5-enoyl-pyruvylshikimate 3- phosphate synthase (EPSPS) in the shikimic acid pathway.** Due to it's structural similarity with the substrate phosphoenol pyruvate, glyphosate binds more tightly with EPSPS and thus blocks the shikimic acid pathway involved in the aromatic acid synthesis (Figure 25.1). The biological manipulations using genetic engineering to develop herbicide resistant plants can be done by four different mechanisms: (a) over-expression of the target protein by integrating multiple copies of the gene or by using a strong promoter, (b) modification of the target protein by mutation, (c) enhancing the plant detoxification system which helps in reducing the effect of herbicide, (d) detoxifying the herbicide by using a foreign gene.

Strategies to Develop Herbicide Resistance Plants

a. Over Expression of Target Protein

Over expression of target protein has generated tolerance in the case of some herbicides *e.g.* glyphosate, sulphonyl urea compounds and imidazolinones. EPSPS gene was over expressed in ***Petunia*** **and over expressed EPSPS gene was isolated from** ***Petunia*** introduced in to the other plants. These plants could tolerate glyphosate at a dose of 2-4 times higher than that required to kill wild type plants.

b. By using Mutant EPSPS Genes

A single base substitution from C to T resulted in the change of an amino acid from **proline to serine in EPSPS**. The modified enzyme cannot bind to glyphosate and thus provides resistance.

c. Enhancement of Plant Detoxification Mechanism

Many xenobiotic compounds are detoxified in plants involving hydroxylation and conjugation of those compounds. **Hydroxylation of herbicides involves cytochrome P450 monooxygenases**. Conjugation of herbicide compounds is done by glutathione-S-transferases into the vacuoles. Atrazine tolerance in maize involves a two-step pathway involving both hydroxylation and conjugation.

d. Detoxifying the Herbicide by using a Foreign Gene

1. Glyphosate Resistance

Detoxification of glyphosate by introducing the ***gox*** **gene**(isolated from soil organism- ***Ochrobactrum anthropi***) encoding for glyphosate oxidase into crop plants. The enzyme glyphosate oxidase converts glyphosate to glyoxylate and aminomethyl phosponic acid. The transgenic plants exhibited very good glyphosate resistance in the field.

Transgenic plant developed with ***cp4 epsps*** **gene (*aroA:CP4*)**from ***Agrobacterium tumefaciens*** strain ***CP4*** conferring more tolerance to the glyphosate herbicide. Efficiency of herbicide binding affinity towards bacterial enzyme 5-enolpyruvulshikimate-3-phosphate synthase (***EPSPS***) is significantly decreased so the transgenic crop enable to synthesize aromatic amino acid with out any herbicide interfierence (Figure 25.2).

2. Phosphinothricin Resistance

Phosphinothricin is a broad spectrum herbicide and is effective against broad-leafed weeds. It acts as a **competitive inhibitor of the enzyme glutamine synthase** which results in the inhibition of the enzyme glutamine synthase and accumulation of ammonia and finally the death of the plant. The disturbance in the glutamine synthesis also inhibits the **photosynthetic activity**.

The enzyme phosphinothricin acetyl transferase (which was first observed in ***Streptomyces*** **sp.** in natural detoxifying mechanism against phosphinothricin) acetylates phosphinothricin, and thus inactivates the herbicide. The gene encoding for phosphinothricin acetyl transferase (***bar* gene**) was introduced in transgenic maize and oil seed rape to provide resistance against phosphinothricin.

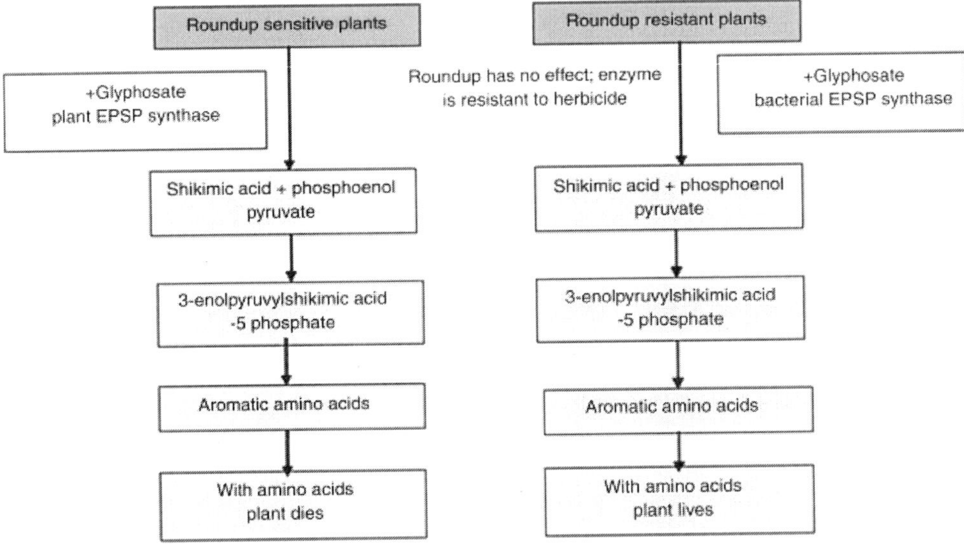

Figure 25.2. Glyphosate Resistant Mechanism in Transgenic Plant.

Biotic Stress Resistant Transgenic Plants

1. Insect resistance plants
2. Virus resistance plants
3. Fungal and bacterial disease resistance

Insect Resistance

A variety of insects, mites and nematodes significantly reduce the yield and quality of the crop plants. The conventional method is to use synthetic pesticides, which also have severe effects on human health and environment. The transgenic technology uses an innovative and eco-friendly method to improve pest control management. About 40 genes obtained from microorganisms of higher plants and animals have been used to provide insect resistance in crop plants. The first genes available for genetic engineering of crop plants for pest resistance were *cry* genes (popularly known as Bt genes) from a bacterium *Bacillus thuringiensis*. Transgenic crops with Bt genes (*e.g.* cotton, rice, maize, potato, tomato, brinjal, cauliflower, cabbage, *etc.*) have been developed. This has proved to be an effective way of controlling the insect pests and has reduced the pesticide use. The most notable example is **Bt cotton bollgard I (which contains *crylAc* gene**) that is resistant to a notorious insect pests belong to Lepidoptera *i.e.*, ***Helicoperpa armigera,***

Spodoptera litura etc. There are certain other insect resistant genes from other microorganisms which have been used for this purpose. ***Isopentenyl transferase*** gene from ***Agrobacterium tumefaciens*** has been introduced into tobacco and tomato. The transgenic plants with this transgene were found to reduce the leaf consumption by tobacco hornworm and decrease the survival of peach potato aphid.

Certain genes from higher plants were also found to result in the synthesis of products possessing insecticidal activity. One of the examples is the **Cowpea trypsin inhibitor gene** (CpTi) which was introduced into tobacco, potato, and oilseed rape for developing transgenic plants. Earlier it was observed that the wild species of cowpea plants growing in Africa were resistant to attack by a wide range of insects. It was observed that the insecticidal protein was a trypsin inhibitor that was capable of destroying insects belonging to the orders Lepidoptera, Orthaptera *etc.* Cowpea trypsin inhibitor (CpTi) has no effect on mammalian trypsin, hence it is non-toxic to mammals.

Table 25.1. Genes Conferring Insect Resistance to Plants from Various Sources

Sl.No.	*Gene/Protein*	*Source*	*Organism*
1	*Cry*/δ-endotoxin	*Bacillus thuringiensis*	Bacteria
2	*ipt*/Isopentyl transferase	*Agrobacterium tumefaciens*	Bacteria
3	Ph toxin	*Photorhabdus luminescens*	Bacteria
4	Cholesterol oxidase	*Streptomyces spp.*	Fungus
5	Proteinase inhibitors	*Nicotiana alata*	Plant
6	*CpTI*/Cowpea trypsin inhibitor	*Vigna unguiculata*	Plant
7	α-Amylase inhibitor	*Phaseolus vulgaris*	Plant
8	Lectins	*Galanthus nivalis*	Plant
9	Bovine pancreatic trypsin inhibitor	*Bos taurus*	Animal

Bt ToGin gene – Bacterial Insecticidal Gene

Bacillus thuringiensis (*Bt*) is an insect killing bacterium that produces and insect control protein. Bt was first discovered by **Ishiwata in 1901 from diseased silkworms**, and was subsequently classified and named by Berliner. The *cry* genes from Bt, code for the crystal proteins **(δ-endotoxin)which forms crystalline inclusion in the bacteria during sporulation**. These crystal proteins are responsible for the insecticidal activities of this bacterium. The crystal proteins are converted to active form upon ingestion by insect, thereby killing the insect by disruption of ion transport across the gut membranes of insect. The *cry* genes [or Cry proteins] have far been grouped into 16 groups, which either code for a 130 kDa protein or a 70 kDa protein. These proteins are solublized in the **alkaline environment of insect midgut** and are then proteolytically processed to yield a 60 kDa toxic core fragment.

Table 25.2. The Crystal Proteins have a Specific Activity Spectrum to the Insect Orders

Cry Protein Class	*Insect Order*
Cry1	Lepidoptera
Cry2	Lepidoptera and Diptera
Cry3	Coleoptera
Cry4	Diptera
Cry5	Coleoptera and Lepidoptera

Mode of Action of Cry Proteins

1. Ingestion of the Bt toxin protein by an insect larva;
2. Dissolving the Bt toxin protein in the insect midgut;

(A) Larvae ingest Bt spores and Cry proteins

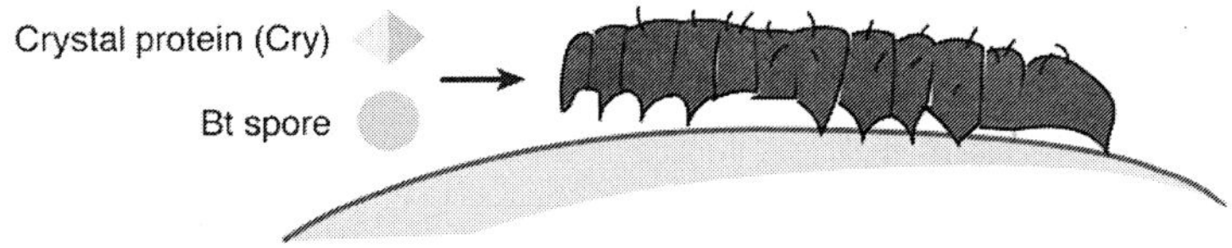

(B) In larval midgut, proteolytic digestion of proteins release Cry toxins, which bind to epithelial receptors

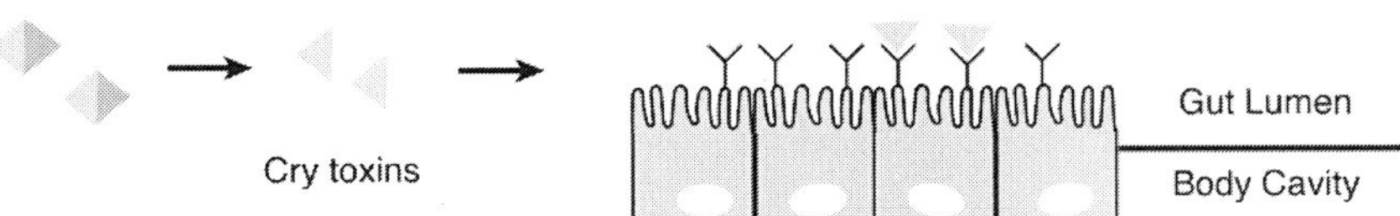

(C) Toxin binding causes cell lysis destroying barrier to body cavity

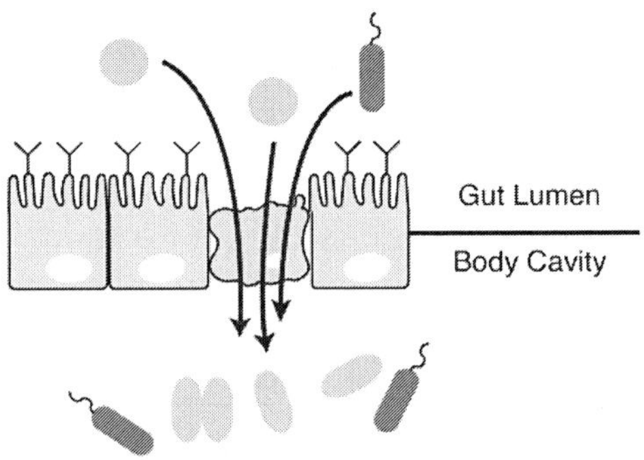

Figure 25.3. Mode of Action of Crystal Protein against Insects.

3. Activation of the Bt toxin protein by protease enzymes;
4. Binding of the activated protein to specific receptors on the cell membrane in the midgut;
5. Insertion of the protein into the cell membrane and formation of a pore into the body cavity;
6. Starvation, destruction of cell tissue and septicaemia and resultant death of the insect larvae (Figure 25.3).

Expression of Cry Genes in Plants (Bollgard II cotton)

Bollgard II cotton contains the genes encoding for the Cry1Ac and Cry2Ab proteins. This proteins possesses specific toxicity to certain species of Lepidoptera that includes *H. armigera* and *H. punctigera*. Control of *Pectinophora gossypii*, rough bollworm and some other Lepidoptera spp. has also been seen. Cry2Ab gene has been inserted into cotton already containing the cry1Ac gene (Bollgard cotton) to form Bollgard II cotton.

Table 25.3. Commercialized Bt Crops

Sl.No.	*Crop*	*Bt Protein*	*Trade Name*	*Resistant to the Insects and Pests*
1	Cotton	Cry 1 Ac	Bollgard	Tobacco budworm, Cotton bollworm and Pink bollworm
2	Cotton	Cry 1 Ac + Cry 2 Ab	Bollgard II	Tobacco budworm, Cotton bollworm and Pink bollworm
3	Cotton	Cry 1 Ac + Cry 1 Fa	Wide strike	Tobacco budworm, Cotton bollworm and Pink bollworm
4	Maize	Cry 1 Ab	Yieldgard	European Corn borer
5	Maize	Cry 1 Fa	Herculex 1	European Corn borer

Insect Resistance to Cry Proteins

There are some reports on development of resistance in some insects to Cry proteins. For example, *Plodia interpunctella* and *Cadra cautella* were selected by continuous exposure to high levels of *B. thuringiensis.* There was a >250-folds increase in resistance in *P. interpunctella* after 36 generations, and a seven fold increase in *C. cautella* after 21 generations. The problem of development of insect resistance to Cry proteins may be managed by (i) combining or (ii) alternating two or more kinds of these proteins, and by (iii) reducing the selection pressure on insects by limiting cry gene expression to only the economically important plant parts.

Virus Resistance

There are several strategies for engineering plants for viral resistance, and these utilizes the genes from virus itself (*e.g.* the viral coat protein gene). The virus-derived resistance has given promising results in a number of crop plants such as tobacco, tomato, potato, alfalfa, and papaya. The induction of virus resistance is done by employing virus-encoded genes-virus coat proteins, movement proteins, transmission proteins, satellite RNA, antisense RNAs, and ribozymes. The virus coat protein-mediated approach is the most successful one to provide virus resistance to plants. **It was in 1986, transgenic tobacco plants expressing tobacco mosaic virus (TMV) coat protein gene were first developed**. These plants exhibited high levels of resistance to TMV. The transgenic plant providing coat protein-mediated resistance to virus are rice, potato, peanut, sugar beet, alfalfa *etc.* The viruses that have been used include alfalfa mosaic virus (AlMV), cucumber mosaic virus (CMV), potato virus X (PVX), potato virus Y (PVY) *etc.*

Resistance against Fungal and Bacterial Infections

As a defense strategy against the invading pathogens (fungi and bacteria) the plants accumulate low molecular weight proteins which are collectively known as **pathogenesis-related (PR) proteins.** Several transgenic crop plants with increased resistance to fungal pathogens are being raised with genes coding for the different compounds. One of the examples is the **Glucanase enzyme that degrades the cell wall of many fungi**. The most widely used glucanase is **beta-1,4-glucanase.** The gene encoding for beta-1,4 glucanase has been isolated from barley, introduced, and expressed in transgenic tobacco plants. This gene provided good protection against soil-borne fungal pathogen *Rhizoctonia solani*. Lysozyme degrades chitin and peptidoglycan of cell wall, and in this way fungal infection can be reduced. **Transgenic potato plants with lysozyme gene providing resistance to *Erwinia carotovora*** have been developed.

Development of Virus Resistant Plants

Several approaches have been used to engineered plants for virus resistance, which are as follows:

I. Pathogen Derived Resistance (PDR) Approach

Pathogen genomic sequences are engineered into the host plant's genome. The pathogen genes like coat protein encoding gene, viral replication related genes, movement protein encoding genes *etc.*,may be expressed in the plant. So the plant can able to produce some form of resistance by inhibition the virus multiplication during the infection cycle.

Out of these strategies, use of **coat protein** mediated cross protection has been the most successful. PDR approach is based on the viral cross protection in plants. It is known as an acquired immunity phenomenon, where a mild virus isolate/strain can protect plants against economic damage caused by a severe challenge strain/isolate of the same virus. Most likely the resistance generated by CP is due to the blocking of the process of uncoating of virus particles, which is necessary viral genome replication as well as expression. Transgenic plants having virus coat protein gene linked to a strong promoter have been produced in many crop plants, *e.g.*, tobacco, tomato, alfalfa, sugarbeet, potato *etc.* (Figure 25.4).

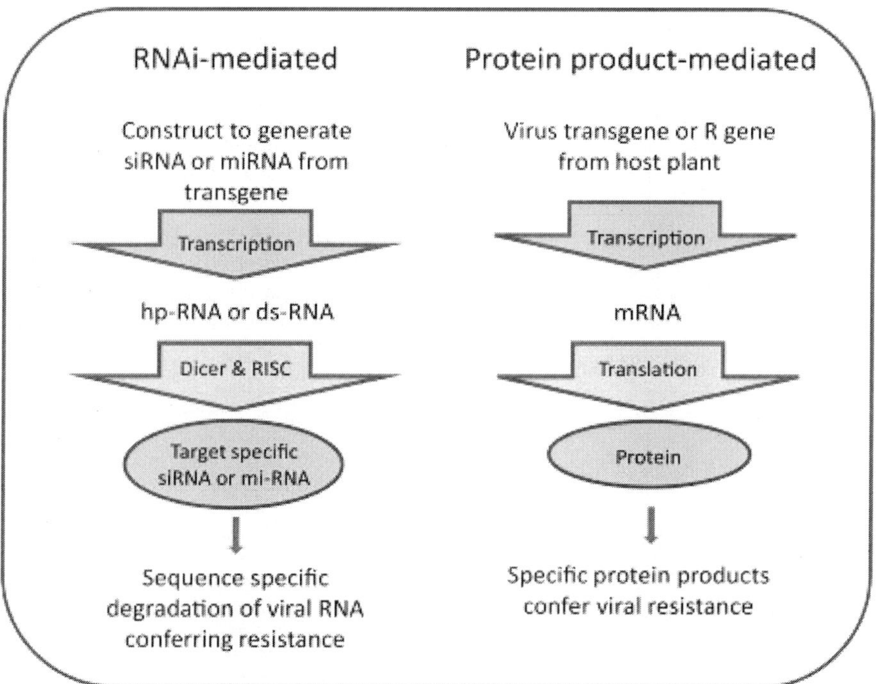

Figure 25.4. Ways of Virus Resistance Transgenic Crop Production.

The first transgenic plants of this type were tobacco produced in 1986; it contained the **coat protein gene of tobacco mosaic virus (TMV) strain U1.** When these plants were inoculated with TMV U1, symptoms either failed to develop or were considerably delayed. Further, there was much less accumulation of virus than in the control plants in both inoculated and systemically infected leaves. In addition, these plants showed delayed expression of disease symptoms when inoculated with the related tomato mosaic virus (ToMV) and with tobacco mild green mosaic virus (TMGMV). It appears to be a common feature that PDR approach not only confers resistance to the concerned virus but also gives a measure of resistance to related viruses.

Table 25.4. Commercialised Virus Resistant Crops by PDR Approach

Crop	*Commercial Cultivars*	*Viral Diseases Controlled*
Zucchini and Squash	Freedom III and Destiny III	Zuchini Yellow Mosaic Virus (ZYMV) and Cucumber Mosaic Virus (CMV)
Papaya	SunUp and Rainbow	Papaya Ring Spot Virus (PRSV)
Potato	NewLeaf	Potato Leaf Roll Virus (PLRV) and Potato Virus Y (PVY)

II. RNA Based Approaches

(1) Antisense RNA approach

(2) Ribozyme mediated resistance

1. *Antisense RNA Approach*

To bring an antisense-mediated resistance to viral disease in transgenic plants, sequences are designed that expresses negative-sense RNA molecule that will bind to the infecting viral RNA sequence and inhibit it to infect the plant. This method specifically interferes with viral replication (Figure 25.5).

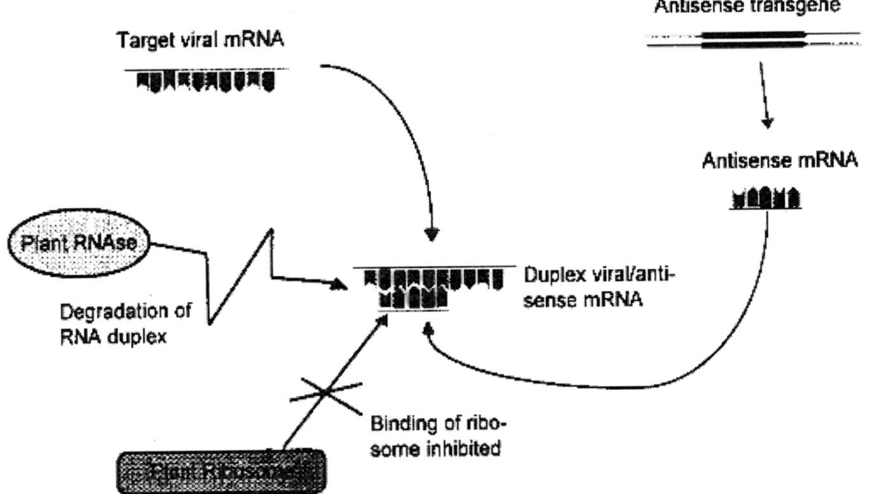

Figure 25.5. Virus Resistance Transgenic Crop Production through Antisense RNA Method.

2. *Ribozyme Mediated Resistance*

Ribozymes are antisense catalytic RNA molecules capable of cleaving the target sense viral RNA sequences. This method gives resistance by both blocking the replication and also by cutting the viral RNA.

Resistance to Bacterial and Fungal Diseases

In case of bacterial and fungal pathogens, resistance has been sought to be generated by expression of plant defense response genes which may include (i) Pathogenesis related proteins, (ii) Antimicrobial proteins (iii) phytoalexins (iv) Race-specific resistance genes (Pto gene against Tomato bacterial wilt (*Pseudomonas syringae*) and (v) HR and SAR inducing genes (NPR1 from *Arabidopsis thaliana*)

(i) Pathogenesis Related (PR) Proteins

They are low-molecular weight proteins, which accumulate to significant levels in infected plant tissues. **Major classes of PR proteins are β 1-3 glucanases, chitinases and ribosome inactivating proteins (RIPs).** β 1-3 glucanases and chitinases are hydrolytic enzymes which break chitin and glucan in the cell walls of the fungal pathogen. RIPs are enzymes that remove an adenine from ribosomal RNA of the pathogens, thus inhibiting their protein synthesis (*e.g.* Type I barley RIP).

(ii) Antimicrobial Proteins

They are proteins from plants, animals and microorganisms, which are not necessarily associated with induced defense response, but their presence exhibit resistance to pathogens. Some of the antimicrobial proteins are **Defensins (Alfalfa defensin), Lysozyme (T4 lysozyme), Thionins (barley α-thionin), Cecropin (Insect anti microbial protein), Temporin (European Red Frog)** *etc.*

(iii) Phytoalexins

They are anti-microbially active secondary metabolites synthesize by the plant in response to an infection, which contribute to the resistance of plants to diseases. During infection, the stored pytoalexins are mobilized. **Resveratrol is the most common phytoalexin**. The key enzyme in **resveratrol synthesis is resveratrol synthase or stilbene synthase**.

Table 25.5. Transgenic Plants Engineered for Enhanced Resistance against Biotic Stresses like Virus, Bacteria and Fungi

Sl.No.	*Transgenic Plant*	*Gene/Product*	*Resistance to*
1	Tomato	N gene	Tomato spotted wilt virus
2	Papaya	Coat protein (CP)	Papaya ringspot virus
3	Tobacco	Coat protein (CP)	Tobacco mosaic virus
4	Cucumber	Coat protein (CP)	Cucumber mosaic virus
5	Potato	*Sarco* gene coding for sarcotoxin IA	*Erwinia carotovora*
6	Apple	Attacin E gene(att E)	*Erwinia amylovora*
7	Cotton	N*PR1*	*Fusaium oxysporum* f.sp.
8	Tobacco	hrp N	*Botrytis cinerea*

Abiotic Stress Tolerance

Abiotic Stress Resistant Transgenic Plants

Plants respond to their changing environment in a complex, integrated way that allows them to react to the specific set of conditions and constraints present at a given time. Therefore, the genetic control of tolerance to abiotic stresses is not only very complex, but is also highly influenced by other environmental factors and by the developmental stage of the plant. Almost all the abiotic stresses such as drought, low temperature, salinity and alkalinity adversely influence growth and induce senescence, leading to cell death or reduced crop yield. Several abiotic stresses such as drought, salinity and extreme temperatures have a common consequence of causing cellular water deficit or osmotic stress.

Genetic Engineering Abiotic Stress Tolerant Plants

The strategies for genetic engineering abiotic stress tolerance can be broadly classified into two groups,

I. Genetic manipulation of genes involved in the stress responsive pathways
II. Genetic manipulation of genes involved in the production and accumulation of osmoprotectants

I. Genetic Manipulation of Genes involved in the Stress Responsive Pathways

The plant's response to abiotic stress is accompanied by the activation of genes involved in the perception of drought stress and in the transmission of the stress signal.

i. Abscisic Acid (ABA) Dependant Gene Regulation

Endogenous ABA levels in the plant greatly increase in response to water stress, resulting in the closure of stomata thereby reducing the level of water loss through transpiration from leaves and activate stress response genes. The reaction is reversible: once water becomes available again, the level of ABA drops, and stomata re-opens. The ABA regulates this process through some transcription factors known as **Abscisic acid Responsive Element Binding (AREB)** which activates **Abscissic acid Responsive Element (ARE)** present in the promoter of dehydration responsive genes. The ability to regulate ABA synthesis and response makes this hormone an excellent target for improving drought tolerance in crop species.

ERA1*, a gene identified in *Arabidopsis, encodes the β-subunit of a **farnesyl-transferase**, and is involved as a negative regulator of ABA signaling. So, plants lacking *ERA1* activity have increased tolerance to drought, however are also severely compromised in growth and yield. Genetic manipulation of ABA signaling, using a drought-inducible promoter to drive the antisense expression of *ERA1*, in both *Arabidopsis* and canola plants was done. Transgenic plants performed significantly better under water stress, with consistently higher yields over conventional varieties. Commonly used drought inducible promoters are *Oryza sativa Dehydrin 1* (*OsDhn1*) and Arabidopsis Responsive to dehydration 29a (*rd29a*) (Figure 25.6).

ii. ABA-Independent Gene Regulation to Drought Stress

The *DREB1* and *DREB2* are *Dehydration Responsive Element Binding* (DREB) transcription factors, which are important in the ABA-independent drought tolerant pathways that induce the expression of stress response genes. DREB induce the expression of drought responsive genes by binding to the ***Dehydration Responsive Element* (*DRE*)** present in the promoter of drought responsive genes. **Over-expression of the native form of *DREB1*, and of a constitutively active form of *DREB2*, increases the tolerance of transgenic *Arabidopsis* plants to drought, high salinity and cold.** Although these genes were initially identified in *Arabidopsis* plants, their presence and role in stress tolerance have been reported in many other important crops, such as rice, tomato, barley, canola, maize, soybean, rye, wheat and maize, indicating that this is a conserved, universal stress defense mechanism in plants. This functional conservation makes the *DREB* genes important targets for crop improvement for drought tolerance through genetic engineering. Scientists also developed cold-tolerant genes (around 20) in *Arabidopsis* when this plant was gradually exposed to slowly declining temperature. By introducing the coordinating gene (it encodes a protein which acts as transcription factor for regulating the expression of cold tolerant genes), expression of cold tolerant genes was triggered giving protection to the plants against the cold temperatures (Figure 25.6).

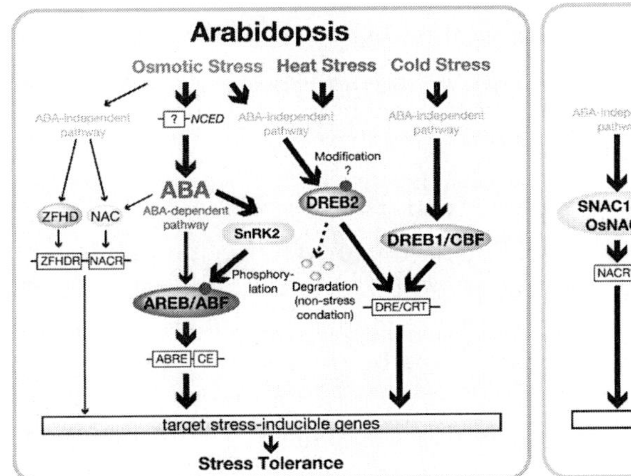

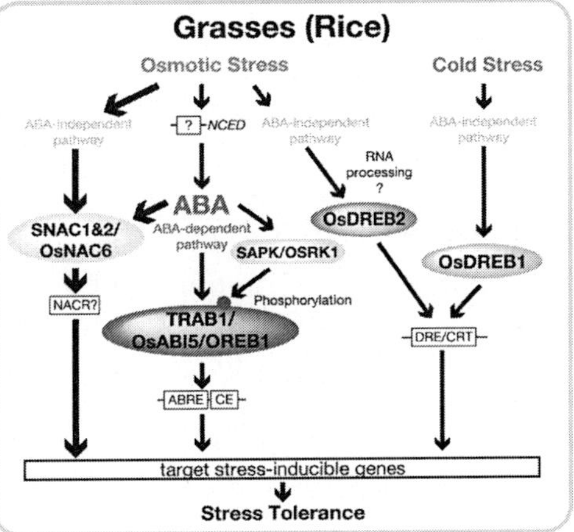

Figure 25.6. Drought Tolerant Transgenic Crop Production.

II. Genetic Manipulation of Genes Involved in the Production and Accumulation of Osmoprotectants

Resistance to abiotic stresses includes stress induced by temperature (heat, chilling, freezing), drought, salinity, and intense light. These environmental stresses result in the destruction, deterioration of crop plants which leads to low crop productivity. The plants show their abiotic stress response reactions by the **production of stress related osmolytes like sugars** (*e.g.* trehalose and fructans), **sugar alcohols** (*e.g.* mannitol), **amino acids** (*e.g.* proline, glycine betaine) and **certain proteins** (*e.g.* antifreeze proteins). These osmoprotectants with in cells lower the osmotic potential and helps maintain turgor. Compatible solutes form a diverse group of compounds, encompassing sugars, sugar alcohols, amino acid and quaternary ammonium compounds. Transgenic plants have been produced which over express the genes for one or more **osmoprotectants (*e.g.* trehalose, fructans, mannitol, proline, glycine betaine *etc.*)** show increased tolerance to environmental stresses. Several plant genes that encode key enzymes of osmoprotectant biosynthetic pathways have been cloned. The attempts are on to use genetic engineering strategies to increase the production of osmoprotectants in the plants.

Sugars (Trehalose)

Trehalose-6-phosphate synthase (*tps1*) from yeast is involved in the accumulation of treahalose sugars. *Tps1* was introduced into tobacco and potato. The transgenic plants showed tolerance to drought condition.

Sugar Alcohols (Mannitol)

An *E.coli* bacterial gene **mt1D (Mannitol-1-phosphate dehydrogenase)** involved in the biosynthesis of mannitol was introduced into tobacco and *Arabidopsis*. The transgenic plants were tested for salt resistance. After 30 days of exposure to salinity, transgenic plants producing mannitol had a greater shoot height and initiated new and longer roots, while those of the control plants turned brown and did not elongate or branch.

Amino Acid (Proline)

A strong correlation has been reported between proline accumulation with tolerance to drought and salinity stress conditions. **γ-Pyrroline-5-carboxylate synthetase (P5CS)** is the important enzyme in the synthesis of proline. Transgenic tobacco and rice plants were generated with **Mothbean P5CS enzyme** and they showed enhanced expression of this enzyme and 10-18 fold more proline. The increase in proline concentration correlated with enhanced growth under salt and drought conditions.

Quartenary Amino Compound (Gycine betaine)

The ability to synthesize and accumulate glycine betaine is widespread among angiosperms and contributes towards drought and salt tolerance. In plants, glycine betaine is synthesized by the two step oxidation of choline via the intermediate betaine aldehyde, the reaction being catalysed **by choline monooxygenase (CMO) and betaine aldehyde dehydrogenase (BADH).** A gene from ***Arthrobacter globiformis* known as Choline Oxidase (*codA*)** has shown more successful production and accumulation of betaine aldehyde in transgenic plants. Transgenic plants of ***Arabidopsis* with *CodA*** have shown increased tolerance to salt, chilling, freezing and heat. The choline oxidase gene from *Arthrobacter* sp. was used to produce transgenic rice with high levels of glycine betaine giving tolerance against water deficit stress.

The biosynthetic pathways for the production of many osmoprotectants have been established and genes coding the key enzymes have been isolated. *e.g.* Glycine betaine is a cellular osmolyte which is produced by the participation of a number of key enzymes like choline dehydrogenase, choline monooxygenase *etc.*

Table 25.6. Transgenics Produced for Various Abiotic Stresses

Plant	*Gene*	*Transgenic over Expressing*	*Claim*
Tobacco	Mannitol 1-phosphate dehydrogenase (mtlD) from *E.coli*	Mannitol	Tolerance to salinity
Arabidopsis	MtlD from *E.coli*	Mannitol	Tolerance to salinity
Tobacco	SacB from *Bacillus subtilis*	Fructan	Resistance to drought
Tobacco	TPS1 encoding trehalose synthase from Yeast	Trehalose	Tolerance to drought
Potato	TPS1 encoding trehalose synthase from Yeast	Trehalose	Tolerance to drought
Sugarbeet	sacB from *Bacillus subtilis*	Fructans	Tolerance to drought
Tobacco	Mothbean Pyrroline-5-carboxylate synthetase	Proline	Tolerance to salt
Rice	Mothbean Pyrroline-5-carboxylate synthetase	Proline	Tolerance to drought, salt, oxidative stress
Rice	Arginine decarboxylase	Polyamines	Tolerance to drought
Soybean	Mothbean Pyrroline-5-carboxylate synthetase	Proline	Tolerance to osmotic pressure, heat
Rice	Barley lea gene (HVAI)	LEA	Tolerance to water deficit and salinity
Rice	CodA from *Arthrobacter globiformis* encoding choline oxidase	Glycine betaine	Tolerance to salt and chilling
Rice	GS2	glutamine	Tolerance to salt and chilling
Arabidopsis	CodA from *Arthrobacter globiformis* encoding choline oxidase	Glycine betaine	Tolerance to salt, freezing, heat and chilling
Tobacco	9-desaturase (Des9) from *Anacystis nidulans*	Desaturase enzyme	Tolerance to cold
Tobacco	ω-3 fatty acid desaturase (Des9)	Desaturase enzyme	Chilling stress
Tobacco	o-3 fatty acid desaturase (Fad7)	Desaturase enzyme	Tolerance to cold
Tobacco	Cu/zn superoxide dismutase from rice	Scavenge toxic oxygen species	Oxidative and chilling stress
Tobacco	Mn-SOD from *N. plumbaginifolia*	Scavenge toxic oxygen species	Oxidative stress
Tobacco	Antifreeze protein (Afp) from winter flounder fish	Inhibits the formation of ice	Freezing stress
Maize	Hemoglobin (Hb) gene from barley	Promote glycolytic flux through NADH oxidation	Hypoxia stress and anoxia stress

Temperature Tolerant Plants

- High temperature stress tolerant transgenic Arabidopsis plants were produced by altering the level of **expression of heat shock proteins (HSPs)** by changing the expression levels of the ***Arabidopsis*** **heat shock protein transcription factor (AtHSF).**
- Transgenic carrot cell lines and plants with constitutive expression of carrot hsp 17.7 showed increased thermotolerance.
- Cold tolerant transgenic tobacco was produced by expression of *chloroplast* ω*-3 fatty acid desaturase.*

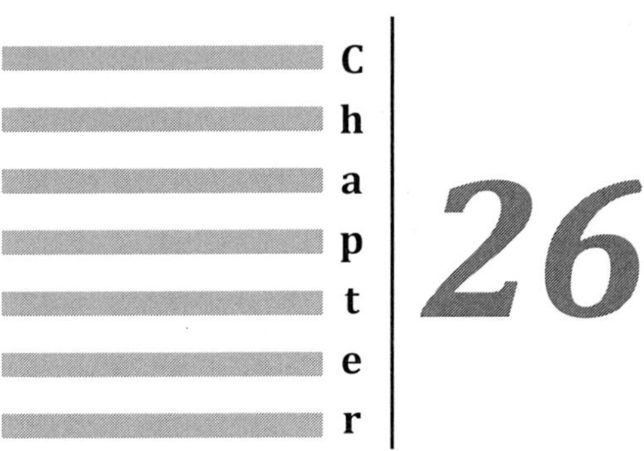

Transgenic Plants: Nutritional Enhancement and Traits for Improved Quality

Enhancement of Nutrition Quality

Modification of Seed Protein Quality

Pulses seed storage proteins are deficient in sulphur containing amino acids, *e.g.* methionine, and tryptophan. This limits their nutritional value for human since these amino acids are essential for human. A gene encoding a storage protein, which is rich in the deficient amino acids, is introduced into the crop to correct its amino acid deficiency. The transgene is linked to a seed-specific promoter to ensure its expression only in seeds. The pea is a rich source of protein which is free of anti-nutritional factors but it is a poor dietary source of the essential sulphur-containing amino acids (**methionine and cysteine**). A sunflower gene encoding a **seed albumin (*SFA8*), which contains 24 per cent methionine and cysteine, was modified for expression in pea.** A chimeric *SFA8* gene along with a pea seed specific **promoter (Vicillin (Vc))** was transferred to peas and was expressed in transgenic pea seeds. A number of transgenic pea lines showed a modest increase in **methionine and cysteine of 17 to 22 per cent** in seed storage proteins.

Metabolic Engineering

Golden Rice (Vitamin A)

Vitamin A content in the diet plays a major role in preventing disorders such as **color blindness.** Rice, which is the staple food for billions of people, does not contain any provitamin A (beta carotene) in the endosperm. Carotenoid biosynthesis begins with a small (C5) compound, isopentenyl-diphosphate (IPP). Chain elongation by C5 units leads to the formation of the C20-compound geranylgeranyl-diphosphate (GGPP), precursor of beta carotene. Upto this stage of carotenoid biosynthesis pathway present in the immature rice endosperm. The synthesis of beta carotene in rice endosperm from GGPP requires four more enzymes: **(i) phytoene synthase (ii) phytoene desaturase iii) (Zeta) ζ-carotene desaturase and (iv) lycopene cyclase** (Figure 26.1).

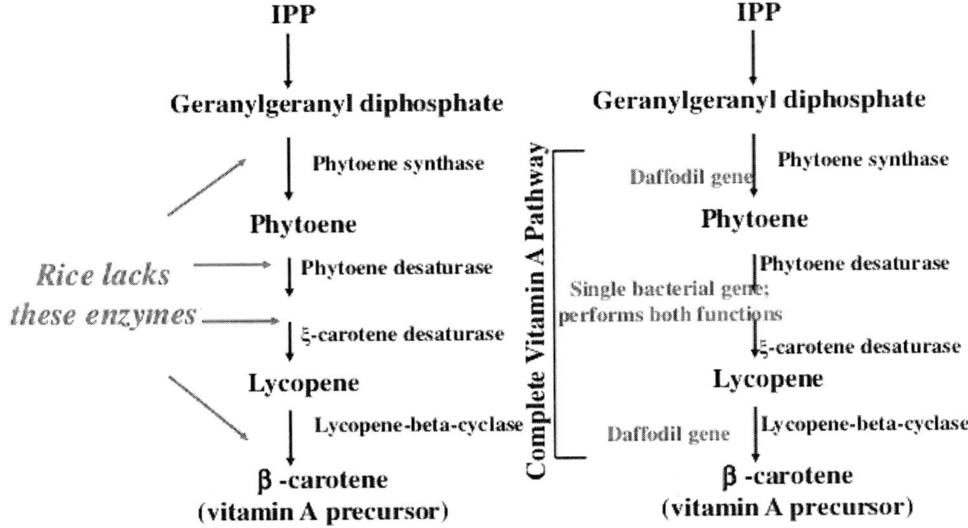

Figure 26.1. Pathway of Production of Provitamin A in Golden Rice.

Among four, the function of two enzymes i.e phytoene desaturase and (Zeta) ζ-carotene desaturase can be done by single enzyme carotene desaturase, so both the enzyme is replaced by carotene desaturase. These three genes phytoene synthase (phy) gene and lycopene cyclase (Lcy) originated from **daffodil (*Narcissus pseudonarcissus*),** carotene desaturase gene originating from ***Erwinia uredovora*** **were introduced into rice endosperm**. The resulting transgenic rice plants produced sufficient β-carotene which can be converted to vitamin A and the rice has been named as golden rice. A second generation of Golden Rice lines were produced, often referred to as Golden Rice 2, with a phytoene synthase gene from ***Zea mays*** **replacing the gene isolated from *Narcissus pseudonarcissus*. Golden Rice 2 contains approximately 20-fold more carotenoids than Golden Rice 1** (Figure 26.2).

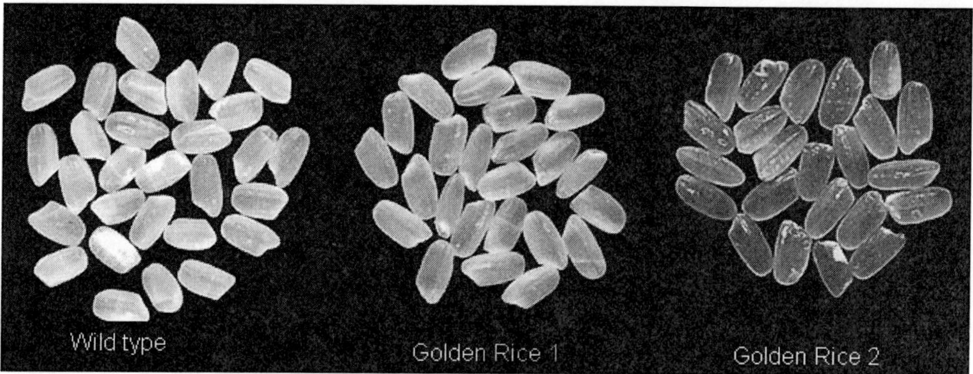

Figure 26.2. Variation of Normal Rice, Golden Rice 1 and 2.

High Iron Rice

Iron deficiency is the most widespread micronutrient deficiency world-wide. A major cause is the poor absorption of iron from cereal and legume-based diets **high in phytic acid**. An approach with introduction of three genes for increasing the amount of iron absorbed from rice-based meals was explored.

a. **Ferritin gene from *Phaseolus vulgaris* or *Glycine max***is introduced into rice grains, increasing their iron content up to two-fold.
b. To increase iron bioavailability, a **thermotolerant phytase from *Aspergillus fumigatus***is introduced into the rice endosperm. The phytase level in the grains increased about 130-fold, giving a phytase activity sufficient to completely degrade phytic acid in a simulated digestion experiment.
c. **Cysteine-rich metallothionein-like protein** (endogenous) is overexpressed, as cysteine peptides are considered a major enhancer of iron absorption.

Shelf Life Improvement

Delayed Fruit Ripening

Antisense RNA Approach

In any gene, the **DNA strand oriented as 3' →5' in relation to its promoter is transcribed**; this strand is called the antisense strand. The mRNA base sequence, therefore, is complementary to that of the antisense strand. The other DNA strand of the gene, called sense strand, is naturally complementary to the antisense strand of the gene. Therefore, the base sequence of sense strand of a gene is the same as that of the mRNA produced by it. Hence, the mRNA produced by a gene in normal orientation is also **known as sense RNA**.

An antisense gene is produced by inserting, *i.e.* reversing the orientation of, the protein encoding region of a gene in relation to its promoter. As a result, the natural sense strand of the gene becomes oriented in the 3' → 5' direction with reference to its promoter, and is transcribed (usual transcribing antisense strand is not transcribed now since its orientation is 5' →3'). The RNA produced by this gene has the same sequence as the antisense strand of the normal gene (except for T in DNA in the place of U in RNA), and is therefore **known as antisense RNA** (Figure 26.3).

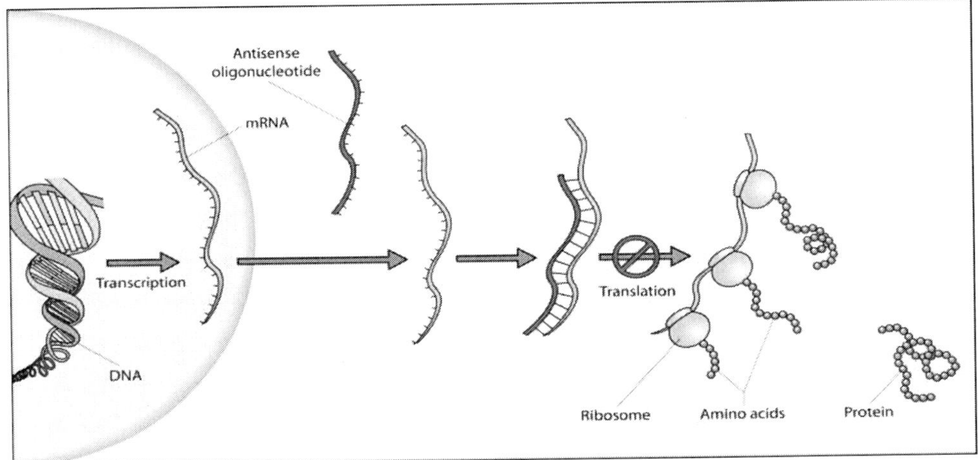

Figure 26.3. Antisence RNA Technology.

When an antisense gene is present in the same nucleus as the normal endogenous gene, transcription of the two genes yields antisense and sense RNA transcripts. Since the sense and the antisense RNAs are complementary to each other, they would pair to produce double-stranded RNA molecules. This event makes (1) the mRNA unavailable for translation. At the same time, (2) the RNA double-strand is attacked and degraded by double-stranded RNA specific RNases. Finally, (3) these events may somehow lead to the methylation of the promoter and coding regions of the normal gene resulting in silencing of the endogenous gene. For example in tomato plant, the PG gene (for the enzyme polygalacturonase) encodes a normal mRNA that produces the enzyme polygalacturonase which is involved in the fruit ripening. The complimentary DNA of PG encodes for antisense mRNA, which is complimentary to normal (sense) mRNA. The hybridization between the sense and antisnse mRNAs renders the sense mRNA ineffective. Consequently, polygalacturonase is not produced causing delay in the fruit ripening.

Shelf Life Improvement in Tomato

Shelf live improvement in fruits can be approached by manipulating the delayed softening and delayed ripening characteristics. **The most common example is the 'Flavr Savr' transgenic tomatoes, which were commercialized in U.S.A in 1994.**

1. Delayed Softening Character - Flavr Savr Tomato

The **softening** of the protein is largely the result of the cell wall degrading activity of the enzymes **polygalacturonase (PG) and Pectin Methylesterase (PME).** In tomato, polygalacturonase (PG) enzyme degrades pectin which is the major component of fruit cell wall. This leads to the softening of fruits and deterioration in fruit quality. The slow ripening tomato is an example of application of antisense RNA technology. Transgenic tomatoes have been produced, which **contain antisense construct of the gene encoding polygalacturonase (PG).** These transgenics show a drastically reduced expression of PG and markedly slower ripening and fruit softening. This has greatly improved the shelf-life and the general of tomato fruits. Such tomatoes were marketed in U.S.A. under the name **'FlavrSavr'.**

2. Delayed Ripening Character

The gas hormone, **ethylene regulates the ripening of fruits, therefore, ripening can be slowed down by blocking or reducing ethylene production.** This can be achieved by introducing ethylene forming gene(s) in a way that will suppress its own expression in the crop plant. Such fruits ripen very slowly (however, they can be ripen by ethylene application) and this helps in exporting the fruits to longer distances without spoilage due to longer-shelf life. The main strategy used was the antisense RNA approach. Similarly strategies have been developed to block the ethylene biosynthesis thereby reducing the fruit ripening. In these plants, production of ethylene was reduced by about 97 per cent with a significant delay in the fruit ripening.

Manipulation of Ethylene Biosynthesis

Ethylene is an important phytohormone and is involved in fruit ripening. It is produced from amino acid methionine. The reactions involved in ethylene biosynthesis are as follows (Figure 26.4).

Regulation of Ethylene Production

The amount of ethylene produced can be controlled primarily by "switching off" or decreasing the production of ethylene in the fruit and there are several ways to do this. They include:

a. **Suppression of *ACC synthase* gene expression.** ACC (1-amino-cyclopropane-1-carboxylic acid) synthase is the enzyme responsible for the conversion of S-adenosylmethionine (SAM) to ACC; the second to the last step in ethylene biosynthesis. Enzyme expression is hindered when an antisense ("mirror-image") or truncated copy of the synthase gene is inserted into the plant's genome.

b. **Suppression of *ACC oxidase* gene expression.** ACC oxidase is the enzyme which catalyzes the oxidation of ACC to ethylene, the last step in the ethylene biosynthetic pathway. Through anti-sense technology, down regulation of the ACC oxidase gene results in the suppression of ethylene production, thereby delaying fruit ripening.

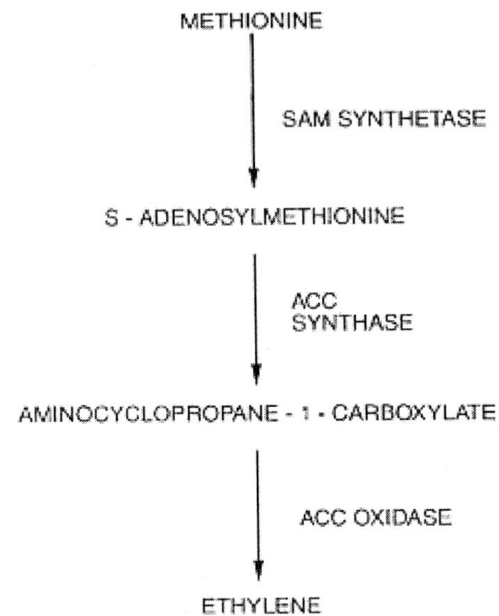

Figure 26.4. Ethylene Synthesis Pathway.

c. **Insertion of the *ACC deaminase* gene.** The gene coding for the enzyme is obtained from *Pseudomonas chlororaphis*, a common nonpathogenic soil bacterium. It converts ACC to a different compound thereby reducing the amount of ACC available for ethylene production.

d. **Insertion of the *SAM hydrolase* gene.** This approach is similar to ACC deaminase wherein ethylene production is hindered when the amount of its precursor metabolite is reduced; in this case SAM is converted to homoserine. The gene coding for the enzyme is obtained from *E. coli* T_3 bacteriophage.

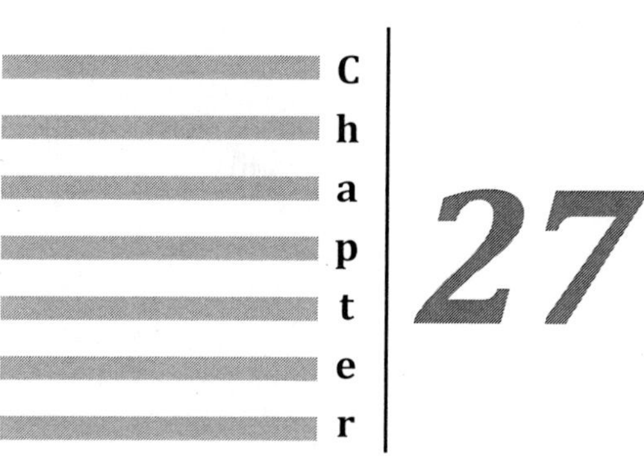

Detection of GMOs: Regulations and Biosafety

Detection of a GMO or a derivative of a GMO can be done by detecting a molecule (DNA, RNA or protein) that is specifically associated with or derived from the genetic modification of interest. The majority of the methods hitherto developed for detection of GMO and GMO-derivatives focus on detecting DNA, while only a few methods have been developed for detecting proteins or RNA. This has various reasons. DNA can be purified and multiplied in billions of copies in just a few hours with a technique called PCR (polymerase chain reaction). Multiplication of RNA and proteins is a more complicated and slow process. DNA is a very stable molecule, while RNA is unstable. The stability of a protein varies and depends on the type of protein. Finally, the genetic modification itself is done at the DNA level.

Protein based methods rely on a specific binding between the protein and an antibody, a molecule related to those protecting our own organism against infections from bacteria and virus. The antibody recognizes the foreign molecule, binds to it, and in GMO detection assays the bound complex is successively detected in a chromogenic (colour) reaction (ELISA). RNA based methods rely on specific binding between the RNA molecule and a synthetic RNA or DNA molecule (called a primer). The primer must be complementary to the nucleotide sequence at the start of the RNA molecule. The result is a double stranded molecule similar to DNA. Usually binding between the RNA molecule and the primer is followed by conversion of the RNA to a DNA molecule through a process called reverse transcription (RT-PCR).

Direct Assays

Detection of the Presence of Exogenous DNA

1. PCR (Polymer Chain Reaction)

The polymerase chain reaction (PCR) was developed by **Mullis and Faloona** in **1987**, and it is the main technique used in molecular biology laboratories to detect GMOs. The technique is based on the replication of specific sequences of exogenous DNA. For this purpose, small pieces of DNA known as primers bind to exogenous DNA present in the GMO, and during the PCR amplification process, which is catalyzed by the DNA polymerase enzyme, thousands copies of the specific sequence are produced. Copies of DNA produced by PCR are easily visualized by electrophoresis in agarose gels. A DNA intercalating agent (*e.g.* Ethidium bromide) is used for visualization of DNA bands present in the gel. If the same primers are used in a non-transgenic organism, the band will not displayed in an agarose gel, as there will be no detection of copies of exogenous DNA because it is not present in the wild or conventional organism.

2. Real-Time PCR

Real-time qPCR is used not only for the detection of specific DNA but also for the quantification of copy number of a particular target DNA sequence inserted in a GMO. The difference between conventional PCR and qPCR is the specificity and sensitivity of the latter method. In real-time qPCR, equipment capable of detecting the fluorescence emitted by the reaction during each cycle of amplification of the target DNA molecule is used. Then, it is possible to recognize the exact time (*i.e.*, cycle) at which the amplification of the target molecule can be detected.

3. Southern Blotting

The Southern blot technique, described by Southern in 1975, is also frequently used in laboratories to detect specific fragments of exogenous DNA integrated into the genomic DNA of a transgenic organism and its products. This technique essentially consists of five steps: 1) extraction and digestion of genomic DNA with one or more restriction enzymes 2) separation of DNA fragments by electrophoresis in an agarose gel 3) transfer and fixation of DNA present in the gel to a nitrocellulose or nylon membrane 4) hybridization of DNA present in the membrane against a DNA probe that has sequence homology to the target DNA 5) visualization by autoradiography or colorimetry. Southern blot analysis is very reliable and is considered molecular evidence of the integration of exogenous elements in a GMO genome. In addition, it is also possible to estimate the number of copies that were introduced into the genome of the recipient organism with this method.

Indirect Assays

Detection Based on the Presence of RNA

1. Northern Blotting

The northern blot technique, also referred to as an RNA blot and was developed to study gene expression through the detection of RNA molecules present in a sample. One of the most important steps in this technique is the extraction of total RNA from the sample because to obtain reliable results, it is necessary to obtain intact and pure RNA. Exercising care during the technique is much more critical than in Southern blotting because RNA degrades easily. To prevent its degradation, it is necessary to treat all objects with specific solutions to eliminate or minimize the presence of RNases, which are enzymes that are very effective in degrading RNA molecules.

2. RT-PCR

RT-PCR is widely used to verify gene expression by detecting mRNA molecules. This technique is based on reverse transcription of mRNA followed by PCR amplification. The reverse transcription reaction is based on the synthesis of complementary DNA (cDNA) from an mRNA molecule template by the reverse transcriptase enzyme. The product of this amplification is visualized in an agarose gel. The intensity of the bands visualized in the gel provides some indication of the amount of target mRNA present in the sample.

Detection Based on the Presence of Protein

Bioassays

The bioassay technique for the detection of GMOs is relatively simple, inexpensive and easy to establish in both laboratories and greenhouses, but a relatively long time is required to obtain results (the results are usually obtained after a week). Bioassays for herbicide tolerance can be conducted using a plant or even seeds. In case of plants, a dose of the herbicide is sprayed on the leaves. Then, the plants are monitored daily to verify the presence or absence of any phenotype (*i.e.*, symptoms) resulting from the application of the herbicide. The leaves of plants with no tolerance to the herbicide initially become yellow and then dry (*i.e.*, the tissue undergoes necrosis). The leaves of herbicide-tolerant plants exhibit no or few symptoms of necrosis, and the plants continue to look as healthy as before the herbicide application

Immunoassays

Immunoassays are ideal methods for the qualitative and/or quantitative detection of specific proteins produced from an exogenous DNA sequence introduced into a GMO.

a) ELISA

An ELISA identifies a target protein present in a protein extract containing a population of other proteins by using specific antibodies that bind to the target protein. The antigen antibody reaction identifies the presence of exogenous protein in a qualitative and even quantitative form. There are several types of ELISA, including direct ELISA, indirect ELISA, sandwich ELISA and competitive ELISA.

b) Western Blotting

The western blot technique is based on the separation of proteins present in the protein extract from a sample in non-denaturing polyacrylamide gels and subsequent transfer to nitrocellulose or nylon membranes. Detection of the target protein is performed by means of specific antibodies that recognize epitopes of the protein of interest. Visualization of the assay occurs through a colorimetric reaction or radiographic detection.

Regulatory Mechanism

India has a well-defined regulatory mechanism for development and evaluation of GMOs and the products thereof. **The Department of Biotechnology (DBT) and the Ministry of Environment and Forests (MoEF) are the two apex regulatory bodies. Rules have been notified by MoEF in 1989 under Environmental Protection Act, 1986 (EPA),** as the production and preservation of the environment is vested upon the government. These rules cover procedures for the manufacture, import, use, research and release of GMOs as well as products made by the use of such organisms. The objective of the rule is to ensure that the use of such products or life forms is safe to the environment and beneficial to the human beings. The competent authorities and their composition for dealing with all aspects of GMOs and products thereof has also been defined.

Guidelines for safety have been issued by the Department of Biotechnology (DBT) in 1990 covering research in biotechnology, field trials and commercial applications. DBT had also brought out separate guidelines for research in transgenic plants in 1998 and for clinical products in 1999. Activities involving GMOs are also covered under other policies such as the Drugs and Cosmetics Act (8th Amendment), 1988, the Drug Policy, 2002, and the National Seed Policy, 2002.

Presently, there are six competent authorities for implementation of regulations and guidelines in the country:

1. rDNA Advisory Committee (RDAC)
2. Institutional Biosafety Committee (IBSC)
3. Review Committee on Genetic Manipulation (RCGM)
4. Genetic Engineering Appraisal Committee (GEAC)
5. State Biotechnology Coordination committee (SBCC)
6. District Level Committee (DLC)

While the RDAC is advisory in function, the IBSC, RCGM, and GEAC are responsible for regulating function. SBCC and DLC are for monitoring purposes. The role of each of the committees is summarized in detailed below (Figure 27.1).

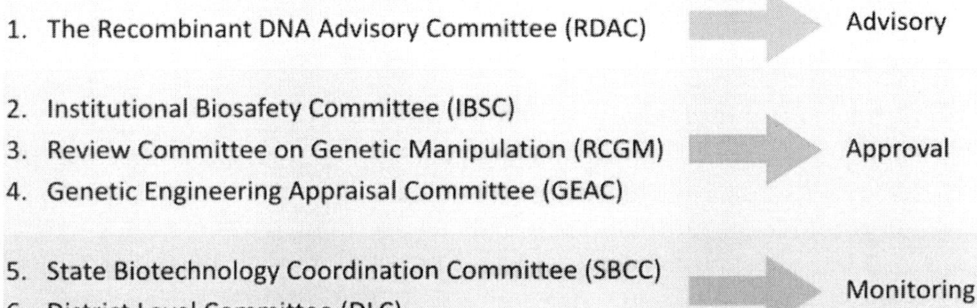

Figure 27.1. Regulatory Organization for GMO in India.

(i) Recombinant DNA Advisory Committee (RDAC)

This committee constituted by the DBT takes note of developments in biotechnology at national and international levels. The RDAC is advisory in nature and expected to give recommendations from time to time on safety regulations in research and applications of GMOs and products thereof. This Committee prepared the Recombinant DNA Biosafety Guidelines in 1990, which were adopted by the Government for conducting research and handling of GMOs in India.

(ii) Institutional Biosafety Committee (IBSC)

It is necessary that each institution intending to carry out research activities involving genetic manipulation of microorganisms, plants or animals should constitute the IBSC. The IBSCs comprise of the head of the organization, three or more scientists engaged in DNA work, a medical expert and a nominee of the DBT. Responsible for ensuring adherence to rDNA safety guidelines, experimentations carried out at designed locations as per approved protocols and prepare onsite emergency plans according to manuals/guidelines of RGCM. The IBSC is the nodal point for interfacing with other regulatory bodies regarding ongoing research within the institution and implementation of the guidelines. Review experiments falling risk category III or above and recommended to RCGM.

(iii) Review Committee on Genetic Manipulation (RCGM)

The RCGM functions as a body under the DBT to monitor the safety related aspects in respect of on-going research projects and activities involving GE organisms/hazardous microorganisms. RCGM is also mandated to bring out manuals of guidelines specifying procedure for regulatory process with respect to activities involving GE organisms in research, use and applications with a view to ensure environmental safety and lay down procedures restricting or prohibiting production, sale, import and use of GMO. The RCGM includes representatives of scientific departments/organizations in the country *viz.* Indian Council of Medical Research (ICMR), Indian Council of Agricultural Research (ICAR), Council of Scientific and Industrial Research (CSIR) and other experts multi-disciplinary fields in their individual capacity.

(iv) Genetic Engineering Appraisal Committee (GEAC)

GEAC is the apex committee functioning in MoEFCC and has representatives from concerned ministries/agencies and experts. GEAC is chaired by a Special Secretary/Additional Secretary of MoEFCC and co-chaired by expert nominated by DBT. GEAC is responsible for approval of activities involving large scale use of hazardous microorganisms and recombinant products in research and industrial production from the environment angle.

(v) State Biotechnology Coordination Committee (SBCC)

SBCC is constituted in each State where research and applications of GMOs are underway. SBCC is headed by the Chief Secretary of the State and comprises of Secretaries from the State Department of Environment and Forest, State Department of Health, State Department of Agriculture, State Department of Industries and Commerce, State Department of Public works, Chairman, State Pollution Control Board, Expert in the field of Microbiology and Pathology as Members. The committee may co-opt other Experts/Members as necessary. Empowered to inspect, investigate and to take punitive action in case of violations of statutory provisions through the Nodal Department and the State Pollution Control Board (SPCB) or the Directorate of Health/Medical Services. Authorized to review periodically the safety and control measures in various industries/institutions handling Genetically Engineered/hazardous organisms. Serve as a nodal agency at the State level for coordinating activities related to GMOs in the State with the Central Ministers including monitoring of conditions stipulated by the RCGM/GEAC.

(vi) District Level Committee (DLC)

DLC is a Regulatory Committee set up in each District where research and applications of GMOs are contemplated. Each DLC is headed by the District Collector of the District and comprises of Factory Inspector, Representative of State Pollution Control Board, Chief Medical Officer, District Agricultural Officer, Representative of Public Health, Engineering Department, Commissioner, Municipal Corporation and Technical Experts in the field of Microbiology and Pathology as Member. The committee may co-opt other Experts/Members as necessary. Authorized to monitor and inspect the safety regulations in installation engaged in the use of GMOs/ hazardous microorganisms and its applications, formulate information chart, identify hazards and risk associated with each of these installation and coordinate activities with a view to meeting emergency. Serve as a nodal point at district level for coordinating activities related to GMOs in the District with the SBCC and GEAC including monitoring of conditions stipulated by the RCGM/GEAC

Biosafety

Approvals and Prohibitions

Rules, 1989 provide for compliance of the biosafety safeguards and any violation and non-compliance in this area attracts punitive actions provided under the EPA, 1986. The approvals and prohibitions under Rules 1989 are summarized below:

- No person shall import, export, transport,
- manufacture, process, use or sell any GMOs,
- substances or cells except with the approval of
- the GEAC.
- Use of pathogenic organisms or GMOs or cells
- for research purpose shall only be allowed in
- laboratories or inside laboratory areas notified for
- this purpose under the EPA, 1986.
- Any person operating or using GMOs for scale up
- or pilot operations shall have to obtain permission
- from GEAC.
- Experiments for the purpose of education involving
- GMOs can be undertaken with the oversight
- of IBSCs.
- Deliberate or unintentional release of GMOs
- not allowed.
- Production in which GMOs are generated or used
- shall not be commenced except with the approval of
- GEAC All approvals shall be for a period of 4 years at first instance renewable for 2 years at a time
- GEAC shall have powers to revoke approvals in case of:
    i. Any new information on harmful effects of GMOs.
    ii. GMOs cause such damage to the environment as could not be envisaged when approval was given.
    iii. Non-compliance of any conditions stipulated by GEAC.

Biosafety and Bioethics

Biosafety refers the policies and procedures adopted to ensure the environmentally safe and responsible application of biotechnology. Biosafety competence is considered as paramount importance even for technologically less developed countries and one of the top concerns of countries world over.

Biotech products are being introduced in a growing number of developing countries plus a range of products are expected from national and international programs *e.g.* transgenic plants, recombinant livestock vaccines *etc.*, that require biosafety reviews.

Three important Biosafety-Related Needs are

1. Develop biosafety guidelines
2. Establish a responsive national system
3. Increase capabilities to perform risk analysis of GMOs

Biosafety Risks and Concerns

There is no evidence that unique hazards exist either in the use or rDNA techniques or in the transfer of genes between unrelated organisms. It is not true that all GMOs are toxic or are likely to proliferate in the environment. However, specific GMOs may be harmful by virtue of the novel combinations of traits they possess. This means that the concerns associated with use of GMOs can differ greatly, depending on the particular gene-organism combination and therefore, a case-by-case approach is required for assessment of safety concerns.

Downstream from the laboratory, the GMOs have found applications in agriculture and healthcare industry, often claiming better value and quality of the products. However, there are some key differences between the two sectors. Healthcare is a highly regulated domain and the products address often life threatening situations in a context where risk and benefits must be balanced. All the key players including the medical practitioner, drug industry and the regulatory authority are often equipped with the latest knowledge.

Further, transgenic plants and animals are exposed to the open environment and the interaction takes place with other organisms in the field. Therefore, genetic modification in agriculture has become a more sensitive issue than advances in healthcare.

Risk to Human Health

Risks of GMOs to human health are related mainly to toxicity, allergenicity and antibiotic resistance of the new organisms/products.

Risk of toxicity: The risk of toxicity may be directly related to the nature of the product whose synthesis is controlled by the transgene or the changes in the metabolism and the composition of the organisms resulting from gene transfer.

Risk of allergies: Production of GMOs sometimes includes the introduction of newer proteins from the organisms which have not been consumed as foods. There is a risk of such proteins becoming allergens since virtually all known food allergens are proteins.

Antibiotic resistance: Production of GMOs generally involves use of genes for antibiotic resistance as selectable markers. Early in the modification process in the laboratory, these markers help in selecting cells that have taken up foreign genes. The use of these antibiotic resistance markers has raised the concerns that eating foods carrying antibiotic resistance marker would reduce the effectiveness of antibiotic to fight disease than these antibiotics are taken with meals.

Eating foreign DNA: There have been apprehensions about danger from eating the foreign DNA in GM foods *i.e.* the pieces of DNA that did not originally occur in that food plant. DNA being present in all living things such as plants, animals, microorganisms is eaten by human beings with every meal.

Changes in nutritional level: There have been concerns about the accidental changes in the nutritional components of transgenic crops while incorporating other traits.

Influence of GMOs on Environments

The gene transferred into an organism or the resultant products can actually remain in environmental leading to environmental problems. The intentional release of GMOs into the environment has led to an increased interest in possible interactions that may occur between other organisms in the environment. Unintended genomic changes can occur as a secondary consequence of genetic modification. Such changes can lead to production of new proteins that may be toxic or allergenic or may disrupt or alter metabolic pathways that play a role in making the GMO successful.

Gene Flow

Accidental cross breeding between GMO plants and traditional varieties through pollen transfer can contaminate the traditional local varieties with GMO genes resulting in the loss of traditional varieties of the farmers.

Resistance/Tolerance of Target Organisms

The potential benefits of planting insect-resistant transgenic crops include decreased insecticide use and reduced crop damage. However, the innate ability of insect populations to rapidly adapt to environmental pressures poses a serious threat to the long-term efficacy of insect-resistance. Adaptation by insects and other pests to pest protection mechanisms can have environmental and health impacts.

Increased Weediness

Weediness means the tendency of the plant to spread beyond the field where it was first planted. There are apprehensions about GM crops becoming weeds. For example, a salt tolerant GM crop if escapes into marine areas could become a potent weed there.

There is also fear about the development of superweeds *i.e.* a weed that has acquired the herbicide tolerant gene due to genetic contamination with a herbicide tolerance GMO through in field cross breeding to related species or through horizontal gene transfer.

Loss of Biodiversity/Reduction of Cultivars

There have been concerns about reduction in the genetic diversity in cropping systems by the development and global spread of improved crop varieties to the green revolution. This genetic erosion has occurred as the farmers have replaced the use of traditional varieties with monocultures. This is expected to further intensify as more and more transgenic crops are introduced which bring in considerable economic benefits to the farmers. The relative rate of susceptibility to any unforeseen infections or destructive situations increases when single varieties are used in cropping system in place of multiple varieties.

Changes in the Soil Ecology

Many plants leak chemical compounds into the soil through their roots. There are concerns that transgenic plants may leak different compounds than conventional plants, as and unintended sequence of their changed DNA. Speculations are that this may change the ecology of the soil in terms of functional composition and biodiversity. The interaction between plants and solid microorganisms is very complex, with the microorganisms living around plant roots also secreting chemical compounds into the soil.

Status of GEAC Approvals

A. Commercial Release of Transgenic Crops

Bt cotton is the only transgenic crop approved for commercial cultivation in India, produced genetic engineering techniques for control of bollworms the major pest thereby reducing the risk of crop failures and use of pesticides. The GEAC approved introduction of Bt cotton in 2002 in the nine cotton growing states namely Andhra Pradesh, Gujarat, Haryana, Karnataka, Madhya Pradesh, Maharashtra, Punjab, Rajasthan and Tamil Nadu after extensive biosafety and agronomic testing.

As of date the GEAC has approved Bt cotton hybrids expressing Cry 1 Ac gene (MON 531 event) and stacked genes Cry1 Ac and Cry 2Ab (MON 15985 event) BG-II developed by M/s Mahyco, encoding fusion genes (cry 1Ab+Cry Ac) GFM developed by M/s Nath Seeds and cry 1Ac gene (Event-1) developed by M/s J. K. Agrigenetics Ltd during 2002 to 2007.

In addition the GEAC also approved the commercial release of BN Bt (variety) developed by **CICR, Nagpur**. For the first time Bt technology has been introduced in a **varietal background** whereby the farmers can save seeds.

B. Status of Approval of GM Food Crops in India

The large scale field trials of Bt brinjal developed by M/s Mahyco expressing *cry 1Ac* gene from *Bacillus thuringiensis* tolerant to the fruit and shoot borer is under progress at 11 locations within the research farms of Indian Institute of Vegetable Research(IIVR)/State Agricultural Universities/Indian Council of Agriculture Research. The trials are being conducted under the supervision of Director IIVR, Varanasi.

Table 27.1. List of Genetic Engineering Plants Approved for Confined Trails in India

Plant	Trait	Organization
Brinjal	Insect resistance	- Indian Agricultural Research Institute - Maharashtra Hybrid Seeds Company Limited (MAHYCO) - Bejo Sheetal Seeds
Cabbage	Insect resistance	- Sungro Seeds
Castor	Insect resistance	- Indian Institute of Oilseeds Research
Cauliflower	Insect resistance	- Sungro Seeds
Chickpea	Abiotic stress tolerance, insect resistance	- Indian Institute of Pulses Research - International Crops Research Institute for the Semi-Arid Tropics (ICRISAT) - MAHYCO
Corn	Insect resistance, herbicide tolerance	- Monsanto - Pioneer - Dow Agrosciences
Cotton	Insect resistance, herbicide tolerance	- Central Institute of Cotton Research - MAHYCO - Dow Agrosciences
Groundnut	Virus resistance, abiotic stress tolerance	- ICRISAT
Mustard	Hybrid seed production	- University of Delhi South Campus
Okra	Insect resistance	- MAHYCO
Papaya	Virus resistance	- Indian Institute of Horticultural Research
Pigeon pea	Insect resistance	- Indian Institute of Pulses Research - MAHYCO
Potato	Tuber sweetening, fungal resistance	- Central Potato Research Institute
Rice	Insect resistance, diseases resistance, hybrid seed production, nutritional enhancement	- Indian Agricultural Research Institute - Tamil Nadu Agricultural University - Bayer Bioscience - MAHYCO - BASF India Ltd.
Rubber	Abiotic stress tolerance	- Rubber Research Institute of India
Sorghum	Insect resistance, abiotic stress tolerance	- Indian Institute of Millets Research
Sugarcane	Insect resistance	- Sugarcane Breeding Institute
Tomato	Insect resistance, virus resistance, fruit ripening	- Indian Institute of Vegetable Research - National Research Centre on Plant Biotechnology - MAHYCO
Watermelon	Virus resistance	- Indian Institute of Horticultural Research
Wheat	Effect of mutant strains Azotobacter	- National Research Centre on Plant Biotechnology

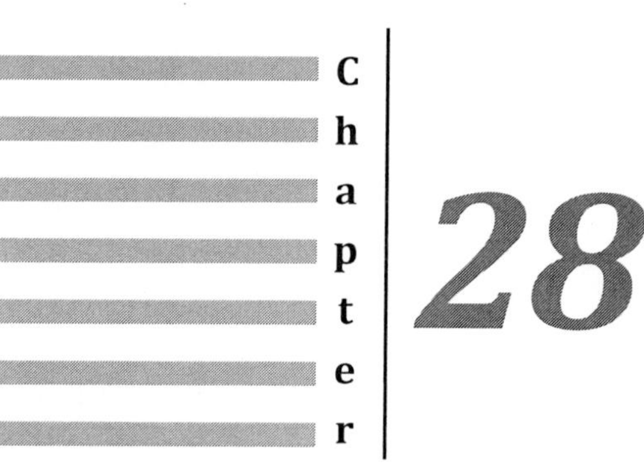

DNA Markers-Hybridization Based Markers (RFLP) and PCR Based Markers: RAPD, SSR, AFLP and SNPs

A molecular marker is defined as a particular segment of DNA that is representative of the differences at the genome level. They may or may not correlate with phenotypic expression of a trait. Molecular markers offer numerous advantages over conventional phenotype-based alternatives as they are stable and detectable in all tissues regardless of growth, differentiation, development, or defense status of the cell. Further, these are not confounded by the environment, pleiotropic and epistatic effects. Due to the rapid developments in the field of molecular genetics, a variety of techniques have emerged to analyze genetic variation during the last few decades. These genetic markers may differ with respect to important features, such as genomic abundance, level of polymorphism detected, locus specificity, reproducibility, technical requirements, and financial investment. No marker is superior to all others for a wide range of applications. The most appropriate genetic marker depends on the specific application, the presumed level of polymorphism,the presence of sufficient technical facilities and know how, time constraints, and financial limitations.

An Ideal Molecular Marker Technique Should

(1) Be highly polymorphic and evenly distributed throughout the genome (2) provide adequate resolution of genetic differences (3) generate multiple,

independent and reliable markers (4)be simple, quick, and inexpensive (5) need small amounts of tissue and DNA samples (6) have linkage to distinct phenotypes (7) require no prior information about the genome of an organism.

Molecular Marker Techniques

A vast array of DNA-based genetic markers for the detection of DNA polymorphism have been discovered since 1980 and new marker types are developed every year. There are several DNA marker types, which may be classified broadly into two groups based on their detection method, (1) Non PCR based or those based on DNA–DNA hybridization and (2) PCR based or those based on amplification of DNA sequences using the polymerase chain reaction (PCR).

Non PCR Based or DNA–DNA Hybridization

1. Restriction Fragment Length Polymorphism

Restriction fragment length polymorphism markers were the first DNA-based genetic markers developed by **Botstein *et al.*, 1980**. Eukaryotic genomes are very large and there was no simple way to observe genetic polymorphisms of individual genes or sequences.

RFLP refers to a difference between two or more samples of homologous DNA molecules arising from differing locations of restriction sites. **If two organisms differ in the** distance between sites of cleavage of particular restriction endonucleases, the length of the fragments produced will differ when the DNA is **digested with a restriction enzyme.** The dissimilarity of the patterns generated can be used to differentiate species (and even strains) from one another.

In RFLP analysis, the DNA sample broken into pieces (digested) by restriction enzymes that are separated according to their lengths on agarose gel electrophoresis. It is possible to visualize DNA within such a gel by staining it with ethidium bromide, however, due to typically so many restriction fragments of all possible sizes, discrete fragments cannot be seen. To overcome this problem, the fractionated DNA is transferred and chemically bound to a nylon membrane by a process called Southern blotting, named after its inventor E. M. Southern (1975). Specific DNA fragments are visualized by hybridizing the DNA fragments bound to the nylon membrane with a radioactively or fluorescently labeled DNA probe. Different sizes or lengths of restriction fragments are typically produced when different individuals are tested. Such a polymorphism can be used to distinguish plant species, genotypes and, in some cases, individual plants. Labeling of the probe may be performed with a radioactive isotope or with alternative non-radioactive stains, such as digoxigenin or fluorescein. These probes are mostly species-specific single locus probes of about 0.5–3.0 kb in size, obtained from a cDNA library or a genomic library. Though genomic library probes may exhibit greater variability than probes from cDNA libraries, a few studies reveal the converse. In addition to genetic fingerprinting, RFLP is an important tool in genome mapping, localization of genes (Figure 28.1).

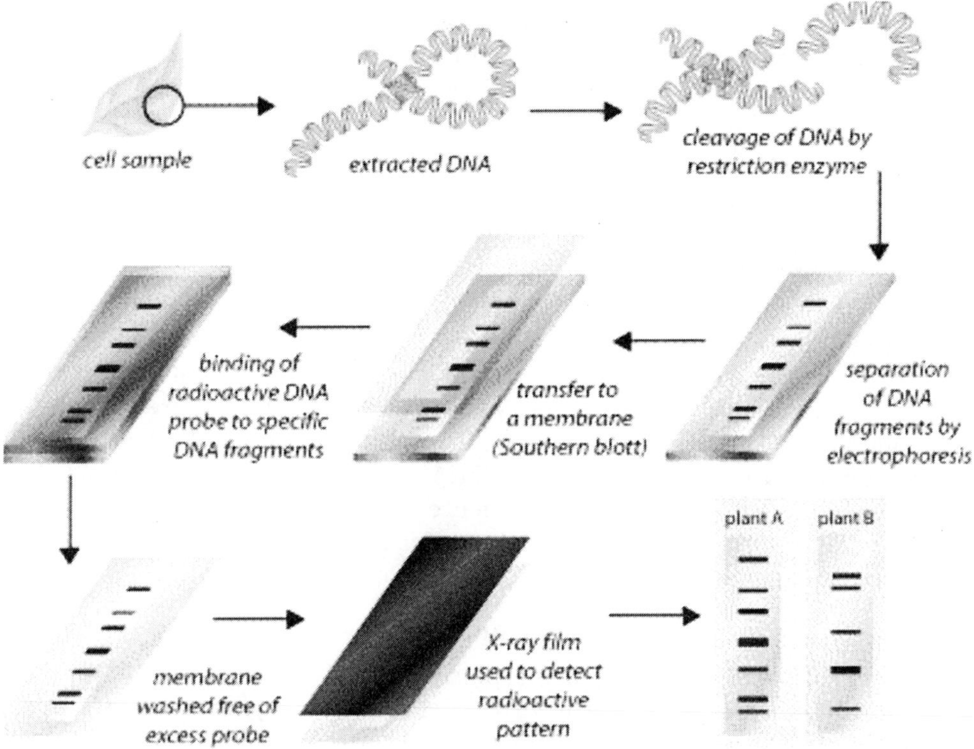

Figure 28.1. Restriction Fragment Length Polymorphism.

Applications

- ☆ Restriction Fragment length polymorphism is a powerful tool for the identification of organisms to the level of species, strains, varieties, or individuals.

Table 28.1. Advantage and Disadvantage of RFLP

Restriction fragment length polymorphism	Sequence information not required	Large amount of good quality DNA required
	High genomic abundance	
	Codominant markers	
	High reproducibility	Labour intensive (in comparison to RAPD)
	Can use filters many times	
	Good genome coverage	Difficult to automate
	Can be used across species	Need radioactive labeling
	Needed for map-based cloning	Cloning and characterization of probe are required

- ☆ RFLPs have been widely used in population genetics to determine slight differences within populations, and in linkage studies to generate maps for quantitative trait locus (QTL) analysis.
- ☆ They also have been used to investigate relationships of closely related taxa or intraspecific level, as fingerprinting tools for diversity studies, and for studies of hybridization.

PCR-Based Marker

After the invention of polymerase chain reaction (PCR) technology, a large number of approaches for generation of molecular markers based on PCR were detailed, primarily due to its apparent simplicity and high probability of success. Before PCR, the analysis of a specific DNA fragment generally required cloning of the fragment and amplification in a plasmid or compatible vector. PCR enables the production of a large amount of specific DNA sequence without cloning, starting with just a few molecules of the target sequence. Usage of random primers overcame the limitation of prior sequence knowledge for PCR analysis and facilitated the development of genetic markers for a variety of purposes.

Amplified Fragment Length Polymorphism (AFLP)

Amplified fragment length polymorphism is a PCR-based tool used in genetics research, DNA fingerprinting and in the practice of genetic engineering. **Developed by Vos *et al.* (1995)**, **AFLP** is essentially an intermediate between RFLP and **PCR**. AFLP selectively amplifies a subset of restriction fragments from a complex mixture of DNA fragments obtained after digestion of genomic DNA with restriction endonucleases. Polymorphisms are detected from differences in the length of the amplified fragments by polyacrylamide gel electrophoresis (PAGE) or by **capillary electrophoresis.** AFLP uses restriction enzymes to cut genomic DNA, followed by ligation of adaptors to the sticky ends of the restriction fragments. A subset of the restriction fragments are then amplified using primers complementary to the adaptor and part of the restriction site fragments. The amplified fragments are visualized on denaturing polyacrylamide gels either through autoradiography or fluorescence methodologies. AFLPs are DNA fragments (80–500 bp) obtained from digestion with restriction enzymes, followed by ligation of oligonucleotide adapters to the digestion products and selective amplification by the PCR. AFLPs, therefore, involve both RFLP and PCR. The AFLP banding profiles are the result of variations in the restriction sites or in the intervening region. The AFLP technique simultaneously generates fragments from many genomic sites (usually 50–100 fragments per reaction) that are separated by polyacrylamide gel electrophoresis and that are generally scored as dominant markers (Figure 28.2).

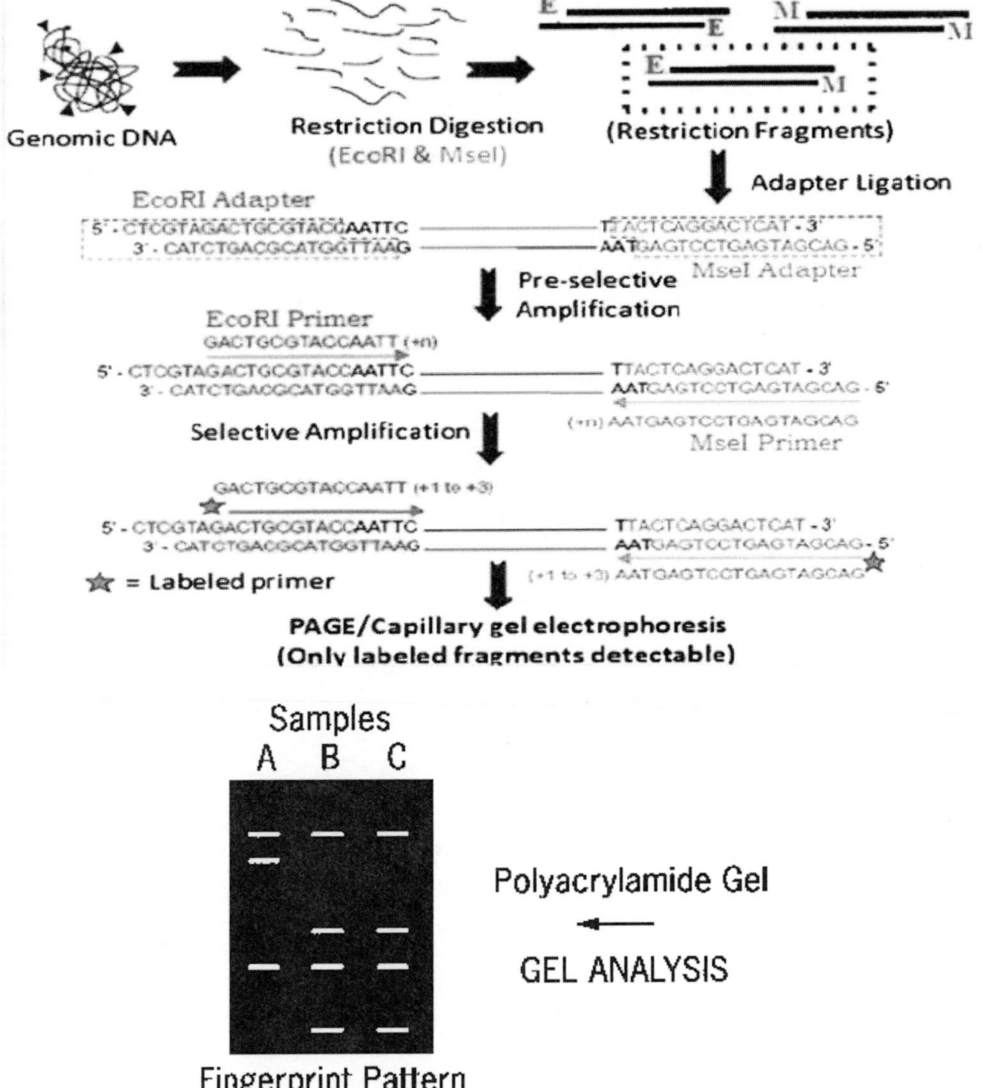

Figure 28.2. Amplified Fragment Length Polymorphism (AFLP).

Applications

- ☆ Most AFLP fragments correspond to unique positions on the genome and have the capability to detect various polymorphisms in different genomic regions simultaneously and hence can be exploited as land marks in genetic and physical mapping.
- ☆ The technique can be used to distinguish closely related individuals at the subspecies level and also for gene mapping.

- ☆ Applications for AFLP in plant mapping is assessing the degree of elatedness or variability among cultivars.
- ☆ AFLP is considered more applicable to intra specific than to inter specific studies due to frequent null alleles.
- ☆ AFLP markers are useful in genetic studies, such as biodiversity evaluation, analysis of germplasm collections, genotyping of individuals, and genetic distance analysis.
- ☆ The availability of many different restriction enzymes and corresponding primer combinations provides a great deal of flexibility, enabling the direct manipulation of AFLP fragment generation for defined applications (*e.g.* polymorphism screening, QTL analysis, and genetic mapping).

Table 28.2. Advantage and Disadvantage of AFLP

Marker	Advantages	Disadvantages
Amplified fragment length polymorphism	Sequence information not required	Very tricky due to changes in patterns with respect to materials used
	Can be used across species	
	Work with smaller RFLP fragments	Low reproducibility
	Useful in preparing contig maps	Need to have very good primers
	High genomic abundance	
	High polymorphism	

Random Amplified Polymorphic DNA (RAPD)

The basis of randomly amplified polymorphic DNA technique is differential PCR amplification of genomic DNA. **This procedure detects nucleotide sequence polymorphisms in DNA by using a single primer of arbitrary nucleotide sequence (10bp primer).** In this reaction, a single primer anneals in arbitrary manner (randomly) to the genomic DNA at two different sites where it finds complementary bases of DNA template. If these priming sites are within an amplifiable range of each other, a discrete DNA product is formed through PCR. On an average, each primer directs amplification of several discrete loci in the genome, making the assay useful for efficient screening of nucleotide sequence polymorphism between individuals. As the approach requires no prior knowledge of the genome that is being analyzed, it can be employed across species using universal primers. The amplification products are separated on agarose gels in the presence of ethidium bromide and viewed under ultraviolet light. The banding patterns distinguish organisms according to the presence or absence of bands (polymorphism). These polymorphisms are considered to be primarily due to variation in the primer annealing sites (inverted repeates in the genome), but they can also be generated by length differences in the amplified sequence between primer annealing sites. Each product is derived from a region of the genome that contains two short segments in inverted orientation, on opposite strands that are complementary to the primer (Figure 28.3).

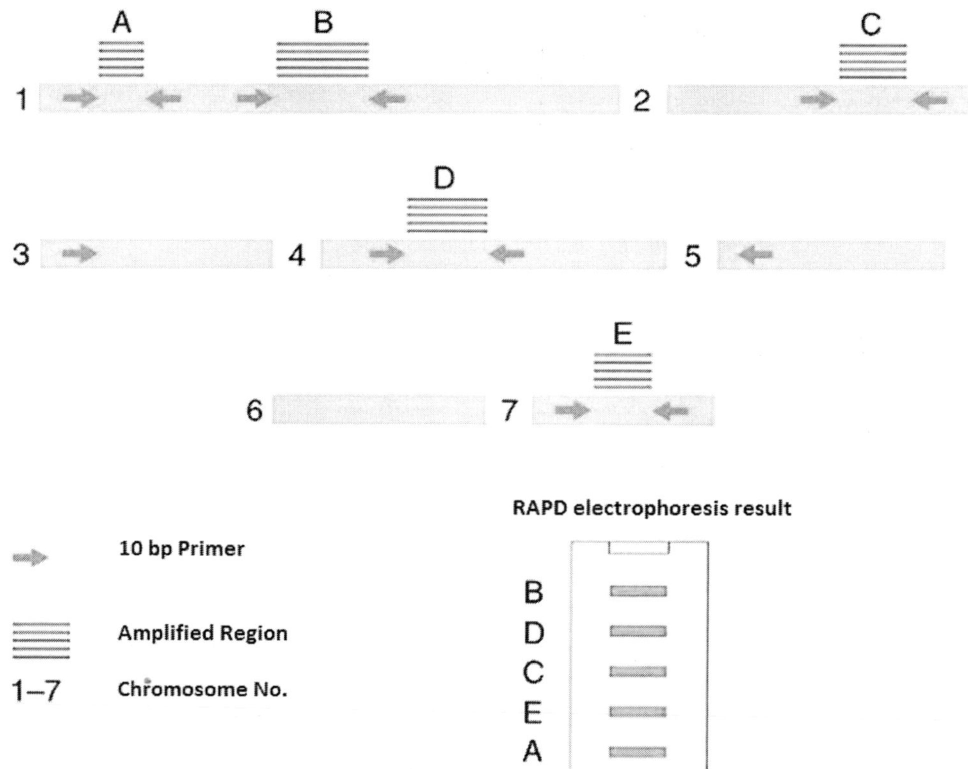

Figure 28.3. Random Amplified Polymorphic DNA.

Table 28.3. Advantage and Disadvantage of RAPD

Marker	Advantages	Disadvantages
Randomly amplified polymorphic DNA	Sequence information not required	No probe or primer information
		Dominant markers
		Very low reproducibility
	Good genome coverage	Cannot be used across species
	Ideal for automation	Not well established
	Less amount and poor quality DNA acceptable	
	No radioactive labeling	
	Relatively faster	
	High genomic abundance	

Applications

- ☆ The application of RAPDs and their related modified markers in variability analysis and individual-specific genotyping has largely been carried out, but is less popular due to problems such as poor reproducibility, faint or fuzzy products, and difficulty in scoring bands, which lead to inappropriate inferences.

- RAPDs have been used for many purposes, ranging from studies at the individual level (*e.g.*, genetic identity) to studies involving closely related species and determination of genetic diversity.
- RAPDs have also been applied in gene mapping studies to fill gaps not covered by other markers.

Sequence Characterized Amplified Region (SCAR)

SCARs are DNA fragments amplified by the use of PCR using specific 20–30 bp primers. The primers are designed from terminal ends of a RAPD marker. **RAPD marker fragments associated** with a phenotypic condition of interest are **cloned and sequenced**. This nucleotide sequence is then used for designing of unique primers for specific amplification of a particular locus. Use of unique primers decreases site competition for specific regions among primers, making the results less sensitive to reaction conditions. Use of longer primers also increases the reproducibility of the results by increasing specificity of template binding by the primer. PCR products obtained after amplification are analyzed for the presence of length polymorphism by gel electrophoresis. Conversion of RAPDs into SCARs may have additional advantage of obtaining a codominant marker, although dominance may be exhibited by SCARs when one or both primers partially overlap the site of sequence variation.

Advantages

- Due to the application of PCR, low amounts of genomic or template DNA is required (10–50 ng per reaction) for analysis of the marker.
- The major advantage of SCARs is the ease of their use, and requirement of relatively less time for the analysis.
- SCAR markers are locus specific and the results obtained from analysis of SCARs are highly reproducible.

Disadvantages

Major limitation lies in the fact that analysis of SCARs can be done only for organism, species, or DNA fragment with known sequence; as knowledge of sequence data is required for designing of the PCR primers.

Applications

- Major application of SCAR makers has been found in gene mapping studies as they are locus specific.
- They are also used in marker assisted selection, where presence of a specific genotype and expression of its corresponding phenotype can be correlated to the presence or absence of a SCAR marker.

Minisatellites, Variable Number of Tandem Repeats (VNTR)

The term 'minisatellite' was introduced by Jeffrey ***et al.* (1985).** These loci contain tandem repeats that vary in the number of repeat units between genotypes and are referred to as variable number of tandem repeats (VNTRs) (*i.e.*, a single locus that contains variable number of tandem repeats between individuals) or hypervariable regions (HVRs) (*i.e.*, numerous loci containing tandem repeats within a genome generating high levels of polymorphism between individuals). Minisatellites are a conceptually very different class of marker. They consist of chromosomal regions containing tandem repeat units of a **10–50 base motif**, flanked by conserved DNA restriction sites. A minisatellite profile consisting of many bands, usually within a **4–20 kb size range,** is generated by using common multi locus probes that are able to hybridize to minisatellite sequences in different species. Locus specific probes can be developed by molecular cloning of DNA restriction fragments, subsequent screening with a multi locus minisatellite probe and isolation of specific fragments. Variation in the number of repeat units, due to unequal crossing over or gene conversion, is considered to be the main cause of length polymorphisms. Due to the high mutation rate of minisatellites, the level of polymorphism is substantial, generally resulting in unique multilocus profiles for different individuals within a population.

Advantages

The main advantages of minisatellites are their high level of polymorphism and high reproducibility.

Disadvantages

- Disadvantages of minisatellites are similar to RFLPs due to the high similarity in methodological procedures.
- If multilocus probes are used, highly informative profiles are generally observed due to the generation of many informative bands per reaction. In that case, band profiles cannot be interpreted in terms of loci and alleles and similar sized fragments may be nonhomologous.
- Minisatellites are of reduced value for taxonomic studies because of hyper variability.

Applications

- The term DNA fingerprinting was introduced for minisatellites, though DNA fingerprinting is now used in a more general way to refer to a DNA-based assay to uniquely identify individuals.
- Minisatellites are particularly useful in studies involving genetic identity, parentage, clonal growth and structure, and identification of varieties and cultivars and for population-level studies.

Simple Sequence Repeat (SSR) or Microsatellites

The simple sequence repeats (SSR) are also referred to as microsatellites. 'Microsatellites' **coined by Litt and Lutty (1989),** consist of tandemly repeating units of DNA ubiquitous in prokaryotes and eukaryotes, scattered throughout most eukaryotic genomes. **Microsatellites can comprise repetition of mono-, di-, tri-, tetra- or penta-nucleotide units.** Simple sequence repeat polymorphism is detected by the use of PCR, in conditions when nucleotide sequences of the flanking regions of the microsatellite are known, or by Southern hybridization using labeled probes. Unlike minisatellites, which also represent tandem repeats, microsatellites consist of short tandem repeat motifs of 1–6 base pair (bp) long units. Knowledge of nucleotide sequence is used to design specific primers (generally 20–25 bp) for amplification of the microsatellite region along with flanking sequences by PCR. In conditions where sequence of the microsatellite region is unknown, primers are designed from genomic regions adjacent to the SSR sequences. The amplified genomic fragment thus obtained is cloned and sequenced to obtain specific sequence of the microsatellite region. Primers are designed using this microsatellite sequence for specific amplification using PCR. This approach is termed as sequence-tagged microsatellite site (STMS) (Figure 28.4).

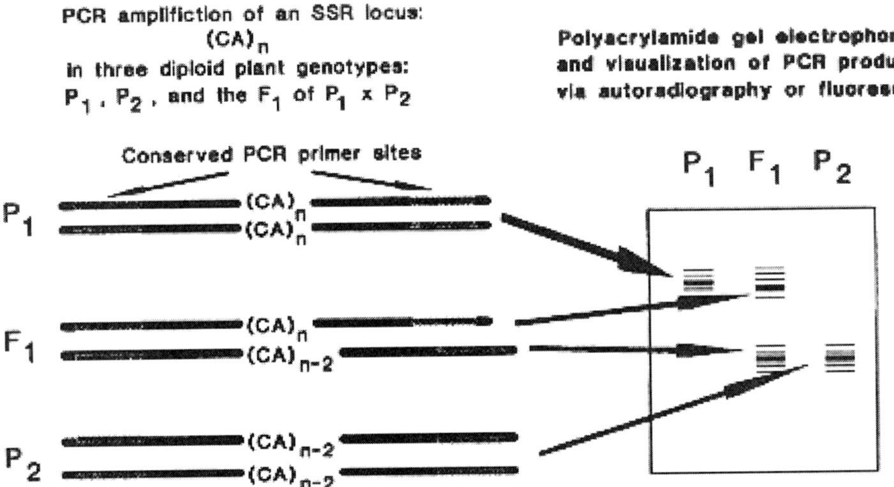

Figure 28.4. Generation and Visualization of Simple Sequence Repeat or Microsatellites.

Advantages

- ☆ High number of alleles and their co-dominance, along with widespread distribution throughout the genome, are the most significant features of microsatellites which make them important molecular markers.
- ☆ As the analysis of SSRs is PCR based, low quantities of template DNA (10–50 ng per reaction) are required.

- In comparison to other markers, such as RAPD, longer primers can be designed and used for microsatellites, thus, increasing reproducibility of the results obtained.
- The analysis of microsatellite can be semi-automated and does not necessitate the use of radioactive isotopes.
- Microsatellite analysis allows identification of multiple alleles at a single locus.

Disadvantages

- Principal draw back of microsatellites lies in their high development costs.
- Sequence information of the template or genomic DNA is required for designing and synthesis of primers.
- Thus, study or analysis of microsatellites is extremely difficult to apply for any unstudied group of species or organism of interest.
- Although SSRs are codominant in nature, mutations in the primer binding sites may result in false-negative result because of non amplification of the intended PCR product (occurrence of null alleles), which may lead to errors in genotype analysis.

Applications

- Microsatellites have high degree of mutability, hence are thought to play a significant role in genome evolution by creation and maintenance of quantitative genetic variation.
- Thus, high level of polymorphism shown by microsatellites makes them informative markers for population genetics studies, ranging from the individual level (*e.g.*, strain identification) to that of closely related species level.
- SSR markers have been useful for genetic variation studies in germplasm collections and are considered to be ideal molecular markers for gene mapping studies
- SSRs are molecular markers used for recombination mapping studies, to verify parental relationships and population genetic studies.
- They are the only molecular marker to provide information about presence or absence of closely related alleles.
- SSRs have been shown to be useful for study of functional diversity among closely related species, in relation to adaptive changes.

Single Nucleotide Polymorphism (SNPs)

Single nucleotide polymorphism describes polymorphisms caused by point mutations that give rise to different alleles containing alternative bases at a given **nucleotide position within a locus.** SNPs are becoming a focal point in molecular marker development since they are the most abundant polymorphism in any organism, adaptable to automation, and reveal hidden polymorphism not detected with other markers and methods. Theoretically, a SNP within a locus can produce as many as four alleles, each containing one of four bases at the SNP site: A, T, C, and G. Practically, however, most SNPs are usually restricted to one of two alleles (most often either the two pyrimidines C/T or the two purines A/G) and have been regarded as biallelic. Once the location of SNPs is identified and appropriate primers designed. Despite technological advances, SNP genotyping is still a challenging endeavor and requires specialized equipment, most expensive, prior genome sequencing or genome information is required for analysis. These are major drawbacks of this markers (Figure 28.5).

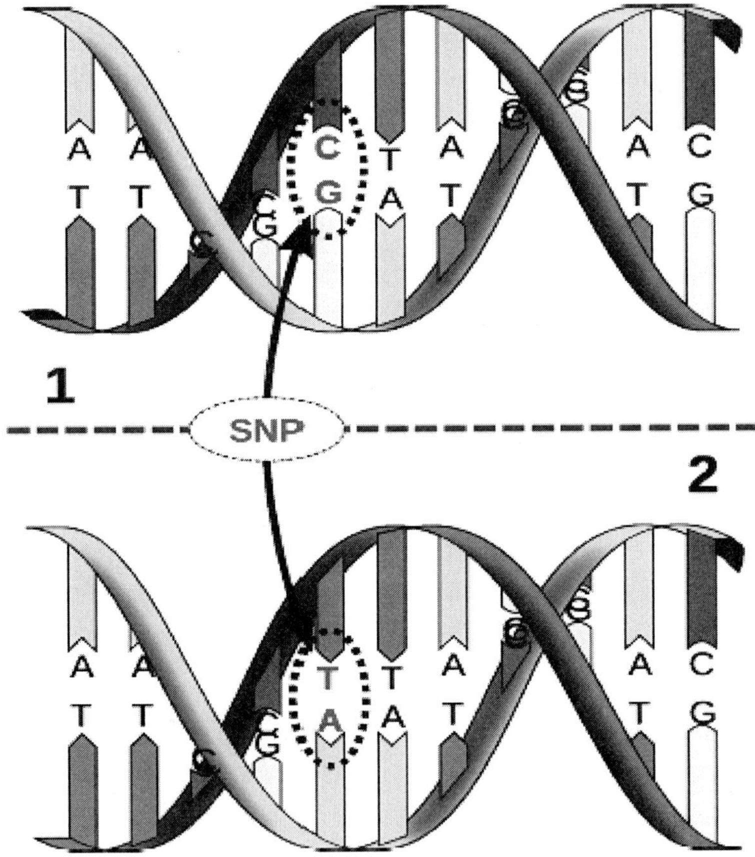

DNA molecule 1 differs from DNA molecule 2 at a single base-pair location (a C/T polymorphism).

Figure 28.5. Single Nucleotide Polymorphism.

Application

(1) highly useful for marker assisted and genomic selection (2) involved in association and QTL mapping, positional cloning (3) haplotype and pedigree analysis (4) seed purity testing (5) variety identification (6) monitoring the combinations of alleles that perform well in target environments.

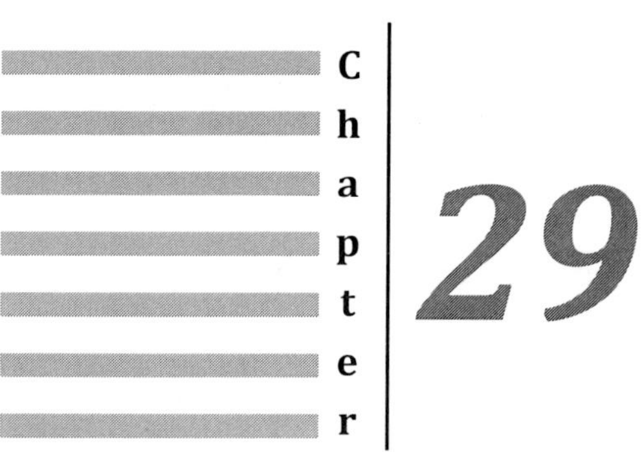

DNA Fingerprinting of Crop Varieties

DNA Fingerprinting of Plant Varieties

The DNA fingerprinting methodology was first introduced to plant genome analysis in 1988 using RFLP technique. Since then, DNA fingerprinting has become an immensely important instrument for genotype identification in both wild plant species and their cultivated relatives. Plants differ widely in life history traits including reproductive parameters such as propagation method, for those that propagate by seed, also in breeding system (selfing or cross-pollinated), in the mode of pollen and seed dispersal. All these factors have profound influence on the amount and partitioning of genetic variability between and within various entities such as cultivars and populations. These differences influence the utilization of DNA markers for fingerprinting individual plants or genotypes. The very first DNA fingerprint report dealing with plants was demonstrated by DNA fragment pattern differences between two varieties of barley, following Southern blot hybridization of HaeIII-digested DNA samples with the MI3 probe. In 1989, synthetic oligonucleotides that recognize microsatellites were introduced to plant DNA fingerprinting.

The introduction of PCR-based methods constituted a new milestone in the field of DNA fingerprinting. The random amplified polymorphic DNA (RAPD) approach using arbitrary primers were shown to generate anonymous PCR amplicons from genomic DNA, resulting in polymorphic banding patterns after gel electrophoresis and staining. A few years later, a promising new method, coined amplified fragment length polymorphism (AFLP) analysis, was introduced. This method incorporated elements of both RFLP and RAPD and, although technically more demanding than RAPD, produced very high numbers of polymorphic bands. Inter-simple sequence repeat (ISSR)-PCR technique, a third group of PCR-based DNA profiling techniques guides the PCR amplification to certain types of (mostly repetitive) DNA, without the need to develop species-specific primers.

The rapidity with which large numbers of samples can be processed made PCR-based methods increasingly popular. AFLP, RAPD, and ISSR are still broadly used, although RAPDs in particular have sometimes been criticized for problems with reproducibility and competitive priming. These problems are less pronounced for AFLP, which is currently regarded as the method of choice when high numbers of bands are desired. All three methods usually arrive at very similar estimates of genetic diversity and genetic distances, when applied to the same plant material (Figure 29.1).

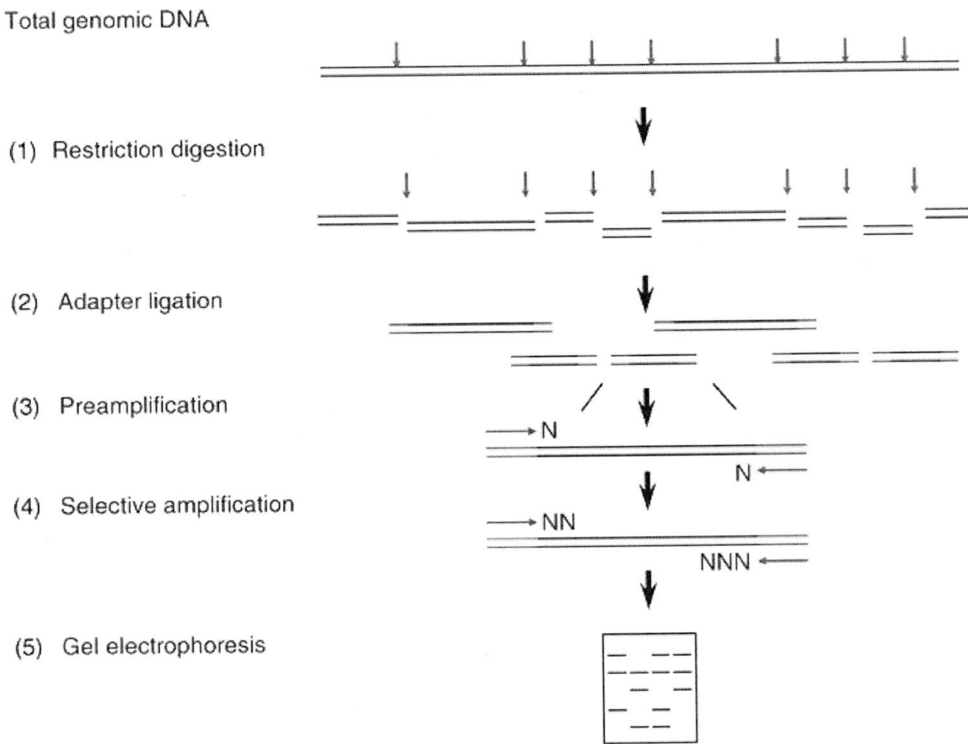

Figure 29.1. AFLP Based DNA Fingerprinting.

Genesis of DNA Fingerprinting

Interest in nucleic acid markers was created by the introduction of restriction fragment length polymorphisms (RFLPs) and sequencing, which gained popularity in the late 1970s. The advent of polymerase chain reaction exponentially increased the availability and affordability of different molecular marker techniques. However, **DNA fingerprinting all started in 1985, when Alec Jeffreys and co-workers in a series of publications reported the simple tandem-repetitive regions of DNA (also called minisatellites) capable of producing somatically stable DNA fingerprints completely specific to an individual.** By April 1985, the first legal case, involving an UK immigration dispute, had been satisfactorily resolved by DNA fingerprinting. By 1987, DNA fingerprinting results had been admitted in evidence in criminal courts in the UK and USA. A new technology was born. Soon after, minisatellites were reported in plants in 1988 and by 1993, **plant minisatellites were demonstrated to be useful markers for variation between and within species.**

Stages of Development

Like human DNA fingerprints, DNA profiles could be obtained in plants led to plant DNA fingerprinting

- ☆ The first stage was made through attempts to identify sequences in the genome that differ between individuals and to establish a set of protocols, which could be used to visualise the differences.
- ☆ The second stage was marked by the demonstration of power of various techniques in plants like Isolation of plant-specific probes/primers and optimisation of molecular profiling to discriminate species and varieties.
- ☆ The third stage is characterised by attempts to optimise sampling methods, sample size, minimum number of primers and probes, mode of depiction, *etc.*

Molecular Basis of DNA Fingerprinting

Unlike the fingerprints with which human beings are born, DNA fingerprints need to be generated, confirmed and assigned. These fingerprints are possible due to the existence of differences in the nucleotide sequence between individuals. Due to the enormous size of the genome, comparison between sequences of genomes in entirety is impractical. Therefore, genomic fragments are generated and cultivars are discriminated by differences in number, size and sequence of such specific DNA fragments.

A variety of genomic fragments are employed as markers. While some occur once in genome, others are repeated. Known gene sequences are used as **unique sequence markers**. However, coding sequences have highly conserved regions and not polymorphic enough to use routinely in fingerprinting (Figure 29.2). Tandemly repeated sequences such as mini- and microsatellites are frequently used markers in DNA fingerprinting.

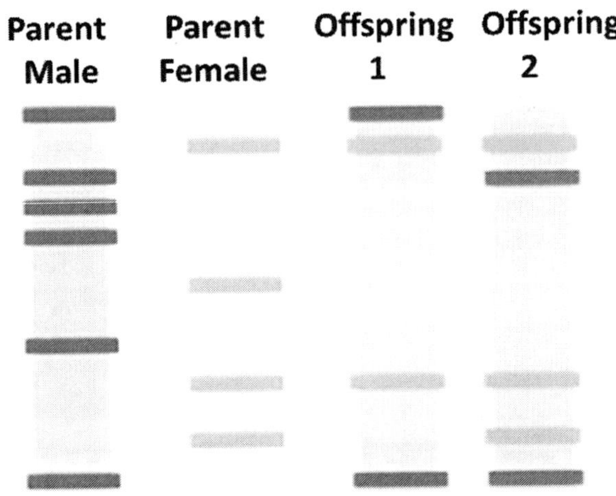

Figure 29.2. DNA Fingerprinting (Polymorphic Band).

Techniques in Plant DNA Fingerprinting

A typical fingerprinting technique generates molecular markers that should be polymorphic enough to discriminate between cultivars but not too polymorphic to throw up differences within individuals of a cultivar. Fingerprinting techniques differ depending on how the DNA fragments are generated and assayed. Numerous profiling techniques are available; all involve detecting fragments that differ in presence, size, or quantity between accessions. Fragments are generated by either restriction digestion or by polymerase chain reaction. The fragments are separated by agarose or polyacrylamide gel electrophoresis and detected by various approaches. All fragments on the gel are directly visualised by staining with ethidium bromide or silver nitrate. Alternatively, specific target fragments are detected by hybridisation with probes carrying radioactive, colorimetric, fluorescent or chemiluminescent label. When single or low-copy number fragments are evaluated, variation in fragment length is referred to as restriction fragment length polymorphism. To analyse repetitive DNA, target fragments are probed by known repeat sequences. This is called as multilocus fingerprinting since the assay produces information about many loci simultaneously. Single locus RFLP markers are co-dominant, genetically defined and highly reproducible, whereas multilocus markers are not genetically defined and dominant.

PCR-based marker techniques are grouped based on sequence, length and number of primers, and size range of the amplified products. With prior knowledge of the single copy target sequence, (homologous or heterologous) primer pairs can be designed to amplify target loci. In assays of these designed primer PCR loci, differences in the fragment length can often be analysed as codominant alleles in diploid genomes. However, these loci are better employed in phylogenetic studies rather than in fingerprinting. Amplification using designed primers flanking microsatellites (SSRs), display polymorphism in length and number of amplicons. Polymorphisms appear because of variation in the number of tandem repeats in a given motif. Polymorphic multiband patterns can be produced based on microsatellites (SSRs) by amplifying inter-SSR DNA sequences (Figure 29.3).

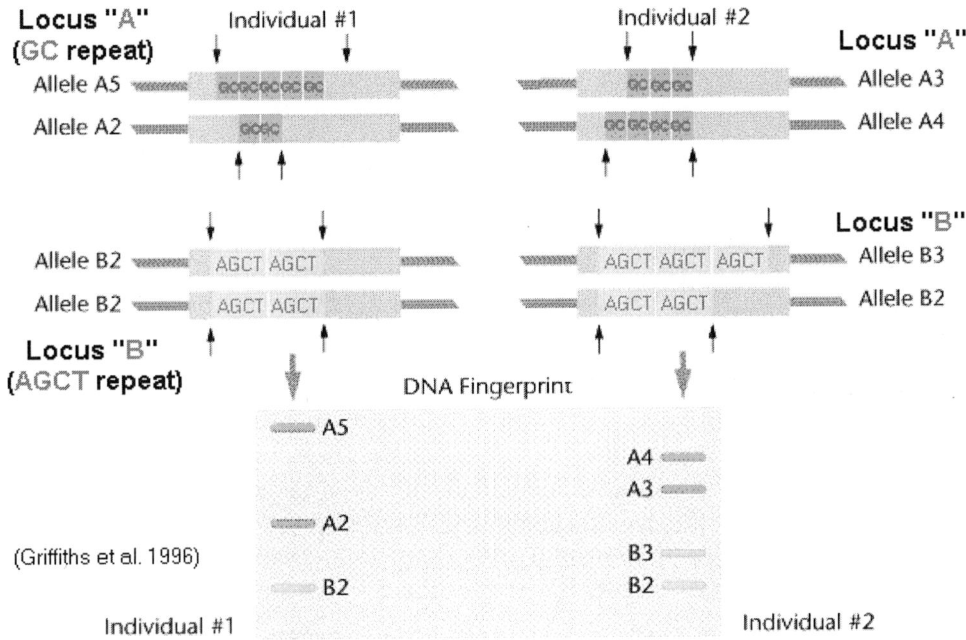

Figure 29.3. SSR Based DNA Fingerprinting.

Randomly amplified polymorphic DNA analysis (RAPD) requires no prior sequence information. A single short arbitrary sequence (usually ten nucleotides) is used as both forward and reverse primer to generate a set of fragments within amplification range. The number and length of the fragments vary between primers and genotypes. Many PCR assays are minor modifications or combinations of designed-primer and random primer PCR. These were developed to increase the reproducibility of the results and to enhance the resolution power of the techniques to discriminate close relatives. The utility of a desired RAPD marker can be increased by sequencing its termini and designing longer primers (*e.g.* up to 24 bases) for specific amplification of markers. Amplification yields sequenced characterised amplified regions (SCARs) that are more reproducible than RAPDs. Production of amplified fragment length polymorphism (AFLP) is based on selective amplification of restricted enzyme digested DNA. Multiple bands are generated in each amplification reaction that contains DNA markers of random origin. Analysis of DNA on polyacrylamide gels typically results in 50-100 bands per sample. AFLP has advantages of high resolution and higher number of markers per assay, which make it a robust fingerprinting technique.

Importance of DNA Fingerprinting

The World Trade Organisation (WTO) requires its member countries to accord protection to plant varieties under Trade-Related Intellectual Property Rights (TRIPs) agreement. Convention on Biological Diversity (CBD) provides sovereign rights to nations over their genetic resources. Countries can regulate access to their genetic resources and demand equitable sharing of benefits arising out of commercial exploitation of the genetic resources. Enforcement of both these international agreements is possible only if the identity and the ownership of the plant genotypes are established. Therefore, a perfect system to identify parental lines, landraces and wild relatives along with released varieties is the most fundamental requirement to enforce the propriety over plant varieties and germplasm.

Variability in morphological and biochemical characters has been useful in this regard because the scoring is easy, economical and practical. However, morphological and biochemical markers suffer from drawbacks such as low variability, environmental influence, epistasis, and their quantitative nature and complex inheritance pattern. Molecular markers, on the other hand, exhibit a high degree of non-tissue-specific polymorphism and simple inheritance patterns with minimal influence of environment and epistasis. DNA fingerprinting is the application of molecular marker techniques for the identification of cultivars.

Application of DNA Fingerprinting in Plants

- DNA fingerprinting it is to provide propriety rights and to settle disputes with commercial stakes in case of plants.
- Plant DNA fingerprinting deals with more number of species with different mating systems and genetic structure, and in-depth genetic studies (structural genomics) for many crops (except for a few such as maize, rice and tomato) are yet to begin.
- In plants populations are identified (a population may be a variety, a species, a landrace, a breeding line or a parent in hybrid production with varying genetic structure with respect to uniformity and stability).
- During the dispute between two biotech companies, traits of the transgenic crops like resistance to biotic and abiotic stress are difficult to identify and characterize. But using DNA fingerprinting it can be quickly identified the
- variety and settle the issue without disclosing the information about the transgene.

Table 29.1. List of Varieties and Germplasm Fingerprinted

S. No.	Crop	Varieties / elite germplasm Fingerprinted	Techniques
1.	Rice	274	STMS. AFLP. RAPD
2.	Wheat	153	STMS, AFLP, RAPD
3.	Sorghum	65	STMS, AFLP, RAPD
4.	Barley	54	STMS, RAPD
5.	Pearl millet	17	AFLP. RAPD
6.	Finger millet	94	ISSR
7.	Chickpea	72	STMS. AFLP. ISSR. RAPD
8.	Mungbean	96	AFLP. RAPD
9.	Urdbean	54	AFLP
10.	French bean	26	AFLP. STMS
11.	Pigeonpea	96	AFLP, RAPD
12.	Peas	38	AFLP
13.	Lentil	41	AFLP
14.	Niger	30	AFLP. RAPD
15.	Brassica	42	ISSR, AFLP, RAPD
16.	Soybean	75	AFLP. RAPD. STMS
17.	Safflower	14	AFLP
18.	Sesame	67	AFLP. RAPD
19.	Cotton	94	AFLP. RAPD
20.	Tomato	27	RAPD
21.	Chillies	42	ISSR, AFLP. STMS, RAPD
22.	Brinjal	19	ISSR. RAPD
23.	Banana	243	AFLP. STMS, RFLP. RAPD
24.	Mango	30	ISSR. AFLP. RAPD
25.	Citrus	34	AFLP. ISSR
26.	Cashew	140	ISSR. AFLP. RAPD
27.	Neem	69	AFLP. ISSR. RAPD
28.	Vetiver	24	AFLP. RAPD
29.	Saffron	13	AFLP
30.	Plantago	48	ISSR. AFLP. RAPD
31.	Palmarosa	34	ISSR. RAPD
32.	Chlorophytum	21	ISSR. RAPD

Gene-tagging

The process of locating genes of importance via linkage to RFLP or isozyme markers is referred to as gene-tagging. Tagging projects are a prerequisite to the use of marker-based selection schemes, and to cloning genes of interest.

The information that emerges from tagging projects includes: (i) the number of genes controlling a phenotypic character of interest; (ii) the map location of those genes; and (iii) in the case of quantitative characters, the relative size of the contribution to trait expression (phenotype) of each.

In plants, a number of reports of successful gene-tagging and monitoring of inheritance of both monogenic and polygenic characters in maize, tomato, and lettuce are available. The ability to detect tight linkage between markers and genes of interest depends on: (i) the number of mapped markers that is available for a given species; and (ii) the level of polymorphism detectable by those markers in the plant material used in the tagging project. Tagging is more reliable when the genetic distance between a marker and the target gene is small because the probability of a crossover event separating a marker from the locus governing the trait diminishes with decreasing distance.

Two approaches are commonly used in gene-tagging experiments. One depends upon the availability of isolines and is useful in tagging single genes, such as those conferring disease and insect resistance. The second approach is based directly on a segregating population. The population must: (i) segregate for the trait(s) of interest; and (ii) segregate for enough molecular markers to have a reasonable probability of detecting linkage with the genes for the trait of interest, no matter where they are located in the genome.

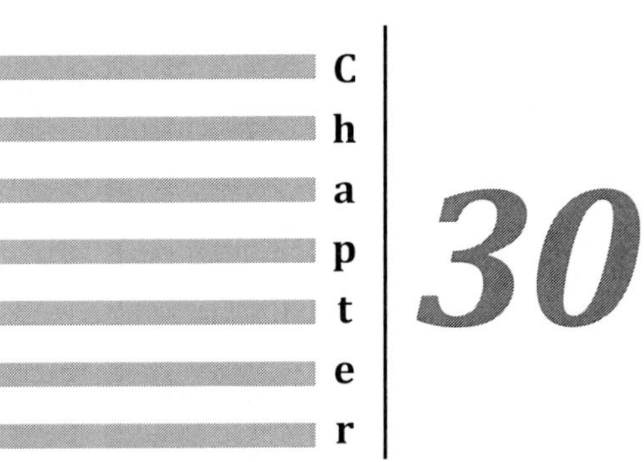

Development of Mapping Populations

Mapping Population

Mapping populations is a population usually created from F1 lines that are derived from two parents that show differing phenotypes for a target trait, suitable for linkage mapping of genetic markers including DNA based molecular markers.

Types of Mapping Populations

There are three primary types of mapping populations used for molecular mapping. F_2 population, backcross population and recombinant inbred lines (RILs). An F_2 population is developed by selfing (or intermating for cross pollinated species) among F_1 individuals. These F_1 individuals are developed by crossing two parents that show significant polymorphism for whichever type of loci you are going to score. Backcross populations are developed by crossing the F_1 with one of the two parents used in the initial cross. It would be always advantageous using populations of early generations such as F_2, F_3, BC population *etc.*, since these populations are amenable to make accurate predictions. However, the predictions made involving early generations would be misleading because of hide or disguise the presence of the major gene on many other minor genes in early generation. Continuous inbreeding to evolve recombinant inbred lines (RILs) can eliminate this problem. Thus, RILs can remain as the best choice of population for QTL analysis. As an alternative doubled haploid (DH) lines can also be used. The inherent homozygosity prevailing in the individuals of these two populations make the RILs and DHLs as immortals and help to have as many replications as required by the experiment.

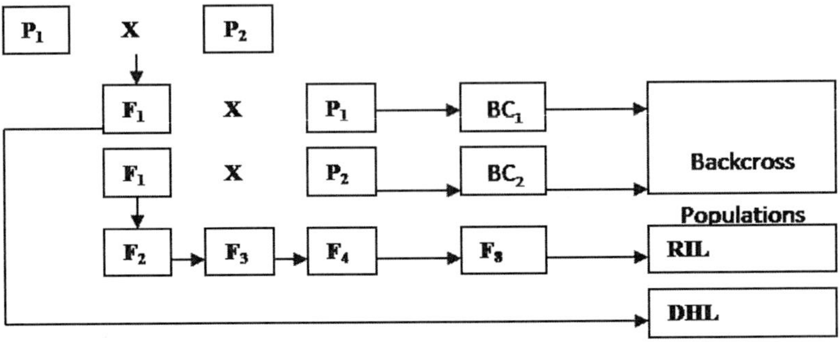

Figure 30.1. Mapping Populations for QTL Mapping.

Developing of F_2 Mapping Population

A segregating F_2 population is formed from the F_1 individuals either by randomly crossing these individuals or allowing them to self. Homozygous (fixed) lines can be produced from F_2 individuals using single seed descent. One seed is harvested from each F_2 individual - grown into an F_3 plant - a single seed is harvested and grown into an F_4 plant and so on until F_8 to F_{10} generations were the lines will be virtually homozygous at all loci. Pockets of heterozygocity sometimes persist, however if these are identified, more rounds of selfing may eliminate these. The end result is a set of recombinant inbred lines (RILS). This can take up to 5 years depending on the species. If lines are intercrossed (sibling mating) in the F_2, F_3 and F_4 generations Advanced Intercross Lines (AILs) can be generated, these are then maintained by single seed descent.

Doubled Haploid Lines

The F_1 individuals will be heterozygous these lines are also used to produce doubled haploid lines (DH lines) using microspore culture. Haploid plantlets produced from embryos usually undergo spontaneous doubling producing DH lines (this can be achieved using colchicines. Doubled haploid lines are advantageous since they are homozygous or fixed lines, and as such can be replicated in trials allowing better estimates of within and between line variation. Plus, they can be produced in a relatively short period (1-2 yrs).

Developing of Recombinant Inbred Lines (RILs)

Recombinant inbred lines are developed by single-seed selections from individual plants of an F_2 population. (Because of this procedure, these lines are also called F_2-derived lines) Single-seed descent is repeated for several generations. At this point, all of the seed from an individual plant is bulked. For example, a F_3: F_4 RI population underwent single-seed descent through the F3 generation, and was bulked to develop the F_4. This population of seed can then be grown to obtain a large quantity of seed of each individual line. Importantly, each of the lines is fixed for many recombination events.

Uses of Recombinant Inbred Lines

1. First, they can be used to derive a map because it essentially is an eternal F_2 population with unlimited mapping possibilities.
2. These lines can be scored for morphological traits (such as disease resistance or flower color) or quantitative traits (such as yield or maturity).
3. This morphological trait data can then be compiled and those traits can be placed on the developing molecular map.
4. These lines are especially powerful for analyzing quantitative traits because replicated trials can be analyzed using identical genetic material.
5. The quantitative trait data can then be used to determine if any molecular markers are closely associated with those traits.

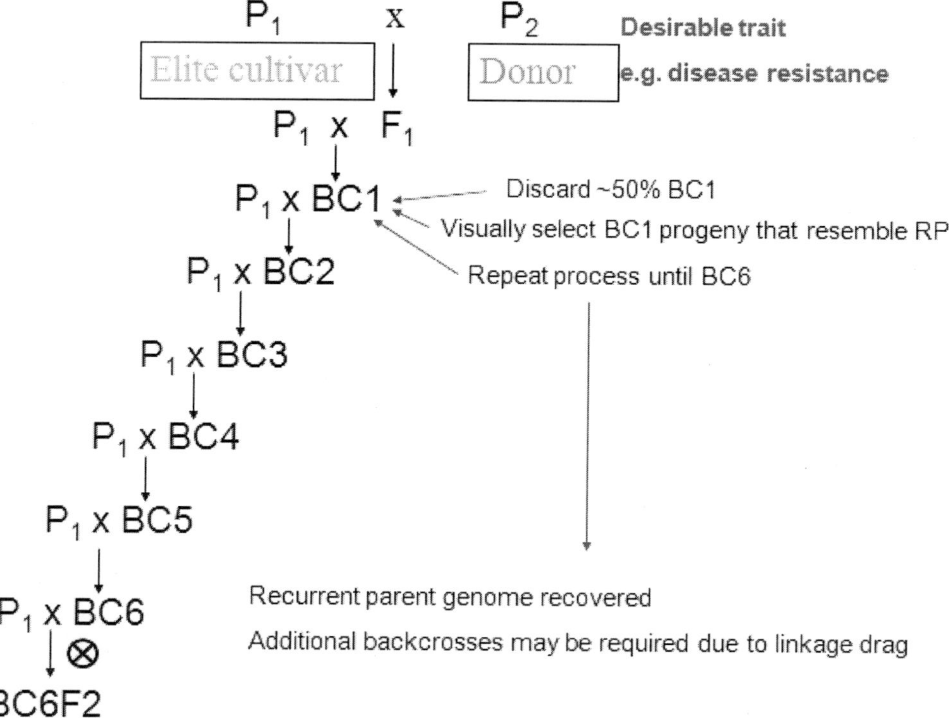

Figure 30.2. Conventional Backcrossing.

Backcross (BC) and Advanced Backcross Lines (ABLs)

Once a particular line or lines have been selected based on the presence of a favorable genotype linked to a trait of interest, then the donor can be backcrossed to the recurrent parent to produce a backcross (BC_1) generation. Subsequent rounds of backcrossing to the recurrent parent in combination with the use of genetic markers that allow selection of only lines containing the favorable genotype (foreground selection), in combination with markers to select for the recurrent parent genotype elsewhere in the genome (background selection) allow lines to be created that contain a small region of the beneficial genotype in virtually homogenous background. The resulting progeny are called Advanced Backcross lines (AB lines) or Backcross Inbred Lines (BILs).

Near Isogenic Lines (NILs)

Depending upon the donor parent, this method can be used to generate a population that have introgressed segments of the donar parent in the background of the recurrent parent that overlap to provide coverage across all chromosomes. If a RIL was used than the resulting progeny may be classed as Near Isogenic Lines (NILs); in this case the desired population will consist of lines that contain small overlapping segments of a particular target region.

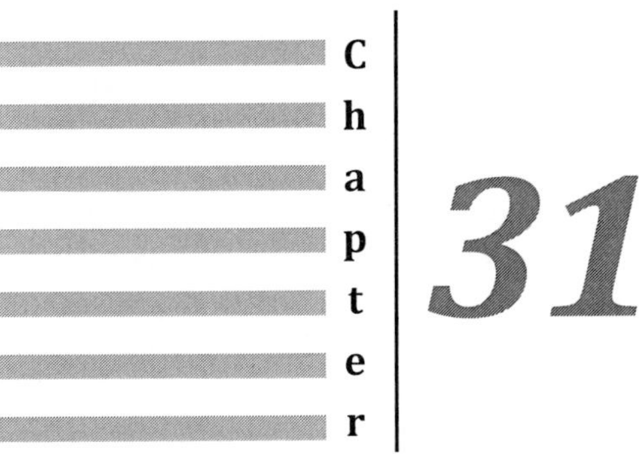

Linkage and QTL Analysis

Japonica rice has 32,000 to 50,000 genes, Indica rice has between 46,022 and 55,615 genes in 24 chromosomes (2n), 13,600 genes for the fruit fly *Drosophila melanogaster* within 8 chromosomes (2n) and 26,000 genes for the flowering plant *Arabidopsis thaliana* chromosomes10 (2n). So the number of genes are more when compared to the chromosomes number in all organisms. Hence to accommodate all the genes, genes are linked together and placed on chromosomes.

Linkage

The tendency of two or more genes to stay together during inheritance is known as linkage. Linked genes do not show independent segregation. Group of genes situated on the same chromosome is known as linkage group. The number of linkage group is equal to the number of haploid chromosome present in the particular organism.

Linkage analysis is used to determine the arrangement of genes on the chromosomes of an organism. How often different forms of two variable traits are co-inherited, that can infer whether the genes for the traits are on the same chromosome (such genes are said to be linked) or different chromosome. If the genes for the trait linked, the genetic distance separating the loci of the linked genes can be calculated. The order and pairwise distances between the loci of three or more linked genes are displayed as a genetic-linkage map.

Concept Behind the Genetic Map Construction

Genes located on the same chromosome tend to remain together and all the genes do not assort independently as Mendel proposed. These genes on the same chromosome that do not show independent assortment are said to be linked.

The strength of linkage between a pair of genes can be determined based on the recombination between genes by a process **called crossing over between two homologous chromosomes.** This results in the production of gametes similar to parental types and some not similar to parental types in a heterozygous organism. The non-parental type of gametes are called **recombinant types**. The frequency of recombinants is a measure of whether genes are linked or not, if linked, how close together they are on the chromosome and this process is called as **linkage analysis**. Based on the linkage analysis one can determine the distance between two genes on a chromosome and establish the order of genes with other genes. Two-point analysis is a method by which the genetic distance between two linked genes is determined. The order of genes is established based on three-point analysis. When many genes are involved it is called multipoint analysis.

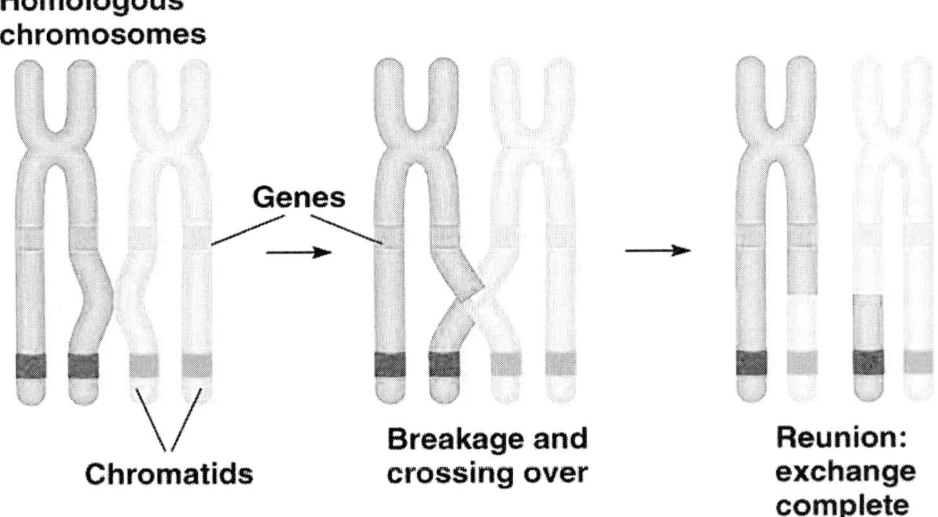

Figure 31.1. Diagrammatic Representation of Crossing Over and Recombination between Two Homologous Chromosomes.

Construction of a Linkage Map

The construction of a genetic map involves the linkage analysis of genes segregating among the progenies of a sexual cross. According to the Mendel's Law of Independent Assortment, members of different pairs of alleles assort independently of each other when the germ cell is formed. This is only true if the genes are on different chromosomes. If they are on the same chromosome and inherited together to the progenies then they are said to be linked. The frequency of recombination of a pair of linked gene is constant and characteristic for that pair of genes. The strength of linkage and recombination observed is a function of the distance on the chromosome between the genes in question. The frequency of recombinants (not similar to both the parents) determines the distance between genes. The early work on linkage map construction was mainly based on the segregation of easily observable morphological traits among the progenies of a cross.

There are several examples of linkage maps resulted from the morphological traits, otherwise called as morphological markers. Morphological markers are easily observable traits with discrete phenotype. Though these markers are highly advantageous but also having number of drawbacks, as follows.

- ✰ Morphological marker less in number
- ✰ Interact with the environment
- ✰ Show differential expression across genotypes
- ✰ Not distributed throughout the genome
- ✰ Expression depends on the ontogeny of the individual
- ✰ Dominant-recessive expression

DNA Markers Hastened the Process of Genetic Map Construction

The advent of DNA markers - polymorphic and locus characterized by a number of variable lengths paved the way for easy and faster linkage map construction. These DNA markers *i.e.* RFLP, SSR, RAPD, AFLP *etc.* possess several positive features over the morphological markers. Demonstration of the role of DNA markers in the construction of genetic maps has been done in major crop species such as tomato maize, lettuce, potato and rice. The recent developments in molecular biology simplified many aspects in the genome mapping based on the position of certain land marks (often referred to as genetic markers) in the genome.

Advantage of Molecular Markers

- ✰ More in number
- ✰ No environmental influence
- ✰ Phenotypically neutral
- ✰ Distributed throughout the genome
- ✰ Possibility of using these markers at any growth stage of the individual
- ✰ Codominant or dominant

Construction of genetic maps using molecular markers generally involves the following steps *viz.*, 1) Identifying suitable DNA marker system for the map construction, 2) Parental survey to identify polymorphic DNA markers, 3) Establishing a suitable mapping population, 4) Segregation analysis of polymorphic markers on the individuals of the mapping population, 5) Linkage analysis to establish linkage map of each chromosome based on marker-segregation data and 6) Assigning chromosome numbers to linkage groups.

Linkage in Maize

In maize, gene C for coloured aleurone is dominant over its allele c for colourless aleurone and gene Sh (denoted for the sake of simplicity as S) for full endosperm is dominant over its allele sh (denoted as s) for shrunken endosperm. In a cross between a plant having coloured and full seeds and one having colourless and shrunken seeds, the following results were obtained:

Table 31.1. Linkage Analysis in Maize

P	*Colourfull CCSS*	*X*	*Colour Shrunkenccss*
F_1		Colourfull CcSs	
F_2	Observed numbers (Hypothetical)	Excepted ratio	Excepted numbers
Coloured full	7300	9	5625
Coloured shrunken	200	3	1875
Colourless full	200	3	1875
Colourless shrunken	2300	1	625

The F_2 did not the 9 : 3 : 3 : 1 ratio. There were greater number of coloured full and colourless shrunken seeds and less number of coloured shrunken and colourless full seeds than the excepted.

If coloured and colourless aleurone are considered alone, the observed numbers of 7500 for coloured and 2500 for colourless seeds fit with the expected 3 : 1 ratio. Similarly, if full and shrunken endosperm are considered alone, the observed numbers of 7500 for full and 2500 for shrunken seeds fit with the expected 3 : 1 ratio.

The large deviation of the observed F_2 population from the expected segregation is therefore not because the members of each pair of alleles do not segregate from each other but because the separation in one pair of alleles is not independent of the separation in the other pair of alleles.

Quantitative Trait Locus (QTL)

A quantitative trait locus (QTL) is a region of DNA which is associated with a particular phenotypic trait, which varies in degree and which can be attributed to polygenic effects, *i.e.*, the product of two or more genes, and their environment.

(or)

A quantitative trait locus (QTL) is a section of DNA (the locus) which correlates with variation in a phenotype (the quantitative trait) or Usually the QTL is linked to, or contains, the genes which control that phenotype.

QTLs are mapped by identifying which molecular markers (such as SNPs or AFLPs) correlate with an observed trait. This is often an early step in identifying and sequencing the actual genes that cause the trait variation. These QTLs are often found on different chromosomes. The number of QTLs which explain variation in the phenotypic trait indicates the genetic architecture of a trait. It may indicate that plant height is controlled by many genes of small effect, or by a few genes of large effect. Typically, QTLs underlie continuous traits (those traits which vary continuously, *e.g.* height) as opposed to discrete traits (traits that have two or several character values, *e.g.* smooth vs. wrinkled peas used by Mendel in his experiments). Moreover, a single phenotypic trait is usually determined by many genes. Consequently, many QTLs are associated with a single trait. Another use of QTLs is to identify candidate genes underlying a trait. Once a region of DNA is identified as contributing to a phenotype, it can be sequenced. The DNA sequence of any genes in this region can then be compared to a database of DNA for genes whose function is already known.

QTL Analysis

The idea of using genetic markers to locate the individual quantitative trait locus (QTL) responsible for variation in quantitative traits goes back nearly to the beginning of modern genetics. With the availability of dense highly informative marker maps, it has recently become feasible to map genes or QTL accounting for part of the heritability of continuously distributed traits in experimental crosses as well as outbred populations. The most extensive comparative data set available at this point probably comes from QTL mapping efforts in plants. Interestingly, an unexpectedly high proportion of QTL affecting seed size, height, flowering and other complex traits do correspond among different taxa. The process of QTL analysis requires 1) a suitable mapping population of phenotypically contrasting parents, 2) a linkage map of molecular markers, 3) mapping methods and software and 4) reliable phenotypic screening methods and generation of phenotypic data. The main practical limitation in localizing QTL, seems to be the non-availability of suitable markers. This limitation was remedied by the construction of complete Restriction Fragment Length Polymorphism (RFLP) linkage maps, permitting systematic searches of an entire genome for QTL influencing a trait. The Amplified Fragment Length Polymorphism (AFLP) markers, the markers of choice, remain the best alternative to construct the linkage maps in a very short period based on the existing RFLP maps. Several linkage maps of molecular markers have been constructed exclusively for QTL analysis of various agronomic traits in crop species such as tomato, maize, rice and soybean.

QTL Mapping Methods

Conceptually, QTL mapping amounts to a three-step recipe: scan the entire genome with a dense collection of genetic markers; calculate an appropriate linkage statistic $S(x)$ at each position x along the genome; and identify the regions in which the statistic S shows a significant deviation from what would be expected under independent assortment. The underlying assumptions of QTL mapping involving molecular markers are : 1) genes controlling quantitative traits are located on the genome, just like simple genetic markers, 2) if the markers cover a large portion of the genome then there is a large chance that some of the genes controlling the quantitative traits are linked with some of the genetic markers and 3) if the genes and markers are segregating in a genetically defined population, then the linkage relationship among them may be resolved by studying the association between trait variation and marker segregation pattern. The association between quantitative trait variation and marker segregation pattern can be carried out by the following methods. The basis of all QTL detection, regardless of the crop to which it is applied, is the identification of association between genetically determined phenotypes and specific genetic markers. The possible methods of analysis to detect QTL include: 1) single marker analysis (otherwise called as Marker-Trait (MT) Method) and 2) interval analysis.

Single Marker Analysis

The single marker analysis (SMA) is a good start not only for learning QTL mapping, but also for practical data analysis. Single marker analysis is the method used in earliest studies on QTL mapping. In this, one marker is involved at a time to find the QTL-marker association (Figure 31.2). The single marker analysis can be implemented as a simple t-test, ANOVA, linear regression, and likelihood ratio test and maximum likelihood estimation. It can be performed using common statistical software. Gene orders and complete linkage map are not required.

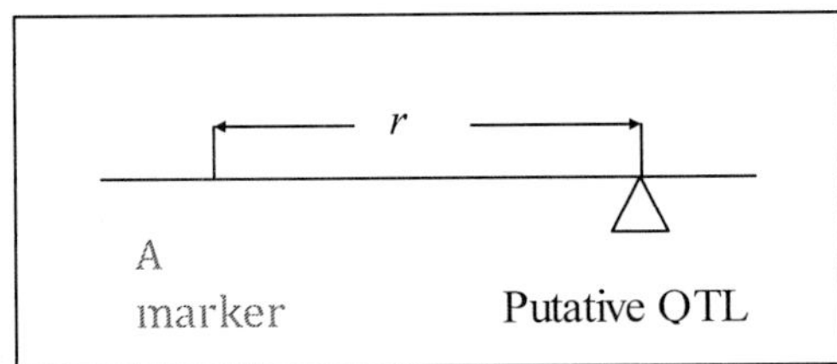

Figure 31.2. Association of a Marker with a Putative QTL.

The disadvantages of the single marker analysis are: 1) the putative QTL genotypic means and QTL positions are confounded. These confounding cause the estimated QTL effects to be biased and the statistical power to be low particularly when linkage map density is low and 2) QTL positions cannot be precisely determined, due to the non-dependence among the hypothesis tests for linked markers that confound QTL effect and position.

Single Interval Mapping (SIM)

Single Interval mapping (SIM) is considered as a second level of QTL mapping. QTL mapping by this method requires prior construction of a marker genetic map. The interval mapping approach is based on the joint frequencies of a pair of adjacent markers and a putative QTL flanked by the two markers (Figure 31.3).

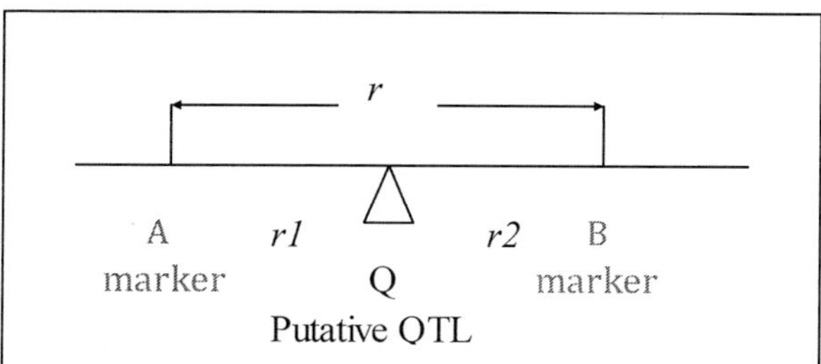

Figure 31.3. Association of a Putative QTL to Two Flanking Markers.

Composite Interval Mapping (CIM)

CIM evaluates the possibility of a target QTL at multiple analysis points across each inter-marker interval. However, at each point it also includes the effect of one or more background markers, as defined in SIM. The inclusion of a background marker in the analysis helps in one of two ways, depending on whether the background marker and the target interval are linked. If they are not linked, inclusion of the background marker makes the analysis more sensitive to the presence of a QTL in the target interval. If they are linked, inclusion of the background marker may help to separate target QTL from other linked QTL on the far side of the background marker.

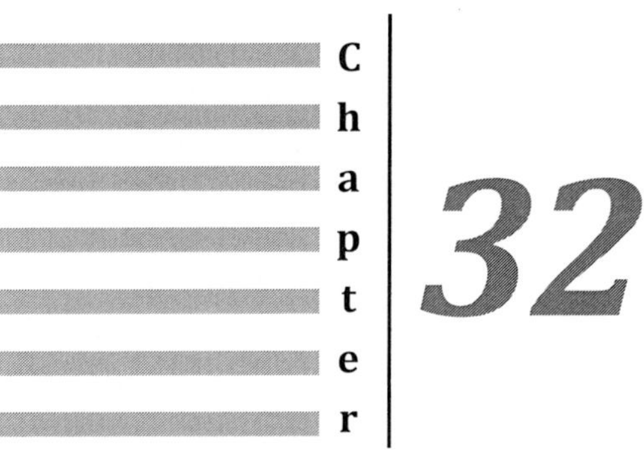

Principles, Methods and Applications of Marker Assisted Selection in Crop Improvement

Marker assisted selection (MAS) is a process whereby a marker (morphological, biochemical or one based on DNA/RNA variation) is used for **indirect selection of a genetic determinant or determinants of a trait of interest** (*i.e.* productivity, disease resistance, abiotic stress tolerance, and/or quality). **Simply MAS refers to indirect selection for a desired plant phenotype based on the banding pattern of linked molecular (DNA) markers.** MAS is based on the concept that it is possible to infer the presence of a gene from the presence of a marker which is tightly linked to the gene of interest. Marker assisted selection (MAS) is also termed as marker aided selection and marker assisted breeding (MAB). Considerable developments in biotechnology have led plant breeders to develop more efficient selection systems to replace traditional phenotypic-pedigree-based selection systems. In MAS trait of interest is selected not based on the trait itself but on a marker linked to it. **So it can be useful for traits that are difficult to measure, exhibit low heritability, and/or are expressed late in development.**

Types of different Markers

Morphological Markers

First markers loci available that have obvious **impact on morphology of plant**. Genes that affect form, colouration, male sterility or resistance among others have been analyzed in many plant species. Examples of this type of marker may include the presence or absence of awn, leaf sheath colouration, height, grain colour, aroma of rice *etc.* In well-characterized crops like maize, tomato, pea, barley or wheat, tens or even hundreds of such genes have been assigned to different chromosomes.

Morphological markers are associated with several general deficits that reduce their usefulness including:

- ✰ The delay of marker expression until late into the development of the organism
- ✰ Dominance
- ✰ Deleterious effects
- ✰ Pleiotropy
- ✰ Confounding effects of genes unrelated to the gene or trait of interest but which also
- ✰ Affect the morphological marker (epistasis)
- ✰ Rare polymorphism
- ✰ Frequent confounding effects of environmental factors which affect the morphological
- ✰ Characteristics of the organism

To avoid problems specific to morphological markers, the DNA-based markers have been developed. They are highly polymorphic, simple inheritance (often codomimant), abundantly occur throughout the genome, easy and fast to detect, minimum pleiotropic effect and detection is not dependent on the developmental stage of the organism.

Numerous markers have been mapped into different chromosomes in several crops including rice, wheat, maize, soybean and several others. Those markers have been used in diversity analysis, parentage detection, DNA fingerprinting, and prediction of hybrid performance. Molecular markers are useful in indirect selection processes, enabling manual selection of individuals for further propagation.

Biochemical Markers

A gene that encodes a protein that can be extracted and observed; for example, isozymes and storage proteins.

Cytological Markers

The chromosomal banding produced by different stains; for example, G banding.

Biological Markers

Different pathogen races or insect biotypes based on host pathogen or host parasite interaction can be used as a marker since the genetic constitution of an organism can affect its susceptibility to pathogens or parasites.

DNA-based and/or Molecular Marker

A unique DNA sequence, occurring in proximity to the gene or locus of interest, can be identified by a range of molecular techniques such as RFLPs, RAPDs, AFLP, DAF, SCARs, microsatellites *etc.*

Gene vs Marker

The gene of interest is directly related with production of protein(s) that produce certain phenotypes whereas markers should not influence the trait of interest but are genetically linked and so go together during segregation of gametes and can be identified in the next generation too. If marker is very close to the gene then accuracy of that marker is too high, increasing the distance between marker and gene the specificity also reduce according to that (**generally distance between marker and gene should be less then 5cM**). In many traits genes are discovered and can be directly assayed for their presence with a high level of confidence. However, if a gene is not isolated marker's help is taken to tag a gene of interest. In such case there may be some false positive results due to recombination between marker of interest and gene (or QTL). A perfect marker would elicit no false positive results.

Important Properties of Ideal Markers for MAS

An ideal marker should be

- ☆ Easy recognition of azl possible phenotypes (homo and heterozygotes) from all different alleles
- ☆ Demonstrates measurable differences in expression between trait types and/or gene of interest alleles, early in the development of the organism
- ☆ Has no effect on the trait of interest that varies depending on the allele at the marker Loci
- ☆ Low or null interaction among the markers allowing the use of many at the same time in a segregating population
- ☆ Abundant in number
- ☆ Polymorphic

Selection for Major Genes Linked to Markers

The major genes which are responsible for economically important characteristics are frequent in the Plant Kingdom. Such characteristics include disease resistance, male sterility, self-incompatibility; others related to shape, colour, and architecture of whole plants and are often of mono- or oligogenic in nature. The marker loci which are tightly linked to major genes can be used for selection and are sometimes more efficient than direct selection for the target gene. The target gene of interest differs between two alleles by a difficult-to-detect single nucleotide polymorphism, an external marker (be it another gene or a polymorphism that is easier to detect, such as a short tandem repeat, RFLP, SCAR *etc.*) may present as the most realistic option (Figure 32.1).

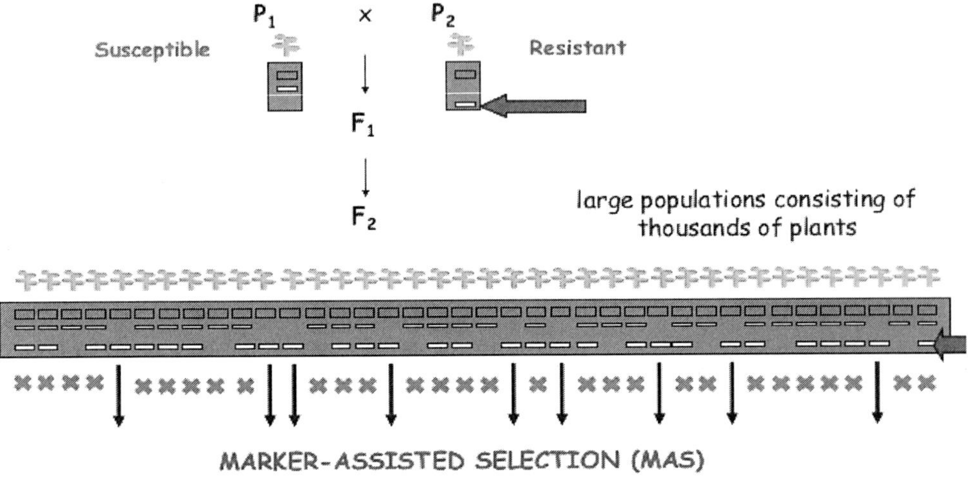

Figure 32.1. Marker Assisted Breeding Method.

Prerequisites for an Efficient Marker-Assisted Selection Program

A. High throughput DNA Extraction

Most breeding programs would need to screen hundreds to thousands of plants for desired marker patterns. In many cases, the results will be needed quickly to allow the breeder to make selections in a timely manner. Both of these considerations demand a DNA extraction system that can handle a large number of samples in a streamlined operation. Many labs conducting MAS extract DNA from small tissue samples in 96- or even 384-well plates.

B. Genetic Markers

The species of interest should have available a technology that allows detection of markers along all of the plant's chromosomes. Although DNA markers have received the most attention, other types of markers (protein, morphological, cytological) can also be used in MAS programs. DNA polymorphisms as markers have the advantages that large numbers are available throughout the genome, their presence or absence is unaffected by environment, and they usually do not directly affect the phenotype. Commonly used DNA markers are referred to by their acronyms: RFLP, SSR, RAPD, AFLP, SCAR, and SNP. Each type of marker has advantages and disadvantages for specific purposes. For efficient MAS, important attributes of markers include:

- ☆ Ease of use

- ☆ Small amount of DNA required
- ☆ Low cost
- ☆ Repeatability of results
- ☆ High rate of polymorphism
- ☆ Occurrence throughout the genome
- ☆ Codominance

This last term (codominance) is the ability to detect both parental forms of a marker in heterozygotes. It is an advantage when heterozygous individuals are screened, such as in backcross breeding programs or in an F_2 population. SSRs, also known as microsatellites, combine the desirable features listed above and are the current marker of choice for many crop species. SNPs require more detailed knowledge of the specific, single nucleotide DNA changes responsible for genetic variation among individuals.

C. Genetic Maps

Linkage maps provide a framework for detecting marker-trait associations and for choosing markers to employ in MAS. Once a marker is found to be associated with a trait in a given population, a dense molecular marker map in a standard reference population will help identify markers that are closer to, or that flank, the target gene

D. Knowledge of Associations between Molecular Markers and Traits of Interest

The most crucial ingredient for MAS is knowledge of markers that are associated with traits important to a breeding program. This information might come from gene mapping or QTL studies, bulked segregant analysis, classical mutant analysis, or some other means.

E. Data Management System

Large numbers of samples are handled in a MAS program, with each sample potentially evaluated for multiple markers. This situation requires an efficient system for labeling, storing, retrieving, and analyzing large data sets, and producing reports useful to the breeder.

Important Steps in Marker Aided Selection

The marker aided selection consists of five important steps, *viz.*: (i) Selection of parents, (ii) Development of breeding population, (iii) Isolation of DNA from each plant, (iv) Scoring RFLPs, and (v) Correlation with morphological traits. In the marker aided selection, among many markers RFLP markers are widely used for genetic improvement of crop plants for various economic characters.

i. Selection of Parents

Selection of suitable parents is an important step in marker aided selection. The parents should be such so that we can get usable level of polymorphism (variation) in the RFLP markers. In other words, parents with contrasting characters or divergent origin should be chosen. This will help in identification of DNA of both the parents and also their segments in F_2 generation in various recombination's. For selection of parents, we have to screen germplasm and select parents with distinct DNA. The parents that are used for MAS should be pure (homozygous). In self- pollinated species, plants are usually homozygous. In cross-pollinated species, inbred lines are used as parents.

ii. Development of Breeding Populations

This is the second important step for application of marker aided selection. The selected parents are crossed to obtain F_1 plants. F_1 plants between two pure-lines or inbred lines are homogeneous (alike phenotypically) but are heterozygous for all the RFLPs of two parents involved in the F_1. The F_2 progeny is required for the study of segregation pattern of RFLPs. Generally 50-100 F_2 plants are sufficient for the study of segregation of RFLP markers.

iii. Isolation of DNA

The third important step is isolation of DNA from breeding population. The main advantage of MAS is that DNA can be isolated even from the seedlings and we need not to wait for flowering or seed development stage. The DNA is isolated from each plant of F_2 population. Standard procedures are available for DNA isolation. The isolated DNA is digested with specific restriction enzyme to obtain fragments of DNA. The DNA fragments of different sizes are separated by subjecting the digested DNA to agarose gel electrophoresis. The gel is stained with ethidium bromide and the variation in DNA fragments can be viewed in the ultraviolet light. The DNA of chloroplasts, when digested with specific enzyme, produces about 40 fragments of different sizes. The nuclear DNA of higher plants, when digested with specific restriction enzymes, produces millions of fragments in a continuous range of sizes. It is a tedious job to identify individual DNA fragment in such cases.

iv. Scoring RFLPs

The polymorphism in RFLPs between the parents and their involvement in the recombinants in F_2 population is determined by using DNA probes. The labelled probes are used to find out the fragments having similarity. The probe will hybridize only with those segments which are complementary in nature. Generally P^{32} is used for radioactive labelling of DNA probe. Now non-radioactive probe labelling techniques are also available. In this way RFLPs are determined.

v. Correlation with Morphological Traits

The DNA marker (say RFLPs) are correlated with morphological markers and the indirect selection through molecular markers is confirmed. Once the correlation of molecular markers is established with morphological markers, MAS can be effectively used for genetic improvement of various economic traits.

Types of Marker Assisted Selection (MAS)

Marker assisted selection (MAS) can be divided into two categories, 1.marker-assisted backcrossing or introgression for a single gene 2. marker-assisted recurrent selection for multiple gene or population improvement. The goal is to incorporate one or few major genes or QTL into elite breeding lines (or in some situations, a breeding population). The second case involves using markers to improve the overall genetic value of a population with respect to some traits. Of the two, marker-assisted backcrossing, particularly of a single gene, is the easiest to put into practice; strategies to use markers in recurrent selection are still being developed and the best strategy for a given situation is not clear at the current time.

1. Marker-Assisted Backcrossing for a Single Gene

Marker-assisted backcrossing is the simplest form of MAS, in which the goal is to incorporate a major gene from an agronomically inferior source or wild relatives (the donor parent) into an elite cultivar (the recurrent parent). The desired outcome is a line containing only the major gene from the donor parent, with the recurrent parent genotype present everywhere else in the genome. Two types of selection are recognized.

Foreground Selection

Foreground selection refers to using markers that are tightly linked to the gene of interest in order to select for the target allele or gene. In which the breeder selects plants having the marker allele of the donor parent at the target locus. The objective is to maintain the target locus in a heterozygous state (one donor allele and one recurrent parent allele) until the final backcross is completed. Then, the selected plants are self-pollinated and progeny plants identified that are homozygous for the donor allele (Figure 32.2).

Background Selection

Background selection refers to using markers that are not tightly linked to the gene of interest to select for recurrent parent alleles at other loci than the target. In which the breeder selects for recurrent parent marker alleles in all genomic regions except the target locus, and the target locus is selected based on phenotype. Background selection is important in order to eliminate potentially deleterious genes introduced from the donor. So-called ‘ linkage drag ’, the inheritance of unwanted donor alleles in the same genomic region as the target locus, is difficult to overcome with conventional backcrossing, but can be addressed efficiently with the use of markers.

In practice, both foreground and background selection are often conducted in the same backcross program, either simultaneously or sequentially. An example of the combined use of foreground and background selection is shown in Figure

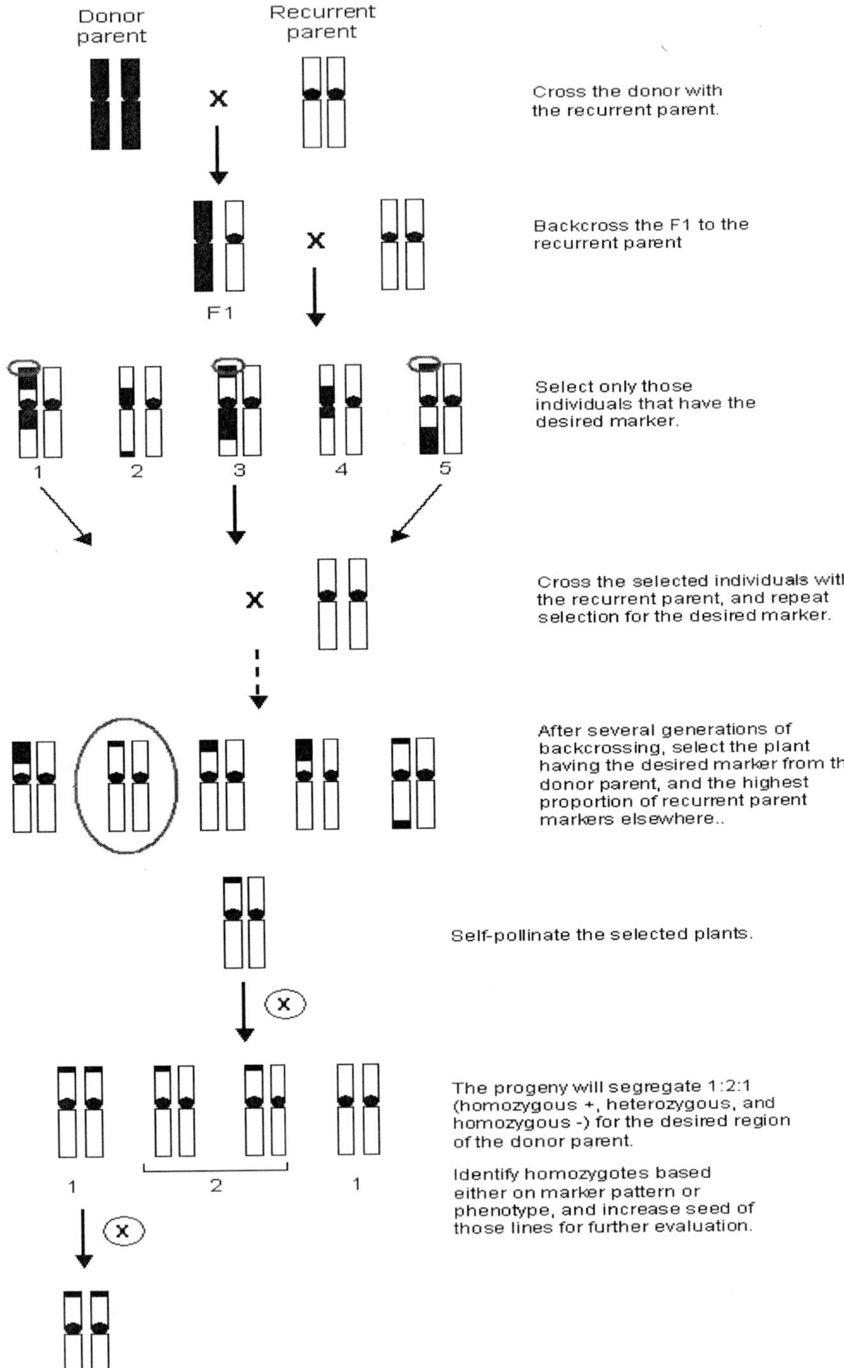

Figure 32.2. Marker-Assisted Backcrossing for Single Gene into an Elite, Recurrent Parent Line.

32.2. For example application of marker-assisted backcrossing has been the introgression of transgenes into an adapted variety or line (*e.g.*, introgression of the Bt insect resistance transgene into different maize genetic backgrounds). Often the target gene can be detected phenotypically, and markers are used to select for the recurrent parent genome. The technique has reportedly accelerated the recovery of the recipient genome by about two backcross generations.

The efficiency of marker-assisted backcrossing depends on a number of factors, including the population size of each backcross generation, distance of markers from the target locus, and number of background markers used. Expected results of a typical marker-assisted backcrossing program, based on simulations of 1000 replicates in table 32.1. In each backcross generation, heterozygotes were selected at the target locus. Recurrent parent alleles were selected at markers flanking the target locus (2 cM on either side) and at three markers on each non-target chromosome.

Table 32.1. Expected Results of a Typical Marker-Assisted Backcrossing Program

Backcross Generation	*Number of Individuals*	*Per cent Homozygosity of Recurrent Parent Alleles at Selected Markers*		*Recurrent Parent Genome*	
		Chromosome with Target Locus	*All other Chromosomes*	*Marker-Assisted Backcross*	*Conventional Backcross*
BC_1	70	38.4	60.6	79.0	75.0
BC_2	100	73.6	87.4	92.2	87.5
BC_3	150	93.0	98.8	98.0	93.7
BC_4	300	100.0	100.0	99.0	96.9

2. Marker-Assisted Selection for Multiple Genes or Population Improvement

Using markers to select for multiple genes is more complex, and less proven, than selection for a single gene. Population sizes required to recover individuals with all the desired marker patterns increase exponentially with the number of genes involved. In a backcrossing scheme, there may be little opportunity to select for the recurrent parent genome, because very few individuals will have the desired marker pattern at all the target loci. If some of the genes are QTLs, whose locations and effects are often imprecisely estimated, then there is uncertainty that the results of MAS will meet expectations. Finally, the more genes undergoing selection, the greater the chance of incorporating unfavorable alleles through linkage drag.

Applications of Marker Assisted Selection (MAS)

MAS in Crop Improvement

MAS has been used for genetic improvement of various characters in different crops. Important characters which have been improved through MAS in different crops include disease resistance, insect resistance, salinity resistance, shattering resistance. MAS has several useful applications in plant breeding. Important applications of MAS in plant breeding are briefly presented below:

1. MAS is very effective, efficient and rapid method of transferring resistance to biotic and abiotic stresses in crop plants.
2. It is useful in gene pyramiding for disease and insect resistance.
3. It has also been used for transfer of various characters such as male sterility, photoperiod insensitivity, earliness, and improvement of protein contents in some crop plants
4. MAS is being used for improvement of quality characters in different crops such as for protein quality in maize, fatty acid (linolenic acid) content in soybean and storage quality in vegetables and fruit crops.
5. MAS can be successfully used for transferring desirable transgene (such as Bt gene) from one cultivar to another.
6. MAS is very effective in introgression of desirable genes from wild into cultivated genotypes.
7. MAS is equally effective in genetic improvement of plants and animals.
8. MAS is useful in genetic improvement of tree species where fruiting takes very long time (say 20 years) because for application of phenotypic selection we have to wait for such a long time.
9. MAS is also being used for genetic improvement of forage and fruit crops. Among fruit crops MAS has been extensively used in pomegranate, apple and pear. In fruit crops MAS is based on RFLP, RAPD, SSR and AFLP markers. In these fruit crops MAS is being used for higher fruit production, better keeping quality for storage and disease resistance.
10. In vegetable crops MAS is being used in tomato and potato based on RFLP, RAPD and AFLP markers mainly for disease resistance. MAS has been found useful for genetic improvement of tree crops such as coconut and rubber.
11. MAS has wide application for genetic improvement of oligogenic traits as compared to polygenic traits.

Achievements of Marker Assisted Selection (MAS)

MAS has been used for genetic improvement of different field crops such as maize, barley, rice, wheat, sorghum, soybean, chickpea, pea, sunflower, tomato, potato and some fruit crops for various economic characters. MAS has been mainly used for developing disease resistant cultivars in different crops. Some notable examples of the use of MAS are given below:

i. Rice

In rice MAS has been successfully used for developing cultivars resistant to bacterial blight and blast. For **bacterial blight resistance four genes (Xa4, Xa5, Xa13 and Xa21)** have been pyramided using STS (sequence tagged site) markers. The pyramided lines showed higher level of resistance to bacterial blight pathogen. In Indonesia, two bacterial blight resistant varieties of rice *viz.*, Angke and Conde have been released through MAS. For blast resistance, three genes (Pil, Piz5 and Pita) have been pyramided in a susceptible rice variety Co 39 using RFLP and PCR based markers.

ii. Maize

In maize, normal lines have been converted into **quality protein maize (QPM) lines through MAS using opaque 2 recessive allele**. This work has been done at CIMMYT (International Centre for Wheat and Maize Improvement, Mexico). Three SSR markers (Umc 1066, Phi 057 and Phi 112) present within opaque 2 gene have been used for this purpose. The MAS used for conversion of normal maize lines into QPM is simple, rapid and accurate.

iii. Soybean

In soybean cyst nematodes pose serious problem and most of the varieties are susceptible to this parasite. The resistant gene (*rhg 1*) is available. In soybean, nematode resistant lines have been developed through MAS using SSR marker (Sat 309).

Advantages of Marker Assisted Selection (MAS)

i. Accuracy

The accuracy of MAS, is very high because molecular markers are not affected by environmental conditions. It is very effective even with the characters having low heritability.

ii. Rapid Method

A minimum of five or six-backcross generations are required to transfer a gene of interest from a donor (may not be adapted) to a recipient (recurrent – adapted cultivar). MAS is a rapid method of crop improvement. The recovery of the recurrent genotype can be accelerated with the use of molecular markers. If the F_1 is heterozygous for the marker locus, individuals with the recurrent parent allele(s) at the marker locus in first or subsequent backcross generations will also carry a chromosome tagged by the marker. It takes 3-5 years for developing a new cultivar against 10-15 years taken by the conventional method of breeding (Figure 32.3).

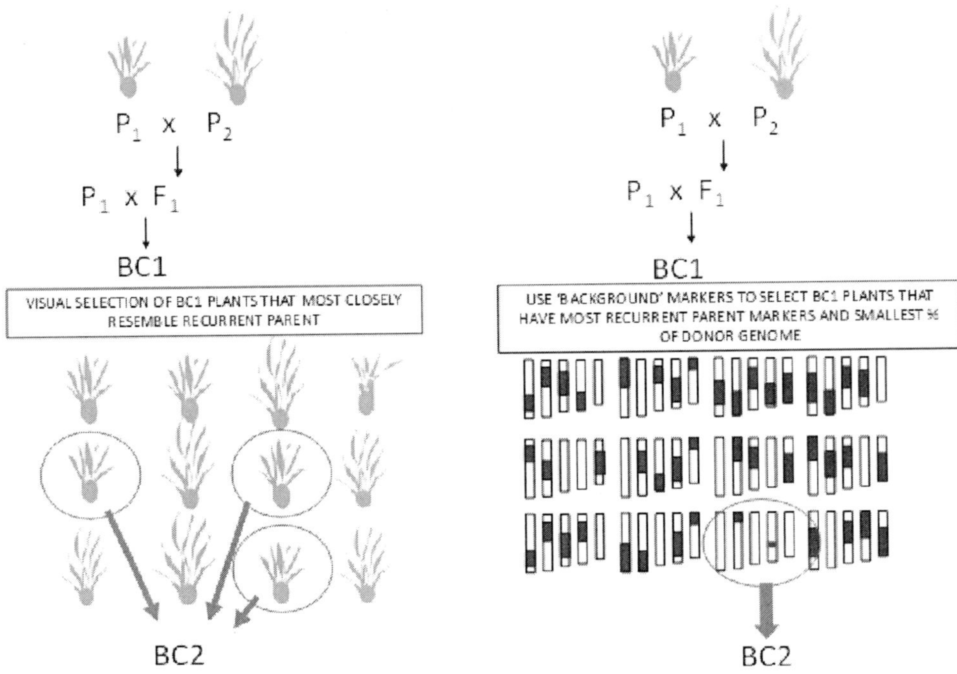

Figure 32.3. Difference between Conventional and Marker Assisted Selection Method.

iii. Non-transgenic Product

MAS leads to development of non-transgenic cultivars which are acceptable to everybody. In other words, it does not involve transgene. Hence there is no question of gene silencing.

iv. Identification of Recessive Alleles

MAS permits identification of recessive alleles even in heterozygous condition and thus speeds up the progress of crop improvement programmes. In other words, it is equally effective for the genetic improvement of recessive characters.

v. Early Detection of Traits

MAS permits early detection of traits that are expressed late in the life of plant. For example characters such as grain or fruit quality, flower colour, male sterility, photoperiod sensitivity that express late in the life of a plant can be screened in the seedling stage. In other words, DNA tested at seedling stage can through light about the trait which are expressed later on.

vi. Screening of Difficult Traits

MAS permits screening traits that are extremely difficult expressive and time consuming to score phenotypically. For example, screening for traits such as root morphology and resistance to biotic (insects and diseases) and abiotic stresses (drought, salinity, heat, frost *etc.*) is very easy through MAS.

vii. Gene Pyramiding

MAS is very effective method in accumulating multiple genes for resistance to specific pathogens and pests within the same cultivar. This process is called gene pyramiding. Gene pyramiding has been proposed and applied to enhance resistance to disease and insects by selecting for two or more than two genes at a time. For example in rice such pyramids have been developed against bacterial blight and blast. The advantage of use of markers in this case allows selecting for QTL-allele-linked markers that have same phenotypic effect. Maker assisted backcrossing is routinely applied in breeding programmes for gene introgression. MAS can provide an effective and efficient breeding tool for detecting, tracking, retaining, combining and pyramiding genes for disease resistance.

viii. Small Sample for Testing

MAS requires only a small amount of plant tissue for DNA testing. In other words, MAS can be carried out with small breeding populations. Moreover, MAS can be applied at any stage of plant growth.

ix. Permits QTL Mapping

MAS permits mapping or tagging of quantitative trait loci (QTL) which is not possible by conventional method.

x. Highly Reproducible

The MAS is based on DNA fingerprinting technique and the results of DNA fingerprinting pattern are highly reliable and reproducible.

Limitations of Marker Assisted Selection (MAS)

1. MAS is a costly method. It requires well equipped laboratory *viz.* expensive equipment's, glassware and chemicals.
2. MAS requires well trained manpower for handling of sophisticated equipments, isolation of DNA molecule and study of DNA markers.
3. The detection of various linked DNA markers (AFLP, RFLP, RAPD, SSR, SNP *etc.*) is a difficult, laborious and time consuming task.
4. MAS sometimes involves use of radioactive isotopes in labelling of DNA, which may lead to serious health hazards. This is a major disadvantage of RFLP based markers. The PCR, markers are safe in this regard.
5. It has been reported that MAS may become less efficient than phenotypic selection in the long term.
6. The use of MAS is more difficult for QTL because they have minor cumulative effects and are greatly influenced by environmental conditions and genetic background.

Table 32.2 .Commercially Available MAS-Varieties Developed in India

Plant	*Cultivar/ Breeding Line*	*Trait*	*Year of Release*	*Institute*
Maize	Vivek QPM 9	High-Quality Protein	2008	ICAR
Pearl Millet	HHB 67-2	Disease resistance	2005	HAU/ICRISAT
Rice	MAS 946-1	Drought- tolerance	2007	UAS
Rice	Pusa 1460	Disease resistance	2007	IARI
Rice	RP Bio 226	Disease resistance	2007	DRR

Table 32.3. Genetic Improvement through MAS in Different Crops

Crop	*Disease Resistance*	*Insect Resistance*	*Other Traits*
Rice	Bacterial blight Blast Rice Tungro virus Gall midge	Brow plant hopper Green leaf hopper	Submergence tolerance Salt tolerance Temperature sensitivity Male sterility Photoperiod sensitivity Semidwarf stature Shattering resistance Grain Aroma Amylose content
Maize	Northern corn blight	–	Cytoplasmic male sterility QPM Days to pollen shed
Wheat	Leaf rust Powdery mildew Loose smut	Hessian fly	Cyst rematode Root lesion nematode Earliness Vernalization requirement Coleoptile colour Flour colour
Sorghum	Head smut	–	Fertility restoration
Soybean	Cyst nematode Mosaic Virus	–	Linolenic acid Content
Pea	Fusarium wilt Powdery mildew	–	Nodulation ability
Tomato	Yellow leaf curl virus Black mold Bacterial wilt	–	–
Potato	Cyst nematode Potato virus x Late blight	–	–
Sunflower	Downy mildew	–	–
Chick pea	–	–	Double podding
Barley	Powdery mildew Stripe rust	– –	–
Mung bean	Powdery mildew	–	–

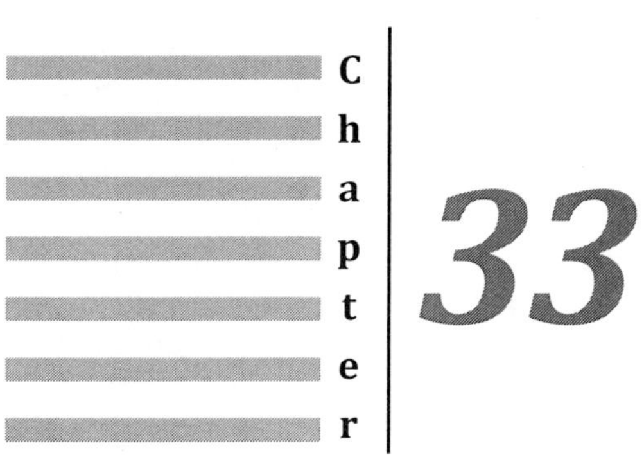

Applications of Plant Genomics and Genome Databases

Genomics

Studying and characterizing the physical nature and function of whole genome of an organism is called as genomics. Based upon the nature of analysis it is divided into two groups 1. Structural genomics; 2. Functional genomics.

Structural Genomics

The prime directive of structural genomic analysis is the complete and accurate elucidation of the DNA sequence of a representative haploid genome of a given species.

Functional Genomics

Functional genomics is the branch studying and characterizing the **transcriptome** *i.e.*, the entire range of transcripts produced by a given organism.

When the sequence is known, it opens the door to numerous possibilities. Development of genomic technologies that ultimately permitted sequencing of complex genomes, inturn it helped step-by-step progression in genome-wide map resolution, development of high-resolution genetic and physical mapping. Computational analysis of the sequence, transcripts and proteins based upon the principles developed by genetic, molecular and biological analysis, it is possible to make predictions of all of the encoded proteins. The available information in database helps us to analyze other haploid genomes from the same species and develop a statistical picture of the genetic variation within populations of that species. Also by comparison of the genomic sequence of different species can be able to understand, how the genome has been remodeled in the course of evolution. Studies of comparative genomics have already proceeded far enough to reveal that, in related species, there is considerable synteny (conserved gene location within large blocks of the genome). Studies of comparative genomics also offer a powerful opportunity to identify highly conserved and functionally important sequence motifs in coding and noncoding genomic DNA. This identification helps researchers confirm predictions of protein-coding regions of the genome and identify important regulatory elements within DNA.

Application of Genomics in Crop Improvement

Genomics is playing an increasing role in plant breeding and this is accelerating with the rapid advances in genome technology. Translating the vast abundance of data being produced by genome technologies requires the development of custom bioinformatics tools and advanced databases. These range from large generic databases which hold specific data types for a broad range of species, to carefully integrated and curated databases which act as a resource for the improvement of specific crops. Plant genomics will revolutionize the study of the molecular basis of plant biology. The traditional hypothesis-driven approach will be gradually transformed into an unbiased data collection at the tissue/organism level approach followed by bioinformatic analyses. Some of the important applications of genomics in crop improvement are listed below,

1. Construction of Genetic Map

The development of molecular markers has allowed for constructing complete genetic maps for most economically important plant species. **A genetic map represents the ordering of molecular markers along chromosomes as well as the genetic distances, generally expressed as centi Morgans (cM), existing between adjacent molecular markers.** Genetic maps contribute to the understanding of how plant genomes are organized and once available they facilitate the development of practical applications in plant breeding, such as the identification of Quantitative Trait Loci (QTL) and Marker Assisted Selection (MAS). Genetic maps are also an important resource for plant gene isolation, establish the extent of genome colinearity and duplication between different species.

2. Physical Maps

Physical maps can be defined as a set of large insert clones with minimum overlap encompassing a given chromosome. Physical maps provide the bridge needed between the resolution achieved by genetic maps and that needed to isolate genes. Although genetic maps provide much-needed landmarks along chromosomes, they are still too far apart to provide an entry point into genes, since even in model plants the kilobases per cent iMorgan (kb/cM) ratio is large, from 120 to 250 kb/cM in *Arabidopsis* and between 500 and 1.500 kb/cM in corn. Therefore, a 1 cM interval may harbor ~30 to 100 or even more genes. Physical maps bridge such gaps, representing the entire DNA fragment spanning the genetic location of adjacent molecular markers.

3. Whole Genome Sequencing

Genetic and physical maps represent a key layer of genomic information at the inter- or intra-species level. However, sequence data represents the ultimate level of genetic information. Three major breakthroughs have allowed the sequencing of complete genomes: 1) The development of fluorescence-based DNA sequencing methods that provide at least 500 bases per read; 2) The automation of several processes such as picking and arraying bacterial subclones, purification of DNA from individual subclones and sample loading among others; and 3) The development of software and hardware able to handle massive amounts (Giga bytes) of data points.

4. Development of ESTs

Large scale sequencing facilities allow the development of ESTs, **also known as single pass sequences of random cDNAs. ESTs are derived from the 3' end of transcripts and are expected to contain sequences including 3' untranslated regions (UTR) and to extend toward the 5' end,** thus reaching exons. Their average length in plant species is ~350-650 bp. Searches for homology with known genes from other species allows the assignment of putative biological functions to ESTs. The use of ESTs also permits the identification of genes encoding functionally unknown proteins. A comparison of EST databases from different species and tissues reveals the diversity in coding sequences between plants and a global perspective on the similarities in genes for specific tissues or conditions. ESTs are also important in establishing expression/transcription maps, since their placement on a genetic map provides the precise location of genes. This helps us understand how genes belonging to a pathway or a given gene family are distributed across the genome. Furthermore, they provide anchors by which physical and genetic maps can be aligned.

Research focusing on improving the nutritional quality of plant products reflects the value of EST programs in plant gene discovery. An EST from *Arabidopsis* allowed for the isolation of the gene *p*-hydroxyphenylpyruvate dioxygenase in *Synechocystis* PCC6803. This enzyme enables the first committed step in the synthesis of plastoquinones and tocopherols in plants and subsequently other steps of vitamin E synthesis. This led to the development of transgenic *Arabidopsis* plants with increased levels of vitamin E levels in oil. For species other than rice or *Arabidopsis*, large-scale EST sequencing provides an excellent and cost-effective way of obtaining valuable information on transcribed genes. ESTs are a highly effective gene discovery tool, and approximately 60 per cent of putatively identified *Arabidopsis* genes have been tagged with ESTs. Furthermore, they have provided the platform necessary for transcriptional profiling experiments. EST sequencing programs, therefore, provide a powerful lead into genomic approaches in plants

5. Quantitative Trait Loci Analysis

Most economically important plant traits such as yield; plant height and quality components exhibit a continuous distribution rather than discrete classes and are regarded as quantitative traits. These traits are controlled by several loci each of small effect and different combinations of alleles at these loci can give different phenotypes. **Quantitative Trait Loci (QTL) analysis refers to the identification of genomic regions associated with the phenotypic expression of a given trait.** Once the location of such genomic regions is known they can be assembled into designer genotypes, *i.e.* individuals carrying chromosomic fragments associated with the expression of a given phenotype. The most important feature of Marker Assisted Selection (MAS) is that once a molecular marker genetically linked to the expression of a phenotypically interesting allele has been detected, an indirect selection for such allele based upon the detection of the molecular marker can be accomplished, since little or any genetic recombination will occur between them. Therefore, the presence of the molecular marker will always be associated with the presence of the allele of interest.

6 Comparative Genome Mapping

A remarkable feature of plant genomics is its ability to bring together more than one species for analysis. **The comparative genome mapping of related plant species has shown that the organization of genes is highly conserved during the evolution of members of taxonomic families.** This has led to the identification of genome colinearity between the well-sequenced model crops and their related species (*e.g. Arabidopsis* for dicots and rice for monocots). Colinearity overrides the differences in chromosome number and genome size and can be defined as conservation of gene order within a chromosomal segment between different species.

7. Parallel Analysis of Gene Expression

While molecular biology generally analyzes one or a few genes simultaneously, recent developments allow the parallel analysis of thousands of genes. **This area of genomics involves the study of gene expression patterns across a wide array of cellular responses, phenotypes and conditions.** The expression profile of a developmental stage or induced condition can identify genes and coordinately regulated pathways and their functions. This produces a more thorough understanding of the underlying biology. There are several systems available to analyze the parallel expression of many genes such as macroarrays, microarrays and **Serial Analysis of Gene Expression (SAGE),** which consists of identifying short sequence tags from individual transcripts, their concatenation, sequencing and subsequent digital quantitation. SAGE provides expression levels for many transcripts across different stages of development.

8. Genome-Wide Expression Profiling

Microarray applications are broadly classified as expression-specific and genome-wide expression studies. In specific expression studies, **they are used**

as a functional genomics tool to address the biological significance of genes discovered through large scale sequencing, as well as a means to understanding the genetic networks explaining biological processes or biochemical pathways. The value of using microarrays to identify novel response genes has been demonstrated by studying the gene expression patterns during corn embryo development, the response to drought and cold stresses, herbivory, and nitrate treatments. Genome-wide arrays are mostly designed for model organisms such as *Arabidopsis* or rice, as there are many genes available to select from, either as clones or as annotated genomic sequences for model species. They are also available to species such as corn that have extensive EST collections. **Genome-wide expression profiles are the ultimate tool to integrate all genes existing in an organism into a series of experiments.** They also help to elucidate the coordinate expression of different genetic networks and document how changes in one would impact others. It is expected that such genome-wide approaches will be particularly useful in identifying new regulatory sequences and master switches that affect distinct but apparently unrelated genetic networks.

9. Transcriptional Profiling

Transcriptional profiling technologies play a central role in predicting gene function since sequence comparison alone is insufficient to infer function. They also help to detect phenomena such as gene displacement non-homologous genes coding for proteins that serve the same function- and gene recruitment genes with identical sequences coding for completely different functions. Unlike animals, plants cannot move and have developed exquisite mechanisms to cope with changing environmental conditions and biotic challenges, since these directly or indirectly affect most biological processes occurring in plants. Therefore, a significant proportion of the information gathered by specific and genome wide transcription profiling processes should have practical applications and facilitate the development of plants more resilient to biotic and abiotic stimuli.

10. Reverse Genetics

Traditional genetic analysis aims to **identify the DNA sequences associated with a given phenotype. Reverse genetics determines the function of a gene for which the sequence is known, by generating and analyzing the phenotype of the corresponding knockout mutant.** Unlike yeast, in which gene disruption is available through homologous recombination, transposon and T-DNA tagging are the best methods available for developing mutagenized plant populations suitable for reverse genetics studies.

Genome Databases

Genomics is playing an increasing role in plant breeding and this is accelerating with the rapid advances in genome technology. Translating the vast abundance of data being produced by genome technologies requires the development of custom bioinformatics tools and advanced databases. These range from large generic databases which hold specific data types for a broad range of species, to carefully integrated and curated databases which act as a resource for the improvement of specific crops.

Genome Databases for Multiple Plant Species

- Gramene (http://www.gramene.org/) is an EnsEMBL-based genome viewer and database hosting information on a variety of crop species, but based around the rice, maize and Arabidopsis genomes.
- PlantGDB is a resource for comparative plant genomics and hosts sequence data for >70,000 plant species with a focus on complete sequencing of reference species, *Arabidopsis*, rice, maize and *Medicago truncatula.*
- Plaza (http://bioinformatics.psb.ugent.be/plaza/) hosts pre-computed comparative genomics data sets for a range of plant species.
- Panzea (http://www.panzea.org/) which hosts data on genomic diversity in a large germplasm collection including genetic data, trait phenotypes, allele frequencies, phenotyping environments, genetic analysis tools and so on. The Panzea databases comprises the genotypic and phenotypic data and genetic marker information. This database design is based on the Genomic Diversity and Phenotype Data Model (GDPDM) (http://www.maizegenetics.net/gdpdm/).

Expressed Sequence Tag

CR-EST

An expressed sequence tag (EST) represents a short sub-sequence of a cDNA sequence. EMBL or GenBank have sub-sections for EST sequences. The crop expressed sequence tag database, CR-EST(http://pgrc.ipk-gatersleben.de/cr-est/), provides access to more than 2,00,000 sequences derived from 41 cDNA libraries of four species: barley, wheat, pea and potato.

Simple Sequence Repeat (SSR)

SSR Primer

SSRs are short stretches of DNA sequence occurring as tandem repeats of mono-, di-, tri-, tetra-,penta- and hexa-nucleotides. They are highly polymorphic due to mutation affecting the number of repeat units. The value of SSRs is due to their genetic co-dominance, abundance, dispersal throughout the genome, multi-allelic variation and high reproducibility. The hypervariability of SSRs among related organisms makes them excellent markers for genotype identification, analysis of genetic diversity, phenotype mapping and marker assisted selection. SSRs demonstrate a high degree of transferability between species, as PCR primers designed to an SSR within one species frequently amplify a corresponding locus in related species, enabling comparative genetic and genomic analysis. SSR Primer (http://flora.acpfg.com.au/ssrprimer2/) is a web-based tool that enables the real time discovery of SSRs within submitted DNA sequences, with the concomitant design of PCR primers for SSR amplification.

SSR Taxonomy Tree

Alternatively, users may browse an SSR Taxonomy Tree http://appliedbioinformatics.com.au/projects/ssrtaxonomy/php/) to identify pre-determined SSR amplification primers for species represented within the GenBank database.

Single Nucleotide Polymorphism (SNPs)

autoSNP

SNPs are the ultimate form of molecular genetic marker, as a nucleotide base is the smallest unit of inheritance, and a SNP represents a single-nucleotide difference between two individuals at a defined location. SNPs are direct markers as the sequence information provides the exact nature of the allelic variants. Furthermore, this sequence variation can have a major impact on how the organism develops and responds to the environment. SNPs represent the most frequent type of genetic polymorphism and may therefore provide a high density of markers near a locus of interest. The high density of SNPs makes them valuable for genome mapping, and in particular they allow the generation of ultra-high density genetic maps and haplotyping systems for genes or regions of interest, and map-based positional cloning. SNPs are used routinely in crop breeding programs, for genetic diversity analysis, cultivar identification, phylogenetic analysis, characterization of genetic resources and association with agronomic traits. mThe SNP discovery software autoSNP identifies SNPs and insertion/deletion (indel) polymorphisms from bulk sequence data using two measures of confidence; redundancy, defined as the number of times a polymorphism occurs at a locus in a sequence alignment; and co-segregation of SNPs to define a haplotype.

autoSNPdb

AutoSNP software has recently been extended to database format, autoSNPdb, which permits complex queries and provides detailed genomic and functional information. Where the sequence trace files are available.

PolyPhred

The SNP discovery tool PolyPhred can make use of the base pair quality scores to further differentiate between true SNP polymorphisms and random sequence error. The recent developments in next-generation sequence data have led to the identification of large numbers of SNPs in a range of plant genomes and these approaches are likely to dominate SNP discovery in the coming years. The increased throughput for the discovery and application of molecular genetic markers has led to the requirement for databases hosting the results of molecular marker analysis.

These maybe integrated within other database systems such as Gramene, the Legume Information System (LIS) or Graingenes.

Mendel - Plant Gene Nomenclature Database

The Mendel database project aims to develop a common nomenclature for sequenced genes, based on gene families, for all photosynthetic organisms, the organelle genomes of both photosynthetic and non-photosynthetic organisms (fungi, algae, and protozoa) and plant viruses.

The Mendel database contains information on:

- Gene Name
- Gene synonym
- Accession number
- Gene product name and synonym
- Information on expression (in a few cases at present)

NCBI

The National Center for Biotechnology Information (NCBI) provides access to genomic information in order to advance science. The genome database currently comprises of 16,326 species and can be sorted by kingdom, group and subgroup.

PGDJ DNA Marker and Linkage Database

The Plant Genome Database Japan's DNA Marker and Linkage Database brings together information from smaller databases and literature. Information on the organism, genome (for example, chromosome number and genome size), markers and genome specific databases can be accessed.

Phytozome

Phytozome (http://www.phytozome.net/) is a plant comparative genomics portal wherein families of related genes representing the modern descendants of ancestral genes are constructed at key phylogenetic nodes. Currently *Phytozome* provides access to 58 sequenced and annotated green plant genomes. Phytozome is one of the most comprehensive plant genome databases currently available.

Plant rDNA Database

The Plant rDNA Database comprises of data from over 600 publications and approximately 3000 plant species. It provides information on the numbers and positions of ribosomal DNA signals and their structures. Where possible, information on ploidy level, chromosome number, genome size and life cycle is also available.

PlantGDB Genome Browser

The Plant GDB Genome Browser displays current gene structure models and transcript evidence from spliced alignments of EST and cDNA sequences. If applicable, matched GSS contigs, community annotations, similar proteins, and microarray probes are displayed.

PTGBase

PTGBase is an integrated database to study tandem repeated genes in plants. Currently *PTGBase* comprises of 39 plant species arrayed in 54,130 tandem repeat gene clusters containing 129,652 genes. Scientists can extract the full list of repeat genes, their coding sequences and protein sequences, as well as whole genome sets about sequenced plant species. A search function can be used to find a target gene, tandem array name and gene numbers of tandem array in a specific species.

The International Crop Information System (ICIS)

The linking of genomic data with agronomic traits remains one of the greatest challenges in the application of genome data for crop improvement. Several databases have been developed to assist in this endeavor. The International Crop Information System (ICIS) is a database system that hosts integrated management information for crop improvement, including details on diverse germplasm and traits. One challenge in developing trait databases is the establishment of functional ontologies. The Plant Ontology (http://www.plantontology.org/) is a controlled vocabulary (ontology) that describes plant anatomy and morphology and stages of growth and development for all plants and this database of ontologies is becoming the standard for comparative physiology and for linking genes with potential function.

CMap

One of the principal uses of molecular genetic markers is the production of genetic maps and the mapping of heritable traits. While mapping data may be described as lists, graphical representations are more readily understood. The genetic map viewer CMap, developed by the GMOD consortium is valuable for the validation of traits that map to the same position in different populations and also for the linkage between crop genetic maps and sequenced model genomes, enabling the identification of candidate genes for genetically mapped traits. A recent addition, CMap3D, enables the comparison of a larger number of maps in 3D space.

Species Focused Databases

It would be impossible to detail all available plant genetic and genomic databases, however some of the main ones are listed below along with a brief description of their content.

GrainGenes

GrainGenes (http://wheat.pw.usda.gov/) is a genetic database for Triticeae, oats, and sugarcane. Comprehensive information includes genetic markers, map locations, alleles, key references and disease symptoms.

Maize

The maize genome was sequenced in 2009 and there are several databases hosting information on this important crop. These include MaizeGDB (http://www.maizegdb.org/) based on GBrowse, and maizesequence.org (http://www.maizesequence.org/) based on EnsEMBL.

Rice

Rice was one of the first crop genomes to be sequenced and there are now numerous resources available to mine this genomic information. Oryza base is an integrated rice science database established in 2000 (http://www.shigen.nig.ac.jp/rice/oryzabase/). The database hosts information on genetic resources, chromosome maps, genes and rice mutants. This is complemented by a rice genome annotation project which presents data using GBrowse (http://rice.plantbiology.msu.edu/).

Wheat

Although wheat is an extremely important crop, advances in genomics have been limited by its large and highly complex genome. Assemblies of the gene rich regions for the group 7 chromosomes have been completed and annotated sequences, including a large number of SNP polymorphisms are available at http://www.wheatgenome.info.

Brassica

A central portal for *Brassica* data is maintained at Brassica.info, with links to genetic marker, map and a range of diverse Brassica related information. The recently sequenced *Brassica rapa* genome is hosted at http://brassicadb.org/in a database named BRAD, with a second database which contains *Brassica* repeat information at http://www.BrassicaGenome.net.

Legume

The Legume Information System (http://www.comparative-legumes.org/) supports basic research in the legumes by relating data from multiple crop and model species, and by helping researchers traverse among various data types. It currently hosts data for seventeen species and includes GBrowse databases for *Glycine max* (soybean), *Lotus japonicus* (birdsfoot trefoil), *Medicago truncatula* (barrel medic) and *Cajanus cajan* (pigeonpea). Lis is complemented by detailed soybean data hosted at SoyBase (http://soybase.org/).

Table 33.1. Examples of Genomic Databases Related to Crop Improvement

Database Name	Web Link
autoSNPdb	http://autosnpdb.appliedbioinformatics.com.au/
Brachypodium database	http://www.brachypodium.org/
Brassica genome gateway	http://www.brassicagenome.net
Brassica rapa genome database	http://brassicadb.org/
DNA Data Bank of Japan (DDBJ)	http://ddbj.sakura.ne.jp/
European bioinformatics institute EnsEMBL plants	http://plants.ensembl.org/
European Molecular Biology Laboratory (EMBL) nucleotide sequence database	http://www.ebi.ac.uk/embl/
GenBank	http://www.ncbi.nlm.nih.gov/genbank/
Graingenes	http://wheat.pw.usda.gov/
Gramene	http://www.gramene.org/
International Crop Information System (ICIS)	http://www.icis.cgiar.org
International Nucleotide Sequence Database Collaboration (INSDC)	http://www.insdc.org/
Legume Information System (LIS)	http://www.comparative-legumes.org/
MaizeGDB	http://www.maizegdb.org/
Maize sequence database	http://www.maizesequence.org/
Oryzabase	http://www.shigen.nig.ac.jp/rice/oryzabase/
Panzea	http://www.panzea.org/
Phytozome	http://www.phytozome.net/
PlantsDB	http://mips.helmholtz-muenchen.de/plant/genomes.jsp
PlantGDB	http://www.plantgdb.org/
The Plant Ontology	http://www.plantontology.org/
Plaza	http://bioinformatics.psb.ugent.be/plaza/
Rice Genome Annotation Project	http://rice.plantbiology.msu.edu/
SSR taxonomy tree	http://appliedbioinformatics.com.au/projects/ssrtaxonomy/php/
SOL Genomics Network (SGN)	http://solgenomics.net/
SoyBase	http://soybase.org/
TAGdb	http://flora.acpfg.com.au/tagdb/
The Crop Expressed Sequence Tag database, CR-EST	http://pgrc.ipk-gatersleben.de/cr-est/
The Triticeae Repeat Sequence Database (TREP)	http://wheat.pw.usda.gov/ITMI/Repeats/
Wheat genome information	http://www.wheatgenome.info

Solanaceae

The SOL Genomics Network (SGN) (http://solgenomics.net/) is a clade oriented database containing genomic, genetic, phenotypic and taxonomic information for plant genomes, with a focus on the Euasterid clade, which includes Solanaceae (*e.g.* tomato, potato, eggplant, pepper)

BeanRef

A collection of references about different aspects of research on beans (Phaseolus/Vigna). BeanRef contains addresses, short descriptions, and links to germplasm collections, genetic maps, conferences, organizations, mailing list, and newsletters.

MaizeDB Maize Genome Database

This project is part of the National Agricultural Library's Plant Genome Research Program. This provides access to Maize-related information in a variety of formats.

SoyBase: Metabolic Database

The metabolic component of SoyBase, a soybean genetic database, contains reaction and pathway descriptions and diagrams for a number of basic metabolic pathways.

Genome Size in Asteraceae Database

The Genome Size in Asteraceae Database is an exhaustive catalogue of genome size data for the family Asteraceae, making Asteraceae genome size data easily accessible to scientists. Genome sizes are currently available for 1,219 species based on 2,768 records from 133 publications, covering approximately 5 per cent of species, 10 per cent of genera, 40 per cent of tribes and 50 per cent of subfamilies.

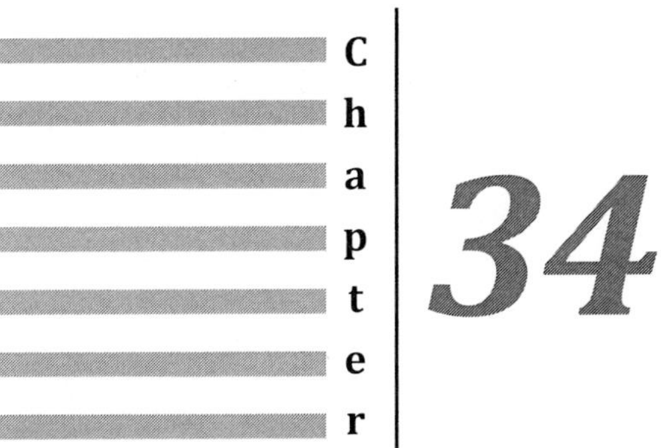

Basics of Bioinformatics

Introduction

Bioinformatics is the application of information technology to the field of molecular biology. **Bioinformatics entails the creation and advancement of databases, algorithms, computational and statistical techniques, and theory to solve formal and practical problems arising from the management and analysis of biological data**. Other terms goes together or close with bioinformatics are computational molecular biology or computational systems biology and computational biology. **Computational biology is a broad term, which covers all efforts of scientific investigations on or related with biology that involve mathematics and computation.** Computational molecular biology, concentrates on the molecular aspects of biology in computational biology, which therefore has more or less the same meaning with bioinformatics. The word "computational" does not only mean "with computers," but it refers **to data analysis with mathematical, statistical, and algorithmatic methods, most of which need to be implemented with computer programs.** As computational biology or bioinformatics mainly studies the biology with quantitative data, sio it also can be called as quantitative biology. Most molecules do not work independently in living cells and most biological functions are accomplished by the harmonic interaction of multiple molecules. In recent years, the new term systems biology also become more related to Bioinformatics**. Systems biology studies cells and organisms as systems of multiple molecules and their interactions with the environment. Bioinformatics plays key roles in analyzing such systems.**

For a certain period, it was thought that bioinformatics as the development of software tools that help to store, manipulate, and analyze biological data. While this is still an important role of bioinformatics, but now realized that bioinformatics should do more. As the advancement of modern biochemistry, biophysics, and biotechnologies is enabling people to accumulate massive data of multiple aspects of biology in an exponential manner. Scientists begin to believe that bioinformatics and computational biology must play a key role for understanding biology. People are studying bioinformatics in different ways. Some people are devoted to developing new computational tools, both from software and hardware viewpoints, for the better handling and processing of biological data. They develop new models and new algorithms for existing questions and propose and tackle new questions when new experimental techniques bring in new data. Other people take the study of bioinformatics as the study of biology with the viewpoint of informatics and systems. These people also develop tools when needed, but they are more interested in understanding biological procedures and mechanisms. They do not restrict their research to computational study, but try to integrate computational and experimental investigations.

The primary goal of bioinformatics is to increase our understanding of biological processes. Major research efforts in the field include sequence analysis, genome annotation, computational evolutionary biology, measuring biodiversity, analysis of gene expression, analysis of gene regulation, analysis of protein expression, prediction of protein structure, comparative genomics, modelling biological systems, high-throughput image analysis and protein-protein docking.

Definitions

Bioinformatics

Bioinformatics is the science concerned with the development and application of computer hardware and software to the acquisition, storage, analysis, visualization, manipulation and interpretation of biological information especially data of nucleic acids, amino acids and studies molecular rules and systems that govern or affect the structure, function and evolution of various forms of life.

Bioinformatics Databases

A database is a collection of information that is organized so that it can be easily accessed, managed and updated. Creation and maintenance of bioinformatics database to store biological information such as nucleotide and amino acid sequences. They offer scientists the opportunity to access and analyze a wide variety of biologically relevant sequence, structural and functional data of an increasingly broad range of organisms. Biological databases play a central role in bioinformatics.

Bioinformatic Tools

Bioinformatic tools are software programs that are designed for extracting the meaningful information from the mass of data stored in bioinformatics databases and to carry out the necessary analysis for better understanding about that particular system.

Major Categories of Bioinformatics Tools

These can be classified as homology and similarity tools, protein functional analysis tools, structural analysis tool, sequence analysis tools and miscellaneous tools.

1. Homology and Similarity Tools

Homologous sequences are sequences that are related by divergence from a common ancestor. Thus the degree of similarity between two sequences can be measured while their homology is a case of being either true of false. This set of tools can be used to identify similarities between novel query sequences of unknown structure and function and database sequences whose structure and function have been elucidated.

2. Protein Function Analysis

This group of programs allow you to compare your protein sequence to the secondary (or derived) protein databases that contain information on motifs, signatures and protein domains. Highly significant hits against these different pattern databases allow you to approximate the biochemical function of your query protein.

3. Structural Analysis

This set of tools allow you to compare structures with the known structure databases. The function of a protein is more directly a consequence of its structure rather than its sequence with structural homologs tending to share functions. The determination of a protein's 2D/3D structure is crucial in the study of its function.

4. Sequence Analysis

This set of tools allows you to carry out further, more detailed analysis on your query sequence including evolutionary analysis, identification of mutations, hydropathy regions, CpG islands and compositional biases. The identification of these and other biological properties are all clues that aid the search to elucidate the specific function of your sequence.

Bioinformatics Databases

In recent years, biological databases have greatly developed, and became a part of the biologist's everyday toolbox. There are several reasons to search databases, for instance:

1. When obtaining a new DNA sequence, one needs to know whether it has already been deposited in the databanks fully or partially, or whether they contain any **homologous sequences** (sequences which are descended from a common ancestor).
2. Some of the databases contain annotation which has already been added to a specific sequence. Finding annotation for the searched sequence or its **homologous sequences** can facilitate its research.

3. Find similar non-coding DNA stretches in the database for instance repeat elements or regulatory sequences.
4. Other uses for specific purpose, like designing oligonucleotide for priming sites for a set of PCR Primars.
5. Search for homologous proteins- proteins similar in their sequence and therefore also in their presumed folding or structure or function

Primary Sequence Databases

In the early 1980's **European Molecular Biology Laboratory (EMBL)** established their DATA library to collect, organize and distribute nucleotide sequence data and related information. This function is now performed by the **European Bioinformatics Institute (EBI)** Hinxton,U.K. During early **1980s the National Centre for Bioinformatics Information (NCBI)** was established in U.S.A.NCBI serves as primary information databank and provider of information. Some time later, **DNA Data Bank Japan (DDBJ) was established in Japan**. The National Biomedical Research Foundation established **Protein Information Resourse (PIR) in 1984**. PIR helps researchers in the identification and interpretation protein sequence information. Several primary database projects evolved in different parts of the world. There are two main classes of databases: DNA (nucleotide) databases and Protein databases.

1. **DNA (Nucleotide) Databases**

   EMBL (UK), GenBank (USA), DDBJ(Japan)

2. **Protein Databases**

   PIR (US), MIPS (Germany), Swiss-Prot (Swiss), TrEMBL(Swiss), NRL_3D (USA) and GenePept (USA).

DNA Databases (Nucleotide Sequences)

The growth rate of DNA databases is much higher than that of the protein databases. This is because most of the DNA is not coding for proteins and because DNA sequencing is the most prominent source of database entries. The large DNA databases are: Genbank (US), EMBL (Europe - UK), DDBJ (Japan). These databases are quite similar regarding their contents and are updating one another periodically. This was is a result of the International Nucleotide Sequence Database Collaboration.

EMBL

EMBL is a DNA sequence database from European Bioinformatics Institute (EBI). EMBL includes sequences from direct submissions, from genome sequencing projects, scientific literature and patent applications. EMBL supports several retrieval tools: SRS for text based retrieval and Blast and FastA for sequence based retrieval. EMBL is divided into several divisions. The division differ by the amount of sequences and by the quality of the data

GenBank

GenBank is a DNA sequence database from National Center Biotechnology Information (NCBI). It incorporates sequences from publicly available sources (direct submission and large-scale sequencing). Like EMBL it is also split into smaller, discrete divisions. This facilitates an efficient search.

Protein Databases (Amino Acid Sequence)

PIR – Protein Information Resource (International Protein Sequence Database)

The Protein Sequence Database was developed in the early 1960's. It is located at the National Biomedical Research Foundation (NBRF). Since 1988 it has been maintained by PIR-International. It is split into four distinct sections, that differ in quality of the data and the level of annotation:

PIR1 - fully classified and annotated entries.

PIR2 - preliminary entries, not thoroughly reviewed.

PIR3 - unverified entries, not reviewed

PIR4- conceptual translations

Swiss-Prot

Swiss-Prot was established in 1986. It is maintained collaboratively by SIB (Swiss Institute of Bioinformatics) and EBI/EMBL. Provides high-level annotations, including description of protein function, structure of protein domains, post-translational modifications, variants, *etc.* It aims to be minimally redundant. Swiss-Prot is linked to many other resources, including other sequence databases.

TrEMBL - Translated EMBL

Translated EMBL was created in 1996 as a computer annotated supplement to Swiss-Prot. It contains translations of all coding sequences in the EMBL nucleotide sequence database. SP-TrEMBL contains entries that will be incorporated into Swiss-ProtREM-TrEMBL contains entries that are not destined to be included in Swiss-Prot, (for example, T-cell receptors, patented sequences). The entries in REM-TrEMBL have no accession number.

GenPept

GenPept is a supplement to the GenBank nucleotide sequence database. Its entries are translation of coding regions in GenBank entries. They contain minimal annotation, primarily extracted from the corresponding GenBank entries. For the complete annotations, one must refer to the GenBank entry or entries referenced by the accession number(s) in the GenPept entry.

NRL 3D

NRL 3D is produced and maintained by PIR. It contains sequences extracted from the Protein DataBank (PDB). The entries include secondary structure, active site, binding site and modified site annotations, details of experimental method, resolution, R factor, *etc.*

Genome Databases of Specific Organisms

These are smaller databases that present an integrated view of a particular biological system.

ESTs (Expressed Sequence Tags)

Short fragments of mRNA samples that are takenf rom a variety of tissues and organisms. These samples are amplified and sequenced. The sequencing is done in one read pass, therefore the ESTs are a non-accurate source of information. There are about 6 million sequenced ESTs (more than 1/3 cloned fromhuman).

STSs (Sequence-Tagged Sites)

Short genomic samples that serve as genomic markers.

HTGS (High Throughput Genomic Sequences)

Sequences obtained in the course of sequencing the whole genome. The records of this databases are classified according to their level of advancement towards sequence completion. Phase 0 - Single or few pass reads of a single clone (not contigs). Phase 1 - Unfinished, may be unordered, unoriented contigs, with gaps.

How to Perform Database-Searching?

As the amount of biological relevant data is increasing so rapidly, knowing how to access and search this information is essential. The two main ways of searching are:

Text based search - Searching the annotations. Examples: SRS, GCG's Lookup, Entrez.

Sequence based search - Searching the sequence itself. Examples: Blast, FastA, SW.

Text Based Retrieval Tools

The listed retrieval systems allow text searching in a multitude of molecular biology database and provide links to relevant information for entries that match the search criteria. The systems differ in the databases they search and the links they have to other information.

SRS (Sequence Retrieval System)

SRS had been developed at the EBI. It provides a homogeneous interface to over 80 biological databases. It includes databases of sequences, metabolic pathways, transcription factors, application results (like BLAST, SSEARCH, FASTA), protein 3-D structures, genomes, mappings, mutations, and locus specific mutations. For each of the 80 available databases, there is a short description, including its last release. Before entering a query, one selects one or more of the databases to search.

It is possible to send the query results as a batch query to a sequence search tool. The SRS is highly recommended for use.

Entrez

Entrez is a molecular biology database and retrieval system, developed by the NCBI. It is an entry point for exploring the NCBI's integrated databases. The Entrez is easy to use, but unlike SRS, the search is limited. It does not allow customization with an institutes preferred databases.

Sequence Based Searching

The straight forward technique to search a DNA sequence is to search it against DNA databases. However, it is possible to translate a coding DNA sequence into a protein sequence, and then search it against protein databases. The main goal in searching is finding the relevant information and avoiding non relevant information. When one chooses which algorithm to use, there is a trade off between these two figures of merit.

- ✰ FastA (better **for nucleotides than for proteins**),
- ✰ BLAST (better for **proteins than for nucleotides**) and
- ✰ SW-search (more sensitive than FastAor BLAST, but much slower).

FastA

FastA is an alignment program for protein sequences created by **Pearsin and Lipman** in 1988. The basic FastA algorithm assumes a query sequence and a database over the same alphabet.

Practically, FastA is a family of programs, allowing also cross queries of DNA versus protein. The program is one of the many heuristic algorithms proposed to speed up sequence comparison. The basic idea is to add a fast pre-screen step to locate the highly matching segments between two sequences, and then extend these matching segments to local alignments using more rigorous algorithms such as Smith-Waterman.

BLAST - Basic Local Alignment Search Tool

BLAST comes under the category of homology and similarity tools. Blast programs use a heuristic search algorithm. The programs use the statistical methods of **Karlin and Altschul**. BLAST programs were designed for fast database searching,with minimal sacrifice of sensitivity for distantly related sequences. Comparison of nucleotide sequences in a database can be performed. Also a protein database can be searched to find a match against the queried protein sequence. The BLAST program compares the query to each sequence in database using heuristic rules to speed up the pairwise comparison. It first creates sequence abstraction by listing exact and similar words. BLAST finds similar words between the query and each database sequence. It then extends such words to obtain high-scoring sequence pairs (HSPs) (BLAST parlance for local ungapped alignments). BLAST calculates statistics analytically, are calculated statistically like in FastA and give output. The BLAST graphical output is similar to FastA output.

Depending on the type of sequences to compare, there are different programs:

- ☆ blastp compares an **amino acid query sequence against a protein sequence database**
- ☆ blastn compares a **nucleotide query sequence against a nucleotide sequence database**
- ☆ blastx compares a **nucleotide query sequence** translated in all reading frames against a **protein sequence database**
- ☆ tblastn compares a **protein query sequence** against a **nucleotide sequence database** dynamically translated in all reading frames
- ☆ tblastx compares the **six-frame translations of a nucleotide query sequence** against the **six-frame translations of a nucleotide sequence database**.

Statistical Estimators

Different types of statistical estimators are used in the analysis to find out the validity of an alignment score.

Z-score

It is defined by the number of standard deviations that separate an observed score from the average random score. In other words, it is the difference between the observed score and the average random score, normalized by the standard deviation of the distribution. **A higher Z-score means that the score can be trusted with a higher confidence level.**

E-value

It is defined as the expected number of false positives with a score higher than the **observed score.** This value is dependant, obviously, on the number of random alignments, determined by the size of the aligned sequences. **A lower E-value indicates that the score** has a higher confidence level.

P-value

The *P-value* is the probability of the observed score. The probability that a certain score occurred by chance. Like the E-value, this value is dependent on the size of the database. A lower P-value means that the score has a higher confidence level. This estimator is not widely used for determining the validity of sequence alignment scores

Multiple Sequence Alignments

Sometimes it is necessary to align a number of sequences, in order to identify regions of homology between them. From the Biologist point of view, this alignment is an important tool in characterizing protein families, determining consensus sequences, finding secondary and tertiary structure of new sequences, and construction of phylogenetic trees according to the similarity level between within the aligned sequences and designing the efficient primar for Polymerase Chain Reaction (PCR).

There are two different approaches to multiple sequence alignment

1. Alignment of similar sequences of nucleotides or amino acids, taking into account physio-chemical properties and mutation data.
2. Alignment of sequences solely according to secondary and tertiary structure. The resulting alignment can, understandably, differ greatly between the two approaches.

Multiple Sequence Alignment Tools

ClustalW

ClustalW is popular software for multiple sequence alignment. It can be used on either DNA or proteins. The output of ClustalW is a multiple alignment, shown graphically, and it can even construct phylogenetic trees according to the alignment. ClustalW creates alignments in a format called GCG. However, most alignment software and viewers uses another format, the Fasta format. The program tofasta converts files from GCG format to fasta format. **The program JalView is an excellent multiple alignment viewer. It uses colors to distinguish regions of homology from regions that are less similar.**

Secondary Databases

Prosite

The Prosite database is based on SwissPort and thus is very well annotated, but small.

Characterization of protein families is done by the single most conserved motif observed in a multiple sequence alignment of known homologous. These conserved motifs usually relate to biological functions such as active sites or binding sites. The search in Prosite does not require an exact match in structure. Prosite enables searches using complex patterns. It is possible to search textually using regular expressions for names of known proteins, *etc.* It is also possible to scan a protein sequence using prosite for structural pattern matches. The database is well cross-linked to SwissProt and TrEMBL.

FingerPrints

Unlike Prosite, FingerPrints has an improved diagnostic reliability which is achieved by using more than one conserved structural motif to characterize a protein family. With FingerPrints, many motifs are encoded using ungapped and unweighed local alignments. The input to Finger Prints is a small multiple alignment, which has some conserved motifs.

These motifs are searched for in the database, and only sequences that match all the motifs are considered for further analysis.

Blocks

Blocks uses multiply aligned ungapped segments corresponding to the most highly conserved regions of proteins. Block Searcher, Get Blocks and Block Maker are aids to detection and verification of protein sequence homology. They compare a protein or DNA sequence to a database of protein blocks, retrieve blocks, and create new blocks, respectively.

Profiles

The Profiles databases uses the notion of profiles to achieve a good detection of distant sequence relationships. **A profile is a scoring table with multiple alignment information for the whole sequences, not just for conserved regions.** Profiles are weighted to indicate:

- What types of residues are allowed at what positions.
- Where insertions and deletions (INDELs) are allowed (not within core secondary structures).
- Where the most conserved regions are located

Pfam

Pfam uses a different method for its database. High quality seed alignments are used to create Hidden Markov Models to which sequences are aligned. Pfam has to classes of alignments, according to their credibility:

- Pfam-a – Non-edited seed alignments which are deemed to be accurate.
- Pfam-b – Alignments derived by automatic clustering of the SwissPort database. These alignments are, of course, less reliable.

eMotif

eMotif, also known as identify, uses data from Blocks and Finger Prints to generate consensus expressions from the conserved regions of sequence alignments.

InterrPro

InterPro is an interface to several secondary databases: ProSite, prints, ProDom and Pfam. It has an intuitive interface both for text and sequence-based searches, and since it incorporates several databases, it is very recommended.

Genome Analysis

Comparative Genomics

Homology refers to two genes sharing a common evolutionary history. Scientists also use the term homology, or homologous, to simply mean similar, regardless of the evolutionary relationship. In comparative genomics one of the major functions is the identification of homologous genes in different organisms. **An important tool which is utilized for this function is BLAST (Basic local alignment search tool).**The **BLAST** algorithm is a heuristic program, which means that it relies on some smart shortcuts to perform the search faster. BLAST performs "local" alignments. Mostproteins are modular in nature, with functional domains often being repeated within the same protein as well as across different proteins from different species. The BLAST algorithm is tuned to find these domains or shorter stretches of sequence similarity. The local alignment approach also means that a mRNA can be aligned with a piece of genomic DNA, as is frequently required in genome assembly and analysis. **If instead BLAST started out by attempting to align two sequences over their entire lengths (known as a global alignment), fewer similarities would be detected, especially with respect to domains and motifs.** When a query is submitted via one of the BLAST Web pages, the sequence, plus any other input information such as the database to be searched, word size, expect value, and so on, are fed to the algorithm on the BLAST server. BLAST works by first making a look-up table of all the "words" (short subsequences, which for proteins the default is three letters) and "neighbouring words", *i.e.* similar words in the query sequence. The sequence database is then scanned for these "hot spots". When a match is identified, it is used to initiate **gap**-free and gapped extensions of the "word".

BLAST Scores and Statistics

Once BLAST has found a similar sequence to the query in the database, it is helpful to have some idea of whether the alignment is "good" and whether it portrays a possible biological relationship, or whether the similarity observed is attributable to chance alone. BLAST uses statistical theory to produce a **bit score** and expect value (**E-value**) for each alignment pair (query to hit). The bit score gives an indication of how good the alignment is; **the higher the score, the better the alignment.** The E-value gives an indication of the statistical significance of a given pairwise alignment and reflects the size of the database and the scoring system used. **The lower the E-value, the more significant the hit**. A sequence alignment that has an E-value of 0.05 means that this similarity has a 5 in 100 (1 in 20) chance of occurring by chance alone.

Phylogeny

With the aid of **nucleotide and amino acid sequences, it should be possible to find the ancestral ties between different organisms**. Thus far, experience has taught us that closely related organisms have similar sequences and that more distantly related organisms have more dissimilar sequences. Proteins that show significant sequence conservation, indicating a clear evolutionary relationship, are said to be from the same protein family. By studying protein folds (distinct protein building blocks) and families, **scientists are able to reconstruct the evolutionary relationship between two species and to estimate the time of divergence between two organisms since they last shared a common ancestor.**

Genetic Variation

Evolution is not always discrete with clearly defined boundaries that pinpoint the origin of a new species, nor is it a steady continuum. Evolution requires genetic variation which results from changes within a gene pool, the genetic make-up of a specific population. Every time a cell divides, cell must make a complete copy of its genome, a process called DNA replication. DNA replication must be extremely accurate to avoid introducing mutations or changes in the nucleotide sequence of a short region of the genome. Inevitably, some mutations do occur, usually in one of two ways; either from errors in DNA replication or from damaging. Mutations in the coding regions of genes are much more important. Those mutations that do have an evolutionary effect in population.

Phylogenetic Trees

Systematics describes the pattern of relationships among taxa and is intended to help us understand the history of all life. But history is not something we can see; it has happened once and leaves only clues as to the actual events. Scientists use these clues to build hypotheses, or models, of life's history. In phylogenetic studies, the most convenient way of visually presenting evolutionary relationships among a group of organisms is through illustrations called **phylogenetic trees**.

Tools for Phylogeny Reconstruction

1. MEGA

MEGA (**Molecular Evolutionary Genetics Analysis**) is a software package for phylogenetic analysis with a graphical user interface. It allows viewing and editing of the aligned input sequence data and provides many tools for phylogenetic and statistical analysis of the alignments.

2. Mesquite

Mesquite is an open source software project designed to deal with comparative data about organisms and evolutionary analyses. Mesquite contains modules for phylogenetic analysis, population genetics, and non-phylogenetic multivariate analysis.

3. MIGenAS Toolkit

Max-Planck Integrated Gene Analysis System (MIGenAS) provides access to many different bioinformatics software tools and databases for sequence similarity searching multiple sequence alignments, phylogenetic analysis, and protein structure prediction. Users can also configure "meta"-tools as a pipeline of individual tools and intermediate filters.

4. MPI Toolkit

Max-Planck Institute Bioinformatics Toolkit provides access to many different bioinformatics software tools and databases for sequence similarity searching, multiple sequence alignments, phylogenetic analysis, and protein structure prediction.

5. NJplot

NJplot is a tool for visualizing binary trees such as the phylogenetic trees output from the PHYLIP programs. Available for several platforms including Windows, MacOS, Linux and Solaris.

6. PHYLIP

Comprehensive set of programs for phylogenetic analyses; available for PC and Mac; source code available for easy compiling in UNIX.

7. PhyloBLAST

BLAST a protein sequence, then perform automated phylogenetic analysis on hits or on uploaded sequences; PHYLIP-based analyses

8. PhyloDome

PhyloDome is a tool with which you can visualize and analyze the phylogenetic distribution of one or more eukaryotic domains.

9. POWER

The Phylogenetic Web Repeater (POWER) allows users to perform phylogenetic analysis using the PHYLIP package. The POWER pipeline can start with processing either **Multiple Sequence Alignments (MSA)** or can proceed directly with aligned sequences.

10. Ribosomal Database Project

Highly curated database of aligned and annotated rRNA sequences with accompanying phylogenies; data available for download.

11. Tree Editors

Tree Editors is an annotated listing of software for the visualization and manipulation of phylogenetic trees.

Protein Modeling

The process of evolution has resulted in the production of DNA sequences that encodeproteins with specific functions. Protein structure has been determined by X-ray crystallography or nuclear magnetic resonance (NMR) spectroscopy. Unknown protein three-dimensional structure of can be predicted using protein or molecular modeling with the reference of already existing close related protein structure in the database. In this method experimentally determined protein structures is called as templates; to predict the structure of another protein that has a similar amino acid sequence is called target. Therefore, scientists have begun to turn toward computers to help predict the structure of a protein based on its sequence. The challenge lies in developing methods for accurately and reliably understanding this intricate relationship.

Databases of Structures from Homology Modeling

Databases are now available that contain large numbers of protein structures that have been obtained by comparative(homology) modeling. Two of these databases are ModBase and 3DCrunch.

Modbase

Modbase was created by Sali and co-workers, using their program Modeller, which creates models based on the satisfaction of spatial restraints. That is, restraints are identified from the alignments of homologues of known structure, and these restraints are then applied to the unknown sequence. Restraints can include distances between alpha carbons, other distances within the main-chain, and main-chain and side-chain dihedral angles. Routines to satisfy the restraints optimally include conjugate gradient minimization and molecular dynamics with simulated annealing.

3DCrunch

3DCrunch is a large scale modeling project that aims to submit all entries from protein sequence databases to SWISS-MODEL. Currently the database contains 64,000 entries.

SWISS-MODEL

It is available through Glaxo Wellcome Experimental Research in Geneva, Switzerland. Web-based tools are now available to generate models of protein 3-dimensional structures using comparative modelling techniques.

WHAT IF

This homology modelling tool available on EMBL servers, includes three components, one to generate the homology models, one to evaluate the quality of the homology models, and one to evaluate models of proteins for which the structure is already known, thereby providing for evaluation of the quality of the modeling program.

Evaluation and Refinement of the Structure

For a homology model from any source,it is important to demonstrate that the structural features of the model are reasonable in terms of what is know about protein structures in general. Several programs are available to assist in this analysis of correctness of a homology model. Programs that provide structure analysis along with output that is useful for publication include PROCHECK and 3D-Profiler

PROCHECK

PROCHECK is based on an analysis of (phi and psi) angles, peptide bond planarity, bond lengths, bond angles, hydrogen-bond geometry, and side-chain conformations of known protein structures as a function of atomic resolution. Thus, the expected values of these parameters are known and can be compared to a modelled structure based on the atomic resolution of the structures from which the model was developed.

3D-Profiler

3D-profiler compares a homology model to its sequence using a 3D profile. The profile is based on the statistical preferences of each of the 20 amino acids for particular environments within the protein. Each residue position in a 3D model can be characterized by its environment. Preferred environments for amino acids are derived from known three-dimensional structures and are defined by three parameters: (1) the area of each residue that is buried, (2) the fraction of side-chain area that is covered by polar atoms (*i.e.* O and N), and (3) the local secondary structure. Based on these environment variables, a 3D structure is converted into a 1D profile that describes each residue in the folded protein structure. Examination of these profiles reveals which regions of a sequence appear to be folded correctly and which do not.

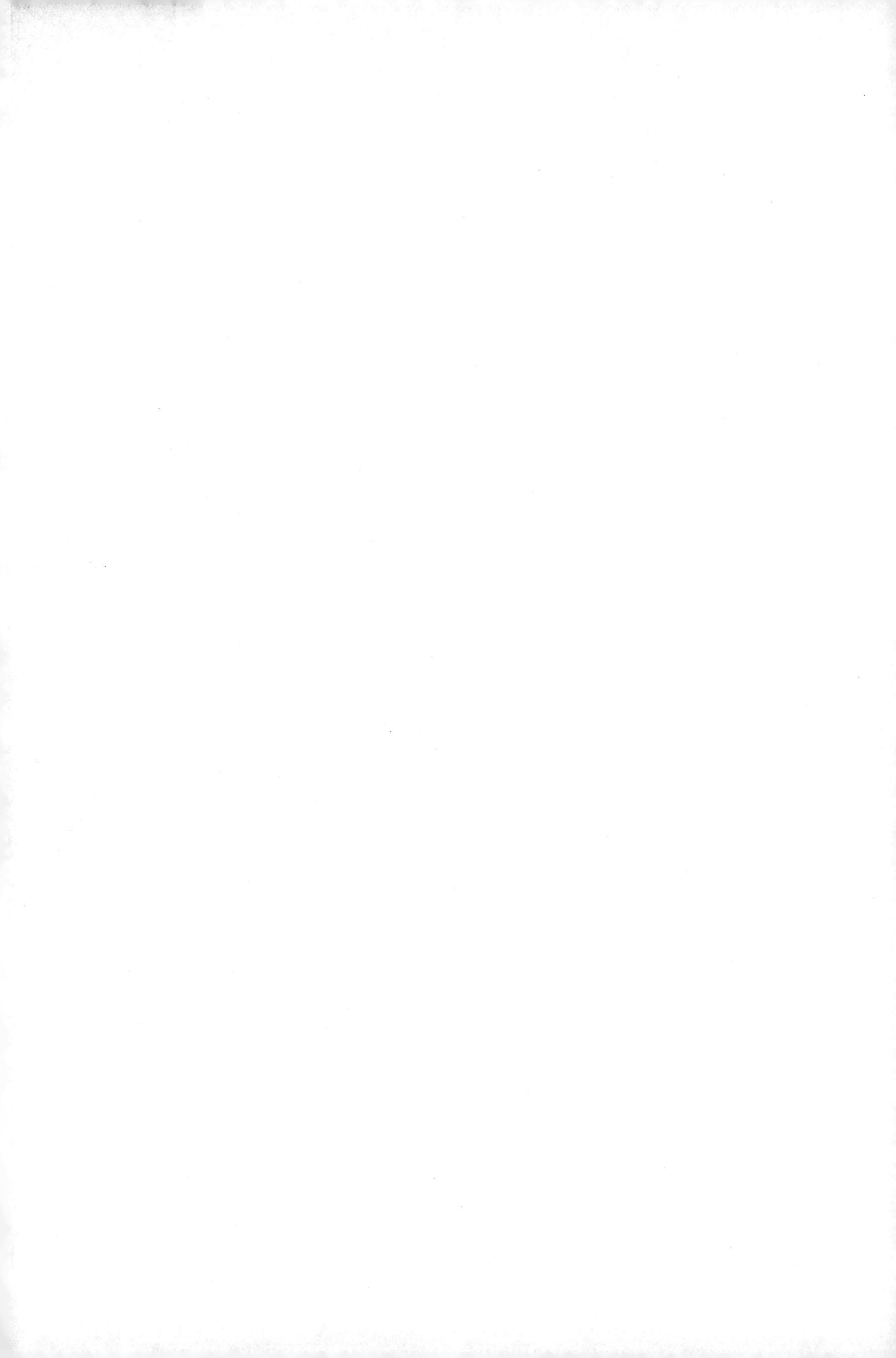

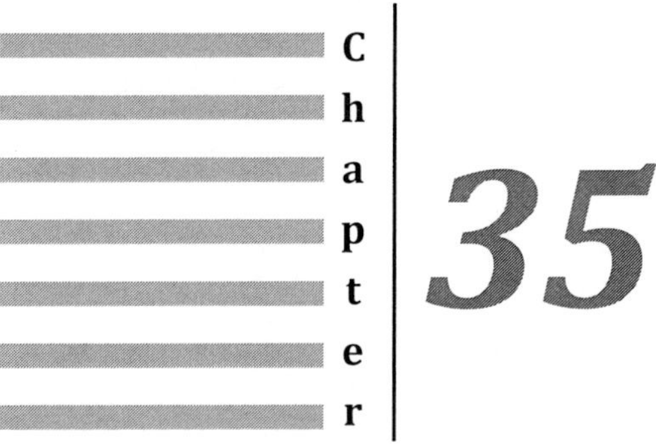

Basics of Nanoscience and Nanotechnology

Nanoscience and nanotechnology are defined differently depending upon the scope and context of each application. The Royal Society of the UK makes the distinction between nanoscience and nanotechnology where the former includes the "study and manipulation" of nanoscale particles and systems, and the latter the "design, characterization, and production of structures, devices and systems" at the nanoscale (1 nm = 10^{-9} meters, or one billionth of a meter).

Nanoscience

Nanoscience is the study of phenomena and manipulation of materials at atomic, molecular and macromolecular scales, where properties differ significantly from those at a larger scale.

To get an idea of how long a nanometer is, this can be compared with a printed page, which is about 75,000 nanometers thick. When structures are made small enough in the nanometer size range they can take on interesting and useful properties. The word nanoscience is a combination of **Nano**, from the Greek "nanos" (or Latin "nanus"), meaning "Dwarf", and the word **Science**, and meaning knowledge. It is an interdisciplinary field that seeks to bring about mature nanotechnology, focusing on the nano scale intersection of fields such as physics, biology, engineering, chemistry, computer science and more (Figure 35.1).

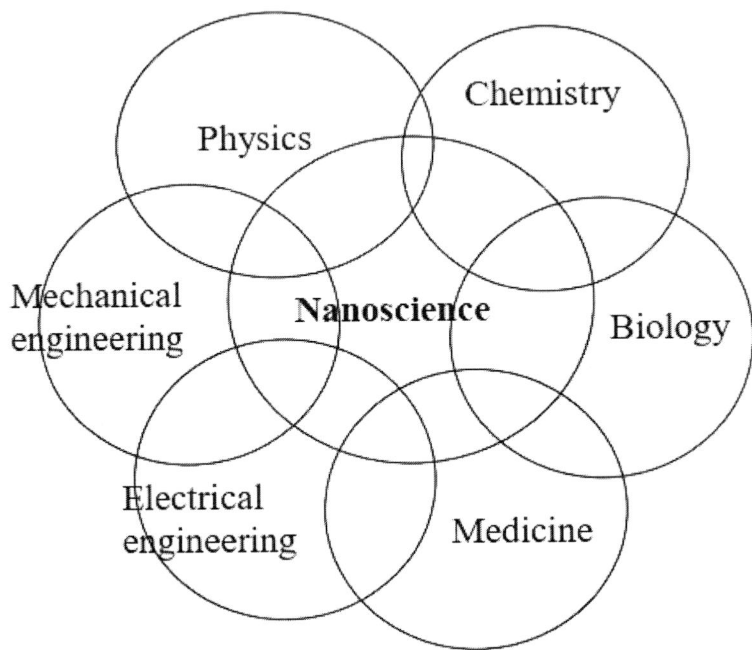

Figure 35.1. Naonscience and its Interdiciplinary Fields.

Nanotechnology

Nanotechnologies are the design, characterization, production and application of structures, devices and systems by controlling shape and size at nanometre scale"

Three requirements are more important in the field of nanoscience and nanotechnology:

1. Ability to control or manipulate on the atomic scale
2. Research and technology development at the atomic, molecular or macromolecular levels, in the length scale of approximately 1-100 nanometer range.
3. Creating and using structures, devices and systems that have novel properties and functions because of their small and/or intermediate size.

Nanoscience and nanotechnology involve research and technology development at the atomic, molecular, or macromolecular level, in the length scale of approximately 1 to 100 nm range. The discovery of novel materials, processes and phenomena at the nanoscale, as well as the development of new experimental and theoretical techniques for research provide fresh opportunities for the development of innovative nanosystems and nanostructured materials. Nanosystems are expected to find various unique applications. Nanostructured materials can be made with unique nanostructures and properties. This may lead to the concept of renaming nanosized objects of biology and chemistry (molecules) as tiny machines.

Nanotechnology is a new word, but it is not an entirely new field. Nature has many objects and processes that function on a micro to nanoscale. The understanding of these functions can guide us in imitating and producing nanodevices and nanomaterials.

Billions of years ago, molecules began organizing themselves into the complex structures that could support life. Photosynthesis harnesses solar energy to support plant life. Molecular ensembles are present in plants, which include light harvesting molecules, such as chlorophyll, arranged within the cells on the nanometer to micrometer scales. These structures capture light energy, and convert it into the chemical energy that drives the biochemical machinery of plant cells. Live organs use chemical energy in the body. The flagella, a type of bacteria, rotates at over 10,000 RPM. This is an example of a biological molecular machine. The flagella motor is driven by the proton flow caused by the electrochemical potential differences across the membrane. The diameter of the bearing is about 20–30 nm, with an estimated clearance of about 1 nm. For instance, ATP synthase which catalyses the synthesis of adenosine triphosphate (ATP) molecule, which is the universal currency of free energy in living systems, can be called a "nanomotor," so are the enzymes which catalyze making, breaking, and rearranging the bonds in other molecules. Another example is the actinmyosin molecular machine which can drive fibers past one another. Similarly DNA serves as a data storage system, transmitting digital instructions to molecular machines, the ribosomes, that manufacture protein and enzyme molecules in turn, make up most of the molecular machineries in living systems.

The Nanometer Scale

The nanometer scale conventionally defines as 1 to 100 nm. One nanometer is one billionth meter (10^{-9}m). The size range is set normally to be minimum 1nm to avoid single atoms or very small groups of atoms being designated as nano-objects. Therefore Nanoscience and Nanotechnologies deal with atleast cluster of atoms of 1nm size. SI units which is used to measure the size of the objects and respective description is given in Table 35.1. Nanoscale and measurements of nano and bulk objects is shown in (Figure 35.2)

Table 35.1. Description of Macro and Nano Units.

SI Unit (Abbreviation)	*Description*
Meter (m)	100 centimeter
Centimeter (cm)	1/100 of a meter,
Millimeter (mm)	1/1,000 of a meter
Micrometer (μm)	1/1,000,000 of a meter also called a micron, this is the scale of most integrated circuits and MEMS devices
Nanometer (nm)	1/1,000,000,000 of a meter; the size scale of single small molecules and nanotechnology

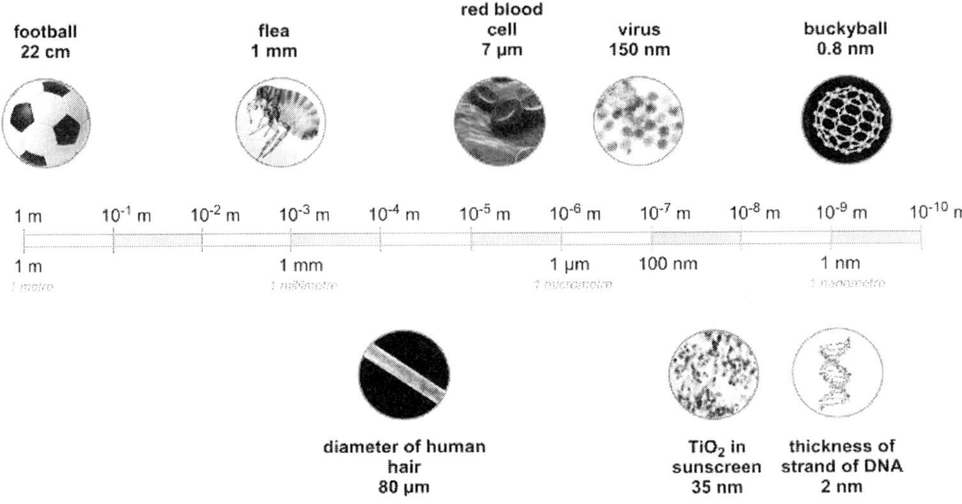

Figure 35.2. Objects and its Measurements of different Scale Range.

Why is Nanoscience Attracting so much Interest?

Elements are made up of atoms, atoms containing proton and electron. More number of atoms are joined together and form molecules and many molecules combine together and form objects (Figure 35.3). The fundamental properties of matter change at the nanoscale. So the properties of atoms and molecules are not governed by the same physical laws as larger objects, but it is governed by quantum mechanics. The physical and chemical properties of nanoparticles can be quite different from those of larger particles of the same substance. Altered properties are colour, solubility, material strength, electrical conductivity, magnetic behavior, mobility (within the environment and within the human body), chemical reactivity and biological activity.

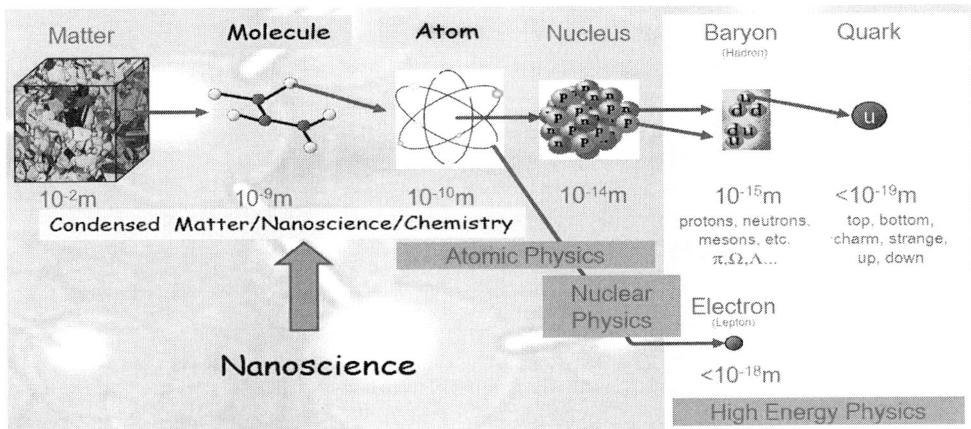

Figure 35.3. Properties of Atoms and Objects and its Measurements.

At the nanometer scale, properties become size dependent. This size-dependent properties enable new applications. Four important ways in which nanoscale materials may differ from macroscale materials.

- ☆ Gravitational forces become negligible and electromagnetic forces dominate
- ☆ Quantum mechanics is the model used to describe motion and energy instead of the classical mechanics model
- ☆ Greater surface area to volume ratios
- ☆ Random molecular motion becomes more important

Changes in Properties

All the materials may be metals, semiconductors or insulators have size dependent physico-chemical properties below a certain critical size depending upon the details of the materials. For most of the materials, it is below 100nm. Thus geometrical structure, chemical bonds, ionization potential, electronic properties, optical properties, mechanical strength, melting point, magnetic properties are all affected by the particle sizes.

1. Physical Properties

In the nanoscale range, surface area to volume enhances. This enhancement transforms the surface pressure and results in a change in the interatomic spacing. The changes happened in interatomic spacing and large volume to surface ratio has a combined effect on the properties of the material.

2. Chemical Properties

- ☆ Based on the surface area to volume effect (Figure 35.4), nanoscale materials have:
  - a) Increased total surface area.
  - b) Increased number of atoms accessible on the surface.
  - c) Increased catalytic activity of those large number surface atoms.
  - d) Different/tunable surface catalytic properties by the change in shape, size and composition.
- ☆ Hence, nanoscale catalysts can increase the rate, selectivity and efficiency of various chemical reactions.

3. Mechanical Properties

Due to the nanometer size, many of the mechanical properties of the nanomaterials are modified to be different from the bulk materials including the hardness, elastic modulus, fracture toughness, scratch resistance and fatigue strength *etc.*

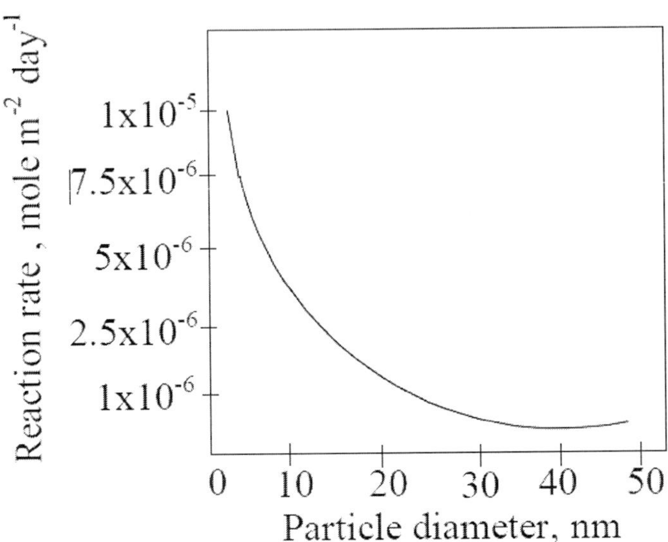

Figure 35.4. Effect of Particle Size on the Reaction Rate.

4. Magnetic Properties

The magnetic behavior of the nanomaterials is size dependent. In the tiny ferromagnetic particles, the magnetic properties are distinct from that of the very large material. In the range of nanoscale, magnetic material has a single magnetic domain and exhibit superparamagnetism. As an outcome, the remanent magnetization and coercive field exhibit a strong dependence on the size of a particle.

5. Optical Properties

The color and transparency of materials change by changing the size of nanoparticles. Hence these can be controlled by processing parameters. Due to the increase in effective band gap of materials, absorption spectra shift towards higher energy and for small particle; it may show stepwise absorption by decreasing size of nanocrystals. Enhanced luminescence with fast response has been observed by decreasing size of nanocrystals; this is because of changes in electronic structure and useful in fast response devices with emission of desired color. Nanoparticles may be used in lasers also since these can operate at lower threshold. Confinement of photons and phonons in nanoparticles also affect the Raman spectra. Nonlinear optical properties are also observed in semiconductor clusters in glass or polymer matrix.

Size-dependent Optical Property

Absorption peak broadens and shifts to longer wavelengths. Reflection, leading to scattering, is weak at small sizes and increases when > 50 nm (Figure 35.5).

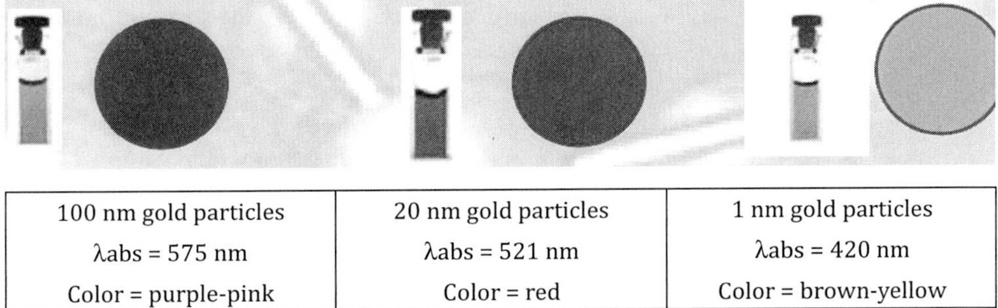

100 nm gold particles λabs = 575 nm Color = purple-pink	20 nm gold particles λabs = 521 nm Color = red	1 nm gold particles λabs = 420 nm Color = brown-yellow

Figure 35.5. Gold Nanoparticles and Colour Variation Based on its Size.

6. Thermal Properties

It is found that melting point is lowered with decreasing particle size. It may be reduced to half of the original. The specific heat and thermal expansion may increase up to 50 per cent or more with reducing particle size. The nanocrystalline materials are expected to have a low conductivity of thermal when compared with the conventional materials.

7. Electrical Properties

Electrical properties are also affected by the size in nanometer range. Electrical conductivity is reduced by decreasing the size of nanocrystals. Ferroelectric materials (*e.g.* $PbTiO_3$) become non-ferroelectric at reduced sizes (20 nm). Transition temperature of superconducting materials (*e.g.* $YBa_2Cu_3O_7$) (Y-*Yttrium*) is reduced and these become non-superconducting for smaller sizes. This has opened up a huge possibility of synthesising and manufacturing the materials with desired characteristics. It should be noted that for a particular material there is always a critical size below which properties are size dependent. In these materials the length of reduced dimension has to be smaller than the phase coherent length or the mean free path scattering length for electrons in the materials.

There are various advantages that nanotechnologies offer due to the unique functional properties of nanomaterials like:

1. Higher charge density and higher reactivity of nanoparticles due to small size.
2. As the surface area increases in comparison to volume, the activity of the atoms on the surface of the particles becomes more than the inside the particles.
3. As a result of large surface to volume ratio, the nanoparticles had more strength, increased heat resistance, decreased melting point and different magnetic properties of Nano-clusters.
4. Differences in the exposed surfaces of different nanoparticles lead to variances in atomic distribution across the nanoparticles, this, in turn,

affect the electron transfer rate kinetics between metal nanoparticles and corresponding adsorbed species.

5. Nanoparticles have higher catalytic activity when they are present in tetrahedral structure followed by cubic and spherical structure, recognized for the improvement of chemical reactivity at the sharp edges and corner of the former.

Reasons for Novel Properties

Nanomaterials exhibit properties often superior to those of conventional coarse-grained materials and in addition, the properties can be tailored by controlling the size. The changes in the properties of nanomaterials are driven mainly by two factors:

a) Increase in Surface Area to Volume Ratio

Atoms and molecules at surface or interface have different environment and bonding configuration, therefore these exhibit different characteristics. In micron size particles, the fraction of surface atoms is less than 10^{-8} and so they cause little effect. As size is reduced, relative number of atoms on surface increases inversely as particle size. For small sizes of the order of few 100 nm, the fraction of surface atoms is large and therefore influences the properties by greater amount making the properties size dependent.

Surfaces and Interfaces Play a Large Role in Material Properties and Interactions

Nanoscale materials have far larger surface areas than similar masses of larger scale materials. As surface area per mass of a material increases, a greater amount of the material can come into contact with surrounding materials, thus affecting reactivity. A simple thought experiment shows why nanoparticles have phenomenally high surface areas. A solid cube of a material 1 cm on a side has 6 square centimeters of surface area, about equal to one side of half a stick of gum. But if that volume of 1 cubic centimeter were filled with cubes 1 mm on a side, that would be 1,000 millimeter-sized cubes (10 x 10 x 10), each one of which has a surface area of 6 square millimeters, for a total surface area of 60 square centimeters about the same as one side of two-thirds of a 3" x 5" note card. When the 1 cubic centimeter is filled with micrometer-sized cubes a trillion (10^{12}) of them, each with a surface area of 6 square micrometers the total surface area amounts to 6 square meters, or about the area of the main bathroom in an average house. And when that single cubic centimeter of volume is filled with 1-nanometer-sized cubes 10^{21} of them, each with an area of 6 square nanometers their total surface area comes to 6,000 square meters. In other words, a single cubic centimeter of cubic nanoparticles has a total surface area one-third larger than a football field (Figure 35.6).

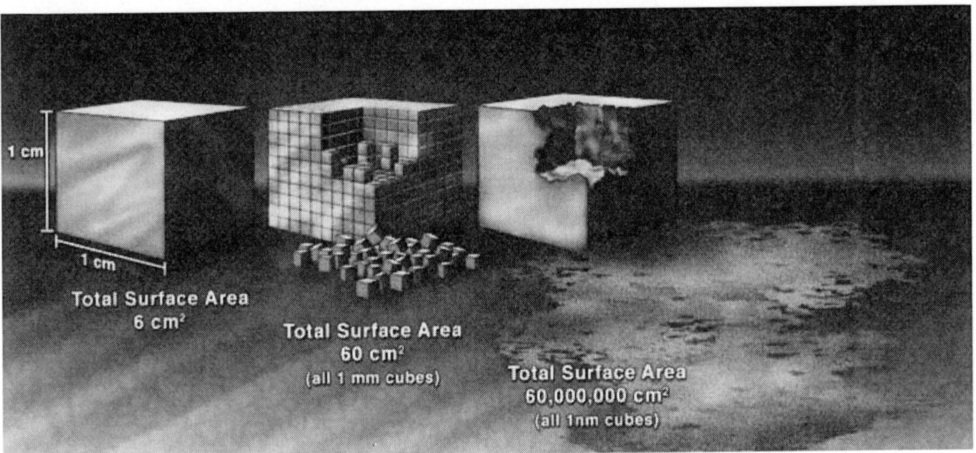

Figure 35.6. Surface Area Comparison of Nano and Bulk Material.

b) Quantum Size Effect

The *quantum size effect* describes the physics of electron properties in solids with great reductions in particle size. This effect does not come into play by going from macro to micro dimensions. However, Quantum effects becomes dominant when the micro dimensions reached nanometer size range. The bulk properties of any material are merely the average of all the quantum forces affecting all the atoms that make up the material. As things become smaller and smaller, it eventually reach a point where the averaging no longer works and have to deal with the specific behavior of individual atoms or molecules - behavior that can be very different to when these atoms are aggregated into a bulk material. Quantum size effect is change of electronic and optical properties when the material sampled is of sufficiently small size - typically 10 nanometers or less. The bandgap increases as the size of the nanostructure decreases. Specifically, the phenomenon results from electrons and holes being squeezed into a dimension that approaches a critical quantum measurement, called the exciton Bohr raduis.

Exciton pair is defined as an electron and the hole that it leaves behind when it is excited up to the conduction band. So valence band electron jumps from there and reach the conduction band with the induction of the external energy and leaves hole, inturn it creates Electron Hole pair. An exciton bohr radius is the distance in an electron-hole pair. A Quantum Dot is a semiconductor so small that the size of the crystal is on the same order as the size of the exciton bohr radius.

Estabilishing of Nanotechnology Field

Nobel Laureate Richard P. Feynman gave a talk on the title "There's Plenty of Room at the Bottom" at the annual meeting On Dec. 29, 1959, of the American Physical Society, California Institute of Technology. He presented a technological vision of extreme miniaturization; the problem of manipulating and controlling things on a small scale. Extrapolating from known physical laws, Feynman envisioned a technology using the ultimate toolbox of nature, building nano-objects atom by atom or molecule by molecule. In mid-**1970s** Idea of molecular nanotechnology, originated in the mind of Eric Drexler, MIT undergraduate. He realized that the biological 'machinery' could be adapted to build non-living products upon common. Since the 1980s, many inventions and discoveries in the fabrication of nanoobjects have become a testament to Feynman vision. In recognition of this reality, the National Science and Technology Council (NSTC) of the White House created the Interagency Working Group on Nanoscience, Engineering and Technology (IWGN) in 1998. In a January 2000 speech at the same institute, former President William J. Clinton talked about the exciting promise of nanotechnology and, more generally, the importance of expanding research in nanoscale science and nanotechnology.

Nanomaterials

Nanomaterials are the pillars or cornerstone of nanoscience and nanotechnology. Nanoscale materials are defined as a set of substances (crystalline or amorphous) of organic or inorganic materials where at least one dimension is less than approximately 100 nanometers. Nanostructure science and technology is a broad and interdisciplinary area of research and development activity that has been growing explosively worldwide in the past few years (Figure 35.7).

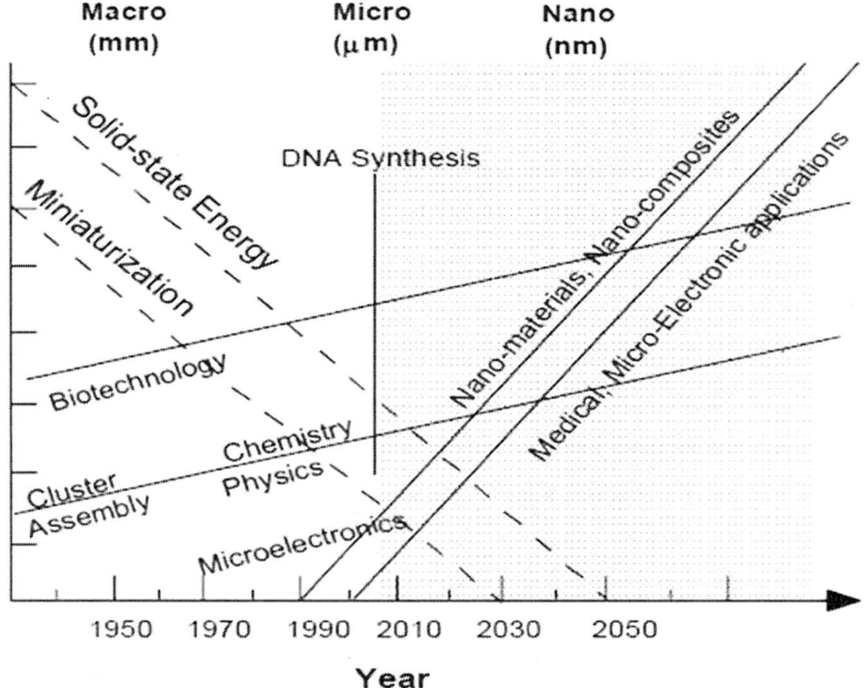

Figure 35.7. Evolution of Science and Technology.

A nanometer is one millionth of a millimeter approximately 1,00,000 times smaller than the diameter of a human hair (Figure 35.8). Precisely speaking nano-scale ranges from about 1 nanometer (nm) to 100 nanometers corresponding to roughly 100 atoms to 10 million atoms. The upper and lower boundaries of this scale are not sharply defined, but are chosen such that one excludes individual atoms on the bottom end and micrometer-scale objects on the top end. This intermediate state of matter lies somewhere between the bulk phase and the atomic or molecular regime. Material properties in nano-sized systems can be controlled appreciably by tuning their size and give rise to potentially new phenomena. Electronic and optical properties of metals and semiconductors depend strongly on the crystallite size once one starts to venture into the nano-scale regime. The evolution of these size dependent fundamental properties can be attributed to the increased surface area in addition to quantum effects that become increasingly important with decreasing size. This change is quite impressive especially in the case of semiconductors. For instance, simply altering the size of CdSe nanocrystals can tune its band gap between 1.7 and 3 eV and hence, the material can absorb and emit across the entire visible spectrum. It is fascinating that the properties in a material of a single chemical composition can be varied so significantly, simply by tailoring bulk material parameters such as size. Nanomaterials are of interest because at this scale unique optical, magnetic, electrical, and other properties emerge. These emergent properties have the potential for great impacts in agriculture, electronics, medicine, and other fields.

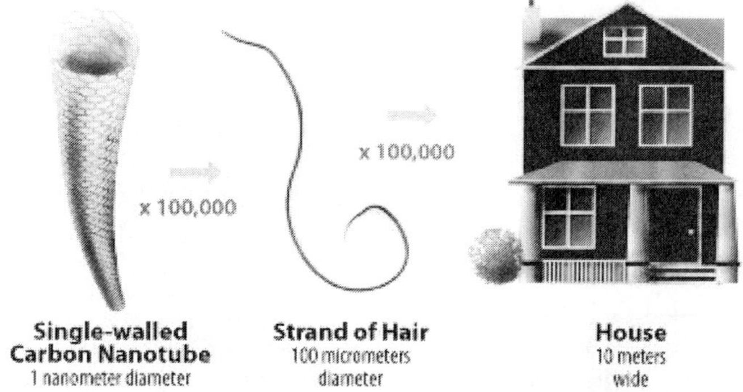

Figure 35.8. Comparison of Carbon Nanotube in to Bulk Material.

Nanostructures and Nano Particles

Nanostructured materials (NSM) and nanophase or nanoparticle (NP)are alltogeter called as nanomaterials. The former refer to condensed bulk materials that are made of grains with grain sizes in the nanometer size range while the latter are usually the dispersive nanoparticles. NPs and NSMs have gained prominence in technological advancements due to their tunable physico-chemical characteristics such as melting point, wettability, electrical and thermal conductivity, catalytic activity, light absorption and scattering based up on the need resulting in enhanced performance over their bulk counterparts.

Classification of Nanomaterials

Molecules are made up of atoms, which are the basic structural components of all living and nonliving organisms in nature. An average molecule can comprise between 1 to 25 atoms, giving it a radius of less than 1 to about 10 nm. A molecule, by definition, must have more than one atom, so the smallest molecule is H_2. Some biomolecules are much, more larger than this, such as DNA, RNA, amino acids *etc.* A nanoparticle contains between 50 and 2,00,000 atoms, so its dimensions can be from a few nanometers to several hundred nanometers. An average bacterial cell, for example, measures a few hundred nanometers across, and a red blood cell is about 6000 nm wide. The smallest parts of a microchip today are around 130 nm across. Nanomaterials can be classified in to many ways, based upon origin, it is classified in to natural, incidental and engineered. Based on the dimension it is classified in to 0D, 1D, 2D and 3D. Based on the material classified in to metal (*e.g.* Au, Ag), non-metal (*e.g.* carbon), semiconductor (*e.g.* CdSe) and a combination. Based on the structure of nanomaterial, it is classified in to amorphous, crystalline, polymeric, and composites; based on their shapes classified in to spheres, tubes, rods, cones and fibers *etc.* Among these some of the important classification are discussed below in more detail.

Classification Based on their Origin

Nanomaterials can be classified into three main categories based on their origin: (i) incidental nanomaterials, which are produced incidentally as a by-product of industrial processes such as nanoparticles produced from vehicle engine exhaust, welding fumes, combustion processes and even some natural process such as forest fires; (ii) engineered nanomaterials, which have been manufactured by humans to have certain required properties for desired applications and (iii) naturally produced nanomaterials, which can be found in the bodies of organisms, insects, plants, animals and human bodies. Incidental and naturally occurring NMs are continuously being formed within and distributed throughout ground and surface water, the oceans, continental soil and the atmosphere. One of the main differences between incidental and engineered NMs is that the morphology of engineered NMs can usually be better controlled as compared to incidental NMs; Out of these three, engineered nanomaterials getting more importance because engineered NMs are purposefully designed to exploit novel features for betterment of the human beings. Atoms and molecules have been naturally manipulated several times to create intricate NPs and NSMs that continually contribute to life on earth.

Classification Based on their Dimensions

Nanomaterials are classified based upon their dimensions such as Zero Dimensional (0D), One Dimensional (1D), Two Dimensional (2D) and Three Dimensional (3D) NMs, as shown in (Figure 35.9). This classification is highly dependent on the electron movement along the dimensions in the nanomaterials. For example, electrons in 0D NMs are entrapped in a dimensionless space whereas as 1D NMs have electrons that can move along the *x*-axis, which is less than 100 nm. Likewise, 2D and 3D NMs have electron movement along the *x*–*y*-axis, and *x*, *y*, *z*-axis respectively. The properties of NMs strongly depend on the grain boundaries, Therefore, the classical inner size effects, such as melting point reduction and diffusion enhancement, will be enhanced by grain boundary engineering. The characteristics of NMs are attributed to the particle shape and dimensionality, as per the "surface engineering" concept, and thereby class of NMs. Thus, these reasons focus on the engineering of particle shape and dimensionality along with grain boundary engineering to extend the application of NSMs.

1. Zero Dimensional nanoparticles (All the three dimensions are under nanoscale) *e.g.* Particles, quantum dots, nanoshells, microcapsules, hollow spheres.
2. One Dimensional nanoparticles (Out of three dimensions 2 dimensions are under nanoscale range) *e.g.* Single-walled carbon Nanotubes, fibers, nanowires.
3. Two Dimensional nanoparticles (Only one dimension is under nanoscale) *e.g.* Anti-adhesive/anti-stain coatings, applied films, viruses applied films, viruses, Thin films.
4. Three Dimensional nanoparticles (All the three dimensions are not under nanoscale) *e.g.* solid crystalline bulk particles.

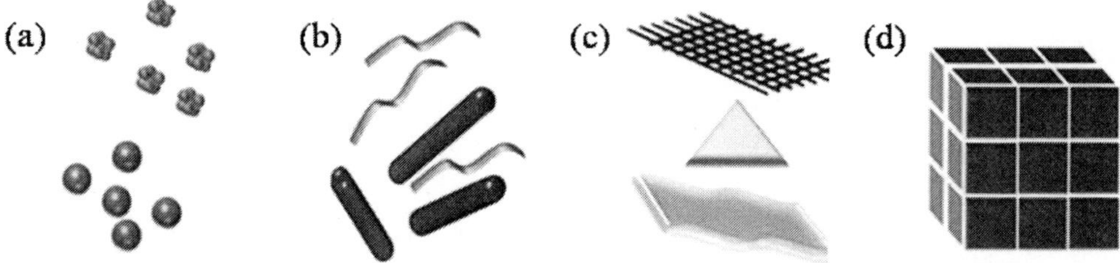

Figure 35.9. Classification of Nanomaterials based on Dimensions (a) 0D spheres and clusters; (b) 1D nanofibers, nanowires, and nanorods; (c) 2D nanofilms, nanoplates, and networks; (d) 3D nanomaterials.

Nanostructured materials occur in the nature as such for example DNA, RNA, proteins, *etc.* Also the deposition of mineral salts under the sea, wings of butterfly, coral reefs, *etc.* everything under goes a natural phenomenon (bio mimetic) where nanostructured materials come into action.

Classification Based on the Material

Most current NPs and NSMs can be organized into four material-based categories

(i) **Carbon-based nanomaterials:** Generally, these NMs contain carbon, and are found in morphologies such as hollow tubes, ellipsoids or spheres. Fullerenes (C60), carbon nanotubes (CNTs), carbon nanofibers, carbon black, graphene (Gr), and carbon onions are included under the carbon-based NMs category. Laser ablation, arc discharge, and chemical vapor deposition (CVD) are the important production methods for these carbon-based materials fabrication (except carbon black).

(ii) **Inorganic-based nanomaterials:** These NMs include metal and metal oxide NPs and NSMs. These NMs can be synthesized into metals such as Au or Ag NPs, metal oxides such as TiO_2 and ZnO NPs, and semiconductors such as silicon and ceramics.

(iii) **Organic-based nanomaterials:** These include NMs made mostly from organic matter, excluding carbon-based or inorganic-based NMs. The utilization of noncovalent (weak) interactions for the self-assembly and design of molecules helps to transform the organic NMs into desired structures such as dendrimers, micelles, liposomes and polymer NPs.

(iv) **Composite-based nanomaterials:** Composite NMs are multiphase NPs and NSMs with one phase on the nanoscale dimension that can either combine NPs with other NPs or NPs combined with larger or with bulk-type materials (*e.g.*, hybrid nanofibers) or more complicated structures, such as a metal-organic frameworks. The composites may be any combinations of carbon-based, metal-based, or organic-based NMs with any form of metal, ceramic, or polymer bulk materials.

Why so much Interest in Nanomaterials?

These materials have created a high interest in recent years by virtue of their unusual mechanical, electrical, optical and magnetic properties. Some examples are given below:

- ☆ Nanophase ceramics are of particular interest because they are more strong and firm at elevated temperatures as compared to the coarse-grained ceramics.
- ☆ Nanostructured semiconductors are known to show various non-linear optical properties.

  Semiconductor quantum dot particles also show quantum confinement effects which may lead to special properties, like the luminescence in silicon powders and silicon germanium quantum dots as infrared optoelectronic devices. Nanostructured semiconductors are used as window layers in solar cells.
- ☆ Nanosized metallic powders have been used for the production of gas tight materials, dense parts and porous coatings. Cold welding properties combined with the ductility make them suitable for metal-metal bonding especially in the electronic industry.

- Single nanosized magnetic particles are mono-domains and one expects that also in magnetic nanophase materials the grains correspond with domains, while boundaries on the contrary to disordered walls. Very small particles have special atomic structures with discrete electronic states, which give rise to special properties in addition to the superparamagnetism behaviour. Magnetic nanocomposites have been used for mechanical force transfer (ferrofluids), for high density information storage and magnetic refrigeration.
- Nanostructured metal clusters and colloids of mono- or plurimetallic composition have a special impact in catalytic applications. They may serve as precursors for new type of heterogeneous catalysts (Cortex-catalysts) and have been shown to offer substantial advantages concerning activity, selectivity and lifetime in chemical transformations and electrocatalysis (fuel cells). Enantioselective catalysis was also achieved using chiral modifiers on the surface of nanoscale metal particles.
- Nanostructured metal-oxide thin films are receiving a growing attention for the realization of gas sensors (NOx, CO, CO_2, CH_4 and aromatic hydrocarbons) with enhanced sensitivity and selectivity. Nanostructured metal-oxide (MnO_2) finds application for rechargeable batteries for cars or consumer goods.
- Nanocrystalline silicon films for highly transparent contacts in thin film solar cell and nano-structured titanium oxide porous films for its high transmission and significant surface area enhancement leading to strong absorption in dye sensitized solar cells.
- Polymer based composites with a high content of inorganic particles leading to a high dielectric constant are interesting materials for photonic band gap structure.

Example of Common Nanomaterials

Some of the commonly used nanomaterials are nanoraods, nanoparticles, carbon nanotube, Dendrimer, liposome, micelle, nanocompositics *etc.* (Figure 35.10). Their nano scaled size emanates novel characteristics such as increased strength, chemical reactivity or conductivity. These unorthodox features put them forth in the list of those recent technological advancements that has led humanity to rethink their limits. The interface of biology/bioengineering and material sciences is one of the most promising areas of nanotechnology. Nano-biomaterials, as they are popularly known, display distinct biological effects when compared with bulk materials having same chemical composition.

Nanorods

The shape of the nano sized materials plays a key role in satisfying the purpose of the nano material. Up till now, out of the many developed different shapes,

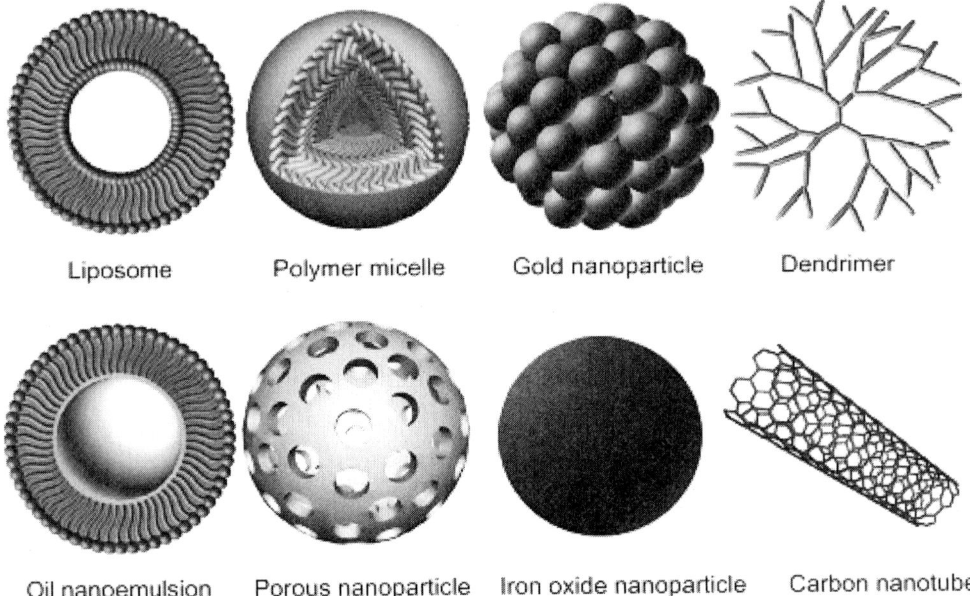

Figure 35.10. Examples of Nanomaterial.

Nanorods are among the most widely used one. Just as the name suggests, these nano rods are the elongated shaped, nano sized objects which have proved to be useful in many technological amelioration (Figure 35.11). These are generally manufactured using metals and semiconductors. The easiest and the most cost effective manufacturing is through direct chemical synthesis using specific chemical reagents which act as ligand during the formation and by their capability to combine specifically, they are the shape governing factor for nanorods. The feature that makes nanorods so special is their anisotropic shape *i.e.* due to their shape,

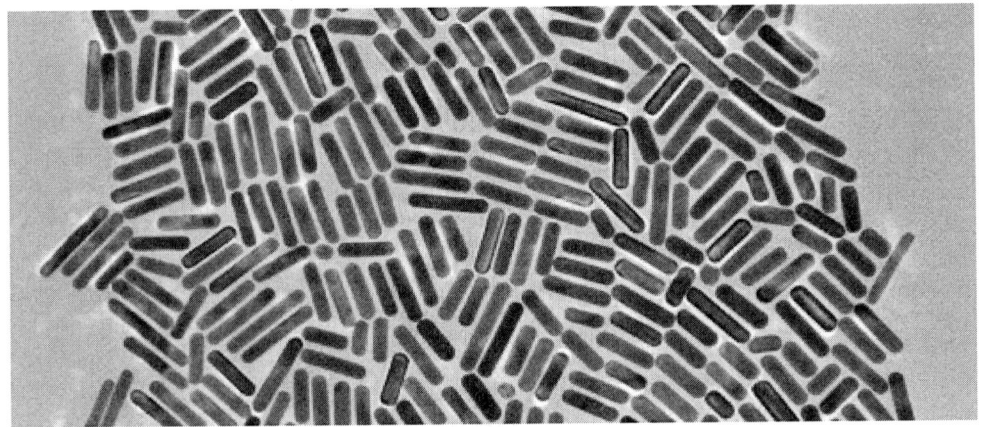

Figure 35.11. Structure and Shape of Nanorods.

various properties like refractive index, adsorption *etc.* differ in different direction. Due to availability of two direction in Rods (transverse direction and longitudinal direction), this phenomenon of change in properties can be used very effectively in Biosensing, Imaging and various other important phenomena. The change in the outer environment leads to aligning of these particles in different ways which leads to change in the wavelength they emit, thus acting as a good sensor which changes the color as soon as there is any change in the environment.

Quantum Dots (QDs)

QDs are inorganic nanocrystals, approximately 1–10 nm in size, with unique optical properties of broad excitation, narrow size-tunable emission spectra, high photochemical stability, and negligible photobleaching (Figure 35.12). They have been widely used, mainly as alternatives to fluorophores, for the development of optical biosensors to detect ions, organic compounds, pharmaceutical analytes, and biomolecules such as nucleic acids, proteins, amino acids, enzymes, carbohydrates,

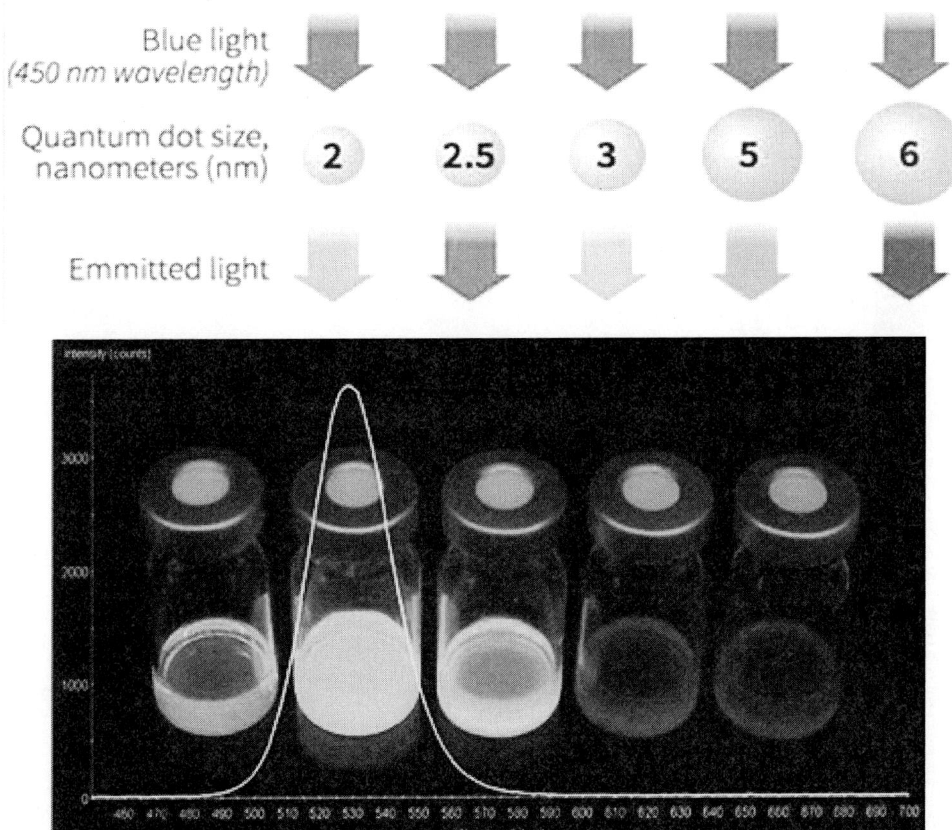

Figure 35.12. Optical Properties Quantum Dots.

and neurotransmitters. They have also been employed for the *in vivo* detection of target sites in cancer. In fact, they are the ideal candidates for multiplexed optical bioanalysis due to their ultra high sensitivity, high specificity, cost effectiveness, miniaturized size, size-dependent emission wavelength, and rapid analyte detection.

Nanoparticles (NPs)

NPs have also been extensively used in various bio-analytical applications, especially for the development of biosensors, diagnostics, imaging, drug delivery, and therapy, due to their unique optical and other properties. They change color in response to the binding of molecules to their surface. The change in the properties of nanoparticles by varying their size or shape has been exploited for various bioanalytical applications. There are many nanoparticles like metal, metal oxide, Magnetic nanoparticles *etc.* (Figure 35.13).

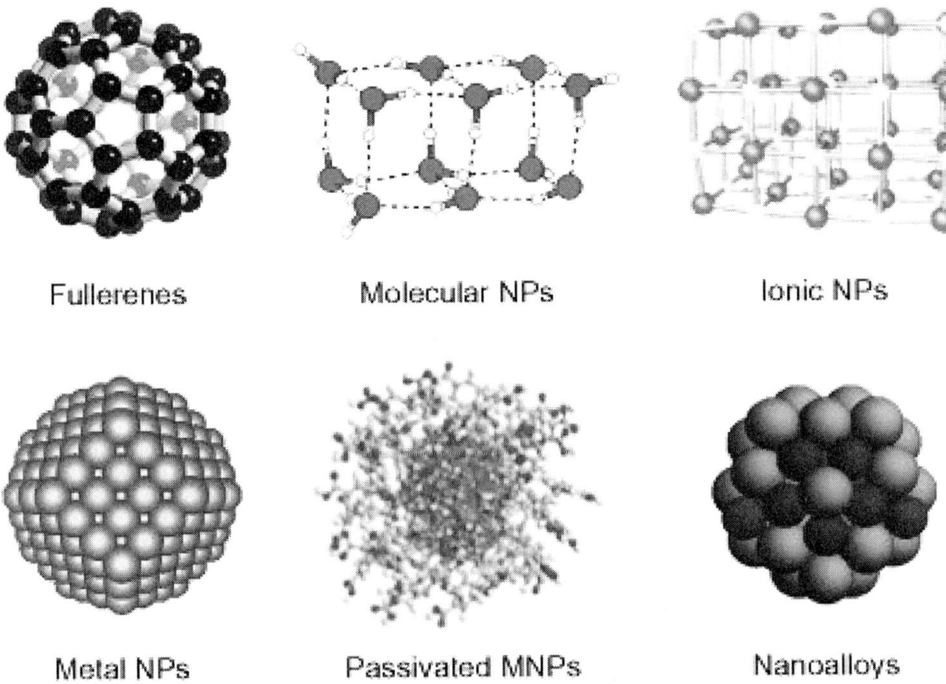

Figure 35.14. Different Type of Nanoparticles

Metal Nanoparticles

Metal nano particles like gold, silver, copper nanoparticles having extraordinary optical properties and this can be tuned by changing the size, shape, local environment, and the synthesis method. The most widely used NPs are GNPs, which have a non- toxic, biocompatible, and inert core. The prominent plasmon absorption and scattering properties of GNPs are highly useful for the early stage detection and photothermal therapy of cancer and other diseases. AuNPs and AgNPs are act as a carriers for the biorecognition element such as antibodies or aptamers and as labels for signal transduction and amplification. AuNPs are highly used in colorimetric and electrochemical assays to detect the pathogenic bacterial contamination in food. AgNPs are comparatively cheaper than AuNPs, mostly used to analyze food products to detect heavy metal ions, toxins and pesticide molecules. They have been used for the development of immunoassays, diagnostics, and biosensors for various analytes. Based on their preferential accumulation at the tumor sites, they have been used for the therapy of cancer and other diseases by acting as nano-carriers for the delivery of drugs, DNA, and genes. The multivalent GNPs facilitate efficient drug delivery to the target sites by shielding the unstable drugs, while their strongly enhanced surface plasmon resonance absorption enables the photothermal therapy of cancer. They have been extensively used in imaging due to their enhancement of the Raman and Rayleigh signals that provide greater chemical information. Therefore, it will be highly useful to combine all the benefits of GNPs, such as diagnostic, specific targeting, and therapeutic, into a single multifunctional GNPs- based platform, which can be chemically tailored for a particular disease.

Cerium Oxide NPs

This is an example of metal oxide nanoparticles, cerium oxide NPs contain dual reversible oxidation state Ce(III)/Ce(IV) on the NP surface has the ability to change redox states and surface properties (Figure 35.15). Cerium Oxide NPs found to possess peroxidase, superoxide and oxidase like activity hence those enzymes can be replaced from the sensing system by using Cerium Oxide NPs. Since Nanoceria is optically active based upon the interaction with the analyte it exhibits specific color patterns. This character of the nanoceria is one of the good choice to be used in the colorimetric sensing assay. Nanoceria's enzyme mimic properties are used to develop an enzyme-less electrochemical aptasensor for detection of food contaminants such as mycotoxins.

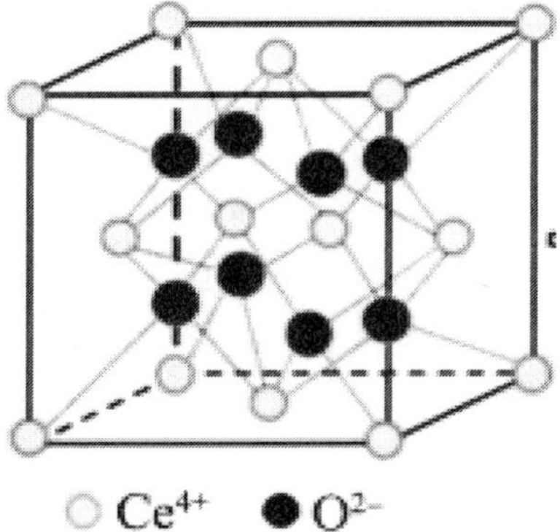

Figure 35.15. Cerium Oxide Nanoparticles.

Magnetic Nanoparticles

Magnetic NPsare the second most widely used NPs, which have been extensively employed in biosensors and diagnostics for the detection of proteins, enzymes, DNA, mRNA, drugs, metabolites, pathogens, and tumor cells. Various types of magnetic sensors based on different signal transduction mechanisms, such as magnetic relaxation switch assay sensors, magnetic particle relaxation sensors, and magnetoresistive sensors, have been developed. The diagnostic magnetic resonance (DMR) technology has also been employed extensively for magnetic biosensing. The development of miniaturized chip-based nuclear magnetic resonance detector (μNMR) has further enhanced the capabilities of DMR for the highly sensitive analyte detection in microliter sample volumes, multiplex analysis, and development of cost-effective, portable, and high- throughput platforms for point-of-care diagnostics.

Dendrimers

Dendrimers are hyperbranched, monodispersed, star-shaped, and nanometer-scale three dimensional macromolecules with a very high density of surface functional groups. They are composed of three distinct components, *i.e.*, the core, the interior dendron, and the exterior surface with terminal functional groups (Figure 35.16). They have been used extensively in various biosensors and diagnostics, such as those based on electrochemistry, fluorescence, surface enhanced Raman scattering, impedimetry, and surface plasmon resonance, mainly as they increase the analytical sensitivity, stability, and reproducibility but reduce the non-specific interactions. They have also been used for other bioanalytical applications such as drug delivery, gene transfection, and catalysis.

Carbon Nanotubes (CNT) and Graphene

Graphene (single atomic layer of graphite) and carbon nanotube having very good electrical conductivity (electron transport property) hence, these are currently utilized in electrochemical analysis (Figure 35.17). Since these carbon nano materials are having very good conductivity, large surface area and easiness of modification with biomolecules, these are applied to a variety of electrochemical biosensing systems based have been for electrochemical detection of Chemical (bisphenol A, hydrazine and nitrite, organophosphorus pesticides melamine, heavy metal ions (and mercury (II) (Hg^{2+}) and silver (I) (Ag^{+}) biological toxin (ochratoxin A) and bacteria have been detected by composite materials made of Graphene biosensor.

Buckyballs or Fullerines

Buckyballs, also called fullerenes, were one of the **first nanoparticles** discovered. Specifically, a **bucky ball is a spherical fullerene** while the **cylindrical fullerene is called a carbon nanotube**. This discovery happened in 1985 by a trio of researchers working out of Rice University named **Richard Smalley, Harry**

Interior with multiple branches (generations **G**), well-suited for encapsulation of drugs and nanomaterials

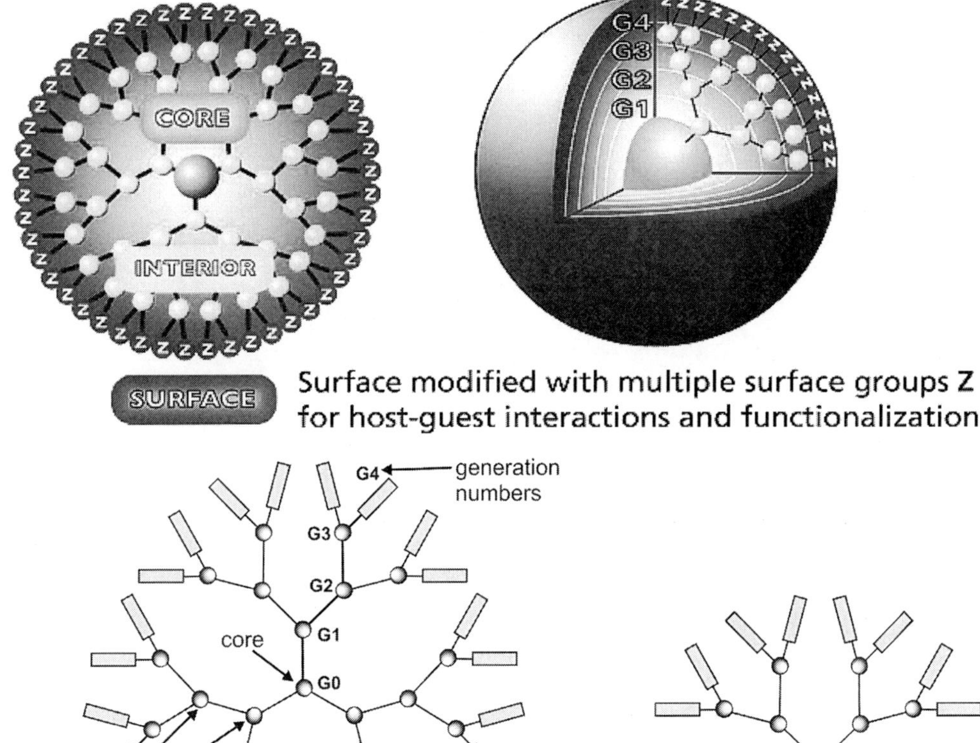

Figure 35.16. Shape and Structures of Dendrimers.

Kroto, and Robert Curl. This nanometer scale structure was named fullerene due to its resemblance to the highly symmetric domes designed by the architect Richard Buckminster Fuller. Buckminster fullerenes or fullerenes are the third allotrope of carbon and consist of a family of spheroidal or cylindrical molecules with all the carbon atoms sp2 hybridized. Buckyballs are composed of carbon atoms linked to three other carbon atoms by covalent bonds. However, the carbon atoms are connected in the same pattern of hexagons and pentagons which looks similar on a soccer ball, giving a buckyball the spherical structure.

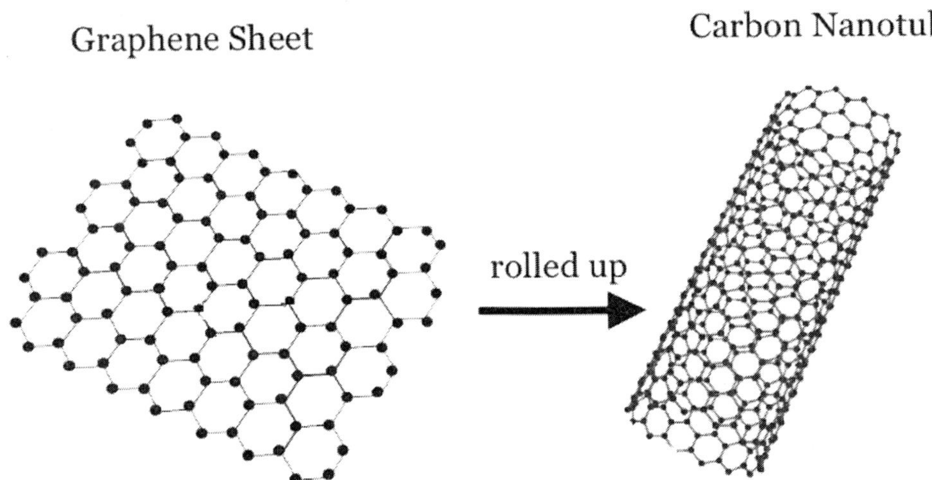

Figure 35.17. Graphene and Carbon Nano Tubes (CNT).

The most common buckyball contains 60 carbon atoms and is sometimes called C60. Other sizes of bucky balls range from those containing 20 carbon atoms to more than 100 carbon atoms. The covalent bonds between carbon atoms make buckyballs very strong, and the carbon atoms readily form covalent bonds with a variety of other atoms. Buckyballs are used in composites to strengthen material. Buckyballs have the interesting electrical property of being very good electron acceptors, which means they accept loose electrons from other materials. This feature is useful, for example, in increasing the efficiency of solar cells in transforming sunlight into electricity.

Nanocomposites

A nanocomposite is a nanomaterial which is incorporates in to the nanomaterial matrix (Figure 35.18). Upon integration of nanocomposite in to biosensor, the sensitivity of the biosensor is enhancing because of its better quenching ability and also it provides better transduction with improved current respons and enhanced storage stability. The porosity of the nanocomposite provides additional stability to the biosensor via eûcient enzyme immobilization. Along with this nanocomposites also has high mechanical strength, resistance to corrosion, high electrical and thermal conduction and long shelf life. Chitosan-TiO_2 graphene nanocomposite has been developed to detect organophosphate pesticides in cabbage. Graphene oxide and gold nanocomposites (GO/AuNCs) has led to ultrasensitive detection of aflatoxin B1 (AFB1) in peanut samples.

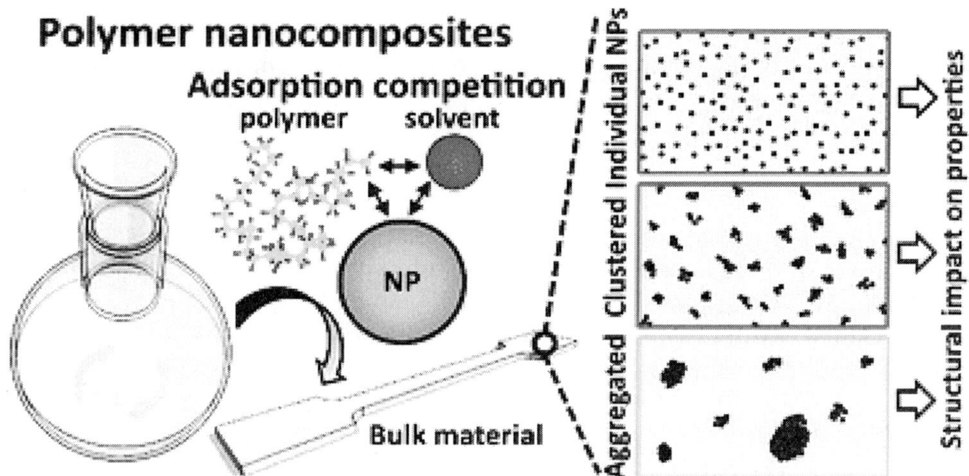

Figure 35.18. Nanocomposites.

Semiconductor

Semiconductor is a solid substance that allows heat or electricity to pass through it or along it in particular conditions (or) Semiconductor is any of a class of crystalline solids intermediate in electrical conductivity between a conductor and an insulator. Semiconductors are employed in the manufacture of various kinds of electronic devices, including diodes, transistors, and integrated circuits. Semiconducting crystallite, which is a few nanometers in scale, with size specific optical and electronic behavior, is referred to as a semiconductor nanocrystal (NC). Semiconductor (SC) NCs are a promising technological material because the ability to control their optical and electronic properties can be exploited for a diverse range of applications, such as light-emitting diodes, bio-labels, single molecule transistors and solar cells. The introduction of trace intentional impurities (or doping) is central to controlling the behavior of SC materials. Dopants possess the ability to modify strongly the optical, magnetic, and electronic properties of bulk SCs. A dopant, with one more valence electron than the host atom it substitutes for, can donate its extra electron to the SC for electronic charge transport. Similarly, an impurity atom with one less electron can donate a hole to the SC. It is the ability to control precisely the number of carriers available in the SC by doping, which has expedited the advance in SC-based electronic and optoelectronic technology. The advantage of doped SCs is that they provide the device engineer with a wide range of mobilities, so that materials are available with properties that meet specific requirements. Hence, it is natural to extend the versatility of nanocrystals by adding dopants. Doping can expand the range of properties in SC NCs substantially.

Diode

Diode, an electrical component that allows the flow of current in only one direction. In circuit diagrams, a diode is represented by a triangle with a line across one vertex.

Micelle

Micelle, in physical chemistry, a loosely bound aggregation of several tens or hundreds of atoms, ions (electrically charged atoms), or molecules, forming a colloidal particle *i.e.*, one of a number of ultramicroscopic particles dispersed through some continuous medium. For example an aggregate of molecules in a colloidal solution formed by detergents.

Polymer

A polymer is a very large, chain-like molecule made up of monomers, which are small molecules. It can be naturally occurring or synthetic.

Synthesis of Nanomaterials

The boundaries between the physical regions of macroscopic, microscopic, and nanoscopic are not well defined and they depend on the effects being considered. Nevertheless, materials of the macro-scale usually exhibit similar physical properties to those of the bulk form. On the other hand, reducing the grain size of a material or synthesizing the material below certain limits results in the appearance of either new or changed chemical and/or physical properties of the material and hence has a dramatic impact on structural, thermodynamic, electronic, spectroscopic, electromagnetic and chemical properties. Nanomaterial can be synthesized by physical, Chemical and biological method. Physical methods for blending nanomaterials include crushing, physical vapor deposition (PVD), ball processing, lithography, pyrolysis and sputtering *etc.*, while chemical method are sol gel synthesis, chemical vapor deposition (CVD), Electrodeposition *etc.* Biological synthesis of nanomaterials includes plants and microbes like yeast, fungi, bacteria and actinomycetes are utilized to syntheize the nanomaterial. It has been found that biological sources act as reducing metal ions from the soil (Figure 35.19). This process is quite safe as comparison to other physical and chemical methods. It is a lesser amount of energy but the nanomaterials produced by these methods have found very reactive.

The physical, chemical and biological method based nanomaterials synthesize grouped in to two basic approaches 1. Top-down method depending on size reduction from bulk materials 2. Bottom-up system where materials are synthesis from atomic level.

1. Top-Down Approach

The top down approach uses natural and man-made chunks or blocks that are cast, sawed or machined into precisely formed products, small or large, ranging

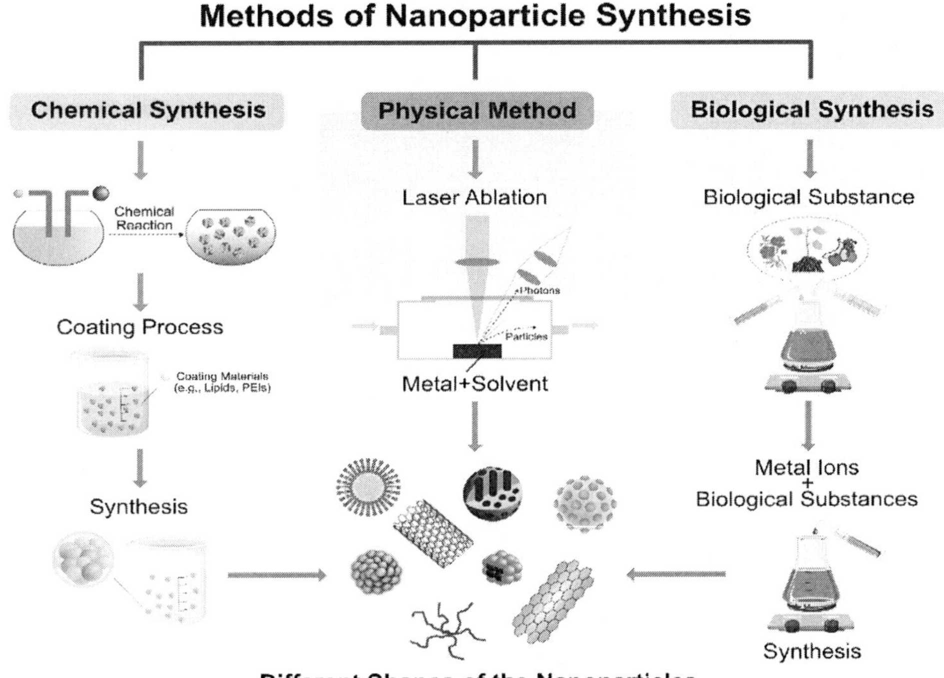

Figure 35.19. Various Methods of Nanomaterial Synthesis.

from integrated circuits to jumbo jets. Methods to produce nanoparticles from bulk materials include high energy ball milling, solution based chemistry, mechano-chemical processing, etching, electro explosion, and sonication. Patterned structures which are grown by suitable lithographic and ion implantation techniques are the cornerstone of silicon integrated chip technology as shown in Figure 35.20.

2. Bottom-Up Approach

Bottom-up approach is the manufacturing of nanomaterials by manipulating and organizing individual atoms and molecules into particular configurations in a fashion similar to processes performed by molecular machines in living organisms. The self-assembly lipid molecules into nanostructure such as liposomes, chemical vapor deposition techniques, Chemical Reduction method, sol-gel method and microbial synthesis are considered as an example of the bottom-up approach for constructing nanomaterials. The key to the application of nanotechnology will be the development of processes that control placement of individual atoms to form products of great complexity at extremely small scale. The advantage of bottom-up approach would be a nearly infinite flexibility to create any substance, object, device, machine or material through atom (or molecule) by atom (or molecule) construction. Also this processing produces more complex structures from atoms or molecules, also, this method produce a uniform controlling sizes, shapes and size ranges of nano materials (Figure 35.20).

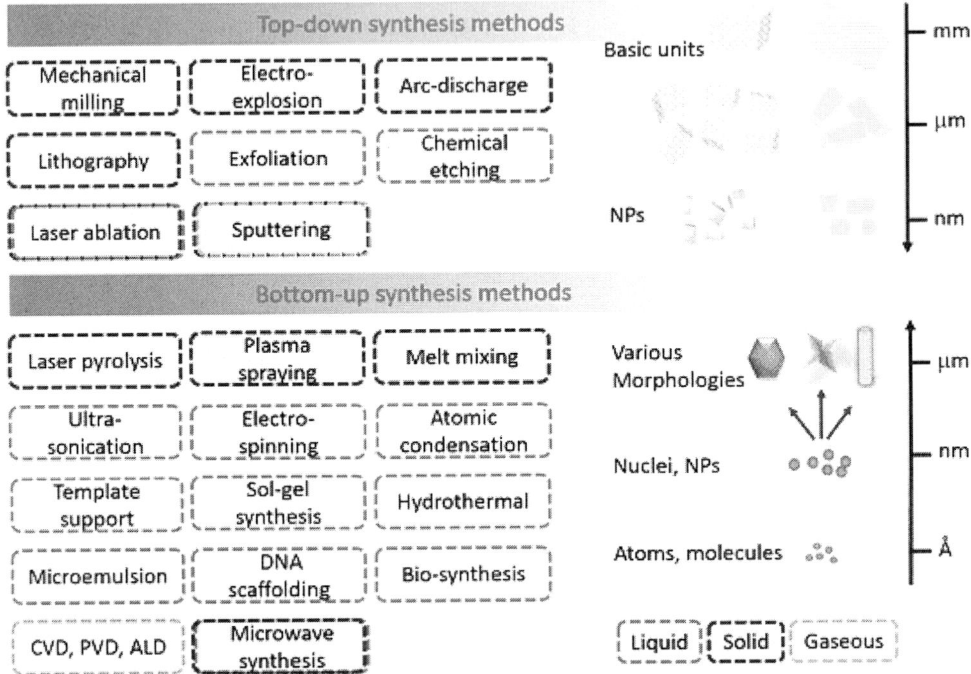

Figure 35.20. Various Methods of Topdown and Bottom Up Approach of Nanomaterial Synthesis.

Applications of Nanomaterials

Nowadays in many aspects of our lives more and more materials with new properties are required to ensure further development of mankind. The appearance of nanomaterials has given a great impulse to further discoveries in various fields of science. Nanomaterials with attractive electronic, optical, magnetic, thermal and catalytic properties have attracted great attention due to their widespread applications in physics, chemistry, biology, medicine, material science and interdisciplinary fields. Some basic distinctive properties of nanomaterials are a very small particle size, the large surface area, accelerating the interaction between nanomaterials and the environment in which they are placed as well as the absence of point defects resulting in strength of nanomaterials ten times the strength of steel. These properties explain the fact that even a gram of a nanomaterial may be more effective than a large number of ordinary matters. Today nanomaterials have been used many areas such as:

- ☆ Agricultural and food technologies

- ☆ Production technologies
- ☆ Military engineering
- ☆ Nuclear power engineering
- ☆ Protection of materials surface
- ☆ Medicine and biotechnology
- ☆ Electronic equipment and other applications

1. Agricultural and Food Technologies

The nanotechnology-aided applications have the potential to change agricultural production by allowing better management and conservation of inputs of plant feed additives and food packaging materials (Figure 35.21). 1. Crop improvement 2. Increase efficient fertilizers and pesticides, 3. Soil management.

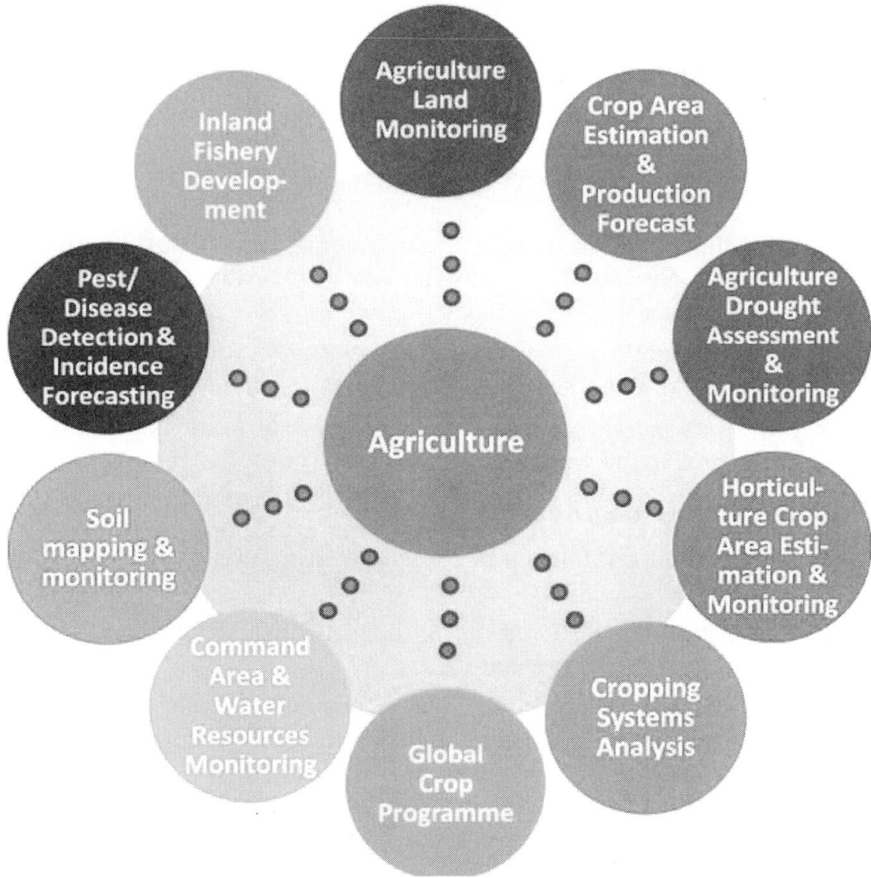

Figure 35.21. A Pictorial Demonstration of Applications of Nanotechnology in Agri-Food Sector.

4. Plant disease detection. 5. Water management and 6. Analysis of gene expression and Regulation, and Posr harvest technology. Different types on nanomaterials also utilized in the following ways (i) Nanoforms zeolites for slow release and efficient dosage of water and fertilizers for plants; drugs for livestock; nanocapsules and herbicide delivery (ii) Nanosensors for soil quality and for plant health monitoring; nanosensors for pests detection (iii) Nanomagnets for removal of soil contaminants and (iv) Nano-particles for new pesticides, insecticides, and insect repellents.

2. Production Technologies

- It is important and perspective now to use nanomaterials in composites as components of various functions.
- In the production of steels and alloys adding nanopowders helps to reduce porosity and improve the range of mechanical properties.
- Manifestation of superplasticity in nanostructured aluminum and titanium alloys makes their use promising in the manufacture of complex shapes details and for using as a connecting layer in welding different solid state materials.
- Very large specific surface nanopowders promote their use in a number of chemical processes as catalysts.

3. Military Engineering

- Ultra-fine powders are used in a number of radar absorbing coatings for aircraft, created with the use of technology "Stealth", and promising types of explosives and incendiary.
- Carbon nanofibers are used in special ammunition intended for the scrapping of the enemy power systems (so-called "graphite bomb").
- Nanosensor used to detect the presence of toxic gases and harmful pathogens in the warfield.

4. Nuclear Power Engineering

- The beginning of nuclear power engineering was given by the ultra-fine powders.
- These powders are commonly used in industrial processes for the separation of uranium isotopes.
- Prospects for the development of nuclear energy by bringing the particles to the nanostate are mainly associated with a decrease in the average consumption of natural uranium.
- This happens mostly at the expense of increasing the depth of the nuclear fuel combustion.
- To do this, scientists are exploring the possibility of the creation of coarse-grained structures of nuclear materials, which can be porous.
- These nanomaterials will promote a high retention of fission products.

5. Material Surface Protection

- ☆ In some cases, for reliable operation, it is necessary to ensure the high water and oil repellency properties of material surface.
- ☆ Some examples of such products may be car windows, glass planes and ships, protective clothing, wall storage tanks for liquids, building construction, *etc.*
- ☆ At present the titanium oxide nanoparticles coating with sizes of 20-50 nm and a polymer binder have been developed. This coating greatly reduces the wettability of the surface with water, oil and alcohol solutions.

6. Medicine and Biotechnology

1. Diagnostics

The development of nanotechnology in biomedicine due to improved technology helps to obtain the images, characterization and analysis of biological material, providing a high degree of resolution. Magnetic nanomaterials are an important source for the production of biosensors. The most commonly used nanoparticles are based on the iron oxide coated with various polymers. The surface can be modified by various biospecific ligands as well. Thus the shell protects the iron oxide nanoparticles from chemical interaction with molecules of cells and tissues. Some nanomaterials are also used as electrochemical sensors (nanotubes and nanoparticles) for diagnostics.

2. Delivery of Drugs (Molecules) to the Target

Targeted drug delivery in cancer therapy will resolve several issues such as protecting drugs from degradation and adversing interactions with biological molecules. Also increasing the selectivity of drug absorption by tumor cells, controlling of pharmacokinetics, increasing bioavailability of drugs into tumor cells. Apart from the drugs nanoparticles can deliver genes into cells.

3. Treatment and Prosthetics using Nanomaterials

The unique properties of nanomaterials allow to produce various implants and dentures. With the use of nanotechnology we can get safe, biocompatible and durable implants.

4. Electronic Equipment

Nanotechnology in Electronics was given a boost by using carbon nanotubes. They are not only able to replace the transistors, but also give the revolutionary electronic circuits their new mechanical and optical properties to create flexible and transparent electronics. The nanotubes are more mobile and do not hold the light in a thin layer, so that the experimental matrix integrated circuit can be bent without loss of the electronic properties.

Another application of nanotechnology in electronics is the creation of a new type of hard disks. In 2007, the Nobel Prize in Physics was awarded to **Peter Grunberg and Albert Fert** for the discovery of the giant magneto resistance effect or, as some authors call it, GMR-effect. On the basis of this effect, it is possible to create magnetic field sensors that can exactly read the information recorded on the hard disk with almost the atomic density.

One more prospective application of nanomaterials is producing solar cells. The solar cells that are made on the basis of nanowires instead of the traditional metal wires can increase fifteen times the amount of energy received by a battery. Conductor nanoscale has unique properties of the light absorption. Using nanostructured materials in the manufacturing of the solar cells can improve their efficiency and reduce their cost.

Various other application of nanomaterials are,

- ✰ Silver nanoparticles have good antibacterial properties are used in surgical instruments, refrigerators, air-conditioners, water purifiers *etc.*
- ✰ Gold nanoparticles are used in catalytic synthesis of silicon nanowires, sensors carrying the drugs and in the detection of tumors.
- ✰ ZnO nanoparticles are used in electronics, ultraviolet (UV) light emitters, piezoelectric devices and chemical sensors.
- ✰ TiO_2 nanoparticles are used as photocatalyst and sunscreen cosmetics (UV blocking pigment).
- ✰ Antimony-Tin-Oxide (ATO), Indium-Tin-Oxide (ITO) nanoparticles are used in car windows, liquid crystal displays and in solar cell preparations.
- ✰ Nanoscale structures and materials such as nanoparticles, nanowires, nanofibers, and nanotubes have been explored in many biological applications *e.g.*, biosensing, biological separation, molecular imaging, and/or anticancer therapy because of their novel properties and functions differ drastically from their bulk counterparts.
- ✰ Their high volume/surface ratio, surface tailorability, improved solubility, and multifunctionality open many new possibilities for biomedicine.
- ✰ The intrinsic optical, magnetic and biological properties of nanomaterials offer remarkable opportunities to study and regulate complex biological processes for biomedical applications in an unprecedented manner.
- ✰ General applications of these materials are found in water purification, wastewater treatment, environmental remediation, food processing and packaging, industrial and household purposes, medicine and in smart sensor development.
- ✰ Nanomaterials prepared from metals, semiconductors, carbon or polymeric species, shaped into nanoparticles and nanotubes have been widely investigated for their ability as electrode modification materials to enhance the efficiencies of electrochemical biosensors.

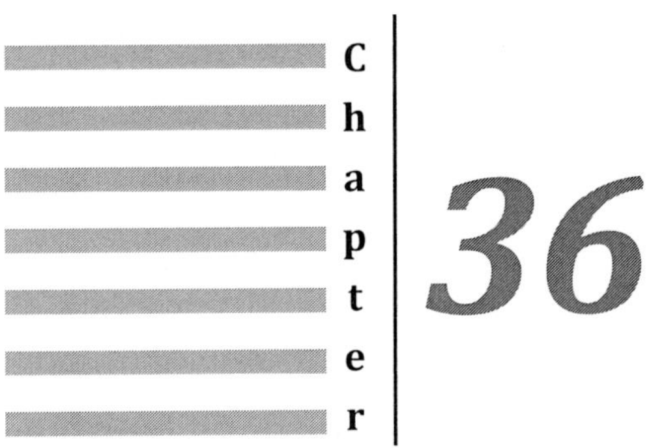

Nanobiotechnology in Agriculture

Nanobiotechnology is a discipline in which tools from nanotechnology are developed and applied to study biological phenomena. Nanobiotechnology employs nanoscale principles and techniques to understand and transform biosystems (living or non-living); utilize biological principles and materials to create new devices and systems which is integrated in the nanoscale. The integration of nanotechnology with biotechnology as well as with cognitive science and infotechnology is expected to expand exponentially in the next few years and give great breakthrough in the scientific field. With the use of nanobiotechnology it is possible to graft small devices closer and closer to reality, which can deliver dynamic molecules easily with enhanced stability. In short, such developments in the field of biotechnology will vastly impact the fields of science and technology. Nanoparticles can serve as probes, sensors or vehicles for biomolecule delivery in cellular systems. Nanobiotechnology offers some unique opportunities in different fields such as agriculture, environment, medicine and biotherapeutics.

Application of Nanobiotechnology in Agriculture

Manipulation of genes in the biological system is the major process of crop improvement through genetic engineering and genome editing. Manipulation of genes would be done in three ways either gene(s) isolated from one organism and transfers them to another organism or puts them back in the original with a different combination or enhance the expression or suppression of certain set of desired genes. In agriculture, gene manipulation mainly involved in development of genetically modified plants or genome edited plants with desired quality. In nutshell it's the manipulation of plants for the benefit of mankind. Genetic engineering of plants is at the core of environmental sustainability efforts, natural product synthesis of pharmaceuticals, and agricultural crop engineering to meet the needs of a growing population in a changing global climate.

Conventional Plant Engineering Techniques

Plant engineering is crucial for ensuring sustainable agricultural production while simultaneously addressing the challenges of growing food demand and improving human nutrition. Genetic engineering can create crops with higher yield under abiotic and biotic stress conditions, and an improved nutrition profile for humans, as well as minimizing the adverse environmental impacts of crop production. Currently, engineering methods mainly comprise; (i) insertion of exogenous genes (ii) protein-level alterations or modifications (iii) RNAi at the mRNA level and (iv) nuclease-based genome-level editing. Unlike mammalian cells, plant cells have rigid and multilayered cell walls that present a substantial barrier to the delivery of exogenous biomolecules (*e.g.*, nucleases, siRNA, proteins/ enzymes) into plant cells. Conventional delivery systems for this purpose include biologically mediated delivery (through *Agrobacterium* or virus infection) and particle bombardment delivery methods (*e.g.*, gene gun). The bacterium/virus-mediated delivery system is the most commonly used tool for plant genetic transformation, but is only applicable to a narrow range of plant species or tissues because of host-range limitations. In addition, this transgenic method often involves the integration of exogenous genes into the host genome. The biolistic method can deliver biomolecules into cells of a wide range of plant species or tissues via a gene gun or external force, but this delivery system is limited to the bombarded sites and often causes tissue damage as a result of external mechanical force.

By using nanomaterials,inserting or tweaking genes and developing genetically engineered or genome edited plants are highly simple and quick with any type of plant. For example a gene bound to a carbon nanotube can easily diffuse into plant cells, where it is expressed as if it were the cell's own gene. To date, most genetic engineering of plants is done by firing genes into the tissue, a process known as biolistics or delivering genes via *Agrobacterium* bacteria. Both the methods are successful only a small percentage, which is a major limitation for scientists seeking to create disease- or drought-resistant crops or to engineer plants for improved quality. Nanotubes, however, are highly successful at delivering a gene into the nucleus and also into the chloroplast that is even harder to target using current methods. An easy gene-delivery technique would be a boon for scientists now trying to improve the efficiency of light energy capture to boost crop yields. The nanotube not only protects the DNA from being degraded by the cell, but also prevents it from being inserted into the plant's genome. So nanobiotechnology not only useful in quick and efficient delivery of genes in to the plants across species and also enable the generation of transgenic plant lines without integration of foreign DNA into the plant genome.

Nanotechnology Renovating Plant Genome Manipulation: Recent Breakthroughs

Nanotechnology-based carriers can deliver a variety of bioactive molecules into cells. Although nanomaterials (NM) have already been utilized extensively in animal cells and organs as delivery vehicles for targeted drug delivery, cancer therapy, and the treatment of genetic diseases, their use in plant systems lags behind. However, results reported recently in plants are proving that NMs may overcome the barrier of the cell wall in adult plants and reduce the drawbacks associated with current transgene delivery systems. Most of the pioneering studies for nanomaterial-based plant genetic engineering are used in plant cell cultures. For example, in plants, nanomaterials are used to deliver plasmid DNA (pDNA), double-standed RNA (dsRNA), Small interfering RNA (siRNA), proteins and phytohormone into either cell wall-free protoplasts or intact cells. A particularly important breakthrough has been the development of honeycomb-like mesoporous silica nanoparticles (MSNs) as a carrier to deliver pDNA and protein into intact cells with the assistance of a biolistic method. In this approach, the pDNA and its chemical inducer are loaded simultaneously into MSNs, and the ends of the MSNs are then capped using gold nanoparticles as a gatekeeper. Once the MSNs are delivered inside the cells, the gold nanoparticles are uncapped by using a gate-opening trigger (*i.e.*, a switch that opens in response to changes in chemical or physiological conditions) to allow controlled release of the biogenic molecules. Further development is on going to develop functionalized MSNs to deliver foreign pDNA into the epidermis, cortex, and endodermis of intact *Arabidopsis* roots without the use of mechanical force. In addition to MSNs, other nanomaterial-based delivery systems have also been developed, such as carbon nanotubes (CNTs), layered double hydroxide (LDH) clay nanosheets, DNA nanostructures, and magnetic nanoparticles. Silicon Carbide-Mediated Transformation is successful approach to deliver DNA in different calli (tobacco, maize, rice, soybean and cotton).

Remarkable progress has been made recently in this respect, although it is still poorly understood how these nanomaterials interact with plant cells and with the series of barriers in plants at the cellular and subcellular levels. For example, functionalized CNTs can be passively internalized into intact and walled cells of a range of plant species. This approach then enables exogenous functional genes in the form of pDNA or siRNA to be delivered into cells, resulting in strong expression of the exogenous gene or highly efficient gene silencing. Meanwhile, CNTs can also protect polynucleotides from nuclease degradation for a desired period, providing a time-window to allow gene expression or silencing in the absence of transgene integration into the plant genome. Such approaches are capable of both subcellular and tissue targeting. CNTs were designed to selectively deliver pDNA into chloroplasts through a lipid exchange envelope-penetration mechanism, without external biolistic or chemical aid. This elegant methodology enables pH-dependent release of loaded pDNA (*e.g.*, only releasing DNA strands at pH >7.5), thereby allowing release in the chloroplast stroma (ca pH 8) but not in the plant cell cytosol (ca pH 5.5). It has also been demonstrated that LDH nanosheets can facilitate delivery of dsRNA into walled plant cells of the model plant *Nicotiana tabacum*, thereby enabling gene silencing of homologous RNA and providing sustained protection against plant viruses. Magnetic nanoparticles can be used to drive exogenous DNA into pollen through pollen apertures in the presence of a magnetic field. This facilitates the creation of transgenic plants, which is particularly useful for plant species that are difficult to genetically transform using conventional methods. These pioneering studies have made important progress in developing nanomaterial-based carrier systems to deliver exogenous biomolecules into intact and walled plant cells, paving the way toward future applications in plant biotechnology.

dsRNA of different plant viruses can be loaded on non-toxic, degradable, layered double hydroxide (LDH) clay nanosheets or BioClay. The dsRNAs and/or their RNA breakdown the viral products provide protection against the Cauliflower Mosaic Virus (CMV) in sprayed tobacco leaves, but they also confer systemic protection to newly emerged, unsprayed leaves on viral challenge 20 days after a single spray treatment in tobacco. More in general, this is a proof of concept for species-independent and passive delivery of genetic material, without transgene integration, into plant cells for different biotechnology applications in plants. A successful stable genetic transformation has been achieved in cotton plants via magnetic nanoparticles (MNPs). β-glucuronidase (GUS) reporter gene- MNP complex were infiltrated into cotton pollen grains by magnetic force, without compromising pollen viability. Through pollination with magnetofected pollen, cotton transgenic plants were successfully generated and exogenous DNA was successfully integrated into the genome, effectively expressed, and stably inherited in the offspring obtained by selfing. Carbon nanotubes scaffolds applied to external plant tissue by infusion were used to deliver linear and plasmid DNA, as well as siRNA, in *Nicotiana benthamiana, Eruca sativa, Triticum aestivum*, and *Gossypium hirsutum* leaves and in *E. sativa* protoplasts, resulting in a strong transgene expression in plants.

In contrast to conventional plant genetic engineering methods (mediated by *Agrobacterium*, viruses, or external biolistic/chemical aid), the use of a nanomaterial-based delivery system can passively traverse intact cell walls to deliver a variety of biomolecule cargos (Figure 36.1). This delivery system provides several benefits for plant genetic engineering. First, it overcomes host-range limitations and is therefore potentially applicable to a wide range of plant species and different tissues, including plants which are difficult to regenerate from tissue culture (a requirement for conventional transgenic methods). Second, it can be easily tailored through functionalization of nanomaterials to enable release of the cargo in a controlled or target-specific manner.

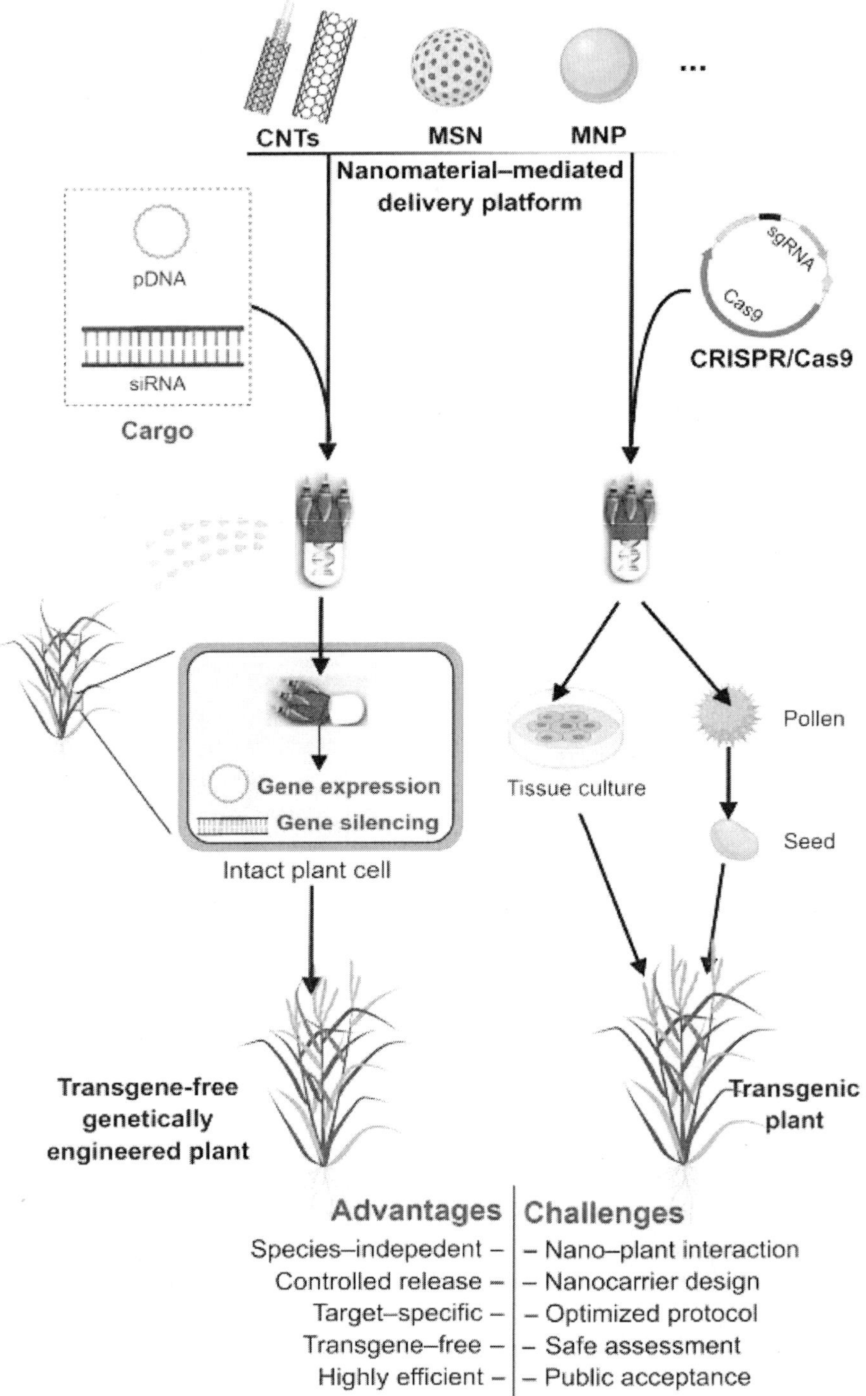

Figure 36.1. Nanomaterial-Mediated Plant Genetic Engineering.

This can be achieved either by an exogenous gate-opening trigger or by a condition-responsive gatekeeper design. These advantages can make this approach 'smarter' for controlled and targeted release of cargo upon reaching a specific target where the required conditions are met (*e.g.*, pH-dependent release. Third, it allows delivery of exogenous functional genes or siRNA/dsRNA into plants to create genetically enhanced plants without transgene integration into the genome (*i.e.*, 'engineered nontransgenic plant'). In this case, the modified traits resulting from transient gene expression or silencing cannot be inherited in the offspring. Finally, the system has higher delivery efficiency. It can load a comparatively large amount of biomolecules and allows codelivery of different biomolecules simultaneously to the target sites.

Chloroplast Transformation

Carbon nanotubes can be used as tools to more easily deliver genes into plant cell nuclei and chloroplasts, by two different approaches. First approach involves grafting DNA onto a carbon nanotube to deliver the biomolecule into plant cells while the second makes use of a mechanism called lipid exchange envelope penetration (LEEP) for delivery into chloroplasts specifically. Both techniques are very different to conventional genetic engineering methods – such as biolistics (which is done by firing genes into plant tissue) or delivering genes using infectious bacteria. It is also possible to make nanoparticles penetrate plant cell membranes by tuning the electrical charge of the particles (so that they had a high enough zeta potential) and their size (so they were of the right dimensions). Getting into chloroplasts carbon nanotubes are interesting because they are among the few nanoparticles that can be made narrow *i.e.*, just 1-nm-wide, which means they are small enough to slip through the plant cell wall. Their exceptionally high strength and needle-like aspect ratio allows them to be passively internalized into the plant cells of many different species. In nanotube grafting technique, the single-walled carbon nanotubes connected to chitosan, a biopolymer that is commonly found in the shells of shrimps and other crustaceans. This chitosan-complexed-SWCNT is positively charged, which allows it to bind to negatively-charged plasmid DNA through electrostatic attraction. The complex enters the leaf through stomata, passes through the cell wall and cell membrane, and finally localizes in the chloroplasts. Since chloroplasts are slightly more basic (pH 8) than the cytosol or the environment outside the plant cell, the chitosan-SWCNT becomes positively charged when it reaches the chloroplasts. Binding with plasmid-DNA is thus weakened and the DNA unloads within the chloroplasts. Once unloaded it can be translated into proteins. Meanwhile, use of the so-called lipid exchange envelope penetration (LEEP) mechanism to deliver nanoparticles with DNA on their surface into plant cells – and more specifically into chloroplasts. Since plant cells have dozens of chloroplasts, those expressing foreign genes could allow for much larger amounts of a desired protein to be generated than is possible in only cell nuclei expressing these genes. Editing chloroplast genes in this way could help increase the amount of energy produced by photosynthesis, which, in turn would allow plants to grow bigger and more quickly, and in greater yield. These two technique works for wide range of plant species.

Nanoparticle-mediated chloroplast transformation approach is a useful complement to the plant biotechnology toolkit. Since the chloroplast genome can only be inherited from maternal cells, the beneficial traits can be passed onto offspring, but, importantly, cannot be transferred to other, nearby, plant species. This means that there is less risk of undesirable gene spread. It could also help optimize pharmaceutical product synthesis in plant chloroplasts – some vaccines are actually produced within the chloroplasts through genetic engineering. So that applications in crop engineering and plant biology studies could also benefit. In the future, it is possible to engineer crops that are resistant to diseases or droughts by delivering the appropriate gene to the chloroplasts."

Nanobiotechnology based Genome Editing

With so many distinct advantages, further development of nanomaterial-based plant genetic engineering will enable a diverse range of applications in plant biotechnology and plant biology. For example, because of the strict regulation of genetically modified organisms (GMOs), there is great interest in creating genetically improved plants in which gene expression is controlled, but in which the exogenous DNA is not integrated into the genome. As a result, this approach may be exempt from the strict regulations that govern the use of GMOs. In addition, the ongoing development of nanomaterial-based plant genetic engineering can be used in plant functional genetic studies by rapidly building RNAi interference or overexpression lines for verifying the functions of specific genes. This will be especially useful for plant species that are difficult to transform genetically using conventional methods. As a high-efficiency and species-independent delivery system, the nanomaterial-based methodology could also be developed as a high-throughput screening tool to identify genotypes that result in desired phenotypes through transient gene overexpression or silencing during a specified period. Similarly, the approach can potentially be extended to carry a nuclease-based genome-editing cargo such as CRISPR/Cas9 for producing stable transgenic plants. A key use would be CRISPR-Cas9 gene editing is delivering the gene for Cas9, which is the enzyme that targets and cuts DNA, along with the DNA encoding guide RNA—Cas9's address label—to edit specific genes with high precision.

The first and promising approach of genome editing mediated by mesoporous silica nanoparticles (MSNs). It has been used as carriers to deliver *Cre recombinase* in *Zea mays* immature embryos, carrying *loxP* sites integrated into chromosomal DNA. After the biolistic introduction of engineered MSNs in plant tissues, the *loxP* was correctly recombined establishing a successful genome editing. Nanotubes can easily slip through plant cell walls, and get in to the nucleous. So packaging of DNA into a single-stranded plasmid then that is attached to a carbon nanotube would make DNA diffused into the cell. Within two or three days after DNA transfer both Cas9 protein and CRISPR guide RNA would be expressed, allowing them to link up to form a ribonucleoprotein complex that edits the genome, permanently.

Double-Strand RNAs to Control Fungal Pathogen

Recent developments in the field of RNA-based fungicides indicate that it is a feasible technology for substituting traditional biochemical fungicides. Double-strand RNAs, designed to hybridize with vital mRNAs of fungal pathogens, are sprayed on leaves or fruits and induce expression silencing in the pathogen. However, the short mean-life of naked RNAs in the environment is an obstacle to overcome. Traditional clay nanosheets were tested as protectants of double-strand RNA and probed to enhance the mean-life of the biomolecules and extend the biocidal actions against the fungal pathogen. Although this technology was created for the protection of aerial plant organs, it has recently been applied in root protection. Several nanoscale encapsulated architectures are tested that ranged from traditional silica particles to recombinant or plant-produced virus capsules. The proof-of-concept was carried out with a nematicide and the biologically derived capsules proved superior in soil penetration and cargo release. These bionanoparticles are biodegradable and leave behind no organic pollution, truly earning the label of ecofriendly. It is expected that this field will highly benefit from next-generation NPs biofunctionalization.

Advances of Nanobiotechnology in DNA Sequencing

Basics of DNA Sequencing

Determination of the precise order of nucleotides in a DNA molecule from biological samples is popularly known as DNA sequencing and it is an integral component of a wide variety of research applications. DNA sequencing is the most powerful method to reveal genetic variations at the molecular level, such as single nucleotide polymorphism, copy number variation, gene fusion, and insertion/deletion, *etc.* The development of DNA sequencing techniques with enhanced speed, sensitivity, high throughput and low cost are of utmost importance to facilitate for studying and exploring of more and more biological systems without any limitations and enhance the basic molecular understanding of biological systems. The efficient sequence technology should have four standards like (1) high accuracy (less than 1 error in 10,000 bases), (2) long read length (essentially no gaps), (3) high throughput (too fast), and (4) low cost.

From the year 1977 to till date DNA sequencing came across much advancement in terms of sequencing tools and techniques *i.e.,* from sanger sequencing to nanophore sequencing techniques. The modern era DNA sequencing are dealing with next generation sequencing and many other advancement are available to the researchers, practitioners, and academicians at a very reasonable cost with highest accuracy. Instruments which are widely used for massively parallel sequencers based DNA sequencing are called as next-generation sequencers. Over the last fifty years large numbers of researchers have applied themselves to the production of techniques and technologies to facilitate this feat, sequencing DNA and RNA molecules. This time-scale has witnessed tremendous changes, moving from sequencing short oligonucleotides to millions of bases, from struggling towards the deduction of the coding sequence of a single gene to rapid and widely available whole genome sequencing. So for sequencing techniques categorized into 3 generations *i.e.*, Sanger sequencing—the first-generation, amplification-based massively parallel sequencing—the second, and single-molecule sequencing—the third generation. The second-generation (2nd-gen) sequencing exploits amplification of target DNA and massively parallelized chips, including arrays of microbeads (Roche and Life Technologies/Thermo Fisher Scientific), DNA nanoballs (Complete Genomics/Beijing Genomics Institute), and DNA clusters. For read length, most of the 2nd-gen sequencers can sequence only a few hundred bases because of gradual intermolecular dephasing among DNA clones within sequencing reaction sites. One of the major breakthroughs brought by the 2nd-gen sequencers is high throughput.

Technologies to sequence DNA at the single-molecule level is coming under third-generation sequencing. In these approaches, the error-prone amplification step is eliminated during sample preparation. Many sequencing techniques are available in the third generation sequencing; among many, nanopore sequencing technique has been expected to potentially accomplish the standards for efficient sequencing method. The biological databases are being flooded with a huge flow of sequences coming out from various organisms across the world. Today the researchers and scientists across the various fields are utilizing these data for a variety of applications including food security by developing better crops and crop yields, livestock, improved diagnostics, prognostics and therapies for many complex diseases. Advancements of nanotechnology highly useful to increase the efficiency of the sequencing with low cost will help to focus more in genomics, transcriptomics of numerous plants and animals. With the development of these high-throughput sequencing technology and advancement of transcriptome and genome analysis of more biological organisms, progressively improving our understanding of genetic base, RNA-based gene regulatory network and important molecular pathways of biological system.

Nanopore Sequencing

Nanopore sequencing is the third generation DNA sequencing technology and the significant advantages of nanopores (biological or solid state) include label-free, ultralong reads (10^4–10^6 bases), high throughput, and low material requirement. Each of these greatly simplifies the experimental process and can be easily used for DNA sequencing applications. In February 2012, Oxford Nanopore Technologies, UK presented initial data of the technology. Nanotechnology is based on microscopic machinery that operates at the level of single molecules. The first example of a single-molecule sequencing method is called nanopore sequencing. As the name implies, the genomic DNA passes through a nanopore, or small opening in a membrane that is approximately 1 nm in diameter. The diameter is so small that it only permits one single strand of DNA to pass through at a time (Figure 36.3). As the single-stranded DNA transits the pore, a detector records how the current changes from the channel. Every base has a slightly different structure, and therefore each base blocks the current differently. The advantages of nanopore technology are its high speed and its ability to handle long DNA molecules. In addition, many nanopores can be assembled into a very small region, and many long fragments of DNA sequence can be determined simultaneously. Nanopore detectors permit a single DNA strand to pass through a tiny pore and sequence it as it passes. A practical nanopore detector consists of a channel in a membrane that separates two aqueous compartments. When a voltage is applied across the membrane, ions flow through the open channel. Since DNA is negatively charged, the DNA is pulled through the nanopore to the positive side. The DNA molecules enter the pore and are pulled through in extended conformation, one at a time (Figure 36.2). During the time the channel is occupied by the DNA, the normal ionic current is reduced. The amount of reduction depends on the base sequence (G > C > T > A); therefore, a computer can measure the current and decipher the sequence based on the differences.

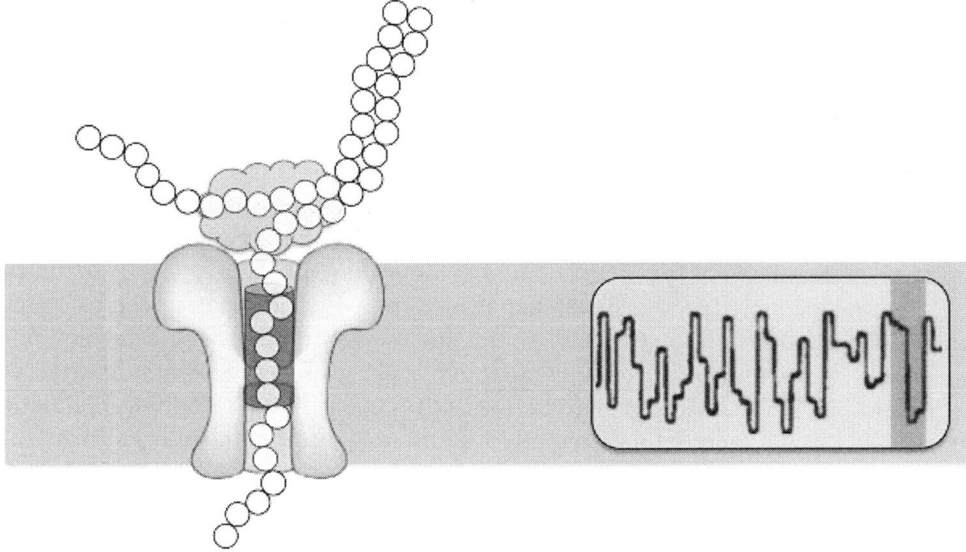

Figure 36.2. Nanopore Sequencing of DNA.

By creating hairpins at the end of DNA fragment, this technology can sequence both sense and antisense strand of a DNA fragment. Hundreds of thousands of nanopores are built on an array chip that is used in these instruments. Although the technology has not been in routine use for sequencing, according to the scientists who developed it, it can sequence the entire 5.4-kilobase genome of the virus in one continuous read. The method has the potency of sequencing the human genome in very short times, reaching even an incredible 15 min.

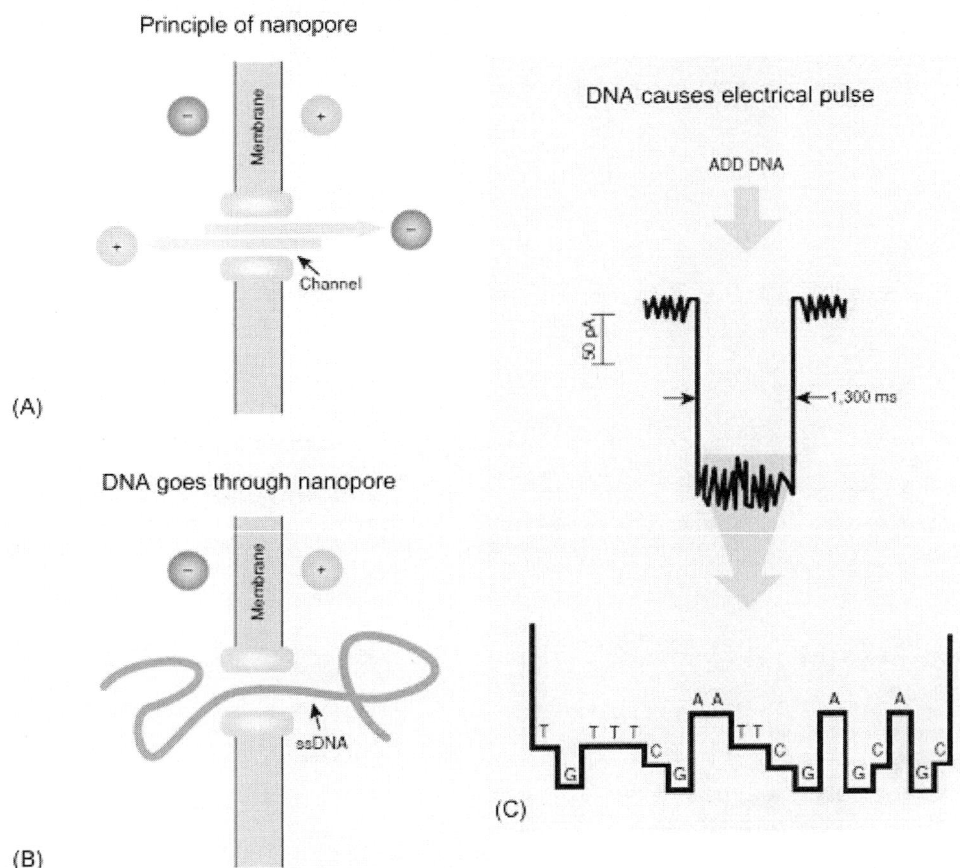

Figure 36.3. Sequences Nanopore Sequencing of DNA and Detection Principle.

Advantages

The potential advantages of the nanopore system are that it could deliver real-time seqeuncing of single molecules at low cost; it is also expected to read very long DNA molecules in a single read. Nanopore technology is expected to provide sequencing at a very low cost, $25 to $40 per gigabase of sequence. That would mean a cost of just a few thousand dollars to sequence a human genome to the standard 30-fold coverage. Being a very fast sequencing process it could be a future choice of sequencing for nearly all applications.

Application of Nanobiotechnology in "Omic" Sciences

Omic sciences attempt to the comprehensive study of the complex interactions between molecules in the different systems biology layers. The main **omic** technologies include genomics, transcriptomics, proteomics, and metabolomics.

Also, the different technologies used in each of the main **omic** studies are introduced (Figure 36.4).

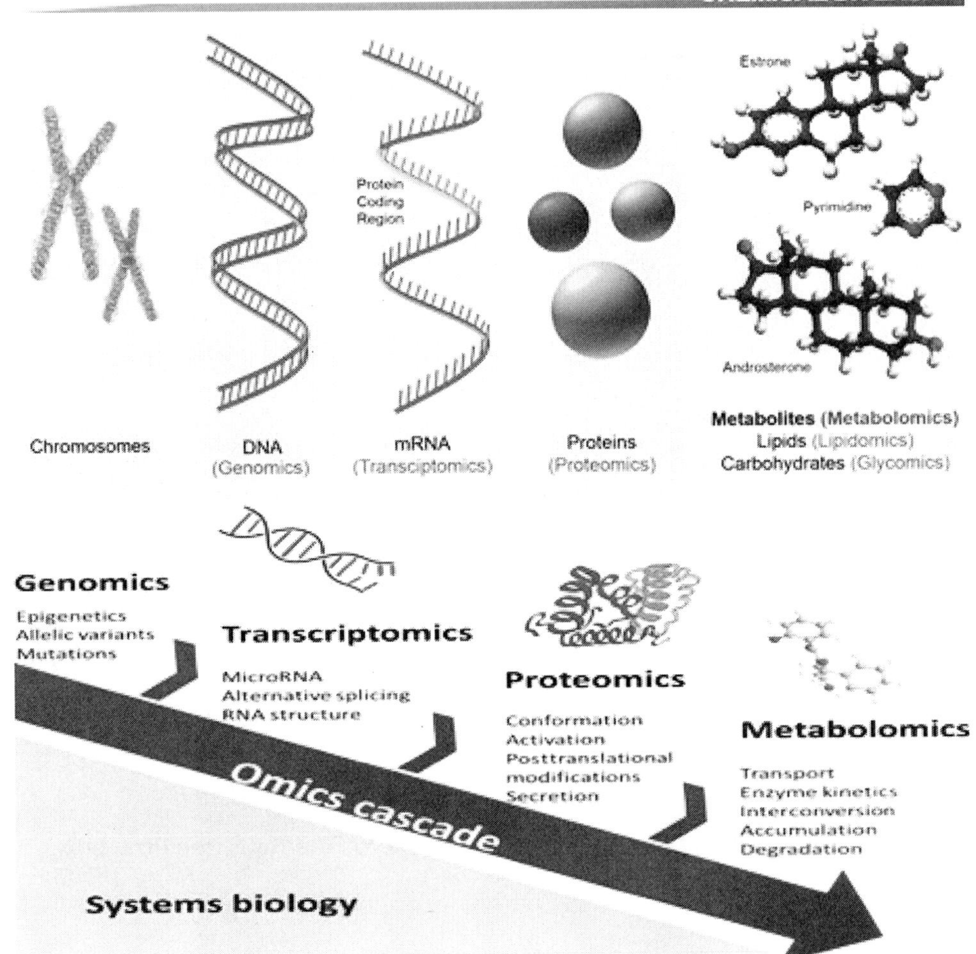

Figure 36.4. Components of "Omic" Sciences.

Genomics

Studying and characterizing the physical nature and function of whole genome of an organism is called as genomics. Based upon the nature of analysis it is divided into two group's 1. Structural genomics; 2. Functional genomics.

Structural Genomics

The prime directive of structural genomic analysis is the complete and accurate elucidation of the DNA sequence of a representative haploid genome of a given species.

Functional Genomics

Functional genomics is the branch studying and characterizing the **transcriptome** *i.e.*, the entire range of transcripts produced by a given organism.

Transcriptomics

Transcriptome is the complete set of RNA transcripts in a specific cell type or tissue at a certain developmental stage and/or under a specific physiological condition, including messenger RNA, transfer RNA, ribosomal RNA, and other non-coding RNAs. Transcriptomics focuses on the gene expression at the RNA level and offers the genome-wide information of gene structure, gene function and its importance in specific biological processes.

Proteomics

Proteomics is a rapidly growing field of molecular biology that is concerned with the systematic, high-throughput approach to protein expression analysis of a cell or an organism. Proteomics involves the applications of technologies for the identification and quantification of overall proteins present content of a cell, tissue or an organism. It supplements the other "omics" technologies such as genomic and transcriptomics to expound the identity of proteins of an organism, and to cognize the structure and functions of a particular protein.

Metabolomics

Metabolomics is the large-scale study of small molecules, commonly known as metabolites, within cells, biofluids, tissues or organisms. Collectively, these small molecules and their interactions within a biological system are known as the metabolome. Nanodevices are used to detect the production of various metabolities produced form different parts of the plants and by plant under different environmental condition. So this data can be correlated with other omics like transcriptomics

Bioinformatics

Bioinformatics is the science concerned with the development and application of computer hardware and software to the acquisition, storage, analysis, visualization, manipulation and interpretation of biological information especially data of nucleic acids, amino acids and studies molecular rules and systems that govern or affect the structure, function and evolution of various forms of life.

Bioinformatics Databases

A database is a collection of information that is organized so that it can be easily accessed, managed and updated. Creation and maintenance of bioinformatics database to store biological information such as nucleotide and amino acid sequences. They offer scientists the opportunity to access and analyze a wide variety of biologically relevant sequence, structural and functional data of an increasingly broad range of organisms. Biological databases play a central role in bioinformatics.

When the sequence is known, it opens the door to numerous possibilities. Development of genomic technologies that ultimately permitted sequencing of complex genomes, in turn it helped step-by-step progression in genome-wide map resolution, development of high-resolution genetic and physical mapping. Computational analysis of the sequence, transcripts and proteins based upon the principles developed by genetic, molecular and biological analysis, it is possible to make predictions of all of the encoded proteins. The available information in database helps us to analyze other haploid genomes from the same species and develop a statistical picture of the genetic variation within populations of that species. Comparison of the genomic sequence of different species can be able to understand, how the genome has been remodeled in the course of evolution. Studies of comparative genomics have already proceeded far enough to reveal that, in related species, there is considerable synteny (conserved gene location within large blocks of the genome). Studies of comparative genomics also offer a powerful opportunity to identify highly conserved and functionally important sequence motifs in coding and noncoding genomic DNA. This identification helps researchers confirm predictions of protein-coding regions of the genome and identify important regulatory elements within DNA.

Plant genomics will revolutionize the study of the molecular basis of plant biology. The traditional hypothesis-driven approach will be gradually transformed into an unbiased data collection at the tissue/organism level approach followed by bioinformatic analyses. DNA sequencing is one of the crucially important tasks in the fields of genetics and cellular biology, which is benefiting from nanotechnology. DNA carries genetic information and sequencing it in a quick way helps researchers in achieving essential goals, including personalized medicine. Solid state nanopores potentially can offer more durability, in sequencing biomolecules, over the protein based nanopores. Fast, cheap, and reliable DNA sequencing could be one of the most disruptive innovations of this decade, as it will pave the way for personalized medicine. In recent years, various ideas are introduced towards the goal of fast and low cost sequencing. In pursuit of such technology, a variety of nanotechnology-based approaches have been explored and established, including sequencing with nanopores. Owing to its unique structure and properties, graphene provides interesting opportunities for the development of a new sequencing technology. In recent years, a wide range of creative ideas for graphene sequencers have been theoretically proposed and the first experimental demonstrations have begun to appear. Different approaches used in graphene nanodevices for DNA sequencing, which involve DNA passing through graphene nanopores, nanogaps, and nanoribbons, and the physisorption of DNA on graphene nanostructures.

DNA Integration and Immobilization for Hybridization and Biosensing Technique

Biological molecules such as deoxyribonucleic acid (DNA) have shown great potential in fabrication and construction of nanostructures and devices. Variety of sequences can be obtained from DNA by convenient solid support synthesis. Besides, DNA modifications with biotin groups and fluorescent labels introduced new applications for DNA in nanobiotechnology. The use of DNA for the fabrication of nanostructures is rapidly expanding in two main different directions. 1. The fabrication of artificial networks consisting of native DNA. 2. The attachment or integration of DNA onto solid state surfaces.

DNA-Naturally Existing Nanomaterial

Biological molecules such as deoxyribonucleic acid (DNA) have shown great potential in fabrication and construction of nanostructures and devices. It is the basic building block of life. DNA is the genetic material of most organisms and organelles, although phage and viral genomes may use single stranded DNA, single stranded RNA (ribonucleic acid) or double stranded RNA. Most hereditary information is encoded in the chemical language of DNA and reproduced in most cells of living organisms. The double stranded helical structure of DNA is a key to its use in self assembly applications. Each strand of the DNA is about 2 nmwide. Each helix or strand of DNA is made up from three components (nucleotides): nitrogen-containing bases, carbohydrate (deoxyribose) and phosphate. There are 4 types of nitrogen-containing base in DNA. They are adenine, guanine, cytosine and thymine. The sugar deoxyribose, forms, with phosphate groups, a very long backbone, alternating sugar-phosphate-sugar-phosphate, and so on. One of the 4 nitrogen containing bases is linked to every sugar molecule. Each unit of a phosphate, a sugar molecule and base is called a nucleotide and is about 0.34 nm long, that is, 10–10.6 nucleotide pairs for a pitch of 3.4–3.6 nm. Thus, constructions made from DNA will have nanoscale features. The specific binding through 3 hydrogen bonds between cytosine (C) and guanine (G) and 2 such bonds between adenine (A) and thymine (T) can result in the joining of two complementary single stranded DNA to form a double stranded DNA. The phosphate ion carries a negative charge in the DNA molecule, which results in electrostatic repulsion of the two strands. To keep the negative charges neutralized, positive ions must be provided by the solution. The joining of two complementary single strands of DNA through hydrogen bonding to form a double stranded DNA is called hybridization. If a double stranded DNA is heated above certain temperature, the two stands will start to dehybridize and eventually separate into single strands. As the temperature is reduced, the two strands will eventually come together and rehybridize to form the double stranded structure. DNA has several advantages to be used for the assembly of devices and computational elements, for the assembly of interconnects or as the device element itself. First, DNA is the molecule whose intermolecular interactions are the most readily programmed and reliably predicted where G pairs with C and A pairs with T. Second, DNA of a variety of sequences can be obtained by convenient solid support synthesis. Besides, DNA modifications with biotin groups and fluorescent labels introduced new applications for DNA in nanobiotechnology. Third, DNA can be modified by a large group of enzymes that include restriction endonucleases, exonucleases, and DNA ligases.

1. The Fabrication of Artificial Networks Consisting of Native DNA

First approach utilizes rigid tetrahedral organic vertices, where the attached oligonucleotides (Short DNA strand) serve as the connectors for the design of more complex architectures. Thus a variable number of oligonucleotide arms could be attached to the core tetrahedral organic linkers, thereby allowing for the construction of different types of DNA structure. One way to exploit this extraordinary precise architectural control is to use self assembled DNA templates to position functional molecules: examples include nanomechanical devices, molecular electronic circuits, near field optical devices and enzyme networks. The simplest active DNA nanostructures are switches that can be driven between two conformations. Motion is induced by changes in ionic conditions, temperature or by the binding of signaling molecule, often a DNA strand.

2. The Attachment or Integration of DNA onto Solid State Surfaces

Attachment of biomolecules such as DNA onto the nanomaterials surface plays a crucial role in the choice of immobilization technique suitable for construction of nanodevices such as bio-electronic devices. Long term use, fast response, operational stability and reproducibility of the electrochemical biorecognition event, are some general aspects for employing the immobilization strategy. Selection of the most appropriate immobilization protocol is strictly dependent on the characteristics of the transducing nanomaterial. Robust immobilization chemistries are usually preferred in order to prevent desorption of the probes from the sensing layer. The first step toward DNA-based technology is to attach DNA molecules to surfaces. Three different methods for such an attachment are used, i. Electrostatic interaction between DNA and a substrate. ii. Covalent binding of a chemical group attached to the DNA end. iii. Binding of a protein attached to the DNA end to the corresponding antibody immobilized at the surface. This integration of DNA onto solid state surfaces is more useful to develop biosensor and microarray.

I. Biosensor

Most widely used method of immobilization is utilizes the covalent bond between sulfur and gold. For example, the DNA molecule can be functionalized with a thiol (S–H) or disulfide (S–S) group at the end. Due to enhanced surface volume or surface area and high surface free energy of nanoparticles can adsorb biomolecules strongly and play an important role in the attachment of biomolecules in the construction of biosensors. Generally, the adsorption of biomolecules directly onto naked surfaces of bulk materials may frequently result in their denaturation and loss of bioactivity. However, the adsorption of such biomolecules onto the surfaces of nanoparticles can retain their bioactivity, because small nanomaterials have ability to reduce the distance between the redox site of immobilized protein or DNA and the working electrode surface which composed of indium-tin-oxide, gold, platinum, glassy carbon, carbon paste, and so forth, since the rate of electron transfer is inversely dependent on the exponential distance between them. Since most of the nanoparticles carry charges, they can electrostatically adsorb biomolecules with different charges (Figure 36.5). Beside the common electrostatic interaction, other strategies to attach DNA to surfaces include covalent binding of DNA oligonucleotide to a preactivated surface and adsorption of biotinylated oligonucleotide on a particle surface coated with avidin.

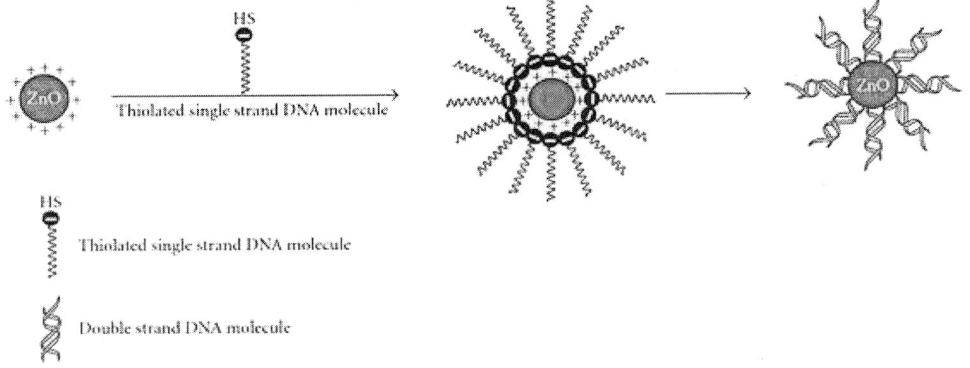

Figure 36.5. Immobilization of Thiolated Single-Stranded Probe DNA on the Surface of ZnO for Hybridization Detection in Double-Stranded DNA (target DNA).

Immobilized probe DNA onto sol-gel derived nanostructured ZnO matrix for the hybridization detection of specific sequnces and investigated the bioactivity of the probe DNA electrode. Many other nanoparticles such as Au, Ag, Pt, CeO_2, TiO_2, ZrO_2 have been reported for the construction of DNA based biosensors for the immobilization of different probe DNA for different biomolecule recognition purposes.

II. DNA Microarray

A DNA microarray is a collection of microscopic DNA spots representing the entire set of genes of an organism, arranged in a grid pattern attached to a solid surface. Scientists use DNA microarrays to measure the expression levels of large numbers of genes simultaneously or to genotype multiple regions of a genome. Each DNA spot contains picomoles of a specific DNA sequence, known as probes.

A microarray is a laboratory tool used to detect the expression of thousands of genes at the same time. DNA microarrays are microscope slides that are printed with thousands of tiny spots in defined positions, with each spot containing a known DNA sequence or gene. Often, these slides are referred to as gene chips or DNA chips. The DNA molecules attached to each slide act as probes to detect gene expression, which is also known as the transcriptome or the set of messenger RNA (mRNA) transcripts expressed by a group of genes.

To perform a microarray analysis, mRNA molecules are typically collected from both an experimental sample and a reference sample. For example, the reference sample could be collected from a healthy individual, and the experimental sample could be collected from an individual with a disease. The two mRNA samples are then converted into complementary DNA (cDNA), and each sample is labelled with a fluorescent probe of a different colour. For instance, the experimental cDNA sample may be labelled with a red fluorescent dye, whereas the reference cDNA may be labelled with a green fluorescent dye. The two samples are then mixed together and allowed to bind to the microarray slide. The process in which the cDNA molecules bind to the DNA probes on the slide is called hybridization. Following hybridization, the microarray is scanned to measure the expression of each gene printed on the slide. If the expression of a particular gene is higher in the experimental sample than in the reference sample, then the corresponding spot on the microarray appears red. In contrast, if the expression in the experimental sample is lower than in the reference sample, then the spot appears green. Finally, if there is equal expression in the two samples, then the spot appears yellow. The data gathered through microarrays can be used to create gene expression profiles, which show simultaneous changes in the expression of many genes in response to a particular condition or treatment.

Common Terminologies Used in Agricultural Biotechnology

Terminologies Used in Tissue Culture Techniques

Adventitious: Developing from unusual points of origin, such as shoots or root tissues from callus, or embryos from sources other than zygotes.

Aneuploid: The state of a cell nucleus that does not contain an exact multiple of the haploid number of chromosomes, one or more chromosomes being present in greater or lesser number than the rest. The chromosomes may or may not show rearrangements.

Asepsis: Without infection or contaminating microorganisms.

Aseptic Technique: Procedures used to prevent the introduction of fungi, bacteria, viruses, mycoplasma, or other microorganisms into cell, tissue, and organ cultures. Although these procedures are used to prevent microbial contamination of cultures, they also prevent cross contamination of cell cultures. These procedures may or may not exclude the introduction of infectious molecules.

Callus: An unorganized, proliferative mass of differentiated plant cells; a wound response.

Cell Culture: Maintenance or cultivation of cells *in vitro,* including culture of single cells. In cell cultures, the cells are no longer organized into tissues.

Cell Hybridization: The fusion of two or more dissimilar cells leading to the formation of a synkaryon.

.**Chemically Defined Medium:** A nutritive solution for culturing cells in which each component is specifiable and, ideally, is of known chemical structure.

Clonal Propagation: Asexual reproduction of plants, the results of which are considered to be genetically uniform and originated from a single individual or explant.

Clone: a group of plants propagated by only vegetative and asexual means, all members of which have been derived from a single individual.

Cryopreservation: Ultralow temperature storage of cells, tissues, embryos, or seeds. This storage is usually carried out using temperatures below –100°C.

Cybrid: The viable cell resulting from the fusion of a cytoplast with a whole cell, thus creating a cytoplasmic hybrid.

Cytoplast: The intact cytoplasm remaining following the enucleation of a cell.

Cytoplasmic Hybrid: Synonymous with cybrid.

Cytoplasmic Inheritance: Inheritance attributable to extranuclear genes; for example, genes in cytoplasmic organelles, such as mitochondria or chloroplasts or in plasmids.

Differentiated: Cells that maintain, in culture, all or much of the specialized structure and function typical of the cell type *in vivo.*

Diploid: The state of a cell in which all chromosomes, except sex chromosomes, are two in number and are structurally identical with those of the species from which the culture was derived.

Electrophoration: Creation, by means of an electrical current, of transient pores in the plasmalemma, usually for the purpose of introducing exogenous material, especially DNA, from the medium.

Embryo Culture: *In vitro* development or maintenance of isolated mature or immature embryos.

Embryogenesis: The process of embryo initiation and development.

Epigenetic Event: Any change in a phenotype that does not result from an alteration in DNA sequence. This change may be stable and heritable and includes alteration in DNA methylation, transcriptional activation, translational control, and post-translational modifications.

Epigenetic Variation: Phenotypic variability that has a nongenetic basis.

Euploid: The state of a cell nucleus that contains exact multiples of the haploid number of chromosomes.

Explant: Tissue taken from its original site and transferred to an artificial medium for growth or maintenance.

Explant Culture: The maintenance or growth of an explant in culture.

Friability: The tendency of plant cells to separate from one another.

Gametoclonal Variation: Variation in phenotype, either genetic or epigenetic in origin, expressed by gametoclones.

Gametoclone: Plants regenerated from cell cultures derived from meiospores, gametes, or gametophytes.

Habituation: The acquired ability of a population of cells to grow and divide independently of exogenously supplied growth regulators.

Heterokaryon: A cell possessing two or more genetically different nuclei in a common cytoplasm, usually a result of cell-to-cell fusion.

Heteroploid: The state of a culture in which the cells possess nuclei containing chromosome numbers other than the diploid number. This term is used to describe only a culture and not individual cells. Thus, a heteroploid culture would be one that contains aneuploid cells.

Homokaryon: A cell possessing two or more genetically identical nuclei in a common cytoplasm, resulting from cell-to-cell fusion.

Hyperhydricity: A condition of plants in cell culture that have abnormal shoot development. The shoots have a glass-like appearance and do not establish well in a potting mix. Generally, this condition is characterized by large intercellular spaces, less epicuticular wax, fewer stomata, chloroplasts with small grana and lacking starch grains. *Vitrification* is another term used to describe this condition.

Induction: Initiation of a structure, organ, or process *in vitro.*

***In vitro* Propagation:** Propagation of plants in a controlled, artificial environment, using plastic or glass culture vessels, aseptic techniques, and a defined growing medium.

***In vitro* Transformation:** A heritable change, occurring in cells in culture, intrinsically or from treatment with chemical carcinogens, oncogenic viruses, irradiation, transfection with oncogenes, and so on and leading to altered morphological, antigenic, neoplastic, proliferative, or other properties.

Juvenile: A phase in the sexual cycle of a plant characterized by differences in appearance from the adult and the lack of ability to respond to flower-inducing stimuli.

Karyoplast: A cell nucleus, obtained from the cell by enucleation, surrounded by a narrow rim of cytoplasm and a plasma membrane.

Liposome: A closed lipid vesicle surrounding an aqueous interior; may be used to encapsulate exogenous materials for ultimate delivery into cells by fusion with the cell.

Meristem Culture: *In vitro* culture of a generally shiny, dome-like structure measuring less than 0.1 mm in length when excised, most often excised from the shoot apex.

Micropropagation: *In vitro* clonal propagation of plants from shoot tips or nodal explants, usually with an accelerated proliferation of shoots during subcultures.

Morphogenesis: (1) The evolution of a structure from an undifferentiated to a differentiated state. (2) The growth and development of differentiated structures.

Mutant: A phenotypic variant resulting from a changed or new gene.

Nurse Culture: In the culture of plant cells, the growth of a cell or cells on a contiguous culture of different origin that in turn is in contact with the tissue culture medium. The cultured cell or tissue may be separated from the feeder layer by a porous matrix such as filter paper or membranous filters.

Organ Culture: The maintenance or growth of organ primordia or the whole or parts of an organ *in vitro* in a way that allows differentiation and preservation of the architecture or function.

Organized: Arranged into definite structures.

Organogenesis: In plant tissue culture, a process of differentiation by which plant organs are formed *de novo* or from preexisting structures. In developmental biology, this term refers to differentiation of an organ system from stem or precursor cells.

Organotypic: Resembling an organ *in vivo* in three-dimensional form or function or both. For example, a rudimentary organ in culture may differentiate in an organotypic manner or a population of dispersed cells may become rearranged into an organotypic structure and may also function in an organotypic manner. This term is not meant to be used with the word *culture* but is meant to be used as a descriptive term.

Passage: The transfer or transplantation of cells, with or without dilution, from one culture vessel to another. Any time cells are transferred from one vessel to another, a certain portion of the cells may be lost and, therefore, dilution of cells, whether deliberate or not, may occur. This term is synonymous with *subculture.*

Passage Number: The number of times the cells in the culture have been subcultured or passaged. In descriptions of this process, the ratio or dilution of the cells should be stated so that the relative cultural age can be ascertained.

Pathogen-Free: Free from specific organisms based on specific tests for the designated organisms.

Plant Tissue Culture: The growth or maintenance of plant cells, tissues, organs, or whole plants *in vitro.*

Population Density: The number of cells per unit area or volume of a culture vessel. Also, the number of cells per unit volume of medium in a suspension culture.

Primary Culture: A culture started from cells, tissues, or organs taken directly from organisms. A primary culture may be regarded as such until it is successfully subcultured for the first time. It then becomes a *cell line.*

Protoplast: A plant, bacterial, or fungal cell from which the entire cell wall has been removed. (See **Spheroplast** for comparison)

Protoplast Fusion: Technique in which protoplasts are fused into a single cell.

Pseudodiploid: The state of a cell that is diploid but in which, as a result of chromosomal rearrangements, the karyotype is abnormal and linkage relationships may be disrupted.

Regeneration: In plant cultures, a morphogenetic response to a stimulus that results in the production of organs, embryos, or entire plants.

Shoot Apical Meristem: Undifferentiated tissue, located within the shoot tip, generally appearing as a shiny, dome-like structure distal to the youngest leaf primordium and measuring less than 0.1 mm in length when excised.

Shoot Tip (Apex): A structure consisting of the shoot apical meristem plus one to several primordial leaves, usually measuring 0.1–1.0 mm in length; when more mature leaves are included, the structure can measure up to several centimeters in length.

Somaclonal Variation: Phenotypic variation, either genetic or epigenetic in origin, displayed among somaclones.

Somaclone: Plants derived from any form of cell culture involving the use of somatic plant cells.

Somatic Cell Genetics: The study of genetic phenomena of somatic cells. The cells under study are most often cells grown in culture.

Somatic Cell Hybrid: The cell or plant resulting from the fusion of plant protoplasts, derived from somatic cells that differ genetically.

Somatic Cell Hybridization: The *in vitro* fusion of plant protoplasts derived from somatic cells that differ genetically.

Somatic Embryogenesis: In plant culture, the process of embryo initiation and development from vegetative or nongametic cells.

Spheroplast: A cell from which most of the cell wall has been removed.

Stage I: A step in *in vitro* propagation characterized by the establishment of an aseptic tissue culture of a plant.

Stage II: A step in *in vitro* plant propagation characterized by the rapid numerical increase of organs or other structures.

Stage III: A step in *in vitro* plant propagation characterized by the preparation of the propagule for successful transfer to soil, involving rooting of shoot cuttings, hardening of plants, and initiating the change from the heterotrophic to the autotrophic state.

Stage IV: A step in *in vitro* plant propagation characterized by the establishment in soil of a plant derived through tissue culture, either after undergoing a Stage III pretransplant treatment or, in certain species, after the direct transfer of plants from Stage II into soil.

Sterile: (1) Without life. (2) Inability of an organism to produce functional gametes.

Subculture: With plant cultures, the process by which the tissue or explant is first subdivided then transferred into fresh culture medium.

Substrain: The result of isolating a single cell or groups of cells in a strain having properties or markers not shared by all cells of the parent strain.

Suspension Culture: A type of culture in which cells, or aggregates of cells, multiply while suspended in liquid medium.

Synkaryon: A hybrid cell that results from the fusion of the nuclei it carries.

Tissue Culture: The maintenance or growth of tissues *in vitro* in a way that allows differentiation and preservation of their architecture or function or both.

Totipotency: The ability of a cell to form all the cell types in the adult organism.

Transfection: The transfer, for the purposes of genomic integration, of naked foreign DNA into cells in culture. The traditional use of this term in microbiology implied that the DNA being transferred was derived from a virus. The definition used here describes the general transfer of DNA irrespective of its source. (See also **Transformation)**

Transformation: In plant cell culture, the introduction and stable genomic integration of foreign DNA into a plant cell by any means, resulting in a genetic modification. This is the traditional microbiological definition.

Undifferentiated: With plant cells, existing in a state of cell development characterized by isodiametric cell shape, very little or no vacuole, and a large nucleus and exemplified by the cells in an apical meristem or embryo.

Variant: With a culture, exhibiting a stable phenotypic change whether genetic or epigenetic in origin.

Vegetative Propagation: Reproduction or plants by a nonsexual process involving the culture of plant parts, such as stem and leaf cuttings.

Virus-Free: Free from specified viruses based on tests designed to detect the presence of the organisms in questions.

Terminologies in Molecular Biology

A site (ribosomal): The ribosomal site to which new aminoacyl tRNAs (except the first one) bind.

A site (RNA polymerase): The site the incoming nucleotide occupies during phosphodiester formation.

Ac: A maize transposon ("activator") that can activate transposition of an inactive transposon like *Ds* by providing the necessary transposase.

Acceptor stem: The part of a tRNA molecule formed by base pairing between the 5'- and 3'-ends of the molecule. The 3'-end can "accept" an amino acid by charging, hence the name.

Accommodation: Unbending of the aminoacyl-tRNA in the A/T state, to allow the aminoacyl-tRNA to bind fully in the A site.

Acidic domain: A transcription-activating domain rich in acidic amino acids.

Activation site: The site on an aminoacyl-tRNA synthetase that activates the amino acid, forming an aminoacyl adenylate.

Activator: A protein that binds to an enhancer (or activator binding region) and activates transcription from a nearby promoter. In eukaryotes, stimulates formation of a preinitiation complex.

A-DNA: A form of DNA found at low relative humidity, with 11 bp per helical turn. The form assumed in solution by an RNA–DNA hybrid.

α**-Amanitin:** A toxin produced by poisonous species of mushrooms in the *Amanita* genus. Inhibits RNA polymerase II at very low concentration, and RNA polymerase III at higher concentration. Usually does not inhibit RNA polymerase I at all.

Alkylation: The addition of carbon-containing groups to other molecules. Alkylation of DNA bases constitutes DNA damage that can lead to mutations.

α**-Complementation:** *In vivo* complementation between the α-peptide and the β -peptide of β-galactosidase to yield an active enzyme. Cloning vectors usually take advantage of α-complementation by having the vector encode the a-peptide and the host encode the β -peptide. Thus, the vector alone will enable a-complementation, but a vector with an insert will not.

Allolactose: A rearranged version of lactose with a b-1, 6-galactosidic bond; the inducer of the *lac* operon.

Allosteric protein: A protein in which binding of a molecule to one site changes the conformation of a remote site and alters its interaction with a second molecule.

Alternative splicing: Splicing the same pre-RNA in two or more ways to yield two or more different mRNAs that produce two or more different protein products.

Amber codon: UAG, coding for termination.

Amino acid: The building block of proteins.

A/T state: The state in which an aminoacyl-tRNA first binds to the bacterial ribosome. Its anticodon is paired with the codon in the A site, but the tRNA is bent to allow the amino acid and acceptor stem to remain bound to EF-Tu and to ribosomal elements to the right of the A site, as the 50S particle is conventionally depicted.

ATPase: An enzyme that cleaves ATP, releasing energy for other cellular activities.

Anabolic metabolism: The process of building up substances from relatively simple precursors. The *trp* operon encodes anabolic enzymes that build the amino acid tryprophan.

Annealing of DNA: The process of bringing back together the two separate strands of denatured DNA to re-form a double helix.

Annotated genes: Genes or gene-like sequences from a genomic sequencing project that are at least partially identified.

Antibody: A protein with the ability to recognize and bind to a substance, usually another protein, with great specificity. Helps the body's immune system recognize and trigger an attack on invading agents.

Anticodon: A 3-base sequence in a tRNA that base-pairs with a specific codon.

Anticodon loop: The loop, conventionally drawn at the bottom of tRNA molecule, that contains the anticodon.

Antigen: A substance recognized and bound by an antibody.

Antiparallel: The relative polarities of the two strands in a DNA double helix; if one strand goes 5'→3', top to bottom, the other goes 3'→5'. The same antiparallel relationship applies to any double-stranded polynucleotide or oligonucleotide, including the RNAs in a codon-anticodon pair.

Antisense RNA: An RNA complementary to an mRNA.

Aporepressor: A repressor in an inactive form, without its corepressor.

Apurinic site (AP site): A deoxyribose in a DNA strand that has lost its purine base.

Apyrimidinic site (AP site): A deoxyribose in a DNA strand that has lost its pyrimidine base.

Archaea: The kingdom of prokaryotic organisms whose biochemistry and molecular biology resemble those of eukaryotes as well as those of bacteria. The archaea typically live in extreme environments that are very hot or very salty. Some of the archaea are strict anaerobes that generate methane.

Autoradiography: A technique in which a radioactive sample is allowed to expose a photographic emulsion, thus "taking a picture of itself."

Autoregulation: The control of a gene by its own product.

Bacterial artificial chromosome (BAC): A vector based on the *E. coli* F plasmid, capable of holding inserts up to 300,000 bp (average insert size, about 150,000 bp).

Barcode: A relatively short DNA sequence from the genome of every species on earth. In principle, reading this barcode would allow the rapid identification of any known species.

Base: A cyclic, nitrogen-containing compound linked to deoxyribose in DNA and to ribose in RNA.

Base pair (bp): A pair of bases (A–T or G–C), one in each strand, that occur opposite each other in a double-stranded DNA.

B-DNA: The standard Watson–Crick model of DNA favoured at high relative humidity and in solution.

β-Galactosidase: An enzyme that breaks the bond between the two constituent sugars of lactose.

β-Galactoside: A complex sugar in which the 1-carbon of galactose is linked through a b-bond to another compound, usually another sugar.

β-Galactosidic bond: The bond linking the 1-carbon of galactose to the other compound in a b-galactoside.

Bidirectional DNA replication: Replication that occurs in both directions at the same time from a common starting point, or origin of replication. Requires two active replicating forks.

Bioinformatics: A field that involves the building and manipulation of biological databases. In the context of genomics, this means managing massive amounts of sequencing data and providing useful access to and interpretation of the data.

Biolistic transformation (or transfection): A method in which tiny metal pellets are coated with DNA and shot into cells.

β-Lactamase: An enzyme that breaks down ampicillin and related antibiotics and renders a bacterium resistant to the antibiotic.

BLAST: A program that searches a database for a DNA or protein sequence and displays how the query sequence lines up with the database sequences.

C-Value: The amount of DNA in picograms (trillionths of a gram) in a haploid genome of a given species.

C-Value paradox: The fact that the C-value of a given species is not necessarily related to the genetic complexity of that species.

cAMP response element (CRE): The enhancer that responds to cAMP.

Cap: A methylated guanosine bound through a 5'-5'triphosphate linkage to the 5'-end of an mRNA, an hnRNA, or an snRNA.

Cap 0: A cap lacking any 2'-O-methylations. Found only on certain viral mRNAs.

Cap 1: A typical cap, with a methyl group on the 2'-hydroxyl group of the penultimate nucleotide.

Cap 2: A cap found in a minority of mRNAs with methyl groups on the 2'-hydroxyl groups of the first two nucleotides.

CAP (catabolite activator protein): A protein which, together with cAMP, activates operons that are subject to catabolite repression.

Carboxyl terminus: The end of a polypeptide with a free carboxyl group.

Catabolic metabolism: The process of breaking substances down into simpler components. The *lac* operon encodes catabolic enzymes that break down lactose into its component parts, galactose and glucose.

Catabolite repression: The repression of a gene or operon by glucose or, more likely, by a catabolite, or breakdown product of glucose.

Catalytic center: The active site of an enzyme, where catalysis takes place.

Catenane: A structure composed of two or more circles linked in a chain.

CCAAT box: An upstream motif, having the sequence CCAAT, found in many eukaryotic promoters recognized by RNA polymerase II.

cDNA: A DNA copy of an RNA, made by reverse transcription.

cDNA library: A set of clones representing as many as possible of the mRNAs in a given cell type at a given time.

Centimorgan (cM): The genetic distance that yields a 1 per cent recombination frequency between two markers.

Centromere: Constricted region on the chromosome where spindle fibers are attached during cell division.

Chaperones: Proteins that bind to unfolded proteins and help them fold properly.

Charging: Coupling a tRNA with its cognate amino acid.

Chloramphenicol: An antibiotic that kills bacteria by inhibiting the peptidyl transferase reaction catalyzed by SOS ribosomes.

Chloramphenicol acetyl transferase (CAT): An enzyme whose bacterial gene is frequently used as a reporter gene in eukaryotic transcription and translation experiments. This enzyme adds acetyl groups to the antibiotic chloramphenicol.

Chromatids: Copies of a chromosomes produced in cell division.

Chromatin: The material of chromosomes, composed of DNA and chromosomal proteins.

Chromatography: A group of techniques for separating molecules based on their relative affinities for a mobile and a stationary phase. In ion-exchange chromatography, the charged resin is the stationary phase, and the buffer of increasing ionic strength is the mobile phase.

Chromodomain: A conserved region found in proteins involved in heterochromatin formation. Probably binds to methylated histones.

Chromogenic substrate: A substrate that produces a colored product when acted on by an enzyme.

Chromosome: The physical structure, composed largely of DNA and protein, the contains the genes of an organism.

Chromosome theory of inheritance: The theory that genes are contained in chromosomes.

cI: The gene that encodes the *lac* repressor.

CI: The *cI* gene product.

***cis*-acting:** A term that describes a genetic element, such as an enhancer, a promoter, or an operator, that must be on the same chromosome in order to influence a gene's activity.

Cistron: A genetic unit defined by the *cis–trans* test. For all practical purposes, it is synonymous with the word gene.

Clone-by-clone sequencing: A systematic method of sequencing large genomes. First the whole genome is mapped, then clones corresponding to known regions of the genome aresequenced.

Clones: Individuals formed by an asexual process so that they are genetically identical to the original individual. Also, colonies of cells of groups of viruses that are genetically identical.

Closed promoter complex: The complex formed by relatively loose binding between RNA polymerase and a prokaryotic promoter. It is "closed" in the sense that the DNA duplex remains intact, with no "opening up," or melting of base pairs.

Co activators: Factors that have no transcription-activation ability of their own, but help other proteins stimulate transcription.

Codon: A 3-base sequence in mRNA that causes the insertion of a specific amino acid into protein or causes termination of translation.

Codon bias: Differences in synonymous codon usage in different organisms.

colE1: A plasmid found in certain strains of *E. coli,* which codes for a bacteriocidal toxin known as a colicin. The colE1 DNA replicates unidirectionally.

Colony hybridization: A procedure for selecting a bacterial clone containing a gene of interest. DNAs from a large number of clones are simultaneously tested with a labeled probe that hybridizes to the gene of interest.

Complementary polynucleotide strands: Two strands of DNA or RNA that have complementary sequences; that is, wherever one has an adenine the other has a thymine, and wherever one has a guanine the other has a cytosine.

Composite transposon: A bacterial transposon composed of two types of parts: two arms containing IS or IS-like elements, and a central region comprised of the genes for transposition and one or more antibiotic resistance genes.

Concatemers: DNAs of multiple genome length.

Consensus sequence: The average of several similar sequences. For example, the consensus sequence of the –10 box of an *E. coli* promoter is TATAAT. This means that if you examine a number of such sequences, T is most likely to be found in the first position, A in the second, and so forth.

Conservative replication: DNA (or RNA) replication in which both parental strands remain together, producing a progeny duplex both of whose strands are new.

Conservative transposition: "Cut and paste" transposition in which both strands of the transposon DNA are conserved as they leave their original location and move to the new site.

Constant region: The region of an antibody that is more or less the same from one antibody to the next.

Constitutive: Always turned on.

Contig: A group of cloned DNAs containing contiguous or overlapping sequences.

Core element: An element of the eukaryotic promoter recognized by RNA polymerase I. Includes the bases surrounding the transcription start site.

Core histones: All the nucleosomal histones except H1. The histones inside the DNA coils of a nucleosome.

Co-repressor: A substance that associates with an aporepressor to form an active repressor (*e.g.*, tryprophan is the corepressor of the *trp* operon). A protein that works in conjunction with other proteins to repress gene transcription. Histone deacetylases can act as co-repressors.

Core promoter: Whatever promoter elements are near (within about 37 bp of) the transcription initiation site.

Core promoter elements (bacterial): The minimal elements of a promoter (*e.g.*, the –10 and –35 boxes).

Core TAFs: The set of 13 TAFs conserved in a wide variety of eukaryotes.

Cos: The cohesive ends of the linear l phage DNA.

Cosmid: A vector designed for cloning large DNA fragments. A cosmid contains the cos sites of l phage, so it can be packaged into l heads, and a plasmid origin of replication, so it can replicate as a plasmid.

CpG island: A region of DNA containing many unmethylated CpG sequences. Usually associated with active genes.

CREB-binding protein (CBP): A coactivator that binds to phosphorylated CREB at the CRE and then contacts one or more general transcription factors to stimulate assembly of a preintiation complex.

CRE-binding protein (CREB): The activator that is phosphorylated and thus activated by cAMP-stimulated protein kinase A. Binds to CRE and, together with CBP, stimulates transcription of associated genes.

Crossing over: Physical exchange between DNAs that occurs during recombination.

Crown galls: Tumorous growths on plants caused by bacterial infection.

Cryptogene: A gene coding for the unedited version of an RNA that requires editing.

α-CTD: The carboxyl-terminal domain of the α-subunit of bacterial RNA polymerase.

Cyanobacteria (blue-green algae): Photosynthetic bacteria. The ancestors of modern cyanobacteria are thought to have invaded eukaryotic cells and evolved into chloroplasts.

Cyclic-AMP (cAMP): An adenine nucleotide with a cyclic phosphodiester linkage between the 3' and 5' carbons. Implicated in a variety of control mechanisms in prokaryotes and eukaryotes.

Cytidine: A nucleoside containing the base cytosine.

Cytidine deaminase acting on RNA (CDAR): An RNA-editing enzyme that deaminates certain cytidines in RNAs, converting them to uridines.

Cytoplasmic polyadenylation element (CPE): A sequence in the 3'-UTR of an mRNA (consensus, UUUUUAU) that is important in cytoplasmic polyadenylation.

Cytosine (C): The pyrimidine base that pairs with guanosine in DNA.

Cytotoxic: Having the ability to kill cells.

***dam* Methylase:** The deoxyadenosine methylase that adds methyl groups to the A in the sequence GATC in the DNA of *E. coli* cells. The mismatch repair system inspects the methylation of GATC sequences to determine which strand is newly synthesized, and therefore unmethylated.

De-adenylation: The removal of AMP residues from poly(A) in the cytoplasm.

Deamination of DNA: The removal of an amino group (NH2) from a cytosine or adenine in DNA, in which the amino group is replaced by a carbonyl group (C–O). This converts cytosine to uracil and adenine to hypoxanthine.

Decatenation: The process of unlinking the circles in a catenane.

Decoding: Interactions between codons and anticodons on the ribosome that lead to binding of the correct aminoacyl-tRNA.

Degenerate code: A genetic code, such as the one employed by all life on earth, in which more than one codon can stand for a single amino acid.

Deletion: A mutation involving a loss of one or more base pairs.

Denaturation (DNA): Separation of the two strands of DNA.

Denaturation (protein): Disruption of the three-dimensional structure of a protein without breaking any covalent bonds.

Densitometer: An instrument that measures the darkness of a spot on a transparent film (*e.g.*, an autoradiograph).

Deoxyribose: The sugar in DNA.

Dicer: The member of the RNase III family that chops the trigger RNA into pieces about 21 bp long during the RNAi process. Also part of the RISC complex that degrades the target mRNA.

Dideoxyribonucleotide: A nucleotide, deoxy at both 2'- and 3'-positions, used to stop DNA chain elongation in DNA sequencing.

Dimer (protein): A complex of two polypeptides. These can be the same (in a homodimer), or different (in a heterodimer).

Dimerization domain: The part of a protein that interacts with another protein to form a dimer (or higher multimer).

Dimethyl sulfate (DMS): An agent used for methylating DNA. After methylation, the DNA can be chemically cleaved at the methylated sites.

Diploid: The chromosomal number of the human zygote and other cells (except the gametes). Symbolized as 2*n*.

Directional cloning: Insertion of foreign DNA into two different restriction sites of a vector, such that the orientation of the insert can be predetermined.

Disintegrations per minute (dpm): The average number of radioactive emissions produced each minute by a sample.

Dispersive replication: A hypothetical mechanism in which the DNA becomes fragmented so that new and old DNA coexist in the same strand after replication.

D loop: A loop formed when a free DNA or RNA end "invades" a double helix, base-pairing with one of the strands and forcing the other to "loop out."

DNA (deoxyribonucleic acid): A polymer composed of deoxyribonucleotides linked together by phosphodiester bonds. The material of which most genes are made.

DnaA: The first protein to bind to *oriC* in forming an *E. coli* primosome.

DnaB: A key component of the *E. coli* primosome. Helps assemble the primosome by facilitating primase hinding. Also has DNA helicase activity to unwind the parental DNA strands prior to primer synthesis.

DNA-binding domain: The part of a DNA-binding protein that makes specific contacts with a target site on the DNA.

DNA fingerprints: The use of highly variable regions of DNA to identify particular individuals.

DNA glycosylase: An enzyme that breaks the glycosidic bond between a damaged base and its sugar.

DNA gyrase: A topoisomerase that pumps negative superhelical turns into DNA. Relaxes the positive superhelical strain created by unwinding the *E. coli* DNA during replication.

DNA ligase: An enzyme that joins two double-stranded DNAs end to end.

DNA microarray: A chip containing many tiny spots of DNA or oligonucleotides. Used as a dot blot to measure expression of many genes at once.

DNA polymerase: An enzyme that synthesizes DNA by linking together deoxyribonucleoside monophosphates (dNMPs) in the order dictated by the complementary sequence of nucleotides in a template DNA strand.

DNA polymerase I (pol I): One of three different DNA synthesizing enzymes in *E. coli;* used primarily in DNA repair.

DNA polymerase II (pol II): Another DNA polymerase in *E. coli.*

DNA polymerase III holoenzyme: The enzyme within the *E. coli* replisome, which actually makes DNA during replication.

DNase: Deoxyribonuclease, an enzyme that degrades DNA.

DNA typing: The use of molecular techniques, especially Southern blotting, to identify a particular individual.

Domain (protein): An independently folded part of a protein.

Domains of life: The three distinct forms of life: bacteria, archaea, and eukarya (or eukaryotes), originally distinguished by their rRNA sequences.

Dominant: An allele or trait that expresses its phenotype when heterozygous with a recessive allele; for example, *A* is dominant over *a* because the phenotypes of *AA* and *Aa* are the same.

Double helix: The shape two complementary DNA strands assume in a chromosome.

Drosophila melanogaster: A species of fruit fly used widely by geneticists.

Ds: A defective transposable element found in corn, which relies on an *Ac* element for transposition.

EF-2: The eukaryotic homolog of EF-G.

EF-G: The bacterial translation elongation factor that, along with GTP, fosters translocation.

EF-Ts: An exchange factor that exchanges GDP for GTP on EF-Tu.

EF-Tu: The bacterial translation elongation factor that, along with GTP, carries aminoacyl-tRNAs (except fMet-tRNAf Met to the ribosomal A site).

eIF1: A eukaryotic initiation factor that stimulates scanning to locate the proper initiation codon.

eIF1A: Acts synergistically with eIF1 to cause 40S ribosomal subunits to scan to the initiation codon.

eIF2: A eukaryotic initiation factor that is responsible for binding Met-tRNAi to the 40S ribosomal subunit.

eIF2A: One of the subunits of eIF2. It is subject to a phosphorylation that can inhibit translation initiation.

eIF2B: A eukaryotic exchange factor that exchanges GTP for GDP on eIF2.

eIF3: A eukaryotic initiation factor that binds to 40S ribosomal subunits and prevents their reuniting prematurely with 60S subunits.

eIF4A: One of the subunits of eIF4F; a DEAD family RNA binding protein with RNA helicase activity. In conjunction with eIF4B, eIF4A can bind to the leader region of an mRNA and remove hairpins in advance of the scanning ribosomal subunit.

eIF4B: An RNA-binding protein that helps eIF4A bind to mRNA during translation initiation.

eIF4E: The cap-binding component of eIF4F.

eIF4F: The cap-binding complex that participates in transcription initiation in eukaryotes.

eIF4G: One of the subunits of eIF4F. Serves as an adapter by binding to two different proteins: Binds to eIF4E, which is bound to the cap; also binds to eIF3, which is bound to the 40S ribosomal particle. In this way, it brings the 40S particle together with the 5'-end of an mRNA, where it can begin scanning. Also binds to PAB I, which binds to poly(A).

eIF5: A eukaryotic initiation factor that promotes association between a 40S initiation complex and a 60S ribosomal subunit.

eIF5B: The eukaryotic homolog of prokaryotic IF2. Helps eIF5 recruit the 60S ribosomal subunit to the initiation complex. Requires GTP hydrolysis to be released from the ribosome.

eIF6: A eukaryotic initiation factor with activity similar to that of eIF3.

Electrophile: A molecule that seeks centers of negative charge in other molecules and attacks them there.

Elctrophoresis: A procedure in which voltage is applied to charged molecules, inducing them to migrate. This technique can be used to separate DNA fragments, RNAs, or proteins.

Electrophoration: The use of a strong electric current to introduce DNA into cells.

Elongation factor: A protein that is necessary for either the aminoacyl-tRNA binding or the translocation step in the elongation phase of translation.

Embryonic stem (ES) cells: Cells that can differentiate into any kind of cell in an organism.

Encode: To contain the information for making an RNA or polypeptide. A gene can encode an RNA or a polypeptide.

Endonuclease: An enzyme that makes cuts within a polynucleotide strand.

Endoplasmic reticulum (ER): Literally, "cellular network"; a network of membranes in the cell on which proteins destined for export from the cell are synthesized.

Enhancer: A DNA element that binds one or more activators and stimulates transcription of a gene or genes. Enhancers are usually found upstream of the genes they influence, but they can also function if inverted or moved hundreds or even thousands of base pairs away.

Enhancer-blocking: The negative action an insulator exerts on an enhancer.

Enzyme: A molecule usually a protein, but sometimes an RNA that catalyzes, or accelerates and directs, a biochemical reaction.

Epigenetic: Not affecting the base sequence of DNA.

Epitope tagging: Using genetic means to attach a small group of amino acids (an epitopic tag) to a protein. This enables the protein to be purified readily by immune precipitation with the antibody that recognizes the epitope tag.

eRF1: The eukaryotic release factor that recognizes all three stop codons and releases the fi nished polypeptide from the ribosome.

eRF3: The eukaryotic release factor with ribosome-dependent GTPase activity that collaborates with eRF1 in releasing finished polypeptides from the ribosome.

***Escherichia coli* (*E. coli*):**An intestinal bacterium; the favourite subject for bacterial molecular biology.

E site (ribosomal): The exit site to which deacylated tRNAs bind on their way out of the ribosome.

E site (RNA polymerase): The site the incoming nucleotide occupies just before moving (including rotation) to the A site.

Essential gene set: The set of genes whose loss is incompatible with the life of an organism.

Euchromatin: Chromatin that is extended, accessible to RNA polymerase, and at least potentially active. These regions stain either lightly or normally with dyes and are thought to contain most of the genes.

Eukaryote: An organism whose cells have nuclei.

Evolutionarily conserved regions (ECRs): Sequences of DNA found in a wide variety of organisms; likely to reside in exons.

Excision repair: Repair of damaged DNA that involves removing the damage and replacing it with normal DNA.

Exon: A region of a gene that is ultimately represented in that gene's mature transcript. The word refers to both the DNA and its RNA product.

Exon junction complex: The complex of an mRNA with proteins added just upstream of the exon-exon junctions at the time of splicing. These proteins facilitate mRNP transport out of the nucleus.

Exonic splicing enhancer (ESE): A region of an exon that stimulates splicing.

Exonic splicing silencer (ESS): A region of an exon that inhibits splicing.

Exonuclease: An enzyme that degrades a polynucleotide from the end inward.

Expect value (E value): The number of matches yielding the corresponding bit score that we would expect to see by chance. The lower the E value, the better the match.

Expressed sequence tag (EST): An STS generated by amplifying cellular mRNA by RT-PCR.

Expression vector: A cloning vector that allows expression of a cloned gene.

F plasmid: An *E. coli* plasmid that allows conjugation between bacterial cells.

F_1: The progeny of a cross between two parental types that differ at one or more genes; the first filial generation.

F_2: The progeny of a cross between two F_1 individuals or the progeny of a self-fertilized F_1; the second filial generation.

50S ribosomal subunit: The large bacterial ribosomal subunit, involved in peptide bond formation.

Ferritin: An intracellular iron storage protein.

Fingerprint (protein): The specific pattern of peptide spots formed when a protein is cut into pieces (peptides) with an enzyme (*e.g.*, trypsin), and then the peptides are separated by chromatography.

FISH: Fluorescence in situ hybridization. A means of hybridizing a fluorescent probe to whole chromosomes to determine the location of a gene or other DNA sequence within a chromosome.

5'-end: The end of a polynucleotide with a free (or phosphorylated or capped) 5'-hydroxyl group.

Fluor: A substance that emits photons when excited by a radioactive emission.

Fluorescent probe: One of the fluorescent molecules in a FRET experiment.

Fluorography: A method for visualizing weak radioactive emissions in a medium, such as a gel, by soaking the medium in a fluor that can convert the radioactive emissions into light.

fMet: *See N*-formyl methionine.

Frameshift mutation: An insertion or deletion of one or two bases in the coding region of a gene, which changes the reading frame of the corresponding mRNA.

Free radicals: Very reactive chemical substances with an unpaired electron. Can attack and damage DNA.

Functional genomics: The study of the pattern of genome-wide gene expression at various times or under various conditions.

Fusidic acid: An antibiotic that blocks the release of EF-G from the ribosome after GTP hydrolysis and thereby blocks translation after the translocation step.

Fusion protein: A protein resulting from the expression of a recombinant DNA containing two open reading frames (ORFs) fused together. One or both of the ORFs can be incomplete.

G protein: A protein that is activated by binding to GTP and inactivated by hydrolysis of the bound GTP to GDP by an inherent GTPase activity.

G-segment: The segment of DNA that breaks to form a gate through which the T segment passes during topoisomerase II activity.

Galactoside permease: An enzyme encoded in the *E. coli lac* operon that transports lactose into the cell.

Galactoside transacetylase: One of the three enzymes encoded by the *lac* operon. It can acetylate a galactoside such as lactose, but its importance to the *lac* operon is unclear.

Gamete: A haploid sex cell.

Gamma rays: Very high energy radiation that ionizes cellular components. The ions then can cause chromosome breaks.

GC box: A hexamer having the sequence GGGCGG on one strand, which occurs in a number of mammalian structural gene promoters. The binding site for the transcription factor Sp1.

Gel electrophoresis: An electrophoretic method in which substances (usually nucleic acids or proteins) are separated on a gel of agarose or polyacrylamide.

Gel filtration: A column chromatographic method for separating substances according to their sizes. Small molecules enter the beads of the gel and so take longer to move through the column than larger molecules, which cannot enter the beads.

Gel mobility shift assay: An assay for DNA–protein binding. A short labeled DNA is mixed with a protein and electrophoresed. If the DNA binds to the protein, its electrophoretic mobility is greatly decreased.

Gene: The basic unit of heredity. Contains the information for making one RNA and, in most cases, one polypeptide.

Gene cloning: Generating many copies of a gene by inserting it into an organism, such as a bacterium, where it can replicate along with the host.

Gene cluster: A group of related genes grouped together on a eukaryotic chromosome.

Gene conversion: The conversion of one gene's sequence to that of another.

Gene expression: The process by which gene products are made.

General transcription factors: Eukaryotic proteins that participate, along with one of the RNA polymerases, in forming a preinitiation complex.

Genetic code: The set of 64 codons and the amino acids (or terminations) they stand for.

Genetic linkage: The physical association of genes on the same chromosome.

Genetic mapping: Determining the linear order of genes and the distances between them.

Genetic marker: A mutant gene or other peculiarity in a genome that can be used to "mark" a spot in a genome for mapping purposes.

Genome: One complete set of genetic information from a genetic system; *e.g.*, the single, circular chromosome of a bacterium is its genome.

Genomic functional profiling: Determining the pattern of expression of all the genes in an organism at all stages of the organism's life.

Genomic library: A set of clones containing DNA fragments derived directly from a genome, rather than from mRNA.

Genomics: The study of the structure and function of whole genomes.

Genotype: The allelic constitution of a given individual. The genotypes at locus *A* in a diploid individual may be *AA, Aa,* or *aa.*

Gigabase pairs (Gb): Billion base pairs.

Glucose: A simple, six-carbon sugar used as an energy source by many forms of life.

Glutamine-rich domain A transcription-activating domain rich in glutamines.

Glycosidic bond (in a nucleoside): The bond linking the base to the sugar (ribose or deoxyribose) in RNA or DNA.

Golgi apparatus: A membranous organelle that packages newly synthesized proteins for export from the cell.

Guanine (G): The purine base that pairs with cytosine in DNA.

Guanine nucleotide exchange protein: A protein that replaces GDP with GTP on a G protein, thereby activating the G protein.

Guanosine: A nucleoside containing the base guanine.

Guide RNAs (editing): Small RNAs that bind to regions of an mRNA precursor and serve as templates for editing a region upstream.

Guide sequences (splicing): Regions of an RNA that bind to other RNA regions to help position them for splicing.

Guide strand (of siRNA): The strand that associates with RISC to degrade cognate mRNA.

Hairpin: A structure resembling a hairpin (bobby pin), formed by intramolecular base-pairing in an inverted repeat of a single stranded DNA or RNA.

Half-life: The time it takes for half of a population of molecules to disappear.

Haploid: The chromosomal number in the gamete (*n*).

Haplotype: A cluster of alleles on a single chromosome.

Haplotype map: A genomic map showing the locations of haplotypes.

Heat shock genes: Genes that are switched on in response to environmental insults, including heat.

Heat shock response: The response of cells to heat and other environmental insults. Cells turn on heat shock genes that encode molecular chaperones that help unfolded proteins refold properly and proteases that degrade hopelessly unfolded proteins.

Helicase: An enzyme that unwinds a polynucleotide double helix.

Helix-loop-helix domain (HLH domain): A protein domain that can cause dimerization by forming a coiled coil with another HLH domain.

Helix-turn-helix: A structural motif in certain DNA-binding proteins, especially those from prokaryotes, that fits into the DNA major groove and gives the protein its binding capacity

and specificity.

Helper virus (or phage): A virus that supplies functions lacking in a defective virus, allowing the latter to replicate.

Hemoglobin: The red, oxygen-carrying protein in the red blood cells.

Heterochromatin: Chromatin that is condensed and inactive.

Heteroduplex: A double-stranded polynucleotide whose two strands are not completely complementary.

Heterogeneous nuclear RNA (hnRNA): A class of large, heterogeneous-sized RNAs found in the nucleus, including unspliced mRNA precursors.

Heteroschizomers: Restriction endonucleases that recognize the same restriction site, but cut at different places within the site.

Heterozygote: A diploid genotype in which the two alleles for a given gene are different; for example, *A*1*A*2.

High-throughput DNA sequencing: *See* sequencing (high throughput, or next generation).

Histone acetyltransferase (HAT): An enzyme that transfers acetyl groups from acetyl CoA to histones.

Histone chaperones: Proteins that load histones onto naked DNA to form nucleosomes.

Histone code: A set of histone modifications in a nucleosome near a gene's control region that have a specific effect on transcription of that gene.

Histone fold: A structural motif found in histones, consisting of three helices linked by two loops.

Histones: A class of five small, basic proteins intimately associated with DNA in most eukaryotic chromosomes.

Homologous chromosomes: Chromosomes that are identical in size, shape, and, except for allelic differences, genetic composition.

Homologous (genes or proteins): Similar because of evolutionary relatedness.

Homologous recombination: Recombination that requires extensive sequence similarity between the recombining DNAs.

Homologs: Genes that have evolved from a common ancestral gene. Includes orthologs and paralogs.

Homozygote: A diploid genotype in which both alleles for a given gene are identical; for example, *A1A1* or *aa.*

Housekeeping genes: Genes that code for proteins needed for basic processes in all kinds of cells.

Hybridization (of polynucleotides): Forming a double-stranded structure from two polynucleotide strands (either DNA or RNA) from different sources.

Hydroxyl radicals: OH units with an unpaired electron. They are highly reactive and can attack DNA and break it. They are therefore useful reagents for footprining.

IF1: The prokaryotic initiation factor that promotes dissociation of the ribosome after a round of translation. Also augments the activities of the other two initiation factors.

IF2: The prokaryotic initiation factor responsible for binding fMet-tRNA fMet to the ribosome.

IF3: The prokaryotic initiation factor responsible for binding mRNA to the ribosome and for keeping ribosomal subunits apart once they have separated after a round of translation.

.**Immunoglobulin (antibody) :** A protein that binds very specifi cally to an invading substance and alerts the body's immune defenses to destroy the invader.

Immunoprecipitation: A technique in which labeled proteins are reacted with a specifi c antibody or antiserum, then cross-linked and precipitated by centrifugation. The precipitated proteins are usually detected by electrophoresis and autoradiography.

***in cis*:** A condition in which two genes are located on the same chromosome.

in silico: Performed by computation only (using the silicon chips of a computer).

***in trans*:**A condition in which two genes are located on separate chromosomes.

Incision: Nicking a DNA strand with an endonuclease.

Inclusion bodies: Insoluble aggregates of protein frequently formed on high-level expression of a foreign gene in *E. coli.* The protein in these inclusion bodies is usually inactive, but can frequently be reactivated by controlled denaturation and renaturation.

Independent assortment: A principle discovered by Mendel, which states that genes on different chromosomes are inherited independently.

Inducer: A substance that releases negative control of an operon.

Initiation factor: A protein that helps catalyze the initiation of translation.

Initiator (Inr): A site surrounding the transcription start site that is important in the efficiency of transcription from some class II promoters, especially those lacking TATA boxes.

Inosine (I): A nucleoside containing the base hypoxanthine, which base-pairs with cytosine.

Insertion sequence (IS): A simple type of transposon found in bacteria, containing only inverted terminal repeats and the genes needed for transposition.

***in situ* hybridization:** Hybridizing labeled probes directly to biological specimens such as sectioned embryos or even chromosome spreads to fi nd genes or gene transcripts.

Insulator: A DNA element that shields a gene from the positive effect of an enhancer or the negative effect of a silencer.

Intercalate: To insert between two base pairs in DNA.

Interferon: A double-stranded RNA-activated antiviral protein with various effects on the cell.

Intrinsic terminator: A bacterial terminator that does not require help from termination factors such as rho.

Intron: A region that interrupts the transcribed part of a gene. An intron is transcribed, but is removed by splicing during maturation of the transcript. The word refers to the intervening sequence in both the DNA and its RNA product.

Intron definition: A splicing scheme in which splicing factors recognize the ends of introns.

Intronic silencing element: A region of an intron that inhibits splicing.

Inverted repeat: A symmetrical sequence of DNA, reading the same forward on one strand and backward on the opposite strand.

For example: **GGATCC**

CCTAGG

Isoelectric focusing: Electrophoresing a mixture of proteins through a pH gradient until each protein stops at the pH that matches its isoelectric point. Because the proteins have no net charge at their isoelectric points, they can no longer move toward the anode or cathode.

Isoelectric point: The pH at which a protein has no net charge.

Isoschizomers: Two or more restriction endonucleases that recognize and cut the same place in the same restriction site.

Kilobase pair (kb): One thousand base pairs.

Klenow fragment: A fragment of DNA polymerase I, created by cleaving with a protease, that lacks the 5'→3' exonuclease activity of the parent enzyme.

Knockouts: Organisms, typically mice, with a gene inactivated by inserting engineered cells into embryos.

Known genes: Genes from a genomic sequencing project whose sequences are identical to previously characterized genes.

Kozak's rules: The set of requirements for an optimal context for a eukaryotic translation initiation signal. The most important of Kozak's rules are that the base at position –3 relative to the AUG initiation codon should be a purine, preferably an A, and that the base at position 14 should be a G.

***lacA*:**The *E. coli* gene that encodes galactoside transacetylase.

***lacI*:**The *E. coli* gene that encodes the *lac* repressor.

***lac* operon:** The operon that encodes enzymes that permit a cell to metabolize the milk sugar lactose.

***lac* repressor:** A protein, the product of the *E. coli lacI* gene, that forms a retramer that binds to the *lac* operator and thereby represses the *lac* operon.

Lactose: A two-part sugar, or disaccharide, composed of two simple sugars, galactose and glucose.

***lacY*:** The *E. coli* gene that encodes galactoside permease.

***lacZ*:** The *E. coli* gene that encodes b-galactosidase.

Lagging strand: The strand that is made discontinuously in semidiscontinuous DNA replication.

λ gt11: An insertion cloning vector that accepts a foreign DNA into the *lacZ* gene engineered into a l phage.

λ phage (lambda phage): A temperate phage of *E. coli.* Can replicate lytically or lysogenically.

Lariat: The name given the lasso-shaped intermediate in certain splicing reactions.

Leader: A sequence of untranslated bases at the 5'-end of an mRNA (the 5'-UTR).

Leading strand: The strand that is made continuously in semidiscontinuous DNA replication.

Leucine zipper: A domain in a DNA-binding protein that includes several leucines spaced at regular intervals. Appears to permit formation of a dimer with another leucine zipper protein. The dimer is then empowered to bind to DNA.

Limited proteolysi:s Mild treatment with a protease that can break a protein down into its component domains.

Linker scanning mutagenesis: Creation of clustered mutations by replacing small segments (roughly 10 bp) of natural DNA with synthetic double-stranded oligonucleotides (linkers).

Liposome: A lipid-bounded vesicle. Can be used to introduce DNA into cells.

Liquid chromatography-mass spectronomy (LC-MS): Separation of substances by liquid chromatography (LC) in a fi ne capillary, followed by MS analysis of each substance as it emerges from the LC.

Locus (loci, pl): The position of a gene on a chromosome, used synonymously with the term gene in many instances.

Long interspersed elements (LINEs): The most abundant non- LTR retrotransposons in mammals.

Luciferase: An enzyme that converts luciferin to a chemiluminescent product that emits light and is therefore easily assayed. The firefly luciferase gene is used as a reporter gene in eukaryotic transcription and translation experiments.

Luxury genes: Genes that code for specialized cell products.

Lysis: Rupturing the membrane of a cell, as by a virulent phage.

Lysogen: A bacterium harboring a prophage.

Marker: A gene or mutation that serves as a signpost at a known location in the genome.

Mass spectrometry: A high-resolution analytical technique that ionizes molecules and shoots them toward a target. Assuming they are all singly charged, their times of fl ight to the target are related to their masses. The masses give important information about the nature of the molecules.

Maternal genes: Genes that are expressed during oogenesis in the mother.

Megabase pair (Mb): One million base pairs.

Meiosis: Cell division that produces gametes (or spores) having half the number of chromosomes of the parental cell.

7-Methyl guanosine (m7G) : The capping nucleoside at the beginning of a eukaryotic mRNA.

Microprocessor: The complex of Drosha and Pasha (or its homolog).

microRNA (miRNA): A short (18–25-nt) RNA produced naturally in cells that can control the expression of cellular genes by causing destruction of specific mRNAs, or blocking their translation.

Microsatellite: A short DNA sequence (usually 2–4 bp) repeated many times in tandem. A given microsatellite is found in varying lengths, scattered around a eukaryotic genome.

Minimal genome: The smallest collection of genes that can sustain life in an organism.

Minisatellite: A short sequence of (usually) 12 or more bp repeated over and over in tandem.

Minus ten box (–10 box): An *E. coli* promoter element centered about 10 bp upstream of the start of transcription.

Minus thirty-five box (–35 box): An *E. coli* promoter element centered about 35 bp upstream of the start of transcription.

Mismatch repair: The correction of a mismatched base incorporated by accident—in spite of the editing system—into a newly synthesized DNA.

Missense mutation: A change in a codon that results in an amino acid change in the corresponding protein.

Mitogen: A substance, such as a hormone or growth factor, that stimulates cell division.

Mitogen-activated protein kinase (MAPK): A protein kinase that is activated by phosphorylation as a result of a signal transduction pathway initiated by a mitogen such as a growth factor.

Mitosis: Cell division that produces two daughter cells having nuclei identical to the parental cell.

Model organism: An organism chosen for study as a surrogate for study on humans because of any or all of the following factors: small genome size, short generation time, and ease of manipulation in genetic experiments.

Molecular chaperone:s *See* chaperones.

mRNA (messenger RNA) : A transcript that bears the information for making one or more proteins.

mRNP (messenger RNP) : The complex of an mRNA and all the proteins that bind to it.

MS/MS: A two-step mass spectronomy technique in which the ions created by the first MS step are manipulated in some way and then subjected to a second MS step.

Multiple cloning site (MCS) : A region in a cloning vector that contains several restriction sites in tandem. Any of these can be used for inserting foreign DNA.

Mutagen: A mutation-causing agent.

Mutant: An organism (or genetic system) that has suffered at least one mutation.

Mutation: The original source of genetic variation caused, for example, by a change in a DNA base or a chromosome. Spontaneous mutations are those that appear without explanation, while induced mutations are those attributed to a particular mutagenic agent.

Negative control: A control system in which gene expression is turned off unless a controlling element (*e.g.*, repressor) is removed.

***Neurospora crassa*:**A common bread mold, developed by Beadle and Tatum as a subject for genetic investigation.

Next-generation sequencing: *See* sequencing (high throughput, or next generation).

***N*-formyl-methionine (fMet) :** The initiating amino acid in bacterial translation.

Nick: A single-stranded break in DNA.

Nick translation: The process by which a DNA polymerase simultaneously degrades the DNA ahead of a nick and elongates the DNA behind the nick. The result is the movement (translation) of the nick in the 39-direction in a DNA strand.

Nitrocellulose: A type of paper that has been changed chemically so it binds single-stranded DNA and proteins. Used for blotting DNA prior to hybridizing with a labeled probe. Also used for blotting proteins prior to probing with antibodies.

Nonautonomous retrotransposon: A non-LTR retrotransposon that encodes no proteins, so it depends on other retrotransposons for transposition activity.

Noncoding base: A DNA base (*e.g.*, 3-methyl adenine) that cannot base-pair properly with any natural base.

Noncoding RNAs (ncRNAs) : Transcripts that do not code for proteins. *See also* transcripts of unknown function.

Nonsense codons UAG, UAA, and UGA: These codons tell the ribosome to stop protein synthesis.

Nonsense mutation: A mutation that creates a premature stop codon within a gene's coding region. Includes amber mutations (UAG), ochre mutations (UAA), and opal mutations (UGA).

Non-stop mRNA: An mRNA with no stop codon.

Nontemplate DNA strand: The strand complementary to the template strand. Sometimes called the coding strand or sense strand.

Nontranscribed spacer (NTS): A DNA region lying between two rRNA precursor genes in a cluster of such genes.

Northern blotting: Transferring RNA fragments to a support medium (*see* Southern blotting).

Nucleic acid: A chain-like molecule (DNA or RNA) composed of nucleotide links.

Nucleo capsid: A structure containing a viral genome (DNA or RNA) with a coat of protein.

Nucleolus: A cell organelle found in the nucleus that disappears during part of cell division. Contains the rRNA genes.

Nucleoside: A base bound to a sugar either ribose or deoxyribose.

Nucleosome: A repeating structural element in eukaryotic chromosomes, composed of a core of eight histone molecules with about 200 bp of DNA wrapped around the outside and one molecule of histone H1, also bound outside the core histone octamer.

Nucleosome core particle: The part of the nucleosome remaining after nuclease has digested all but about 146 bp of nucleosomal DNA. Contains the core histone octamer, but lacks histone H1.

Nucleosome positioning: The establishment of specific positions of nucleosomes with respect to a gene's promoter.

Nucleotide (nt) : The subunit, or chain-link, in DNA and RNA, composed of a sugar, a base, and at least one phosphate group.

Ochre codon: UAA, coding for termination.

Okazaki fragments: Small DNA fragments, 1000–2000 bases long, created by discontinuous synthesis of the lagging strand.

Oligomeric protein: A protein that contains more than one polypeptide subunit.

Oligonucleotide: A short piece of RNA or DNA.

Oncogene: A gene whose product can contribute to the transformation of cells to a malignant phenotype.

One gene–one polypeptide hypothesis: The hypothesis, now generally regarded as valid, that one gene codes for one polypeptide.

Opal codon: UGA, coding for termination.

Open complex: A complex of *dnaA* protein and *oriC* in which three 13-mers within *oriC* are melted.

Open promoter complex: The complex formed by tight binding between RNA polymerase and a prokaryotic promoter. It is "open" in the sense that at least 10 bp of the DNA duplex open up, or separate.

Open reading frame (ORF) : A reading frame that is uninterrupted by translation stop codons.

Operator: A DNA element found in prokaryotes that binds tightly to a specific repressor and thereby regulates the expression of adjoining genes.

Operator constitutive mutation: A mutation in an operator that renders it unable to bind effectively to its repressor. Thus, the operon is constitutive, or somewhat active all the time.

Operon: A group of genes coordinately controlled by an operator.

O region: The small region of homology between *attP* and *attB.*

***oriC*:** The *E. coli* origin of replication.

Origin of replication: The unique spot in a replicon where replication begins.

Orthologs: Homologous genes in different species that have evolved from a common ancestral gene.

P site (ribosomal): The ribosomal site to which a peptidyl tRNA is bound at the time a new aminoacyl-tRNA enters the ribosome.

Palindrome: inverted repeat.

Paper chromatography: A chromatography method that separates molecules based on their relative affinities for paper and for a solvent flowing through the paper.

Paralogs: Homologous genes that have evolved by gene duplication within a species.

Paromomycin: An antibiotic that binds to the A site of the ribosome and decreases accuracy of translation.

Passenger strand: The strand of an siRNA that is discarded from the RISC, leaving the guide strand associated with the RISC.

Pathway (biochemical) : A series of biochemical reactions in which the product of one reaction (an intermediate) becomes the substrate for the following reaction.

Peptide bond: The bond linking amino acids in aprotein.

Peptidyl transferase: An enzyme that is an integral part of the large ribosomal subunit and catalyzes the formation of peptide bonds during protein synthesis.

Phage display: Expression of a foreign gene as a fusion protein with a phage coat protein so the foreign gene product will be displayed on the surface of the phage.

Phagemid: A plasmid cloning vector with the origin of replication of a single stranded phage, which gives it the ability to produce single-stranded cloned DNA on phage infection.

Phage P1: A lytic phage of *E. coli* used in cloning large pieces of DNA.

Pharmacogenomics: Using a patient's SNPs to predict his or her reaction to various drugs so that therapy can be custom designed.

Phenotype: The morphological, biochemical, behavioral, or other properties of an organism. Often only a particular trait of interest, such as weight, is considered.

Phosphodiester bond: The sugar-phosphate bond that links the nucleotides in a nucleic acid.

Phosphorimager: An instrument that performs phosphorimaging.

Phosphorimaging: A technique for measuring the degree of radioactivity of a substance (*e.g.*, on a blot) electronically, without using fi lm.

Photoreactivation: Direct repair of a pyrimidine dimer by DNA photolyase.

Physical map: A genetic map based on physical characteristics of the DNA, such as restriction sites, rather than on locations of genes.

P/I state: A hybrid state in which the initiator aminoacyl-tRNA initially binds, with its anticodon in the P site and its amino acid and acceptor stem in an "initiator" site on the E site side of the P site.

Plaque: A hole that a virus makes on a layer of host cells by infecting and either killing the cells or slowing their growth.

Plaque assay: An assay for virus (or phage) concentration in which the number of plaques produced by a given dilution of virus is determined.

Plaque-forming unit (pfu) : A virus capable of forming a plaque in a plaque assay.

Plaque hybridization: A procedure for selecting a phage clone that contains a gene of interest. DNAs from a large number of phage plaques are simultaneously tested with a labeled probe that hybridizes to the gene of interest.

Plasmid: A circular DNA that replicates independently of the cell's chromosome.

Plasmid: A circular DNA that replicates independently of the cell's chromosome.

Point mutation: An alternation of one, or a very small number, of contiguous bases.

Poly(A): Polyadenylic acid. The string of about two hundred A's added to the end of a typical eukaryotic mRNA.

Poly(A)-binding protein I (PAB I, Pab1p): A protein that binds the poly(A) tails on mRNAs and apparently helps confer translatability on the mRNAs.

polyadenylation: Addition of poly(A) to the 39-end of an RNA.

Polyadenylation signal: The set of RNA sequences that govern the cleavage and polyadenylation of a transcript. An AAUAAA sequence followed 20–30 nt later by a GU-rich region, then a U-rich region is the canonical cleavage signal. After cleavage, the AAUAAA sequence is the polyadenylation signal.

Polycistronic message: An mRNA bearing information from more than one gene.

Polymerase chain reaction (PCR) : Amplifi cation of a region of DNA using primers that flank the region and repeated cycles of DNA polymerase action.

Polynucleotide: A polymer composed of nucleotide subunits; DNA or RNA.

Polypeptide: A single protein chain.

Polyprotein: A long polypeptide that is processed to yield two or more smaller, functional polypeptides; for example, the *pol* polyprotein of a retrovirus.

Polysome: A messenger RNA attached to (and presumably being translated by) several ribosomes.

Positional cloning: Locating genes involved in particular genetic traits.

Positive control: A control system in which gene expression depends on the presence of a positive effector such as CAP (and cAMP).

Positive strand: The strand of a viral genome with the same sense as the viral mRNAs.

Positive strand phage (or virus) : An RNA phage (or virus) whose genome also serves as an mRNA.

Post synapsis: The phase of homologous recombination in *E. coli* in which the single-stranded DNA replaces a strand in the double-stranded DNA to form a new double helix.

Post transcriptional control: Control of gene expression that occurs during the posttranscriptional phase when transcripts are processed by splicing, clipping, and modification.

Post transcriptional gene silencing (PTGS) : *See* RNA interference.

Post translational modification: The set of changes that occur in a protein after it is synthesized.

Predicted genes: Genes from a genomic sequencing project that contain sequences homologous to ESTs.

Pre-initiation complex: The combination of RNA polymerase and general transcription factors assembled at a promoter just before transcription begins.

Pre-insertion state: A hypothetical state in transcription elongation in which the incoming nucleotide can be examined for proper fit with the template base and for the presence of the appropriate sugar.

Pre-miRNA: The stem-loop precursor to an miRNA, cleaved from a pri-miRNA by Drosha.

Pribnow box: *See* minus ten box (-10 box).

Primary structure: The sequence of amino acids in a polypeptide, or of nucleotides in a DNA or RNA.

Primary transcript: The initial, unprocessed RNA product of a gene.

Primase: The enzyme within the primosome that actually makes the primer.

Primer: A small piece of RNA that provides the free end needed for DNA replication to begin.

Primer extension: A method for quantifying the amount of a transcript in a sample, and also for locating the 5'-end of the transcript. A labeled DNA primer is hybridized to a particular mRNA in a mixture, extended to the 5'-end of the transcript with reverse transcriptase, and the DNA product electrophoresed to determine its size and abundance.

Primosome: A complex of about 20 polypeptides, which makes primers for *E. coli* DNA replication.

Probe (nucleic acid) : A piece of nucleic acid, labeled with a tracer (traditionally radioactive) that allows an experimenter to track the hybridization of the probe to an unknown DNA. For example, a radioactive probe can be used to identify an unknown DNA band after electrophoresis.

Processed pseudogene: A pseudogene that has apparently arisen by retrotransposon-like activity: transcription of a normal gene, processing of the transcript, reverse transcription, and reinsertion into the genome.

Processing (of RNA) : The group of cuts that occur in RNA precursors during maturation, including splicing, 5'- or 3'-end clipping, or cutting rRNAs out of a large precursor.

Prokaryotes: Microorganisms that lack nuclei. Comprising bacteria, including cyanobacteria (blue-green algae), and archaea.

Promoter: A DNA sequence to which RNA polymerase binds prior to initiation of transcription-usually found just upstream of the transcription start site of a gene.

Promoter clearance: The process by which an RNA polymerase moves away from a promoter after initiation of transcription.

Proofreading (DNA): The process a cell uses to check the accuracy of DNA replication as it occurs and to replace a mispaired base with the right one.

Proofreading (protein synthesis): The process by which aminoacyl-tRNAs are double-checked on the ribosome for correctness before the amino acids are incorporated into the growing protein chain.

Prophage: A phage genome integrated into the host's chromosome.

Protease: An enzyme that cleaves proteins; for example, the protease that cleaves a retroviral polyprotein into its functional parts.

Proteasome: A collection of proteins (sedimentation coefficient 26S) that proteolytically degrades a ubiquitinated protein.

Protein: A polymer, or polypeptide, composed of amino acid subunits. Sometimes the term *protein* denotes a functional collection of more than one polypeptide (*e.g.*, the hemoglobin protein consists of four polypeptide chains).

Protein sequencing: Determining the sequence of amino acids in a protein.

Proteolytic processing: Cleavage of a protein into pieces.

Proteome: The structures and activities of all the proteins an organism can make in its lifetime.

Proteomics: The study of proteomes.

Proximal promoter: Class II promoter elements lying approximately between positions -37 and -250.

Proximal sequence element: The essential element of a class II snRNA promoter.

Pseudogene: A nonallelic copy of a normal gene, which is mutated so that it cannot function.

Pseudouridine: A nucleoside, found in tRNA, in which the ribose is joined to the 5-carbon instead of the 1-nitrogen of the uracil base.

pUC vectors: Plasmid vectors based on pBR322, containing an ampicillin resistance gene, and a multiple cloning site that interrupts the *lacZ*9 gene, which enables blue/white screening for inserts.

Pulsed-field gel electrophoresis (PFGE): An electrophoresis technique in which the electric field is repeatedly reversed. Allows separation of very large pieces of DNA, up to several Mb in size.

Purine: The parent base of guanine and adenine.

Puromycin: An antibiotic that resembles an aminoacyl-tRNA and kills bacteria by forming a peptide bond with a growing polypeptide and then releasing the incomplete polypeptide from the ribosome.

Pyrimidine: The parent base of cytosine, thymine, and uracil.

Pyrimidine dimers: Two adjacent pyrimidines in one DNA strand linked covalently via a cyclobutane ring, interrupting their base pairing with purines in the opposite strand. The main DNA damage caused by UV light.

Pyrogram: The output of a camera monitoring a pyrosequencing run. Consists of a series of peaks corresponding to the incorporation of nucleotides.

Pyrosequencing: A high-throughput DNA sequencing method that converts inorganic phosphate released at the incorporation of each new nucleotide to light that can be quantified.

Quaternary structure: The way two or more polypeptides interact in a complex protein.

Quenching: Quickly chilling heat-denatured DNA to keep it denatured.

Read (in DNA sequencing) : A contiguous sequence obtained from a single run of a sequencing aparatus.

Reading frame: One of three possible ways the triplet codons in an mRNA can be translated. For example, the message CAGUGCUCGAC has three possible reading frames, depending on where translation begins: (1) CAG UGC UCG; (2) AGU GCU CGA; (3) GUC CUC GAC. A natural mRNA generally has only one correct reading frame.

Real-time PCR: A method that uses fluorescent tags to measure the amplification of a DNA as it happens during PCR.

Recessive: An allele or trait that does not express its phenotype when heterozygous with a dominant allele; for example, *a* is recessive to *A* because the phenotype for *Aa* is like *AA* and not like *aa.*

Recombinant DNA: The product of recombination between two (or more) fragments of DNA. Can occur naturally in a cell, or be fashioned by molecular biologists in vitro.

Recombination: Reassortment of genes or alleles in new combinations. Occurs by crossing over between or within DNAs.

Recombination repair: A mechanism that cells use to replicate DNA containing uninformative lesions such as pyrimidine dimers. First, the two strands are replicated, leaving a gap across from the lesion. Next, recombination between the progeny duplexes places the gap across from normal DNA so it can be filled in.

Recruitment: Encouraging the binding of a substance to a complex. Usually refers to enhancing the binding of RNA polymerase or transcription factors to a promoter.

Regulon: A set of genes that are regulated together.

Related genes: Genes from a genomic sequencing project whose sequences are homologous to known genes, or parts of genes, of the same or other species.

Release factor (RF) : A protein that causes termination of translation at stop codons.

Renaturation of DNA: *See* annealing of DNA.

Repetitive DNA: DNA sequences that are repeated many times in a haploid genome.

Replacement vector: A cloning vector derived from λ phage, in which a significant part of the phage DNA is removed and must be replaced by a segment of foreign DNA of similar size.

Replicating fork: The point where the two parental DNA strands separate to allow replication.

Replicative form: The double-stranded version of a single stranded RNA or DNA phage or virus that exists during genome replication.

Replicative transposition: "Copy and paste" transposition in which the transposon DNA replicates, so one copy remains in the original location as another copy moves to the new site.

Replicon: All the DNA replicated from one origin of replication.

Replisome: The large complex of polypeptides, including the primosome, which replicates DNA in *E. coli.*

Reporter gene: A gene attached to a promoter or translation start site, and used to measure the activity of the resulting transcription or translation. The reporter gene serves as an easily assayed surrogate for the gene it replaces.

Repressed: Turned off. When an operon is repressed, it is turned off, or inactive.

Restriction endonuclease: An enzyme that recognizes specific base sequences in DNA and cuts at or near those sites.

Restriction fragment: A piece of DNA cut from a larger DNA by a restriction endonuclease.

Restriction fragment length polymorphism (RFLP) : A variation from one individual to another in the number of cutting sites for a given restriction endonuclease in a given genetic locus.

Restriction map: A map that shows the locations of restriction sites in a region of DNA.

Restriction–modification system (R-M system) : The combination of a restriction endonuclease and the DNA methylase that recognizes the same DNA site.

Restriction site: A sequence of nucleotides recognized and cut by a restriction endonuclease.

Reverse transcriptase: RNA-dependent DNA polymerase; the enzyme, commonly found in retroviruses, that catalyzes reverse transcription.

Reverse transcriptase PCR (RT-PCR): A PCR procedure that begins with the synthesis of cDNA from an mRNA template, using reverse transcriptase. The cDNA then serves as the template for conventional PCR.

Reverse transcription: Synthesis of a DNA using an RNA template.

Reversion: A mutation that cancels the effects of an earlier mutation in the same gene.

RF (replicative form): The circular double-stranded form of the genome of a single-stranded DNA phage such as xX174. The DNA assumes this form in preparation for rolling circle replication.

Rho (r): A protein that is needed for transcription termination at certain terminators in *E. coli* and its phages.

Rho-dependent terminator: A terminator that requires rho for activity.

Ribonuclease (RNase) : An enzyme that degrades RNA.

Ribonucleoside triphosphates: The building blocks of RNA: ATP,CTP, GTP, and UTP.

Ribose: The sugar in RNA.

Riboprobe: A labeled RNA probe, commonly used in RNase protection assays.

Ribosome: An RNA-protein particle that translates mRNAs to produce proteins.

Ribosome drop-off: Premature release of ribosomes from an mRNA.

Riboswitch: A region of an RNA that can bind to a small molecule that alters gene expression by infl uencing transcription or translation.

Ribozyme: A catalytic RNA (RNA enzyme).

Rifampicin: An antibiotic that blocks transcription initiation by *E. coli* RNA polymerase.

RISC loading complex (RLC): The protein complex that (presumably) separates the two siRNA strands, then delivers the guide strand to the RISC.

RNA (ribonucleic acid): A polymer composed of ribonucleotides linked together by phosphodiester bonds.

RNA-dependent DNA polymerase: *See* reverse transcriptase.

RNA-directed RNA polymerase (RdRP): The enzyme that elongates the siRNA primers, using target mRNA as a template, thus providing more substrate for Dicer and amplifying the siRNA.

RNA helicase: An enzyme that can unwind a double-stranded RNA, or a double-stranded region within an RNA.

RNA-induced silencing complex (RISC): The RNase complex that degrades the target mRNA during RNAi. Includes Dicer, Argonaute, and an unknown RNase that cleaves the target mRNA.

RNA interference (RNAi): Control of gene expression by specific mRNA degradation caused by insertion of a doublestranded RNA into a cell.

RNA ligase: An enzyme that can join two pieces of RNA, such as the two pieces of a pre-tRNA created by cutting out an intron.

RNA polymerase: The enzyme that directs transcription, or synthesis of RNA.

RNA polymerase I: The eukaryotic RNA polymerase that makes large rRNA precursors.

RNA polymerase II: The eukaryotic RNA polymerase that makes mRNA precursors and most snRNAs.

RNA polymerase III: The eukaryotic RNA polymerase that makes 5S rRNA and tRNA precursors, as well as the precursors of several other small RNAs, including U6 snRNA.

RNA polymerase core: The collection of subunits of a prokaryotic RNA polymerase having basic RNA chainelongation capacity, but no specificity of initiation; all the RNApolymerase subunits except the σ-factor.

RNA polymerase II holoenzyme: The combination of polymerase II, transcription factors, and other proteins that can be purified as a unit using mild techniques.

RNA polymerase holenzyme (bacterial) : The collection of polypeptides that make up the whole enzyme.

RNA processing: Modifying an initial transcript to its mature form by cleavage, splicing, capping, polyadenylation, *etc.*

RNA splicing: The process of removing introns from a primary transcript and attaching the exons to one another.

RNA triphosphatase: The enzyme that removes the g-phosphate at the 5'-end of a pre-mRNA prior to capping.

Rolling circle replication: A mechanism of replication in which one strand of a double-stranded circular DNA remains intact and serves as the template for elongation of the other strand at a nick.

rRNA (ribosomal RNA) : The RNA molecules contained in ribosomes.

rRNA precursor: The large rRNA precursor in mammals, which contains the 28S, 18S, and 5.8S rRNA sequences.

rRNA (5.8S): The smallest of the mammalian rRNAs derived from the 45S precursor. Found in the large (60S) ribosomal subunit, base-paired to the 28S rRNA.

rRNA (18S): The mammalian rRNA found in the small (40S) ribosomal subunit.

rRNA (28S): The largest mammalian rRNA. Found in the large (60S) ribosomal subunit, base-paired to the 5.8S rRNA.

Scanning: A model of translation initiation in eukaryotes that invokes a 40S ribosomal subunit binding to the 5'-end of the mRNA and scanning, or sliding along, the mRNA until it finds the first start codon in a good context for initiation.

Secondary siRNAs: Short double-stranded RNAs that lie outside the limits of the original trigger RNA. Always upstream with respect to the sense strand of the trigger RNA.

Secondary structure: The local folding of a polypeptide or RNA. In the latter case, the secondary structure is defined by intramolecular base pairing.

Sedimentation coefficient: A measure of the rate at which a molecule or particle travels toward the bottom of a centrifuge tube under the influence of a centrifugal force.

Seed BAC: A BAC chosen for complete sequencing during shotgun sequencing of a large genome.

Selection: A genetic sorting procedure that eliminates unwanted organisms, usually by preventing their growth or by killing them.

Semiconservative replication: DNA replication in which the two strands of a parental duplex separate completely and pair with new progeny strands. One parental strand is therefore conserved in each progeny duplex.

Semidiscontinuous replication: A mechanism of DNA replication in which one strand is made continuously and the other is made discontinuously.

Sequence-tagged site (STS) : A short stretch of DNA that can be identified by amplifying it using PCR with defined primers.

Sequencing: Determining the amino acid sequence of a protein, or the base sequence of a DNA or RNA.

Sequencing (high throughput, or next generation) : DNA sequencing that uses very rapid automated methods, such as pyrosequencing, to produce relatively short reads of DNA in a massively parallel manner that yields a great deal of sequence in a short time.

Serial analysis of gene expression (SAGE) : A method for determining the levels of expression of many genes at once. Uses short cDNAs, or tags, from many mRNAs that are linked together, cloned, and sequenced. Tags that are most frequently found are expressed most actively.

70S initiation complex: The complex of 70S ribosome, mRNA, and fMet-tRNA f Met that is poised to initiate translation.

Shine–Dalgarno (SD) sequence: A G-rich sequence (consensus = AGGAGGU) that is complementary to a sequence at the 3'-end of *E. coli* 16S rRNA. Base pairing between these two sequences helps the ribosome bind an mRNA.

Shotgun sequencing: Genomic sequencing performed by chopping the genome up into small pieces that are cloned and sequenced at random. Later these sequences are pieced together to give the sequence of the whole genome.

Shuttle vector: A cloning vector that can replicate in two or more different hosts, allowing the recombinant DNA to shuttle back and forth between hosts.

Sickle cell disease: A genetic disease in which abnormal b-globin is produced. Because of a single amino acid change, this blood protein tends to aggregate under low-oxygen conditions, distorting red blood cells into a sickle shape.

Sigma (σ) : The bacterial RNA polymerase subunit that confers specificity of transcription—that is, ability to recognize specific promoters.

Signal peptide: A stretch of about 20 amino acids, usually at the amino terminus of a polypeptide, that helps to anchor the nascent polypeptide and its ribosome in the endoplasmic reticulum. Polypeptides with a signal peptide are destined for packaging in the Golgi apparatus and are usually exported from the cell.

Signal transduction pathway: A biochemical pathway that connects a signal, such as a growth factor binding to the cell surface, with an intracellular effect, usually gene activation (or repression).

Silencer: A DNA element that can act at a distance to decrease transcription from a eukaryotic gene.

Silencing: Repression of eukaryotic gene activity. Can occur by forming heterochromatin in the region of the gene, or by more localized mechanisms, including tightening the binding between particular nucleosomes and DNA.

Single-nucleotide polymorphism (SNP): A single-nucleotide difference between two or more individuals at a particular genetic locus.

siRNAs (short interfering RNAs): The short pieces (21–28 nt) of double-stranded trigger RNA created by Dicer during the RNAi process.

Site-directed mutagenesis: A method for introducing specific, predetermined alterations into a cloned gene.

Site-specific recombination: Recombination that always occurs in the same place and depends on limited sequence similarity between the recombining DNAs.

Sodium dodecyl sulfate (SDS): A strong, negatively charged detergent used to denature proteins in SDS polyacrylamide gel electrophoresis (SDS-PAGE).

Somatic 5S rRNA genes: The 5S rRNA genes (haploid number about 400 in *Xenopus laevis*) that are expressed in both somatic cells and oocytes.

Somatic mutation: A mutation that affects only somatic cells, so it cannot be passed on to progeny.

S1 nuclease: A nuclease specifi c for single-stranded RNA and

Southern blotting: Transferring DNA fragments separated by gel electrophoresis to a suitable support medium such as nitrocellulose, in preparation for hybridization to a labelled probe.

Spacer DNA: DNA sequences found between, and sometimes within, repeated genes such as rRNA genes.

spliced leader (SL) : The independently synthesized 35-nt leader that is *trans*-spliced to surface antigen mRNA coding regions in trypanosomes.

Spliceosome: The large RNA–protein body on which splicing of nuclear mRNA precursors occurs.

Spliceosome cycle: The process of forming the spliceosome, splicing, then dissociation of the spliceosome.

Splicing: The process of linking together two RNA exons while removing the intron that lies between them.

Splicing factors: Proteins besides snRNP proteins that are essential for splicing nuclear pre-mRNAs.

Spore: (1) A specialized haploid cell formed sexually by plants or fungi, or asexually by fungi. The latter can either serve as a gamete, or germinate to produce a new haploid cell. (2) A specialized cell formed asexually by certain bacteria in response to adverse conditions. Such a spore is relatively inert and resistant to environmental stress.

Sporulation: Formation of spores.

SSB: Single-strand DNA-binding protein, used during DNA replication and recombination. Binds to single-stranded DNA and keeps it from base-pairing with a complementary strand.

Sticky ends: Single-stranded ends of double-stranded DNAs that are complementary and can therefore base-pair and stick together.

Stop codon: One of three codons (UAG, UAA, and UGA) that code for termination of translation.

Streptavidin: A protein made by *Streptomyces* bacteria that binds avidly to biotin.

Streptomycin: An antibiotic that kills bacteria by causing their ribosomes to misread mRNAs.

Strong-stop DNA: The initial product of reverse transcription of a retroviral RNA. It initiates at the primer-binding site and terminates about 150 nt later, at the 5'-end of the viral RNA.

Structural genomics: The study of the expression of large sets of genes.

Superhelix: A form of circular double-stranded DNA in which the double helix coils around itself like a twisted rubber band.

Superinfection (λ phage) : Infection of a lysogen of one lambdoid phage with a second lambdoid phage.

Supershift: The extra gel mobility shift observed when a new protein joins a protein–DNA complex.

Superwobble hypothesis: The idea that a tRNA with a U in the fi rst position of its anticodon can, at least under certain conditions, recognize a codon ending in any of the four bases.

Suppression: Compensation by one mutation for the effects of another.

Synapsis: Alignment of complementary sequences in the single stranded and double-stranded DNAs that will participate in strand exchange during homologous recombination in *E. coli.*

Syntenic blocks: Blocks of DNA in which the order of genes has been preserved in different organisms.

Synteny: Preservation of gene order in different organisms. Also, existence of genes on the same chromosome in a given organism.

Tags (in SAGE) : Short cDNAs corresponding to the mRNAs in a cell.

Taq polymerase: A heat-resistant DNA polymerase obtained from the thermophilic bacterium *Thermus aquaticus.*

Target mRNA: The mRNA that is targeted and degraded during RNAi.

TATA box: An element with the consensus sequence TATAAAA that begins about 25–30 bp upstream of the start of transcription in most eukaryotic promoters recognized by RNA polymerase II.

TATA-box-binding protein (TBP) : A subunit of SL1, TFIID, and TFIIIB in class I, II, and III preinitiation complexes, respectively. Binds to the TATA box in class II promoters that have a TATA box.

T loop: A loop formed in the telomere at the end of a eukaryotic chromosome.

TBP-associated factor: A protein associated with TBP in SL1, TFIID, or TFIIIB.

TBP-free TAFII-containing complex (TFTC) : An alternative TFIID that lacks TBP.

T-DNA: The tumor-inducing part of the Ti plasmid.

Telomerase: An enzyme that can extend the ends of telomeres after DNA replication.

Telomere: A structure at the end of a eukaryotic chromosome, containing tandem repeats of a short DNA sequence.

Telomere end-binding protein (TEBP) : A dimeric protein in ciliated protozoa that binds to telomere ends and protects them from degradation and from DNA repair enzymes.

Telomerase reverse transcriptase (TERT) : The subunit of telomerase with the reverse transcriptase active site.

Template: A polynucleotide (RNA or DNA) that serves as the guide for making a complementary polynucleotide. For example, a DNA strand serves as the template for ordinary transcription.

Template DNA strand: The DNA strand of a gene that is complementary to the RNA product of that gene; that is, the strand that served as the template for making the RNA. Sometimes called the anticoding strand or antisense strand.

Terminal transferase: An enzyme that adds deoxyribonucleotides, one at a time, to the 39-end of a DNA.

Terminator: *See* transcription terminator.

Tertiary structure: The overall three-dimensional shape of a polypeptide or RNA.

Tetramer (protein:) A complex of four polypeptides.

TFIIA: A class II general transcription factor that stabilizes binding of TFIID to the TATA box.

TFIIB: A class II general transcription factor that binds to a promoter after TFIID in vitro. Helps TFIIF plus RNA polymerase II bind to the promoter.

TFIIBC: The C-terminal domain of TFIIB, which binds to the TATA box after it is bent by TBP.

TFIIBN: The N-terminal domain of TFIIB, which binds near the active site of RNA polymerase II, positioning it for initiation the correct distance from the TATA box.

TFIID: A class II general transcription factor that binds first to TATA-box-containing promoters *in vitro* and serves as a nucleation site around which the preinitiation complex assembles. Contains TATA-box-binding protein (TBP) and TBP-associated factors (TAFIIs).

TFIIE: A class II general transcription factor that binds to the preinitiation complex after TFIIF and RNA polymerase and before TFIIH *in vitro.*

TFIIF: A class II general transcription factor that binds to the preinitiation complex cooperatively with RNA polymerase II in vitro after TFIIB has bound.

TFIIH: The last class II general transcription factor to bind to the preinitiation complex in vitro. Has protein kinase and DNA helicase activities.

TFIIS: A protein that stimulates transcription elongation by RNA polymerase II by limiting pausing at pause sites.

TFIIIA: A general transcription factor that works with TFIIIC to help activate eukaryotic 5S rRNA genes by facilitating binding of TFIIIB.

TFIIIB: A general transcription factor that activates genes transcribed by RNA polymerase III by binding to a region just upstream of the gene.

TFIIIC: A general transcription factor that stimulates binding of TFIIIB to classical class III genes.

30S ribosomal subunit: The small bacterial ribosomal subunit, involved in mRNA decoding.

3' box: A DNA element near the end of a class II snRNA gene that ensures proper 3' processing of the primary transcript.

3'-end: The end of a polynucleotide with a free (or phosphorylated) 3'-hydroxyl group.

3' tRNase: tRNA 3' processing endoribonuclease.

Thymidine: A nucleoside containing the base thymine.

Thymine (T: The pyrimidine base that pairs with adenine in DNA.

TIF-1B: The homolog of human SL1 in certain lower eukaryotes.

Ti plasmid: The tumor-inducing plasmid from *Agrobacterium tumefaciens.* Used as a vector to carry foreign genes into plant cells.

Tiling array: A DNA microarray containing DNAs with overlapping sequences.

Topoisomerase: An enzyme that changes a DNA's superhelical form, or topology.

Type I topoisomerase: A topoisomerase that introduces transient single-strand breaks into substrate DNAs.

Type II topoisomerase: A topoisomerase that introduces transient double-strand breaks into substrate DNAs.

Trailer: The untranslated region of bases at the 3'-end of an RNA between the termination codon and the poly(A). Also called the 3'-UTR.

***Trans*-acting:** A term that describes a genetic element, such as a repressor gene or transcription factor gene, that can be on a separate chromosome and still influence another gene. These *trans*-acting genes function by producing a diffusible substance that can act at a distance.

Transcribed fragments (transfrags) : Small regions of a genome that are represented by transcripts, as detected by microarrays.

Transcribed spacer: A region encoding a part of an rRNA precursor that is removed during processing to produce the mature rRNAs.

Transcript: An RNA copy of a gene.

Transcription: The process by which an RNA copy of a gene is made.

Transcription-activating domain: The part of a transcription activator that stimulates transcription.

Transcription bubble: The region of locally melted DNA that follows the RNA polymerase as it synthesizes the RNA product.

Transcription factor: A protein that stimulates (or sometimes represses) transcription of a eukaryotic gene by binding to a promoter or enhancer element.

Transcription factor B (TFB) : An archaeal factor homologous to eukaryotic TFIIB.

Transcription factories: Discrete nuclear sites where transcription of multiple genes occurs.

Transcription terminator: A specific DNA sequence that signals transcription to terminate.

Transcription unit: A region of DNA bounded by a promoter and a terminator that is transcribed as a single unit. May contain multiple coding regions, as in the major late transcription unit of adenovirus.

Transcriptome: The sum of all the different transcripts an organism can make in its lifetime.

Transcriptomics: The global study of an organism's transcripts.

Transfection: Transformation of eukaryotic cells by incorporating foreign DNA into the cells.

Transformation (genetic) : An alteration in a cell's genetic makeup caused by introducing exogenous DNA.

Transgene: A foreign gene transplanted into an organism, making the recipient a transgenic organism.

Transgenic organism: An organism into which a new gene or set of genes has been transferred.

Transition: A mutation in which a pyrimidine replaces a pyrimidine, or a purine replaces a purine.

Translation: The process by which ribosomes use the information in mRNAs to synthesize proteins.

Translocation: The translation elongation step, following the peptidyl transferase reaction, in which an mRNA moves one codon's length through the ribosome and brings a new codon into the ribosome's A site.

Transpeptidation: The reaction (formation of peptide bonds) catalyzed by peptidyl transferase.

Transposable element: A DNA element that can move from one genomic location to another.

Transposase: The name for the collection of proteins, encoded by a transposon, that catalyze transposition.

Transposition: The movement of a DNA element (transposon) from one DNA location to another.

***Trans*-splicing:** Splicing together two RNA fragments transcribed from separate transcription units.

***Trans*-translation:** The shift from reading a non-stop mRNA to reading the ORF of a tmRNA that occurs during tmRNA mediated ribosomal rescue.

Transversion: A mutation in which a pyrimidine replaces a purine, or vice versa.

Trigger dsRNA: The double-stranded RNA that initiates the RNAi process.

tRNA (transfer RNA) : A relatively small RNA molecule that binds an amino acid at one end and "reads" an mRNA codon at the other, thus serving as an "adapter" that translates the mRNA code into a sequence of amino acids.

tRNA charging: The process of coupling a tRNA with its cognate amino acid, catalyzed by aminoacyl-tRNA synthetase.

tRNA 3' processing endoribonuclease (3'tRNase): The enzyme that removes excess nucleotides from the 3'-ends of tRNA precursors in eukaryotes.

***trp* operon:** The operon that encodes that enzymes needed to make the amino acid tryptophan.

***trp* repressor:** The repressor of the *trp* operon. Composed of the *trp* aporepressor plus the corepressor tryptophan.

Two-dimensional gel electrophoresis: A high-resolution method for separating proteins. First the proteins are separated in the first dimension by isoelectric focusing. Then they are separated in the second dimension by SDS-PAGE.

2 mm plasmid: A yeast plasmid that serves as the basis for yeast cloning vectors.

Untranslated region (UTR) : A region at the 5'- or 3'-end of an mRNA that lies outside the coding region, so is not translated.

Upstream activating sequence (UASG) : An enhancer for yeast galactose-utilization genes that binds the activator GAL4.

Upstream activating factor (UAF) : The yeast homolog of UBF.

Upstream-binding factor (UBF): A class I transcription factor that binds to the upstream promoter element (UPE). Acts synergistically with SL1 to stimulate polymerase I binding and transcription.

Upstream-binding site (UBS) : A site on the bacterial core RNA polymerase that binds to the upstream half of the RNA hairpin at a terminator and thereby slows down hairpin formation and inhibits transcription termination.

Uracil (U) : The pyrimidine base that replaces thymine in RNA.

Uracil N-glycosylase: An enzyme that removes uracil from a DNA strand, leaving an abasic site (a sugar without a base).

Uridine: A nucleoside containing the base uracil.

UTR: An untranslated region on an mRNA-either at the 5'- or 3'-end.

Variable loop: The loop, or stem, in a tRNA molecule, which lies between the anticodon and T stems.

Variable number tandem repeats (VNTR) : A type of RFLP that includes tandem repeats of a minisatellite between the restriction sites.

Variable region: The region of an antibody that binds specifically to a foreign substance, or antigen. As its name implies, it varies considerably from one kind of antibody to another.

Vector: A DNA (a plasmid or a phage DNA) that serves as a carrier in gene cloning experiments.

Vegetative cell: A cell that is reproducing by division, rather than sporulating or reproducing sexually.

Virulent phage: A phage that lyses its host.

Void volume: The fraction in a gel filtration experiment that contains the large molecules that cannot enter the pores in the gel at all.

Western blotting: Electrophoresing proteins, then blotting them to a membrane and reacting them with a specific antibody or antiserum. The antibody is detected with a labeled secondary antibody or protein A.

Wobble: The ability of the third base of a codon to shift slightly to form a non-Watson–Crick base pair with the first base of an anticodon, thus allowing a tRNA to translate more than one codon.

Wobble base pair: A base pair formed by wobble (a G–U or A–I pair).

Wobble hypothesis: Francis Crick's hypothesis that invoked wobble to explain how one anticodon could decode more than one codon.

Wobble position: The third base of a codon, where wobble base pairing is permitted.

X-Ray crystallography: *See* x-ray diffraction analysis.

X-Ray diffraction analysis: A method for determining the three dimensional structure of molecules by measuring the diffraction of x-rays by crystals of the molecule or molecules.

X-Rays: High-energy radiation that is diffracted by crystals. The pattern of x-ray diffraction can then be used to determine the shape of the molecule(s) in the crystal. X-rays also ionize cellular components and can therefore cause chromosome breaks.

Yeast artificial chromosome: A high-capacity cloning vector consisting of yeast left and right telomeres and a centromere. DNA placed between the centromere and one telomere becomes part of the YAC and will replicate in yeast cells.

Yeast two-hybrid assay: An assay for interaction between two proteins. One protein (the bait) is produced as a fusion protein with a DNA-binding domain from another protein. The other protein (the target, or prey) is produced as a fusion protein with a transcription-activation domain. If the two fusion proteins interact in the cell, they form an activator that can activate one or more reporter genes.

Z-DNA: A left-handed helical form of double-stranded DNA whose backbone has a zigzag appearance. This form is stabilized by stretches of alternating purines and pyrimidines.

Zinc finger: A DNA-binding motif that contains a zinc ion complexed to four amino acid side chains, usually the side chains of two cysteines and two histidines. The motif is roughly finger-shaped and inserts into the DNA major groove, where it makes specific protein–DNA contacts.

Important Questions in Agricultural Biotechnology

1. **The most effective technique to produce virus free plants from infected individuals is**
   A. Shoot tip culture
   B. Protoplast culture
   C. Single cell culture
   D. Meristem culture
2. **Growth hormones are sterilized by using**
   A. Auto clave
   B. Hot air oven
   C. Mercuric chloride
   D. Ultra filtration
3. **The important nutrient medium for the culture of pollen is**
   A. MS medium
   B. SKoog's medium
   C. N6 medium
   D. Camborg medium
4. **Generation of plants with different genomes is possible through**
   A. Endosperm culture
   B. Meristem culture
   C. Protoplast culture
   D. Pollen culture
5. **The most serious objection to micropropagation**
   A. Genetic instability
   B. More expensive
   C. Genetic stability
   D. Less growth

6. **The process of formation of somatic embryos from the callus is referred to as**
   A. Embryogensis B. Organogensis
   C. Sporogensis D. Gametogensis

7. **Which of the following is preferred for making artificial seeds.**
   A. Potassium alginate B. Sodium alginate
   C. Agar D. Gelrite

8. **The scientist regarded as father of plant tissue culture is**
   A. Maheshwari B. Murashige
   C. White D. Haberlandt

9. **Bioreactors are used for the production of**
   A. Enzymes B. Secondary metabolities
   C. Cell culture D. All the above

10. **Which of the following assays involve in an antigen-antibody?**
   A. Southern hybridization B. Dot-blot assay
   C. ELISA D. Colony hybridization

11. **The indispensable component of solid culture media**
   A. Sucrose B. Distilled water
   C. Agar Agar D. None of these

12. **The stage is micropropagation**
   A. Multiple shoots induction B. Establishment of culture
   C. Both A and B D. None of these

13. **Quarantine procedures enable**
   A. Prevent entry of infectious material into the country B. Control of external infection
   C. Aseptic conditions D. None of these

14. **Single cell culture is used in**
   A. Callus culture B. Meristem culture
   C. Protoplast culture D. None of these

15. **Hardening enables the plants to**
   A. Multiplication B. Acclimatization
   C. Sterilization D. None of these

16. Haploid production in *Datura innoxia* was demonstrated by Guha and Maheshwari in

A. 1960 B. 1962

C. 1964 D. 1966

17. Virus free plants are produced by

A. Root tip culture B. Endosperm culture

C. Meristem culture D. Protoplast culture

18. The scientist who first described 'totipotency'?

A. White B. Haberlandt

C. Murashige D. Skoog

19. Ability of individual plant cells to regenerate into whole plants is allied

A. Rhizogenesis B. Totipotency

C. Organogeneisis D. Redifferentiation

20. Bipolar embryo like structures induced from somatic cells through *in vitro* is known as

A. Zygotic embryo B. Synthetic seeds

C. Somatic embryo D. Premature embryo

21. Virus indexing of plants could be analyzed using

A. ELISA B. Electron microscopy

C. Indicator plants D. All the above

22. Embryo rescue refers to

A. Rescuing abortive embryos of wide hybridization

B. Rescuing mature embryos that are not able to germinate

C. Rescuing inherently weak embryos

D. Both A and B

23. The most widely used carbon source in plant tissue culture media is

A. Glucose B. Fructose

C. Sucrose D. Maltose

24. Chromosome doubling is induced by

A. EDTA B. TEMED

C. SDS D. None of the above

25. An example of a fusogenic agent is

A. Methanol
B. Ethyl alcohol
C. Polyethelene alcohol
D. Polyethelene glycol (PEG)

26. The isolated protoplasts are made to fuse to produce a hybrid cell in

A. Tissue culture
B. Genetic engineering
C. Protoplast fusion
D. Gene cloning

27. The rigid plant cell wall is digested by

A. Pectinase
B. Protease
C. Amylase
D. Sucrase

28. Inoculated culture vessels are protected from contamination of other organism by

A. Cleaning
B. Cotton plug
C. Oil cloth
D. Cork plug

29. The isolated protoplasts are grown in

A. Hypotonic culture medium
B. Hypertonic culture medium
C. Isotonic culture medium
D. Agar culture medium

30. Which cell-based plant technology involves the combining of two cells without cell walls from different species?

A. Clonal propagation
B. Cybridization
C. Protoplast fusion
D. Mutant selection

31. Protoplasts can be produced from suspension cultures, callus tissues or intact tissues by enzymatic treatment with

A. Cellulotyic enzymes
B. Pectolytic enzymes
C. Both cellulotyic and pectolytic enzymes
D. Proteolytic enzymes

32. What is meant by 'Organ culture' ?

A. Maintenance alive of a whole organ, after removal from the organism by partial immersion in a nutrient fluid
B. Introduction of a new organ in an animal body with a view to create genetic mutation in the progenies of that animal
C. Cultivation of organs in a laboratory through the synthesis of tissues
D. The aspects of culture in community which are mainly dedicated by the need of a specified organ of the human body

33. Which method of plant propagation involves the use of girdling?

A. Grafting
B. Cuttings
C. Layering
D. Micropropagation

34. Organogenesis is

A. Formation of callus tissue
B. Formation of root and shoots on callus tissue
C. Both A and B
D. Genesis of organs

35. Which of the following is used in the culture of regenerating protoplasts, single cells or very dilute cell suspensions?

A. Nurse medium
B. Nurse or feeder culture
C. Both A and B
D. None of these

36. In a callus culture

A. Increasing level of cytokinin to a callus induces shoot formation and increasing level of auxin promote root formation
B. Increasing level of auxin to a callus induces shoot formation and increasing level of cytokinin promote root formation
C. Auxins and cytokinins are not required
D. Only auxin is required for root and shoot formation

37. Protoplasts are the cells devoid of

A. Cell membrane
B. Cell wall
C. Both A and B
D. None of these

38. Which breeding method uses a chemical to strip the cell wall of plant cells of two sexually incompatible species?

A. Mass selection
B. Protoplast fusion
C. Transformation
D. Transpiration

39. The phenomenon of the reversion of mature cells to the meristematic state leading to the formation of callus is known as

A. Redifferentiation
B. Dedifferentiation
C. Either A or B
D. None of these

40. Cell fusion method includes the preparation of large number of

A. Plant cells stripped of their cell wall
B. Single plant cell stripped of their cell wall
C. Plant cells with cell wall
D. Cells from different species

41. Subculturing is similar to propagation by cuttings because

A. It separates multiple microshoots and places them in a medium

B. It uses scions to produce new microshoots

C. They both use in vitro growing conditions

D. All of the above

42. The process of callus to form a whole plant is known as

A. redifferentiation B. dedifferentiation

C. Either A or B D. None of these

43. What is/are the benefit(s) of micropropagation over to conventional propagation?

A. Rapid multiplication of superior clones

B. Multiplication of disease free plants

C. Multiplication of sexually derived sterile hybrids

D. All of the above

44. When plated only in nutrient medium, how much time is required for the protoplast to synthesize new cell wall?

A. 2-5 days B. 5-10 days

C. 10-15 days D. 15-17 days

45. Cellular totipotency is the property of

A. Plants B. Animals

C. Bacteria D. All of these

46. Establishment of embryogenic cell suspensions with high regeneration potential is a pre-requisite for successful

A. Protoplast culture

B. Detection of nucleic acid sequence

C. Restriction of fragment length polymorphisms

D. Microinjection

47. Meristem culture of banana enables

A. Rapid multiplication

B. Elimination of bunch top virus disease

C. Both A and B

D. Slow growth

48. Protoplast fusion technique generally involves

A. Isolation only

B. Isolation and fusion

C. Isolation, fusion and culturing

D. Hybridization between two species

49. Somatic cell hybridization is the process in which

A. Two protoplast along with their nuclei fuse

B. A normal protoplast along with an enucleated protoplast fuse

C. Both A and B

D. Two enucleated protoplasts fuse

50. Somaclonal variation method refers to

A. Heritable changes

B. Genetic isolation

C. Small number of species having limited commercial potential

D. Large number of plant cells

51. MS medium, is found essential for initial morphogenesis of the immature embryos and to enhance callus development, when supplemented with

A. GA_3

B. GA_3 and coconut milk

C. Adenine

D. Adenine and kinetin

52. Plant tissue culture technique is used to select somaclones that are

A. Resistant to herbicide

B. Not resistant to herbicide

C. Resistant to salinity

D. Both A and C

53. Which of the following constituent/(s) is/are added to help in speedy generation of meristem culture in case of *Ipomoea batatas* improvement?

A. Auxins

B. Cytokinins

C. Both A and B

D. Adenine

54. Which of the following is an ethylene biosynthesis inhibitor?

A. Citric acid

B. Succinic acid

C. Activated charcoal

D. Silver thiosulphate

55. Nitrogen in the plant cell culture media is provided by either ammonia or nitrate salt. In the media

A. Utilization of ammonium cause culture pH to drop while utilization of nitrate cause culture pH to rise

B. Utilization of nitrate cause culture pH to drop while utilization of ammonium cause culture pH to rise

C. Utilization of both ammonium and nitrate result in rise in pH

D. Utilization of both ammonium and nitrate result in drop in pH

56. Which of the following growth regulator is added for short initiation during plant regeneration from callus?

A. Auxins B. Cytokinins

C. Gibberellins D. Brassinosteroids

57. Which of the following growth regulator promote cell division?

A. Auxins B. Cytokinins

C. Gibberellins D. Brassinosteroids

58. Which of the following growth regulator is used to stimulate embryo development?

A. Auxins B. Cytokinins

C. Gibberellins D. Brassinosteroids

59. Which of the following growth regulator cause callus formation in plant?

A. Auxins B. Cytokinins

C. Gibberellins D. Brassinosteroids

60. Silver thiosulphate is added to culture medium as it helps to

A. Maintain the pH

B. Remove toxic phenolics from plant cells

C. Prevent the gaseous plant hormone, ethylene dioxide from accumulating to detrimental condition.

D. All of the above

61. In plant cell culture media, auxins and cytokinins are used in the range of

A. 1-50μM B. 50-100μM

C. 100-125μM D. More than 125μM

62. Concentration of sucrose generally used in plant cell culture media is

A. 10-15 g/l B. 20-30 g/l

C. 40-50 g/l D. 60-70 g/l

63. Which is/are the naturally occurring plant auxins?

A. Indole acetic acid (IAA)

B. Naphthalenacetic acid (NAA)

C. 2,4-dichlorophenoxyacetic acid

D. All of the above

64. Which is/are the disadvantage/(s) of using IAA in plant cell culture media?

A. It is unstable in solution

B. Gets easily oxidized

C. Conjugated to inactive form by plant cells

D. All of the above

65. To maintain the pH of the culture

A. Organic acid such as citric, fumaric, malic and succinic acid is used

B. Synthetic buffers such as Tris, MES or HEPS are used

C. Both A and B

D. Ammonium salts are used

66. Which of the following is not a cytokinin?

A. 2,4-dichlorophenoxyacetic acid

B. 6 benzylaminopurine

C. Zeatin

D. Kinetin

67. Which of the following is example of cytokinin?

A. Naphthalenacetic acid (NAA)

B. Indole acetic acid (IAA)

C. Zeatin

D. Indole butyric acid

68. Synthetic seeds are

A. Artificially synthesized seeds

B. Somatic embryos encapsulated in suitable matrix

C. Seeds of plants modified genetically

D. None of these

69. Somatic embryoids are

A. Identical with zygotic embryos and without seed coats

B. Identical with zygotic embryos and with seed coats

C. Non-identical with zygotic embryos and without seed coats

D. Non-identical with zygotic embryos and with seed coats

70. The production of high quality and uniform embryos has been limited to only

A. Carrot B. Alfalfa

C. Both A and B D. Sandalwood

71. The preserved embryoids are termed as

A. Synthetic seeds B. Semi-synthetic seeds

C. Natural seeds D. Fermented seeds

72. Encapsulation is necessary to produce and protect synthetic seeds. The encapsulation is carried out by various types of hydrogels, which are

A. Soluble in water B. Soluble in organic solvents

C. Insoluble in water D. Insoluble in organic solvents

73. Which of the following is not true about synthetic seeds?

A. Can be stored for a year without the loss of valuables

B. Easy to handle

C. Can be directly sown in the soil like natural seeds

D. Need hardening in the greenhouse

74. Recalcitrant seeds are

A. Resistant to drying and freezing temperature

B. Killed by drying and freezing temperature

C. Both A and B

D. None of the above

75. The technique which is useful in genetic engineering to introduce rDNA and other DNA fragments into higher plant cells in culture is

A. Protoplasmic fusion B. Tissue culture

C. Hardening D. Splicing

76. Several plantlets are developed from the

A. Clone B. Inoculum

C. Callus D. Plasmid

77. Cells of higher plants are grown artificially in laboratory conditions using the technique of

A. Molecular cloning B. Gene cloning

C. Tissue culture D. Hybridzation

78. The cells in tissue culture divide and form a mass of undifferentiated tissue called

A. Inoculum
B. Plasmid
C. Replicon
D. Callus

79. The process of transferring plantlets to pots and subjected gradually to natural environmental conditions is called

A. Hardening
B. Totipotency
C. Cloning
D. Splicing

80. The following ratio of hormonal concentration is required to induce callus to form shoot and root

A. Gibberellins to auxin
B. Auxin to cytokinin
C. Gibberellins to cytokinin
D. Ethylene to auxins

81. Genes are directly introduced into the eukaryotie host for cloning through a

A. Plasmid
B. Vector
C. Endonuclease
D. Hormone

82. Virus free potatoes, tulips, sugarcanes and orchids are obtained by the technique of

A. Meristem culture
B. Shoot tip culture
C. Callus culture
D. Cell culture

83. Very small number of isolated living cells is called

A. Plasmid
B. Vector
C. Auxin
D. Inoculum

84. The instrument used for keeping inoculated vessels at a desired constant temperature is

A. Platinum wire
B. Micropipette
C. Petriplate
D. Incubator

85. The inherent capacity of an isolated plant cell to give rise to a whole plant is called

A. Totipotency
B. Protoplast
C. Hybridization
D. Gene manipulation

86. Plants obtained through tissue culture method constitute genetically uniform population called

A. Clone
B. Callus
C. Inoculum
D. Plasmid

87. The antiviral protein produced by virus infected cells is called

A. Insulin B. Auxin

C. Vaccine D. Interferon

88. The transfer of explant/culture is done under

A. Aseptic condition B. Septic condition

C. Hygenic condition D. Environmental condition

89. Flamed and cooled platinum wire is used to transfer

A. Bacteria B. Fungi

C. Callus D. Inoculum

90. Introducing the nitrogen fixing genes from bacteria to major food crops is possible through

A. Tissue culture B. Hybridization

C. Protoplast D. Genetic engineering

91. Who among the following coined the term Biotechnology?

A. Karl Ereky B. James Clarke

C. Paul Terasaky D. Clarke and Sommer

92. A molecular technique in which DNA sequences between two oligonucleotide primers can be amplified is known as

A. Southern blotting B. Northern blotting

C. Polymerase chain reaction D. DNA replication

93. The Southern blotting technique depends on

A. similarities between the sequences of probe DNA and experimental DNA

B. similarities between the sequences of probe RNA and experimental RNA

C. Similarities between the sequences of probe protein and experimental protein

D. The molecular mass of proteins

94. Charged molecules are separated based on varying rates of migration through a solid matrix when subjected to an electric field. This technique is known as

A. Photoreactivation B. Gel electrophoresis

C. Autoradiography D. Blotting

95. For gene probes to be useful they must

A. Be large enough to contain gene-specific sequences

B. Be labeled in some manner to allow detection

C. Both A and B

D. None of the above

96. A genomic library is

A. A database where the sequence of an organism's genome is stored

B. A collection of many clones possessing different DNA fragments from the same organisms bound to vectors

C. A book that describes how to isolate DNA from a particular organism

D. A place where the information of the genetic organization of organisms are kept.

97. Which of the following enzyme is used to covalently bond foreign DNA to a vector plasmid?

A. DNA polymerase

B. Restriction endonuclease

C. DNA ligase

D. DNA helicase

98. Bacterial cells protect their own DNA from degradation by restriction endonucleases by

A. Methylating the DNA at the sites that the enzyme recognizes

B. Deleting all recognition sites from the genome

C. Not producing any restriction endonucleases

D. Having anti restriction endonucleases

99. Which type of restriction endonuclease cuts the DNA within the recognition site?

A. Type I

B. Type II

C. Type III

D. All of the these

100. The advantage of using DNA polymerases from thermophilic organisms in PCR is that

A. The DNA polymerases of these bacteria are much faster than those from other organisms

B. The DNA polymerases of these bacteria can withstand the high temperatures needed to denature the DNA strands

C. The DNA polymerases of these bacteria never make mistakes while replicating DNA

D. All of the above

101. A micro array is an ordered array of microscopic elements on a planer substrate that allows the specific binding of

A. Gene or gene products
B. Whole genome
C. Both A and B
D. None of these

102. Biochips are made up of

A. Semi-conducting molecules inserted into the protein frame work
B. Conducting molecules inserted into the protein frame work
C. Non-conducting molecules inserted into the protein frame work
D. Any of the above

103. Which of the following technology is used for micro array manufacturing?

A. Photolithography
B. Ink jetting
C. Contact printing
D. All of these

104. Gene banks conserve stocks of

A. Seed only
B. Vegetative material only
C. Seed and vegetative material both
D. None of these

105. To qualify as a micro array the analytical device must be

A. Ordered
B. Microscopic
C. Planer and specific
D. All of these

106. Microarrays are also known as

A. Biochips
B. DNA chips
C. Gene chips
D. All of these

107. Single stranded circular RNA encapsulated with a larger RNA in a plant virus is

A. A virion
B. A viroid
C. A virusoid
D. None of these

108. Microarray analysis involves biological assays based on

A. Gels
B. Filters
C. Purification columns
D. Small glass chips

109. Which of the following is correct about micro biosensors?

A. Implantation in human body and are suitable for in-vivo measurements
B. Can be integrated on one chip and are useful for measuring various substrates in a small amount of sample solution simultaneously

C. It is possible to develop disposable transducers for biosensors through mass production

D. All of these

110. Industrial production of enzymes, vitamins, vaccines and bio-fertilizers are the products of

A. Ploidy
B. Genetics
C. Physiology
D. Biotechnology

111. Restriction endonucleases are discovered in

A. 1910
B. 1906
C. 1966
D. 1970

112. The donor DNA fragments and vector DNA fragments are joined together by

A. DNA ligase
B. Plasmid
C. Auxin
D. Cytokinin

113. The following is used in industrial fermentation to produce food and drinks

A. Yeast
B. Algae
C. Vitamins
D. Vaccines

114. The enzymes that cleave DNA from their ends are called _______

A. Endonucleases
B. Exonucleases
C. Both A and B
D. None of the above

115. The elements of DNA molecule that require the transcription of genes are called

A. Promoters
B. Repressors
C. Both A and B
D. None of the above

116. The number of hydrogen bonds present between adenine and Thymine is

A. One
B. Two
C. Three
D. Four

117. The following does not have nuclease activity

A. DNA polymerases
B. Exonucleases
C. RNA polymerase
D. Endonucleases

118. RNA polymerase synthesizes

A. DNA from RNA
B. RNA from DNA
C. RNA from RNA
D. DNA from DNA

119. Maxam Gilbert and Sanger dideoxy methods are concerned with

A. DNA
B. DNA damage
C. DNA repair
D. DNA sequencing

120. Amplification process was conceived by

A. Welsh
B. McClelland
C. Kary Mullis
D. Fodor

121. Blotting technique that involves protein transfer is

A. Southern blotting
B. Northern blotting
C. Western blotting
D. All the above

122. Electrophoresis of DNA is done to

A. Separate the DNA
B. Quantify the DNA
C. Hydrolyze the DNA
D. Renature the DNA

123. DNA double helix was invented in the year

A. 1954
B. 1953
C. 1956
D. 1955

124. Coding sequences are

A. Introns
B. Exons
C. 5' UTR
D. 3' UTR

125. Replication fork is formed during

A. DNA replication
B. Translation
C. Transcription
D. Cloning

126. Which of the following is true of DNA double helix?

A. The 5' end of one DNA strand is aligned with 5' end of the other strand.
B. Total number of purine bases is equal to the total number of pyrimidine bases
C. The sequence of bases on one strand is identical to the sequence of bases on the other strand
D. None of the above

127. Which of the following approaches for virus resistance has been most successful?

A. Coat protein gene
B. DNA of satellite RNA
C. Antisense RNA approach
D. Ribozyme approach

128. The enzyme that cuts DNA at specific site

A. DNA polymerases
B. Restriction endonucleases
C. Helicase
D. Ligase

129. Nucleotides undergo the process of polymerization to form long chain of

A. Nucleoside
B. Polynucleotide
C. Homonucleotide
D. None of these

130. Jacob and Monad (1961) gave the concept of

A. Gene expression
B. Evolution of split genes
C. Lac operon
D. None of these

131. Extra chromosomal, self replicating and double stranded closed and circular DNA molecules present in the bacteria are called

A. Cosmids
B. Plasmids
C. Viruses
D. None of these

132. A virus which eats upon bacteria

A. Bacteriophage
B. Plasmid
C. Bacteria
D. None of these

133. The following does not have nuclease activity

A. DNA polymerases
B. Endonucleases
C. RNA polymerase
D. Exonucleases

134. RNA polymerase synthesizes

A. DNA from RNA
B. RNA from RNA
C. RNA from DNA
D. DNA from DNA

135. The number of hydrogen bonds present between Guanine and Cytocine is

A. One
B. Two
C. Three
D. Four

136. Electrophoresis of DNA is done to

A. Separate the DNA
B. Quantify the DNA
C. Both A and B
D. None of the above

137. The first therapeutic chemical produced by recombinant DNA technology using *E.coli* is

A. Human insulin
B. Interferon
C. Riboflavin
D. Peptide

138. Transgenic plants are

A. Naturally occurring
B. Both A and B
C. Synthesized artificially
D. None of these

139. Each colony is a collection of bacteria having many copies of rDNA fragments called

A. Molecular cloning
B. Splicing
C. Cloning vehicles
D. Vectors

140. DNA of donor and vector plasmid is cut into pieces using

A. Vector
B. Plasmid
C. Restriction Endonuclease
D. Inoculum

141. The mechanism which has the ability to engineer new organisms is known as

A. Totipotency
B. Molecular cloning
C. Genetic engineering
D. Splicing

142. The production of new characteristics by introducing new genes and altering the genome is known as

A. Recombinant DNA technology
B. Protoplast fusion
C. Totipotency
D. Splicing

143. The molecular scissors which cut DNA at specific sites are

A. Plasmids
B. Fusogenic agents
C. Inoculum
D. Restriction enzymes

144. The extra-chromosomal circular DNA found in the E.coli is

A. Plasmid
B. DNA ligase
C. Vector
D. Cytokinin

145. The other name for hybrid DNA is

A. Recombinant DNA (rDNA)
B. DNA ligase
C. Plasmid
D. Replicon

146. Vectors are also known as

A. DNA ligase
B. Plasmid
C. Cloning vehicles
D. Inoculum

147. The recent and fascinating branch of biology is

A. Physiology
B. Genetics
C. Genetic engineering
D. Ecology

148. Suitable host in genetic engineering to introduce DNA fragments of donor is

A. Yeast
B. *Bacillus subtilis*
C. *Escherichia coli*
D. Bacteriophages

149. DNA ligase and restriction endonucleases are the basic tools required for

A. Genetic engineering
B. Physiology
C. Genetics
D. Totipotency

150. Molecular cloning is also known as

A. Splicing
B. Gene cloning
C. Gene manipulation
D. Hardening

151. In a _______ protocol, plant with engineered abilities to detoxify pollutants are intentionally released in an area.

A. Microcosm establishment
B. Mibridization
C. Bioremediation
D. Rhizosecretion

152. The controversy regarding the use of Bt corn is that it

A. Is potentially harmful to monarch butterflies
B. Is a potential allergen to humans
C. Both A and B
D. Can contaminate groundwater

153. Metabolic interference is a term used to describe a method to metabolize a compound and prevent the synthesis of something that is normally produced. What compound(s) have been targeted for metabolic interference in tomato?

A. ACC (1-aminocyclopropane-1-carboxylic acid)
B. SAM (S-adenosylmethionine)
C. Both A and B
D. AOA (aminooxyacetic acid)

154. Starch content of potatoes can be increased by using a bacterial gene, known as

A. Sucrose phosphate synthase gene

B. ADP glucose pyrophosphorylase gene

C. Polygalactouranase gene

D. None of the above

155. Which tropical fruit crop has been successfully engineered to be protected against a lethal virus?

A. Passion fruit	B. Papaya

C. Papaya	D. Lychee

156. Which of the following metabolites are implicated in stress tolerance?

A. Proline	B. Betaines

C. Both A and B	D. Citrate

157. Which of the agricultural challenges below cannot be solved with transgenic techniques?

A. Crops are damaged by frost

B. Crops are killed by a virus

C. Public concern about safety of synthetic pesticides

D. Public preference for organic vegetables

158. Which of the following statements is true regarding genomics?

A. Plant genomics lags behind similar efforts in animals and microorganisms

B. Researchers can make use of genomic information even if the entire genome of an organism is not known

C. Researchers are busy in trying to determine the genome of the potato plant

D. All of the above

159. Which of the following gene is responsible for resistance against chilling?

A. Glycerol 1 phosphate acyl transferase

B. Polygalactouranase

C. ACC deaminase

D. Sucrose phosphate synthase gene

160. Which of the following gene detoxifies herbicide phosphinothricin?

A. Nitrilase

B. Glutathione S-transferase (GST)

C. Phosphinothricin acetyl transferase

D. All of these

161. Plants derived sexually from the same plant are___ while those derived from somatic tissue from the same plant are___.

A. Identical, different

B. Different, also different

C. Different, identical

D. Plants cannot be derived from somatic tissue

162. Transgenic plants with increased tolerance to aluminum have been produced by making plants that

A. Secrete phytosiderophores into the soil

B. Make more metal-binding peptides like phytochelatins

C. Bind aluminum to the cell wall

D. Secrete citrate into the soil

163. Transplastomics

A. Targets genes in the chloroplast

B. Provides exceptionally low yields of protein products

C. Produces genes that are released in pollen

D. Offers little opportunity for practical use

164. Plants containing genes encoding cytokines and blood clotting factors are used in

A. Nutrition improvement

B. Pharmaceutical production

C. Vaccine production

D. Textile production

165. The first transgenic plants expressing engineered foreign genes were tobacco plants produced by the use of

A. *Agrobacterium tumefaciens*

B. *Bacillus thuringiensis*

C. *Arabidopsis thaliana*

D. *Streptomyces hygroscopicus*

166. Transgenic plants

A. Contain foreign genes in their cells

B. Are used to produce human antibodies

C. Both A and B

D. Are plants that differ in geographical locations

167. Low temperatures induce the expression of many cold-induced genes. Transgenic plants with improved cold tolerance have been produced by

A. Expressing the protein that activates expression of these genes all the time in plants

B. Cooling plants using the Peltier effect

C. Expressing a gene for production of antifreeze (ethylene glycol) in plants

D. Increasing evaporative cooling from leaf surfaces

168. Nitrilase is encoded by

A. Gene bxn in *Klebsiella pneumoniae*

B. Bar gene in *Streptomyces* spp.

C. Both A and B

D. None of these

169. What are the various disadvantages of cross protection?

A. Possibility of mutations in inducing mild virus strain

B. Possibility of synergism between inducing virus and other unrelated virus

C. Possibility of unnecessary spread of mild virus

D. All of the above

170. Which of the following gene is transferred to plants that detoxify the herbicide atrazine?

A. Nitrilase

B. Glutathione S-transferase (GST)

C. Phosphinothrium acetyl transferase

D. All of these

171. Which of the following genes can be used for making resistances against viral infection?

A. Genes for capsid protein

B. Gene for nucleocapsid protein

C. Satellite RNA

D. All of these

172. Which of the following has been widely used to provide resistance against plant viruses?

A. Virus resistance genes from bacteria

B. Expression of virus coat protein genes in transgenic plants

C. Expression of anti-virus genes in vectors that transmit viruses

D. Expression of ribonuclease (RNase) genes in host plants

173. Cross protection against viruses in transgenic plants can be obtained by

A. Inoculating the susceptible strain of a crop with a mild strain of a virus that helps in developing resistance against more virulent strain

B. Inoculating the susceptible strain with the coat proteins of virulent strain

C. Inoculating the susceptible strain with genes of nucleocapsid

D. Any of the above

174. Bruise resistant tomatoes have been developed by the expression of antisense RNA against

A. Glycerol 1 phosphate acyl transferase

B. Polygalactouranase

C. ACC deaminase

D. Sucrose phosphate synthase gene

175. The first field tests were conducted with which of the following genetically altered organism?

A. Bt Corn

B. Vaccinia virus containing a gene from the rabies virus

C. The flavrsavr tomato

D. Strawberry seedlings sprayed with ice-minus bacteria

176. The delayed ripening tomato was created by a biotechnologist who ________ a gene.

A. Altered

B. Silenced

C. Replaced

D. Relocated

177. Antisense technology

A. Selectively blocks expression of a gene

B. Combines genetic material from different species

C. Combines organelles and cells

D. Alters or transfers cells

178. Antisense transgenic plants produced fruit that softened

A. More slowly than the normal fruit

B. More rapidly than the normal fruit

C. As the normal fruits

D. None of these

179. Insect resistance in the transgenic plant has been achieved by

A. Transferring genes for Bt toxins

B. Transferring genes for protease inhibitors

C. Transferring genes for other insecticidal secondary metabolities

D. All of the above

180. Resistance to L-phosphinothrium in tobacco plants is developed by the transfer of

A. Gene for EPSPS (5-enol-pyruvyl shikimat 3 phosphate synthase)

B. Gene for ALS (acetolactate synthase)

C. Gene for GS (glutamine synthase)

D. Any of the above

181. ACC demainase gene is responsible for

A. Synthesis for ethylene

B. Degradation of ACC an immediate precursor to ethylene

C. Both A and B

D. Synthesis of polygalactouranase

182. Two genes from a bacterium (*Alcaligenes eutrophus*) and a cotton gene produce

A. A plastic

B. A vaccine against the bacterium

C. A pharmaceutical product

D. Herbicide resistance

183. Resistance to glyphosphate in transgenic petunia plants has been developed by the transfer of

A. Gene for EPSPS(5-enol-pyruvyl shikimat 3 phosphate synthase)

B. Gene for ALS (acetolactate synthase)

C. Gene for GS (glutamine synthase)

D. Any of the above

184. Which of the following compounds has been produced in transgenic plants to improve tolerance to salt stress and water deficit?

A. Sucrose
B. Mannitol
C. Nicotine
D. Octopine

185. Expression of antisense RNA in transgenic plants is a general method used to

A. Activate the expression of all genes in a biochemical pathway
B. Eliminate the expression of all genes in a biochemical pathway
C. Block the expression of virus coat protein genes
D. Reduce or eliminate the expression of individual genes

186. Tomatoes exhibiting delayed ripening express antisense RNA against

A. Glycerol 1 phosphate acyl transferase
B. Polygalactouranase
C. ACC deaminase
D. Sucrose phosphate synthase gene

187. Given the DNA sequence ATTAAGGC, which sequence would be used by researchers as an antisense molecule?

A. AUUAAGGC
B. UAAUUCCG
C. CGGAATTA
D. TAATTCCG

188. Which of the following gene detoxify herbicide bronoxynil?

A. Nitrilase
B. Glutathione S-transferase (GST)
C. Phosphinothricin acetyl transferase
D. All of these

189. For developing herbicide resistance in transgenic plants which of the following approach/(es) is/are used?

A. Target molecule is made insensitive to herbicide
B. Target protein is overproduced
C. A pathway should be introduced that detoxify the herbicide
D. All of the above

190. Which of the following is not a characteristic of a transgenic crop?

A. Herbicide resistance
B. Bt insect resistance toxin
C. Increased methionine content
D. None of these

191. Phosphinothricin acetyl transferase is encoded by

A. Gene bxn in *Klebsiella pneumoniae*

B. Bar gene in *Streptomyces* spp.

C. Both A and B

D. None of these

192. Reducing the expression of pectin methylesterase (PME) has resulted in

A. Plants with resistance to bacteria and fungi

B. Tomato juice that has higher viscosity

C. Tomato fruit that last longer before they become rotten

D. Tomato fruit that will not ripen

193. Resistance to sulphonyl urea compounds in transgenic tobacco plant has been developed by the transfer of

A. Gene for EPSPS (5-enol-pyruvyl shikimat 3 phosphate synthase)

B. Gene for ALS (acetolactate synthase)

C. Gene for GS (glutamine synthase)

D. Any of the above

194. In transgenic plants that have been manipulated to express pathogenesis-related (PR) proteins all the time it has been shown that

A. These provide no protection at all against pathogens

B. Expression of one PR protein provides high levels of protection against many pathogens

C. Expression of two PR proteins provides some protection against a few pathogens

D. These proteins trigger the production of other antimicrobial defenses

195. Virulence trait of *Agrobacterium tumefaciens* **is borne on**

A. Chromosomal DNA

B. Tumour inducing plasmid DNA

C. Both chromosomal and plasmid DNA

D. Cryptic plasmid DNA

196. The size of the virulent plasmid of *Agrobacterium tumefaciens* **is**

A. 40-80 kb

B. 80-120 kb

C. 140-235 kb

D. >235 kb

197. Which of the following is not true about the helper plasmids?

A. These can replicate in *Agrobacterium*

B. These help in the mediating conjugation of intermediate vectors

C. These can't replicate in *Agrobacterium*

D. All of the above

198. Which technique is used to introduce genes into dicots?

A. Electrophoration

B. Particle acceleration

C. Microinjection

D. Ti plasmid infection

199. Direct DNA uptake by protoplasts can be stimulated by

A. Polyethylene glycol (PEG)

B. Decanal

C. Luciferin

D. All of these

200. In a plant tumour cell

A. Complete Ti plasmid is incorporated in plant nuclear DNA

B. Different parts of the Ti-plasmid are incorporated

C. Only a small specific segment of callus T DNA is incorporated

D. May vary from plant to plant

201. Co-integrating transformation vectors must include a region of homology in

A. The vector plasmid

B. The Ti-plasmid

C. Between vector plasmid and Ti-plasmid

D. None of these

202. Crown gall tissue

A. Can be cultivated in vitro in absence of bacteria

B. Retains tumorous properties when cultivated

C. Both A and B

D. Shows tumorous properties only in presence of bacteria

203. Integrated nopaline T-DNA occurs as

A. Single segment

B. Two segments

C. Three segments

D. Four segments

204. Opines are

A. Amino acid derivatives found in tumor tissues

B. Amino acid derivatives found in normal tissues

C. Amino acid derivatives found in both normal as well as tumor tissues

D. None of the above

205. Which of the following is true about ***Agrobacterium tumefaciens*****?**

A. It causes crown gall disease of plants
B. It infects gymosperms
C. It infects dicotyledonous angiosperms
D. All of the above

206. In the liposome mediated gene transfer in plants, nucleic acids are

A. Protected from nuclease digestion
B. Stable in liposomes
C. Both A and B
D. Not stable in liposomes

207. Advantage of microprojectile method over microinjection method for gene transfer in plants include

A. Intact cells are used
B. Method is universal in its application irrespective of all shape, size, type and presence or absence of cell wall
C. Gene can be transferred to many cells simultaneously
D. All of the above

208. On Ti-plasmid T-region or T-DNA is flanked by a direct repeat of

A. 12 bp
B. 20 bp
C. 25 bp
D. 30 bp

209. ***Agrobacterium tumefaciens*** **is a**

A. gram (+) bacteria
B. gram (-) bacteria
C. a fungi
D. a yeast

210. Microprojectile method of gene transfer in plants involves delivery of DNA

A. With the help of micromanipulator
B. With the help of bolistics
C. With the help of needles
D. Any of the above

211. Which of the following genes are constitutively expressed and control the plant induced activation of other vir genes?

A. vir A and vir G
B. vir C and vir D
C. vir B and vir E
D. vir A and vir B

212. Integrated octopine T DNA occurs as

A. Single segment
B. Two segments
C. Three segments
D. Four segments

213. Liposomes mediated gene transfer in plants involves

A. Plasmid DNA enclosed in a lipid bag
B. Fusion of liposomes with protoplast
C. Use of polyethylene glycol (PEG)
D. All of the above

214. Which of the following plant signal molecules regulate the expression of vir B, C, D and E in case of tobacco?

A. Acetosyringone
B. α-hydroxy syringone
C. Both A and B
D. None of these

215. Opines that are present in crown gall tumour include

A. Octopine
B. Nopaline
C. Agropine
D. All of these

216. Which of the following is true about T DNA?

A. Integration of T DNA can occur at many different, apparently random, sites in the plant nuclear DNA

B. Integration of T DNA occurs only at one specific sites in the plant nuclear DNA

C. Integration of T DNA occurs at two specific sites in the plant nuclear DNA

D. Integration of T DNA occurs at one site that may be random in the plant nuclear DNA

217. Which of the following is not true about the direct repeats flanking T-DNA?

A. They are conserved between nopaline and octopine Ti-plasmids

B. These repeats are transferred intact to the plant genome

C. These are important in integration mechanism

D. All of the above

218. The left segment of octopine T-DNA (TL) is necessary for

A. Enzymes for agropine biosynthesis
B. Tumour formation
C. Conjugative transfer
D. All of these

219. The right segment of octopine T-DNA (TR) is necessary for

A. Enzymes for agropine biosynthesis
B. Tumour formation
C. Conjugative transfer
D. All of these

220. Opine synthesis is the property

A. Conferred to plant cells when it transformed by *Agrobacterium tumefaciens*

B. Determined by the bacteria *Agrobacterium tumefaciens*

C. Both A and B

D. Of normal plant cells

221. The direct repeats flanking the T-DNA of *Agrobacterium tumefaciens* **are known as**

A. Cos site
B. Flanking sequences
C. Border sequences
D. Transfer sequences

222. T-DNA transfer and processing into plant genome requires products of which of the following genes?

A. vir A,B
B. vir G,C
C. vir D,E
D. All of these

223. Because of large size of Ti-plasmid, intermediate vectors (IV) are developed in which T DNA has been subcloned into

A. pBR 322 based plasmid vector
B. pRK 2013
C. pRN 3
D. All of these

224. The transfer of intermediate vectors into *Agrobacterium* **are brought about by**

A. Transformation
B. Biparental mating
C. Triparental mating
D. Transduction

225. In response to the activating signal molecule, an endonuclease is produced that causes nicks in the T-DNA. It is encoded by

A. vir A
B. vir B
C. vir C
D. vir D

226. Which of the following are used as selection marker for the cells transformed with *Agrobacterium***?**

A. Neomycin phosphotransferase
B. Streptomycin phosphotransferase
C. Hygromycin phosphotransferase
D. all the above

227. Vir genes required for the T-DNA transfer and processing are located

A. On the T-DNA
B. Outside the T-DNA region
C. On the plant genome
D. None of these

228.. Problems in obtaining large amounts of proteins encoded by recombinant genes can often be overcome by using

A. BACS
B. Expression vectors
C. YACS
D. All of these

229. *Agrobacterium tumefaciens* is

A. A disease in humans that causes loss of sight

B. A bacterium that can be used to introduce DNA into plants

C. A fungi that is used to produce antibiotics in large amounts

D. A disease in humans that causes loss of weight

230. In genetic engineering, a chimera is

A. An enzyme that links DNA molecules

B. A plasmid that contains foreign DNA

C. A virus that infects bacteria

D. A fungi

231. The deliberate modifications of an organism's genetic information by directly changing its nucleic acid content is a subject matter of

A. Genetic engineering

B. Population genetics

C. Microbiology

D. Protein engineering

232. Electrophoration is

A. The process of separating charged molecules through a gel maintained in an electric field

B. The process of combining foreign DNA to an electrically charged vector molecule

C. The application of high voltage pulses

D. The process of multiplication of the cells

233. Which of the following is obtained using processed mRNA molecules as a template?

A. rDNA

B. mDNA

C. cDNA

D. tDNA

234. Vectors are

A. Molecules that degrade nucleic acids

B. Molecules that help in replication

C. Molecules that are able to covalently bond to and carry foreign DNA into cells

D. Molecules that protect host cells from invasion by foreign DNA

235. What is the normal role of restriction endonucleases in bacterial cells?

A. To degrade the bacterial chromosome into small pieces during replication

B. To degrade invading phage DNA

C. To produce RNA primers for replication

D. All of the above

236. Which of the following is not commonly used as vector?

A. Artificial chromosome

B. Cosmid

C. Fungi

D. Plasmid

237. A short molecule containing 2-20 nucleotide is

A. Plasmid

B. Vector

C. Oligonucleotide

D. Mononucleotide

238. Enzymes that recognize and cleave specific 4 to 8 base pair sequences of DNA are

A. DNA ligase

B. Helicases

C. Restriction endonucleases

D. DNA gyrase

239. Which of the following vector can maintain the largest fragment of foreign DNA?

A. YAC

B. Cosmid

C. Plasmid

D. Phage

240. The piece of equipment, that introduces DNA into cells via DNA-coated microprojectiles is known as

A. Laser

B. DNA probe

C. Gene gun

D. Inoculating needle

241. A plant, that has gained new genetic information from the acquisition of foreign DNA, is considered as

A. A chimera

B. A transgenic plant

C. A vector

D. An enzyme that links DNA molecules

242. *Agrobacterium* based gene transfer is efficient

A. Only with dicots

B. Only with monocots

C. With both monocots and dicots

D. With majority monocots and few dicots

243. Involvement of sugarcane phytoalexins in red-rot resistance has been observed. The phytoalexin compound is reported to be

A. 3-deoxyanthocyanidin
B. luteolinidin
C. Apigeninidin
D. 5-0 apigeninidin

244. Human serum albumin has been synthesized by

A. Transgenic potato and tobacco plants
B. Transgenic maize plants
C. Transgenic wheat plants
D. Any of the above

245. Avermectins (AVM) are macrocyclic lactones which have potent antihelminthic and insecticidal action. They are generally derived from the mycelia of

A. *Streptomyces avermitilis*
B. *B. thrunigiensis*
C. *P. flourescens*
D. *L. peruvianum*

246. The tumor phenotype, which can be maintained indefinitely in tissue culture, results from the expression of genes present in the

A. T-DNA
B. c-DNA
C. r-DNA
D. m-RNA

247. For increased level of mannitol in transgenic tobacco plants which of the following gene is transferred?

A. Mannitol dehydrogenase
B. Mannitol synthease
C. Both A and B
D. Mannitol pyrophosphorylase

248. Wheat variety Rendezvous, with resistance to eye spot (Pseudo-cercosporella herpotrichoides) derived from *Aegilops ventricosa*, **has a chloroplast genome derived from**

A. Aegilops
B. Triticum
C. Both A and B
D. S alleles

249. Human serum albumin in case of transgenic plant is secreted in

A. Transgenic leaf tissues
B. Transgenic root tissues
C. Is not secreted out of plant
D. Transgenic stem tissues

250. α and β cyclo dextrins are produced by

A. Transgenic tomato
B. Transgenic maize
C. Transgenic potato
D. Transgenic wheat

251. α and β cyclo dextrins are used for

A. Pharmaceutical delivery system

B. Flavour and odour enhancement in foods

C. Removal of undesired compounds like caffeine from foods

D. All of the above

252. Microinjection technique of introducing DNA is a

A. Physical method

B. Biological method

C. Combination of physical and biological method

D. Chemical method

253. Which of the following mutant/(s) has/have increased amount of lysine and/or methionine in corn seeds?

A. Opaque-2 B. Sugary-1

C. Flory-2 D. All of these

254. In transgenic plants of *Arabidipsis thaliana* which of the following gene is transferred for the synthesis of PHB (polyhdroxybutyrate)?

A. Acetyl Co A reductase

B. Polyhydroxybutyrate synthease

C. Both A and B

D. Pyrophosphorylase

255. When the transposon jumps into functional gene, it has the effect of

A. Blocking correct transcription

B. Initiating correct transcription

C. Propagating correct transcription

D. Initiating some genetic codes

256. Maximum size of foreign DNA that can be inserted into a replacement vector is

A. 25-30 kb B. 18-20 kb

C. 20-25 kb D. 40-50 kb

257. Which of the following is not true about phagemid?

A. Contain functional origin of replication of the plasmid and λ phage

B. May be propagated as a plasmid or as phage in appropriate strain

C. Contain λ att site

D. Can only be propagated as phage

258. pBR 322 has/have which of the following selection marker(s)?

A. Amp^r
B. Tet^r
C. Both A and B
D. Kan^r

259. A plasmid can be considered as a suitable cloning vector if

A. It can be readily isolated from the cells
B. It possesses a single restriction site for one or more restriction enzymes
C. Insertion of foreign DNA does not alter its replication properties
D. All of the above

260. Difference between λ gt 10 and λ gt 11 vectors is that

A. λ gt 11 is an expression vector
B. λ gt 10 is an expression vector
C. λ gt 10 is a replacement vector
D. λ gt 11 is a replacement vector

261. λ ZAP vector is an example of

A. Phage
B. Phagemid
C. Cosmid
D. Plasmid

262. λ gt 10 and λ gt 11 vectors can propagate cloned fragments up to

A. 6-7 kb
B. 1-2 kb
C. 40-44 kb
D. 20-23 kb

263. Select the wrong? Statement about plasmids

A. It is extrachromosomal
B. It is double stranded
C. Its replication depends upon host cell
D. It is closed and circular DNA

264. Stuffer is

A. The right arm of the vector DNA
B. The left arm of the vector DNA
C. Central fragment of the vector DNA
D. None of the above

265. Conjugative plasmids

A. Exhibit antibiotic resistance
B. Do not exhibit antibiotic resistance
C. Carry transfer genes called the tra genes
D. Do not carry transfer genes

266. Plasmid incompatibility is

A. Inability of a plasmid to grow in the host

B. Inability of two different plasmids to coexist in the same host cell in the absence of selection pressure.

C. Both A and B

D. None of the above

267. P1 cloning vector allow cloning of DNA of the length of

A. 100 kbp
B. 50 kbp
C. 20 kbp
D. 10 kbp

268. Charon 34 and Charon 35 can clone DNA upto

A. 1-2 kb
B. 6-7 kb
C. 9-20 kb
D. 30-35 kb

269. Charon vectors are different from EMBL vectors because

A. They have more extensive range of restriction targets with in their polylinkers

B. Physical separation of lambda arm from central fragment is required

C. Both A and B

D. Physical separation of lambda arm from central fragment is not required

270. P1 cloning vector is the example of

A. Plasmid
B. Cosmid
C. Bacteriophage
D. Phagemid

271. Cos site of the cosmids

A. Consists of 12 bases
B. Helps whole genome in circularization and ligation
C. Both A and B
D. Contains cleavage site

272. M 13 is an example of

A. Filamentous phage
B. Single stranded DNA vector
C. Both A and B
D. Plasmid

273. Phagemid vectors are

A. Combination of plasmid and phage λ

B. Combination of phages and cosmid

C. Phages carrying properties of plasmids

D. All of the above

274. Single stranded vectors are useful

A. For sequencing of cloned DNA

B. For oligonucleotide directed mutagenesis

C. For probe preparation

D. All of the above

275. Inserted DNA in λ gt 11 can be expressed as

A. β-galactosidase fused protein

B. Free protein in the cytoplasm

C. free protein that is secreted out

D. All of the above

276. EMBL 3 and EMBL 4 are replacement vectors, which can clone DNA up to

A. 6-7 kb

B. 15-25 kb

C. 40-44 kb

D. 1-2 kb

277. Size of the DNA that can be packaged into a λ phage is

A. 50 kb

B. 35-53 kb

C. 40-50 kb

D. any size

278. Cosmid vectors are used for

A. Cloning small fragments of DNA

B. Cloning large fragments of DNA

C. Cloning prokaryotic DNA only

D. Cloning eukaryotic DNA only

279. Plasmids which are maintained as limited number of copies per cell are known as

A. Stringent plasmids

B. Relaxed plasmids

C. Cryptic plasmids

D. All of these

280. Cryptic plasmids

A. Do not exhibit any phenotypic trait

B. Exhibit many phenotypic traits

C. Exhibit one phenotypic traits

D. Exhibit antibiotic resistance

281. Phagemid consist of

A. Plasmid vector carrying λ phage's cos site

B. Plasmid vector carrying λ attachment (λ att) site

C. Plasmid vector carrying origin of replication of λ phage only

D. Plasmid vector carrying origin of replication of plasmid only

282. Maximum size of foreign DNA that can be inserted into an insertion vector is

A. 35 kb B. 18 kb

C. 50 kb D. 27 kb

283. Plasmids which are maintained as multiple copy number per cell are known as

A. Stringent plasmids B. Relaxed plasmids

C. Cryptic plasmids D. None of these

284. Cosmid vectors are

A. Plasmids that contain fragment of λ DNA including the cos site

B. Phages that lack cos site

C. Plasmids that have no selection marker

D. Cryptic plasmids

285. Cosmids lack

A. Genes coding for viral proteins

B. Origin of replication

C. Marker genes coding for replication

D. Cleavage site for the insertion of foreign DNA

286. The host bacterium follows the instruction of the

A. DNA ligase B. Foreign recombinant DNA

C. Plasmid D. Auxin

287. Random amplified polymorphic DNA (RAPD) is a method that

A. Stimulate production of sense RNA to compensate

B. Activate the expression of all genes in a biochemical pathway

C. Eliminate the expression of all genes in a biochemical pathway

D. Reveals intra-specific variation and diversity between species

288. Which of the following marker is not a PCR based marker.?

A. RAPD
B. AFLP
C. RFLP
D. SSR

289. Simple sequence length polymorphisms

A. Can be minisatellites
B. Can be microsatellites
C. Are used in genetic mapping
D. All the above

290. Microsatellites

A. Are tandemly repeated sequences
B. Are not very common in the human genome
C. Are usually longer than 200 bp
D. Are normally found at the end of chromosomes

ANSWERS

1	D	31	C	61	A	91	A	121	C
2	D	32	A	62	B	92	C	122	A
3	C	33	C	63	A	93	A	123	B
4	C	34	B	64	D	94	B	124	B
5	B	35	C	65	C	95	C	125	A
6	A	36	A	66	A	96	B	126	B
7	B	37	B	67	C	97	C	127	C
8	D	38	B	68	B	98	A	128	B
9	D	39	B	69	A	99	B	129	B
10	C	40	B	70	C	100	B	130	C
11	C	41	A	71	A	101	A	131	B
12	C	42	A	72	A	102	A	132	A
13	A	43	D	73	D	103	D	133	C
14	C	44	B	74	B	104	C	134	C
15	B	45	A	75	B	105	D	135	C
16	C	46	A	76	C	106	D	136	A
17	C	47	C	77	C	107	C	137	A
18	B	48	C	78	D	108	D	138	C
19	B	49	C	79	A	109	D	139	A
20	C	50	A	80	B	110	D	140	C
21	D	51	B	81	B	111	D	141	C
22	A	52	D	82	A	112	A	142	A
23	C	53	C	83	D	113	A	143	D
24	D	54	D	84	D	114	B	144	A
25	D	55	A	85	A	115	A	145	A
26	C	56	B	86	A	116	B	146	C
27	A	57	B	87	D	117	C	147	C
28	B	58	C	88	A	118	A	148	C
29	C	59	A	89	D	119	D	149	A
30	C	60	C	90	D	120	C	150	B

151	C	181	B	211	A	241	B	271	C
152	C	182	A	212	B	242	A	272	C
153	C	183	A	213	D	243	A	273	A
154	B	184	B	214	C	244	A	274	D
155	B	185	D	215	D	245	A	275	A
156	C	186	C	216	A	246	A	276	B
157	C	187	A	217	B	247	A	277	B
158	D	188	A	218	B	248	A	278	B
159	A	189	D	219	A	249	A	279	A
160	D	190	D	220	C	250	C	280	A
161	C	191	B	221	C	251	D	281	B
162	D	192	B	222	D	252	A	282	B
163	A	193	B	223	A	253	D	283	B
164	B	194	D	224	C	254	C	284	A
165	A	195	B	225	D	255	A	285	A
166	C	196	C	226	D	256	C	286	B
167	A	197	A	227	B	257	D	287	D
168	A	198	D	228	B	258	C	288	C
169	D	199	A	229	B	259	D	289	D
170	B	200	C	230	B	260	A	290	A
171	D	201	C	231	A	261	B		
172	B	202	C	232	C	262	A		
173	A	203	A	233	C	263	C		
174	B	204	A	234	C	264	C		
175	D	205	D	235	B	265	C		
176	B	206	C	236	C	266	B		
177	A	207	D	237	C	267	A		
178	A	208	C	238	C	268	C		
179	D	209	B	239	A	269	C		
180	C	210	B	240	C	270	C		

Fill in the Blanks

1. Tissue culture media is sterilized in **autoclave**
2. Plant growth regulations which promote rooting are known as **auxin**
3. Virus indexing can be done by **ELISA**
4. Micropropagation can be done using the explant **Adventious shoot, Bulb and scales, axillary buds**
5. *In-vitro* culture is an aseptic method of propagation plants **tissue culture**
6. What is the commonly used sterilant for explant- **mercuric chloride**
7. Mention the important component of tissue culture media that provides anchorage to the plants. **Agar**
8. Chemical is used to induce polyploidy in plants **Colchicine**
9. Optimum pH range for plant tissue culture **5.6 to 5.8**
10. **IAA (or) IBA** is an example for natural auxin
11. Heritable variability observed among plants regenerated from tissue culture is called as **Somoclonal variation**
12. Mass multiplication of plants through *in vitro* technology commercial application is called **Micropropagation**
13. **Embryo culture** is developed to overcome Post-fertilization barriers in crop plants
14. Embryo culture was first done by **Hanning 1906**
15. **MS medium** is the most common plant tissue culture medium
16. **Ascorpic acid or citric acid (antioxidant)**is added in plant tissue culture medium to arrest tannin exudation.
17. Name a very strong root inducing growth hormone **IAA (Auxin)**
18. In suspension culture, maximum cell division occurs at **log or exponential phase**
19. Secondary metabolite isolated from Stevia is **sweet stevioside**
20. Media sterilization is done in **121°C** temperature
21. Among fruit crops, commercial scale micropropagation is practiced in **Banana**
22. IAA stands for **Indole-3-acetic acid**
23. Normally **2.4-D** hormone in used for callus induction in tissue culture.
24. Anther culture technique was discovered by **Guha and Maheswari**
25. **Cytokinin**is a growth hormone used for shoot regeneration in plant tissue culture

26. Regeneration of plant from naked single cell in a culture medium is known as **protoplast culture**
27. All those compounds which are not directly involved in the primary metabolic processes **secondary metabolites**
28. Growth hormone cytokines promote **shoot proliferation**
29. Culture are generally initiated from pieces of "whole plant" The pieces are termed **explants**
30. In the initial stage (embryo initiation) a high concentration **of sugar (8-12 per cent)** is used.
31. Male gametophyte is termed as **pollen grain or microgametophyte**
32. Female gametophyte is termed as **embryo sac or megagametophyte**
33. Regeneration of a plant from naked single cell in a culture medium is known as **protoplast culture**
34. The important tissue culture technique used in the development of salinity resistant genotype is **somaclonal variation**
35. The post fertilization barriers can be overcome by **embryo culture**
36. Variability observed among plants regenerated from pollen culture is called **androclonal** variations.
37. The post fertilization barriers can be overcome by **embryo culture or embryo rescue**
38. **Sodium Hypo cholarite** chemical is used for sterilizing explants.
39. In tissue culture medium phenolic exudations can be controlled by addition of **anti-oxidants**
40. The temperature maintained at liquid nitrogen storage is **-196°C**
41. The technique used to get viable embryo in distant hybridization is **fluorescence in diacetate (FDA)**
42. Who coined the term cybrid?**Bunn *et al.*, in 1974**
43. Variability observed among plants regenerated from pollen culture is called_**androclonal variations.**
44. BAP stands for_**Benzyl amino purine**
45. *In vitro* culture of either the polarized egg, zygote, pre-embryo or mature embryo is called **Embryo culture**
46. The phenomenon of the reversion of mature cells to the parenchyma state is called **dedifferentiation**
47. Meristematic state leading to the formation of callus is called **Caulogenesis**
48. Macerozyme is used for **Protoplast**isolation.
49. B5 medium discovered by **Gamborg**
50. The tissue culture technique used to produce triploids is **Endosperm culture**

51. Give an example for auxin type of plant growth regulator **IBA**
52. Shoots developed *in vitro* appear brittle, glassy and water soaked and is called **Vitrification or hyperhydricity**
53. The process of root formation is **Rhizogenesis**
54. In the phrase 'MS medium', MS stands for **Murashige and Skoog**
55. **Colchicine** is used for chromosome doubling.
56. Plants containing nucleus from one plant and cytoplasm from both parent is called **Cybrid**
57. Absence of **Vascula r connections** prevents virus entry in the meristem.
58. The main aim of continuous shaking of suspension culture is to **provide aeration and unifrom nutrition**
59. **Larkin Scowcroft** coined the term Somaclonal variation.
60. Name the type of cell culture that is given a fixed amount of nutrients and could only be used to 'grow' the cells with only one harvest at the end. **Batch culture**
61. The explant used for banana micropropagation is **Pseudo stem**
62. The secondary metabolite obtained from *Datura* is **Hyoscyamine**
63. Name the bio molecule present in *Catharanthus roseus* **Vinblastine, Vincristine**
64. Name any one secondary metabolite that is produced through bioreactors. **Shikonin**
65. Preservation of cells, tissues and organs in liquid nitrogen is called ***in vitro* germplasm conservation**
66. Molecules that stimulate the production of secondary metabolites are called **Elicitors**
67. In some fruit trees, embryos require a period after ripening to germination called **seed dormancy**
68. BAP is an example of **cytokinin**
69. Gautheret published first the handbook on **Plant Tissue Culture**
70. DMSO is a **cryoprotectant**.
71. An example for natural cytokinin **Isopentynal adenine**
72. White's medium used for **Root culture**
73. The most commonly used vitamin in tissue culture is **Thiamine**
74. Anther culture technique was discovered by **Guha and Maheswari** in the year of **1964**
75. **Morel and Martin** discovered the technique to produce **virus free plants**by meristem culture
76. Ascorbic acid and citric acid used as an **antioxidant**

77. The medium should be sterilized in **autoclave** at **121°C** for 15 minutes
78. The process of ovary culture is known as **gynogenesis**
79. A **somatic embryo** is an embryo derived from a somatic cell, other than zygote, usually on *in vitro* culture.
80. The process of somatic embryo development is called as **somatic embryogenesis.**
81. Products of fusion between two or more protoplasts of the same species -**Homokaryon**
82. The process of anther culture otherwise known as **Androgenesis**
83. The phenomenon of mature cell reverting to the meristematic state and forming undifferentiated callus tissue is termed **dedifferentiation**
84. The phenomenon of conversion of component cells of callus tissue to whole plant is called-**Redifferentiation**
85. The first attempt of embryo culture was made by **Hanning** in 1904
86. **Duhamel du Monceau** discovered callus induction in 1756
87. Who observed the phenomenon of somatic embryogenesis in carrot? **Steward**
88. The chemical which is used to induce the polyploidy is **Colchicine**.
89. **Suspension culture** -the cells are cultured in liquid mediumunder the submerged condition
90. The variability observed among plants regenerated from pollen culture is called **Gametoclonal variation**
91. Artificial seed is a product of **Somatic embryogenesis**
92. Attainment of biological organization or form is termed as **morphogenesis**
93. **Caulogenesis** is a type of organogenesis by which only adventitious shoot bud initiation takes place in the callus tissue.
94. When organogenesis leads to root development, then it is known as **rhizogenesis**
95. Heat sensitive compounds are sterilized by **filtration** method
96. **N_6 medium** used for anther culture
97. Enzymatic isolation of protoplast first demonstrated by **E.C. Cocking**
98. The tissue culture technique used to produce triploid is **Endosperm culture**
99. **Synthetic seeds** are encapsulated somatic embryos which functionally mimic seeds and can develop into seedlings
100. Plant tissue culture technique is a redefined method of **Vegetative propagation**
101. A medium which is composed of chemically defined compound is **Synthetic media**

102. The first report of interspecific hybridization through protoplast fusion on two species of Nicotiana was given by **Carlson**
103. The variations arising in cultures of gamete is called **Gametoclonal** variation
104. The ovary culture is most successful for the plants having **Cytoplasmic male sterility**
105. The peak accumulation of secondary metabolites occurs during **Stationary phase**
106. The main function of hormone Gibberlin is **Internode elongation**
107. **NCS-TCP management cell** is responsible for the accreditation of test laboratories.
108. The citronella variety CIMAP/Bio13 was developed by which method **Somaclonal variation**
109. The process of making the *in vitro* plant to get adopted in the *in vivo* condition **Acclimatization**
110. In indirect somatic embryogenesis, Name the third stages of it's? **Torpedo**
111. Optimum pH of plant tissue culture MS medium **5.8 ± 0.2**
112. Optimum temperature of plant growth room **24+-1·C**
113. NCS-TCP strands for **National Certification System for Tissue culture Plants**
114. The first synthetic seeds were produced by **Kitto and Janick.**
115. The first report on gynogenesis was done by **San Noem in 1976**
116. The seed sterility can be overcome by **Embryo culture**
117. Anther culture mainly used for production of **Haploid plants**
118. Which of the crop commercially produced by tissue culture **-Banana**
119. The commercially used surface sterilizing agent is **Ethanol and mercuric chloride**
120. The chemical which is used to kill the virus is **virazole**
121. A localized group of actively dividing cells are known as **meristem**
122. The Ministry of Environment and Forests (MoEF) had enacted Environment and Protection Act in **1986**
123. National Certification System for Tissue Culture Plants was established by **Department of Biotechnology**
124. **CDFD** is the referral laboratory for genetic fidelity testing in tissue culture plants
125. **Bioprospecting**-Discovery of novel compounds from plants
126. **Shikonin** commercially isolated from *Lithospermum erythrorhizon* suspension cultures

127. **Secondary metabolites** are organic compounds that are not directly involved in growth, development or reproduction of an organism
128. **Biotransformation-** chemical conversion of an exogenously supplied substance by living cell cultures
129. **DNA polymerase** enzyme is responsible for DNA synthesis
130. The process of producing DNA from mRNA is called **Transcription**
131. Nucleotides consists of **Ribose sugar, phosphate group and, Nitrogenous base**
132. Semi conservative mode of replication was given by **1958 by Meselson and Stahl**
133. **Okazak**i fragments are found in lagging strand during DNA replication
134. First known restriction enzyme is-**HindII, from the bacterium *Haemophilus influenzae***
135. RNA has **Uracil** instead of thymine in DNA
136. The DNA and histone complex is called_**nucleosome**
137. In the lagging strand DNA synthesis is short, separated segments leads Okazaki fragments
138. **Nirenberg1966**deciphered the genetic code.
139. The enzyme **Reverse transcriptase** is a RNA dependent DNA polymerase.
140. Role of Ligases in DNA Replication **Joining of Okazaki fragments**
141. The mRNA is an exact copy of the genetic message contained in the **Exon** region of the DNA in eukaryotes.
142. .The recognition site of the enzyme EcoRI is made of **six**number of bases.
143. **Ribosome** is the seat of protein synthesis.
144. The **restriction endonuclease** enzymes are called as molecular scissors.
145. **M13** is an example of a phage vector.
146. Scientist who used bacteria and phage to discover DNA **Hershey and Chase**
147. The genetic material is **DNA**
148. **Micro satellite and mini satellite** is a type of repetitive DNA.
149. **AUG** is the initiation codon in translation.
150. **UAG,UGA and UAA** are the stop codon in translation.
151. In a gene the promoter sequence normally present at **3'** terminals of gene
152. **Helicase** is an enzyme that facilitates strand separation in DNA
153. The specific sequences recognized by restriction endonucleases are called **recognition sites**
154. The main enzyme used in cDNA conversion is **reverse transcriptase**
155. The process of producing DNA from mRNA is called **cDNA synthesis**

156. **Promoter** is a region of DNA involved in the binding of RNA polymerase to initiate transcription
157. mRNA in the eukaryotes must undergo further processing to remove **Introns**
158. The term gene was coined by **Wilhelm Johannsen**
159. The genetic material in tobacco mosaic virus is **RNA**
160. Operon concept was put forth by **Francois Jacob** and **Jacques Monod**
161. The double helix model of DNA was proposed by **Watson and Crick**
162. Catalyses the removal of 5' Phosphategroups from DNA is **Alkaline Phosphatese**
163. Enzyme involved in Transcription is **RNA polymerase**
164. **Plant ubiquitin (*Ubi*), rice actin 1 (*Act-1*) and CaMV 35S** _is an examples for constitutive promoter
165. Name the enzyme used in PCR technique **Taq Polymerase**
166. The sequential transfer of information from DNA to protein via RNA is known as**central dogma**
167. Southern hybridization is developed by **E.M. Southern**
168. **Galactosidase** enzyme hydrolyzes lactose to glucose and galactose
169. Introns are not present in **prokaryotes**
170. Pyrimidine bases present in nucleic acid are **cytosine and thymine**
171. The growth of DNA chain is always **5' to 3'** direction
172. Nitrogen bases present in RNA are **AGCU**
173. **Asparagine** is an example of sulphur containing amino acid
174. **Endonucleuses** are enzymes that produce internal cleavage.
175. The 3'ends of DNA strands always bear a **free OH** group
176. Induction of derived mutations at specific sites in gene is called **site directed mutagenesis**
177. Introduction of DNA in to cells by exposing them for very brief period to high voltage pulses is called **electrophoration**
178. RNA molecules that have catalytic action are called **Ribozymes**
179. Adenine and Guanine are **purines**
180. **PCR** is used for *in vitro* DNA amplification
181. **Euchromatin** is not tightly wound and it is active DNA
182. PCR (**Polymerase Chain Reaction**) was invented by **Kary Mullis**.
183. RNA polymerase synthesis **RNA from DNA**
184. Central dogma of life proposed by **Francis Crick**
185. **Exon**- coding sequence present in the gene

186. Intron- non-coding sequence present in the gene

187. Transposable elements otherwise called **jumping genes**

188. Jumping genes discovered by **Mc Clintock**

189. Nucleoside contains **Base +Sugar**

190. Nucleotide contains **Base +Sugar +Phosphate**

191. RNA has a **ribose sugar** instead of a **deoxyribose sugar** in DNA

192. In RNA thymine is replaced by **Uracil**

193. DNA Replication is the process of producing two identical replicas from one original DNA molecule

194. Translation described as synthesizing of protein from mRNA

195. The correct amino acid is added to its tRNA by a specific enzyme called an ***aminoacyl-tRNA synthetase***. The process is called **aminoacylation** or charging.

196. Reverse transcription-cDNA synthesized from mRNA by the enzyme **reverse transcriptase**

197. The lagging stand which having short discontinuous DNA fragments called **Okazaki fragments**

198. Primer – It is a short sequence (often of RNA)/an oligonucleotide that pairs with one strand of template DNA and provides a 3' OH essential for DNA polymerase to extend the primer through DNA synthesis

199. Topoisomerase I-change the degree of supercoiling of DNA by causing single –strand break and re-ligation,

200. Topoisomerases II- cut both strands of the DNA helix simultaneously in order to manage DNA tangles and supercoils

201. DNA ligase is a specific type of enzyme that facilitates the **joining of DNA strands** together by catalyzing the formation of a phosphodiester bond.

202. Helicase is an enzyme that unwinds and separates the two strands of the *DNA* double helix.

203. Under normal physiological condition the dominant form of DNA is **B-DNA**

204. A segment of DNA that is transcribed to produce one RNA molecule is called **Transcription Unit**

205. Activation of amino acid is carried out by **Amino acyle tRNA synthatase** enzyme.

206. Allolactose is an inducer of the lac operon.

207. DNA is composed of repeating units of **Deoxyribonucleotides**

208. Transfer of DNA fragment from an electrophototic gel to the nitrocellulose filter by capillary action is known as **Southern blotting**

209. Southern blotting technique first introduced by **E.M. Southern**.

210. Genetic code was deciphered by **Nirenberg, Korana and Holley.**
211. DNA sequencing methods were devised by **Maxam Gilbert (**chemical method**) and Frederick Sanger** (chain termination method)
212. A ***codon*** is a sequence of three DNA or RNA nucleotides that corresponds with a specific amino acid or stop signal during protein synthesis
213. The Sulphur containing amino acid is **Methionine** is encoded by **AUG** codan
214. In eukaryotes Transcription and RNA processing are completed in **Nucleous**
215. **Phenylalanine** is a Aromatic amino acid.
216. The Structure of tRNA is **Clover leaf**
217. The initiation of Transcription occurs when RNA polymerase binds at specific sequence Called **Promoter**
218. In prokaryotes the initiation factor IF3 binds to the which ribosomal sub unit of **30 S**
219. he nuclear DNA-protein complex is called **Chromatin**
220. The location of the RNA polymerase I enzyme is **Nucleolus**
221. Prokaryotic genome is a **Haploid**
222. The activity of RNA polymerase was first discovered by **Wess**
223. During Transcription only one strand of a DNA molecule is transcribed. This strand is Called **Antisense strand**
224. Transgenic plants **Contain foreign genes in their cells**
225. **Dolly** is the cloned sheep for the first time.
226. In plant transformation the chemical Which gives the signal for infection of the tissue by Agrobacterium is **acetosyringone**
227. The process of incubating leaf discs with Agrobacterium for transformation is called **Co-Cultivation**
228. The most commonly used bacterium as bio-insecticide is ***Bacillus thuringiensis***
229. First transgenic crop released in India was **Bt cotton**
230. The carrier or vehicle molecule that carry DNA fragments into host **Vector**
231. Bacterial cell in recombinant DNA technology is known as **Host**
232. *Agrobacterium tumefaciens* harbours **Ti** plasmid.
233. From the bacterium *Bacillus thuringiensis*, genes (cry genes) for **crystel** proteins used in rDNA technology to generate insect resistant plants
234. Insensitivity to Glyphosate is conferred by bacteria derived ***aroA* gene from *Salmonella typhimurium, ocs* gene from *A. tumafaciens*** gene.

235. Abiotic stress transduction pathway in plants is controlled mainly by **ABA hormone** signaling.
236. Flavr Savr tomato was engineered to increase **Shelf life (Storage)** character.
237. The current generation of Golden rice has the **phytoene synthase** gene from maize.
238. Papaya ring-spot virus can be controlled by using **coat protein** mediated cross protection technique.
239. To control insect pests, **Cowpea trypsin inhibitor, α-Amylase inhibitor and Proteinase inhibitors** inhibitor genes can be used apart from Bt gene.
240. Recombinant proteins can be targeted to **plastid or chloroplast** to avoid plant cytoplasmic toxicity.
241. Planting of untransformed Bt - free plants along with transgenic plants to postpone the evolution of Bf - resistant insects is called **Refugia crop** technique.
242. Genetically modified organisms (GMO) and rDNA products in India are governed by EPA Rule of year **1989**.
243. Golden rice is the genetic engineered rice with enhanced levels of **Vitamin A** in the endosperm.
244. Insulin was the first therapeutic protein to be introduced to treat the **Diabetics** disease
245. The technique of identification of existing DNA or the newly inserted DNA **Polymerase chain reaction and southern blotting**
246. Introduction of new DNA that can function as a tag for the gene of interest is known as **Gene tagging**
247. Hygromycin resistance is an example for **selectable marker**
248. Bt forms crystalline bodies during sporulation that contains **Crystal protein**
249. Transgenic plants technology produces **Genetically Modified Organism**.
250. Enzyme Restriction end nucleases are also called as **molecular scissors**
251. Name the first genetically modified tomato that had delayed ripening due to anti sense technology. **Flavr Savr**
252. Recombinant DNA technology first introduced by **Stanely cohen and Herbert Boyer.**
253. **Restriction endonuclease**-is an enzyme that cuts DNA at or near specific recognition nucleotide sequences known as **restriction sites**.
254. **Type II** restriction enzymes are used for gene cloning.
255. Flavr savr is a **Transgenic Tomato.**

256. The sites recognized by restriction enzymes called **restriction sites.**
257. **Alkaline Phosphatase** catalyses the removal of 5' phosphate groups from the DNA
258. **Poly Nucleotide Kinase** the enzyme add phosphate group in the 5 prime end of the DNA molecule
259. **Fredrick Griffith** was first to demonstrate the transformation in bacteria which causing pneumonia.
260. The first drug produced using recombinant DNA technology was **human insulin.**
261. **Shuttle vector-** A cloning vector that can replicate in cells of more than one type of organism.
262. An **expression vector** is usually a plasmid or virus designed for protein **expression** in cells
263. **Arthur Kornberg** discovered the enzyme **DNA polymerase I.**
264. A ***plasmid*** is a small, circular, double-stranded self-replicating DNA molecule that is distinct from a cell's chromosomal DNA
265. **Recombinant DNA** is DNA that has been created artificially i.e DNA from two or more sources is incorporated into a single recombinant molecule.
266. Which gene is responsible for producing glycine in transgenic tobacco crops **BADH**
267. The **Cry** proteins are solubilized in insect midgut and then proteolytically processed to yield a toxic core fragment of **60 kDa**
268. The insect(s) resistance to cry protein are ***Plodia interpunctella, Cadra cautella***
269. The first flavr savr tomato produced in the year of **1994**
270. The gene responsible for increasing vitamin A in transgenic rice plant are **Phytoene synthasecarotene desaturase, lycopene cyclase**
271. Which enzyme coding by mtl D gene **Mannitol dehydrogenase**
272. The enzyme responsible for Ethylene synthesis from 1-Amino cyclopropane-1-Carboxilic acid (ACC) is **ACC oxidase**
273. The gene which is transferred from one place to another place within a DNA sequence is called **transposable elements**
274. **Methionine** is the precursor of ethylene hormone
275. The **bar** gene containing transgenic plants are resistant to **phosphinothricin** herbicide
276. Drought and water logging tolerant somaclonal plants are checked by adding **PEG** in culture medium
277. Cereals are deficient in the amino acid **lysine**

278. Insensitivity to glyphosate is conferred by bacteria derived from **aro A** gene
279. The amino acid produced from the plants during the stress condition is **proline**
280. Abiotic stress transduction pathway in plants is controlled mainly by **abscisic acid** hormone
281. A second generation of Golden rice lines *i.e.* Golden rice 2 with a phytoene synthase gene isolated from **maize**
282. **Coat protein mediated** method has been the most successful for producing virus resistant transgenic plants.
283. The response of plants to abiotic stresses leads to synthesis and accumulation of low molecular weight compounds called as **osmoprotectants.**
284. ***Aspergillus fumigatus*** is the source of thermo-tolerant phytase gene in high iron rice.
285. Polyhydroxy butyrate (PHB-Bioplastics)-was first isolated and characterized by **Maurice Lemoigne**
286. **Transplastomic engineering-**targeting recombinant proteins to plastid to avoid cytoplasmic toxicity
287. First commercially produced recombinant protein is **Human insulin**
288. **Ri plasmid** isolated from ***Agrobacterium rhizogenes*** is responsible for hairy root culture
289. First recombinant plant derived protein is **Human serum albumin**
290. Example for plant derived antibody (Plantibodies)-**S Ig A**
291. **GEAC-**Genetic Engineering Approval Committee –approval of activities involving GMO and their products
292. Bt Cotton containing Cry1Ac is named as **Bollgard I**
293. Bt Cotton containing Cry1Ac and Cry2Ab is named as **Bollgard II**
294. The most widely used promoter in dicotyledonous plants is **CaMV 35S** promoter.
295. The organism known as natural genetic engineer is ***Agrobacterium tumefaciens.***
296. B-**glucuronidase (GUS)** and **Green fluorescent protein (GFP)** are examples of reporter gene.
297. **Ti plasmid**-tumor inducing plasmid is found in ***Agrobacterium tumefaciens***
298. **Daffodil** is the source of phytoene synthase and lycopene cyclase genes in first generation golden rice.
299. Example of dominant marker is **RAPD**

300. Isozymes is an example for protein markers.

301. Amplification of DNA fragments is carried out by **Thermo cycler** machine.

302. DNA fingerprinting for studying polymorphism was discovered! By British geneticist **Alec Jeffrey** in **1984**

303. SSR stands for **Simple sequence repeat**

304. AFLP is an example of codominant marker system.

305. SSR markers are an example of **co-dominant** markers

306. SNP markers **Single Nucleotide polymorphism**

307. RFLP -**Restriction Fragment Length Polymorphism**

308. RFLPs are **codominant** markers

309. RAPD-**Randomly-Amplified Polymorphic** DNA

310. RAPD is **dominant** marker

311. AFLP-**Amplified Fragment Length Polymorphism**

312. SSRs-**Simple Sequence Repeats**

313. SNP-**Single Nucleotide Polymorphism**

314. The process of locating genes of importance via linkage to RFLP or isozyme markers is referred to as **Gene-tagging**

Write Short Notes (1 mark)

1. Explant
2. Suspension culture.
3. Cybrid.
4. Homokaryon.
5. Differentiation.
6. What is callus?
7. Meristem tip culture
8. Solid and liquid media
9. Synthetic seed
10. Callus culture
11. Embryo rescue
12. Cybrids
13. Wide hybridization
14. Factors influencing plant tissue culture
15. Cytoplasmic male sterile lines
16. Methods of Protoplast isolation.
17. *In vitro* Morphogenesis.
18. Callus Culture.
19. Pollen culture.
20. Endosperm culture
21. Rhizogenesis.
22. Organogenesis.
23. Methods to increase secondary metabolite production in suspension
24. Virus indexing
25. Cybrids Somadonal variation.
26. What are synthetic seeds and its advantages?
27. Different methods of protoplast fusion.
28. What are somatic hybrids?
29. What are doubled haploids?
30. What are Edible vaccines?
31. What are Secondary metabolites?
32. How will prepare synthetic seeds?
33. Somatic embryogenesis.

34. Micropropagation.
35. Indicator plants.
36. What is cybrid?
37. Andronoclonal variation.
38. Androgenesis.
39. Natural cytokinin, Transcription
40. Somatic embryogenesis.
41. Embryogenesis.
42. Advantages of tissue culture
43. Browning of tissue culture
44. Enzymatic isolation of protoplasts.
45. Androgenesis.
46. Auxins
47. Organic additives
48. Filter sterilization
49. Solidifying agents
50. Thermotherapy
51. Cell suspension
52. ELISA test
53. Write the role of Cytokinin in tissue culture.
54. Who coined the term Totypotency and what does it mean?
55. Auxin and its uses
56. Carbon source in plant tissue culture
57. Solidifying agents
58. De-differentiatation
59. Merits and demerits of micropropotion
60. Sterilization techniques in plant tissue culture
61. Commonly used tissue culture media
62. Nutritional requirements for plant tissue culture
63. Advantage of meristem culture
64. Sterilization
65. Protoplast fusion
66. Embryo rescue
67. What are plant tissue, cell and organ cultures? Differentiate between callus and suspension culture.
68. Quote an example for a plant secondary metabolite

69. Cryopreservation
70. Caulogenesis
71. Define biotechnology
72. Write an importance of biotechnology.
73. Secondary metabolioties.
74. Cybridization.
75. Composition of Nucleic acids
76. Promoter;
77. RNA Splicing.
78. DNA ligase.
79. Chargraff s rule.
80. Replicon.
81. Introns and exons.
82. Okasaki fragments.
83. Nucleoside.
84. Post- Transcriptional Gene Silencing.
85. Central dogma of life.
86. Wobble hypothesis.
87. PCR.
88. Southern blotting.
89. Translation.
90. Nucleoside.
91. Mention the steps in PCR reaction.
92. Gene regulation.
93. What is transposon tagging?
94. Edwin Southern
95. Codon.
96. DNA Iigase
97. cDNA library
98. Transcription.
99. Repetitive DNA
100. Describe GMOs, bio-safety and bio-ethics.
101. Risk regulation.
102. Proteomics.
103. Kary Mullis.
104. PCR based and non-PGR based markers.

105. Define plasmid
106. What are biosafety and bioethics?
107. Ti plasmid
108. What do you mean by Bioethics?
109. Mention any two genes used in plant genetic engineering research for disease resistance.
110. Mention any two methods used in detection of GMOs.
111. Expression vector.
112. Competent bacteria.
113. DNA modifying enzymes.
114. Write on type II Restriction enzymes.
115. Gene transfer methods
116. Plasmid vectors
117. Selectable markers
118. Cosmids and phagemids.
119. Electrophoration.
120. Neomycin Phosphotransferase.
121. Cry protein.
122. Mention two bio-safety issues related to GM crops.
123. Bacteriophage
124. Essential features of pBR 322.
125. Phagemid vector.
126. Molecular scissors.
127. SCAR marker.
128. Marker assisted selection.
129. Write a short note on RAPD.
130. Expand SSR (Markers)
131. DNA fingerprinting
132. Name any two PCR based markers

Write Brief Answer (3 marks)

1. What is sterilization? List out differant mathods of starilization.
2. What is anther culture? List its uses,
3. What is the role of plant growth regulators in tissue culture?
4. How will yob process explants before placing in a tissue culture medium?
5. Wet heat sterilization
6. Agencies coordinating tissue culture labs in India
7. Quality control in tissue culture
8. Genetic fidelity testing
9. ELISA technique.
10. Why meristems are mostly free of viruses?
11. Certification system for tissue cultured plants
12. Write a brief note on cryopreservation.
13. Write about protoplast fusion and protoplast culture.
14. Mention the ways to avoid post fertilization barriers.
15. Define Somaclonal variation and its application in agriculture.
16. What do you mean by synthetic seeds. Write the way to achieve it.
17. What is totipotency? Differentiate redifferentiation and dedifferentiation.
18. Somatic hybrids in crop improvement
19. Advantages and limitations of micropropagation.
20. Applications of embryo culture.
21. Write briefly on secondary metabolite production.
22. Various components of tissue culture media
23. Steps in the production of virus free plants
24. Different pathways of androgenesis that lead to haploid plant production
25. Somatic hybrids in crop improvement
26. Write short notes on Micropropagation
27. Ovule culture and applications of embryo culture
28. Give brief answers on Define morphogenesis
29. RFLP markers and enzymatic method of isolation of protoplasts
30. Advantages and disadvantages of cryoprotectants
31. How will you culture protoplasts?
32. What is somatic hybridization? Mention the various steps in somatic hybridization.

33. Define somaclonal variation. Discuss its advantages and limitations?
34. What is homokaryon and heterokaryon?
35. Describe the southern blotting technique.
36. What is a nucleotide?
37. Where do you find DNA In a eurkaryotlc cell? Write a brief note on their organization.
38. Who proved that the DNA is the genetic material and mention the technique in short?
39. Define transcription and steps involved in the same.
40. Write about restriction enymes and their application.
41. Draw the structure of a prokaryotic ribosome and explain.
42. What is repetitive DNA? Give its significance.
43. Differentiate between a genomic DNA library and CDNA library.
44. Who discovered PCR technique? Write its principle.
45. Mention six features of the genetic code.
46. Write short notes on cDNA library construction
47. Process of dedifferentiation and redifferentiation
48. Satellite and repetitive DNA and its significance
49. DNA polymerases
50. Enzymes involved in DNA manipulation with their functions.
51. Explain two mathods uasd for introducing foreign DNA Into living calls.
52. Brief any one promoter that is used for driving DNA expression in specific tissues
53. Differentiate between a selectable and scorable marker.
54. What are phage? How are they exploited in recombinant DNA technology?
55. How will you induce resistance to pests through transgenic technology?
56. What is meant by copy number' of plasmids?
57. What is slow ripening tomato?
58. Define recombinant - DNA technology
59. Write the different methods of gene transfer to plants.
60. What are vectors? Mention the characteristics of vectors.
61. Give two examples of vectors used in bacterial transformation.
62. Direct methods of plant transformation.
63. Recombinant DNA technology and its applications.
64. Golden rice
65. Application of transgenic plants

66. Finger printing
67. Methods of gene delivery
68. Recombinant proteins
69. Reporter genes
70. Gene tagging
71. Plasmid DNA and phage
72. What are restriction endonucleases?
73. What is a promoter?
74. What is a recombinant DNA?
75. Write a short note on current status of transgenic crops at National level.
76. Briefly describe fhe procedure followed in PCR and list the advantages and limitations of this method.
77. Briefly describe the various approaches for the production of virus resistant transgenic plant.
78. Describe the Ti plasmid
79. Name any two 'single-locus' marker systems.
80. Name any one software used for the analysis of marker data.
81. Distinguish between hybridization and PCR based markers.
82. List any four uses of molecular marker technology.
83. Describe the RAPD technique. What is transposon tagging?
84. What are molecular markers? Explain the types of molecular markers.

Essay Type Questions (5 marks)

1. Explain the steps involved in producing secondary metabolites through tissue culture.
2. Discuss on the various approaches adopted for the maintenance of aseptic conditions during tissue culture.
3. Write an essay on micropropagation of ornamental crops. Write a summary about DNA finger printing of varieties.
4. Describe the procedure involved in production of disease free plants by *in vitro* methods. Explain diagrammatically with suitable examples.
5. Mention the advantages of using plant cell culture for production of secondary metabolites.
6. Discuss about ovary and embryo culture and their applications? used with references to industrial application?
7. What is anther and microspore culture? Explain the pathway leading to haploid.
8. Explain in detail the different steps involved in the micropropagation of banana.
9. Give an account on certification system for tissue culture plant
10. What are the different growth regulators added to the plant tissue culture media? Explain their effect on plant tissue culture
11. Describe the composition of plant tissue culture media.
12. Give an account on the scope of Biotechnology in Agriculture, Horticulture and Forestry
13. Write the origin, applications, achievements and limitations of somaclonal variations in crop improvement
14. Different pathways of androgenesis that lead to haploid plant production
15. Explain the steps involved in production of virus free plants
16. Explain about the secondary metabolite production with a classic example
17. Write an essay on the history of plant tissue culture. Acheivements of plan tissue culture
18. Applications of anther and ovule culture,Protoplast isolation
19. *In vitro* germplasm concervation Advantages and disadvantages of cryoprotectants
20. Explain the methods of isolation of ovary and embryo culture
21. Write an essay on the Plant growth regulators used in plant tissue culture and their effects with examples.

22. Describe the large scale production and applications somatic embryos and synthetic seeds.
23. Write the applications of plant tissue culture in crop improvement.
24. Explain the different types of techniques used for sterilization in plant tissue culture, growth room chambers and instruments.
25. Methods used for enhancement and screening of secondary metabolite.
26. Anther culture technique and meristem culture and its applications.
27. What are different classes of secondary metabolites that can be produced in suspension culture? Explain with examples
28. Explain the scope of commercial scale micropropagation and discuss on the low cost alternatives available in micropropagation
29. What is Biotrasformation? Give an example Enumerate Transgenic horticultural crops and Transgenic nutritional enhancement in crops
30. What is gametoclonal selection? Explain the differences between somoclonal and gametoclonal selection.
31. Explain the various methods of virus indexing.
32. Describe the principles and operations of Autoclave. Waht are the materials sterilized in it?
33. Who are pioneers in Operon concept? Write about Lac operon when glucose is present in the media.
34. Explain the translation in prokaryotes
35. Explain in detail the semi-conservative mode of DNA replication.
36. Explain the different blotting techniques
37. Explain Watson and Crick double helical DNA model
38. Explain the Lac Operon Model of Gene Expression in bacteria.
39. Write in detail the Maxam and Gilbert method of gene sequencing.
40. Explain central dogma. Give the structure and function of tRNA.
41. Structure and organization of plant genome
42. Describe the structure of nucleic acids
43. Explain the mechanism of DNA replication? Discuss the role of various enzymes
44. Mention the steps in translation in prokaryotes and explain initiation of translation in detail.
45. Explain regulation of gene expression in prokaryotes with reference to Lac Operon.
46. Write an essay on different sequencing methods.
47. Write on polymerases and write on type II restriction enzymes.

48. What are the direct methods of plant transformation? What is a biolistic gun? Explain briefly.
49. What are vectors? Discuss different methods of plant gene transfer
50. Recombinant DNA technology and its applications Golden rice
51. Explain the different methods of gene transfer in plants
52. Explain about the tools and techniques of DNA recombinant technology
53. Elaborate on biosafety issues related to transgenic plants
54. Distingush selectable marker-and reporter genes.
55. Write an essay on particle bombardment method of gene transformation in plants.
56. Write an essay on bacterial transformation.
57. What are enzymes? Explain type II restriction enzymes used in recombinant DNA technology with examples.
58. What are the applications of transgenic plants? Explain with examples.
59. Write about Agrobacterium mediated transformation in plants
60. Describe the construction of recombinant DNA molecules.
61. Narrate the direct and indirect methods of gene transfer.
62. Describe in detail crop improvement, with an example crop through marker assisted selection.
63. Discuss in-depth the current status of transgenic crops at national and global level.
64. Describe the transformation methods? genes and promoters that can be used for abiotic stress tolerance
65. Elaborate the biosafety measures and, the bioethics, that need to be followed for a transgenic plant
66. Describe in detail atleast three non-transgenic methods of crop improvement
67. Describe the regulatory steps taken for transgenic research at National level
68. Write an essay on development of transgenic plants for insect resistance.
69. Discuss about recombinant DNA technology with reference to features of cloning vectors?
70. Applications of transgenic plants in crop improvement with examples.
71. Discuss the a)direct and indirect gene transfer methods, b) Explain the DNA packaging in the nucleus.
72. Explain how you would transform a crop plant with 'cry' gene using the Ti plasmid and confirm the presence of the gene.

73. Define plasmid. Role of plasmid in genetic engineering and the difference between natural plasmids and the artificial vectors.
74. Explain the role of recombinant DNA technology in Agriculture
75. What are the different types of gene transfer methods? Write in detail about the commonly used one in plants
76. What is marker assisted selection? Explain with example.
77. Explain about DNA markers and their uses in biotechnology
78. Discuss on the applications of molecular markers
79. Explain different markers used in recombinant DNA technology with examples
80. List out the advantages and disadvantages of AFLP and protocol of AFLP Explain MAS.
81. Describe the step in RFLP technique.
82. Explain the procedure of RFLP analysis in detection of polymorphism with suitable examples.

References

Books

Adrian Slater, Nigel W. Scott and Mark R. Fowler. 2008, Plant Biotechnology: The Genetic Manipulation of Plants, Oxford University Press, 2008 -

Bhojwani SS, Razdan MK, 1983. Plant Tissue Culture: Theory and Practice. Elsevier publications.

Brown TA. 2010. Gene cloning and DNA analysis: An Introduction. 6th ed. Wiley Blackwell.

Chawla, HS. 2000, Introduction to Plant Biotechnology. Science Publishers,

David Hames and Nigel Hooper. 2005 Biochemistry. Third ed. Taylor and Francis Group: New York.

Dubey, RC. 2014. A textbook of Biotechnology. S. Chand and Company Limited.

Jiang R, Zhang X, Zhang MQ (Eds). 2013. Basics of Bioinformatics. Springer publishers

Lehninger AL, Nelson DL, Cox MM. 2000. Lehninger principles of biochemistry. New York: Worth Publishers.

Lodge J. 2007. Gene cloning: principles and applications. Taylor and Francis Group.

M.Sivaji, C.Mohan, R.Rasakumar, and S.Sathiyaraj. Basics and application of Nanotechnology, Thannambikkai Puplication, Coimbatore, p304.

Madigan MT, Martinko JM, Bender KS, Buckley DH, Stahl DA. 2015. Brock biology of microorganisms (Fourteenth edition). Boston: Pearson.

Moore DD. 2001. Genomic DNA Libraries. Current Protocols in Molecular Biology.

Nair AJ. Introduction to Biotechnology and Genetic Engineering. 2008.Infinity Science Press

Primrose SB, Twyman RM, Old RW. 2001. Principles of Gene Manipulation. Oxford: Blackwell Scientific.

Rodwell VW, Botham KM, Kennelly PJ, Weil PA, Bender DA. 2015. Harper's illustrated biochemistry (30th ed). New York, N.Y.: McGraw-Hill Education LLC.

Singh BD. 2008. Biotechnology: Expanding Horizons. 2nded. Kalyani Publishers.

Sivaji M, Sathiyaraj S, Mohan C, Vijayaraghavan H. Basic Concepts of Plant Biotechnology, Thannambikkai Publishers.

Internet Sources

http://barc.gov.in/publications/nl/

http://dbtindia.gov.in/regulations-guidelines/regulations/biosafety

http://www.ebi.ac.uk/

http://www.ncbi.nlm.nih.gov/.

https://dbtncstcp.nic.in/About-the-System/NCS-TCP-Guidelines

https://en.wikibooks.org/

https://en.wikipedia.org

https://microbenotes.com/

https://nptel.ac.in/course.php

https://passel2.unl.edu/view/lesson/a7b9c8f0ffa2/7

https://shodhganga.inflibnet.ac.in/

https://www.ncbi.nlm.nih.gov/pmc/articles/

https://www.quora.com/

https://www.researchgate.net/

https://www.sciencedirect.com/

https://www.slideshare.net/

www.biologydiscussion.com

Index

C

D

E

J

K

L

M

N

U

V

W

Z

S

T

O

P

Q

R